Femtosecond Laser Assisted Lenticule Extraction

Walter Sekundo · Felix Mathias Wagner
Editors

Femtosecond Laser Assisted Lenticule Extraction

Principles, Techniques, Complication Management, and Future Concepts in KLEx

Second Edition

Springer

Editors
Walter Sekundo
Department of Ophthalmology
Philipps University of Marburg
Marburg, Germany

Felix Mathias Wagner
Department of Ophthalmology
University Medical Center
Johannes Gutenberg-University Mainz
Mainz, Germany

ISBN 978-3-031-60423-2 ISBN 978-3-031-60424-9 (eBook)
https://doi.org/10.1007/978-3-031-60424-9

This Springer imprint is published by the registered company Springer Nature Switzerland AG
The registered company address is: Gewerbestrasse 11, 6330 Cham, Switzerland

Preface

Dear Reader,

Welcome to the first comprehensive textbook on Keratorefractive Lenticule Extraction!

Thinking back to 2006, when we stood before a small audience at the AAO Meeting in Las Vegas, presenting the first 10 eyes treated with femtosecond laser-only assisted laser-refractive surgery (then known as "femtosecond lenticule extraction" or FLEx), we could scarcely imagine what has now become a major trend in laser vision correction (LVC). For the first time, it became possible to extract corneal tissue without evaporating it. Within a year, it was clear that a flap was not necessary and a small incision sufficed to extract a corneal lenticule. In 2007, the first SMILE surgery was performed. The results of the first prospective study, published a year later, were recently named the "most cited modern article in refractive surgery between 2010 and 2020" [1]. The first edition of this book, *Small Incision Lenticule Extraction (SMILE): Principles, Techniques, Management, and Future Concepts*, appeared 10 years ago as the first English textbook on SMILE. At that time, SMILE was gaining popularity in Europe and Asia but was not yet available in North America. The predominant procedure then was still LASIK. Therefore, our first edition aimed to demonstrate that SMILE was not only comparable to LASIK but also had distinct advantages over flap-based procedures. A decade later, with over 10 million procedures performed, SMILE has gained global acceptance. Furthermore, other renowned refractive laser manufacturers, initially skeptical, have since developed their own refractive platforms, including Smart Sight®, CLEAR®, and SILK®. This development is the best testament to the mainstream acceptance and rapid evolution of femtosecond laser-assisted small incision intracorneal surgery. Consequently, it was logical to gather experts to compile the first comprehensive book on what has been termed "Keratorefractive Lenticule Extraction" (KLEx), as suggested by the editors of the Journal of Refractive Surgery and the Journal of Cataract and Refractive Surgery [2].

The aim of this textbook is to enable readers to easily understand the principles of KLEx surgery, while distinguishing between the sophisticated technologies offered by various manufacturers. The book covers all available KLEx procedures, detailing their clinical results. Dedicated chapters on centration, energy, along with standard operating procedures, are included and partially accompanied by videos. Practical in approach, the contributors share their own protocols, tips, and tricks. Applications such as the treatment of hyperopia, retreatment techniques, and wound healing are described, alongside the latest knowledge on corneal biomechanics and sensitivity. Despite superior corneal biomechanics, KLEx, like other LVC procedures, can result in keratectasia. As a more surgically demanding procedure, KLEx also has its own specific set of complications. Several chapters discuss their prevention and treatment.

The availability of optically shaped human corneal tissue has opened new frontiers in corneal additive refractive surgery, including lenticule implantation and rotation, enriching our armamentarium with combinations of other corneal shaping techniques.

From the depths of my heart, I thank all contributors for their passionate work, done at the cost of personal leisure time and without financial reward. My deepest appreciation, however, goes to my beloved wife, Maria Sekundo, MD, who has provided relentless support throughout my professional journey, inevitably requiring sacrifices in our private life.

Please read, enjoy, reread, and enjoy again this major work of many outstanding scientists and surgeons.

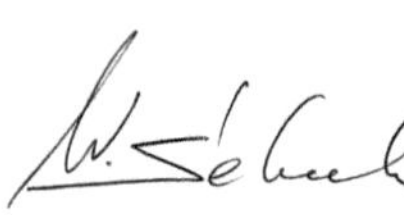

Marburg, Germany

Walter Sekundo, MD, Ph.D.
Senior Editor

References

1. Randleman JB. The most cited articles in refractive surgery (2010-2020). J Refract Surg. 2023;39(11):784–90.
2. Dupps WJ, Randleman JB, Kohnen T, Srinivasan S, Werner L. Scientific nomenclature for keratorefractive lenticule extraction (KLEx) procedures: a joint editorial statement. J Cataract Refract Surg. 2023;49(11):1085.

Contents

Editors and Contributors

About the Editors

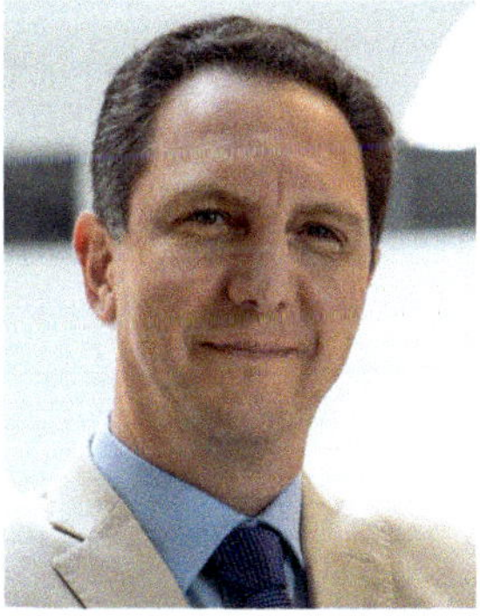

Prof. Walter Sekundo, MD, Ph.D. is Professor and Chairman, Department of Ophthalmology, Philipps University of Marburg, Germany. He studied Medicine in Frankfurt (Germany), New Orleans and Durham (US). He was a resident at the University of Bonn in Germany and a fellow in Corneal and Refractive surgery at Moorfields Eyes Hospital and Ocular Pathology at the University of Glasgow in UK. He received his vitreoretinal training in Marburg and glaucoma training in Mainz (Germany). He also holds a degree of "Health Care Manager" from the Faculty of Economics in Marburg. Prof. Sekundo has published 200+ original papers, over 50 book chapters and edited the first international book on SMILE surgery. He gave countless presentations at national and international meetings. He is a reviewer for 21 Ophthalmic Journals and a board member of "*Die Ophthalmologie.*" Prof. Sekundo is a busy surgeon with over 30,000 procedures in the anterior and posterior segment and has been repeatedly named as one of the 30 top refractive and cataract surgeons in Germany. Together with Marcus Blum he largely contributed to the development of KLEx. In fact, he was the first surgeon in the world who performed FLEx and SMILE. He received several prestigious prizes for the contribution to the field of ophthalmic surgery. In the last 25 years his research has been focused on corneal, cataract and refractive surgery.

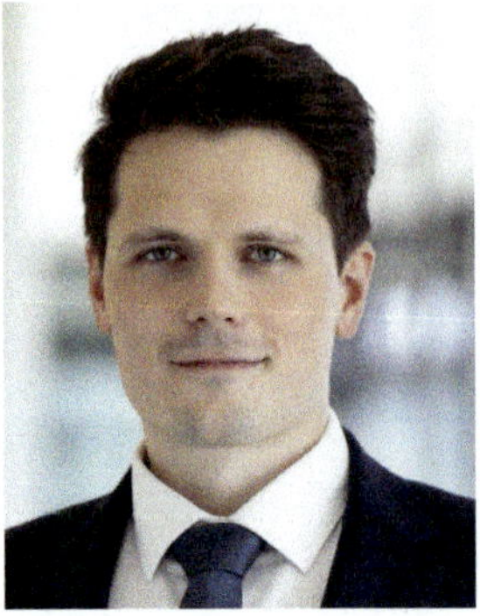

Felix Mathias Wagner is the head of Refractive Laser Surgery and a consultant at the Department of Ophthalmology, University Medical Center of the Johannes Gutenberg University Mainz, Germany. He studied medicine at the Ruperto Carola University Heidelberg and received his doctorate there in 2019. Dr. Wagner completed his residency in ophthalmology at the University Medical Center Mainz, where he became a board-certified ophthalmologist and a fellow of the European Board of Ophthalmology (FEBO) in 2022. He pursued his clinical fellowship in refractive surgery under Prof. Sekundo at the Philipps University of Marburg from 2021 to 2022. Dr. Wagner has published over 30 original research papers.

Contributors

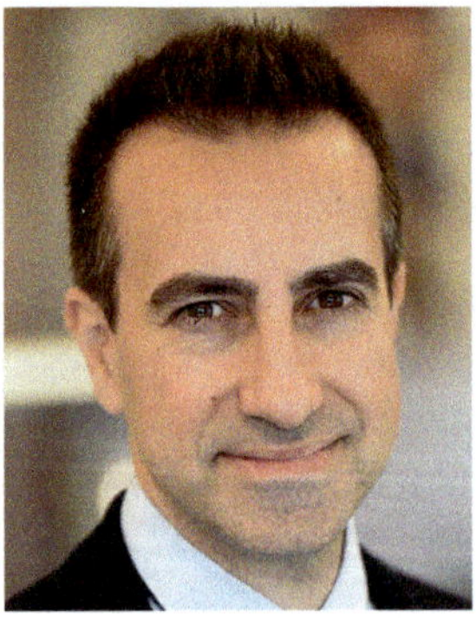

Shady T. Awwad is a professor of Ophthalmology and the head of the cornea and refractive surgery division at the American University of Beirut Medical Center.

He received many international awards including the George Waring Medal for editorial excellence from the *Journal of Refractive Surgery*. He has founded many online analytical tools and software, and has several patents in computer vision machine learning. His clinical interests and research are focused on elective and therapeutic refractive surgery, analytical corneal imaging, machine learning and computer vision, and wavefront technology.

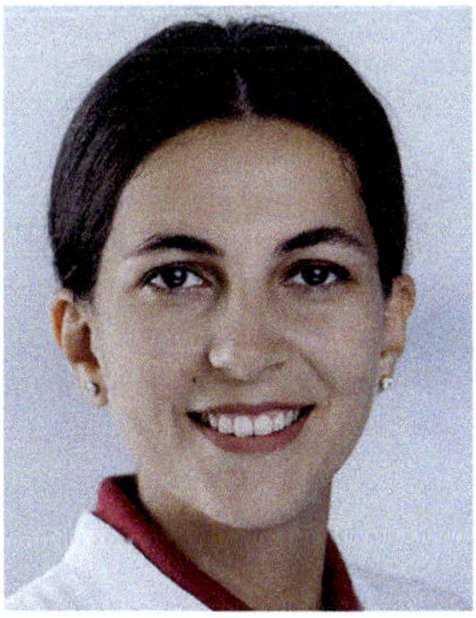

Dr. Beril Tülü Aygün, FEBO, FICO is an Ophthalmologist at Medizentrum Eckert in Karlsruhe, Germany. She studied Medicine at Istanbul University, Cerrahpasa Medical Faculty, and attended an observership in Ophthalmology at Charité Universitätsmedizin Berlin. She completed her residency in Ophthalmology at Beyoglu Eye Hospital of the University of Health Sciences in Istanbul, where she gained significant experience in refractive and cataract surgeries, as well as treating keratoconus patients. Notably, she worked with the team that first performed SMILE surgery in Turkey.

Dr. Tülü Aygün continued her career in Germany at Augenklinik Rendsburg, where she served as a senior physician and specialist. She holds two international titles in ophthalmology, FEBO and FICO. Her research focuses on refractive surgery, keratoconus, and corneal diseases. She has published numerous articles in prestigious international and national journals, received awards for her contributions, presented at international conferences, and contributed to several book chapters.

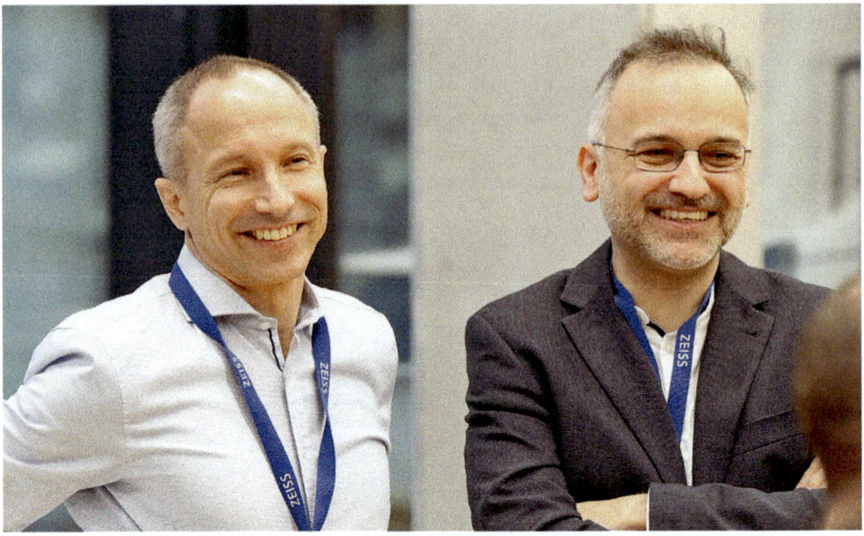

Mark Bischoff earned his Ph.D. in Physics in 2000 from Friedrich-Schiller-University Jena. He worked as post-doctoral scientist at IMRA America, Inc. in Ann Arbor, USA, from 2000 to 2001. Subsequently, he joined the extreme ultraviolet (EUV) radiation source group of the Friedrich-Schiller-University Jena. In 2002, Mark joined Carl Zeiss Meditec's R&D department as a femtosecond laser specialist. He became the general project manager for the development of the VISUMAX femtosecond laser device in 2003. By 2008, he held positions such as Manager of Systems Engineering and Head of R&D Refractive Lasers. From 2016 to 2020, Mark served as a senior manager of Application Research at Carl Zeiss Meditec AG. Since 2021, he has been the Head of the Tissue Engineering Team at the Corporate Research and Technology Department of Carl Zeiss AG.

Mark Bischoff (left) and **Gregor Stobrawa** (right) have collaborated for years, developing ground breaking technology for VISUMAX and SMILE alongside ZEISS colleagues. Their authorship of numerous patents showcases their outstanding contributions to the field.

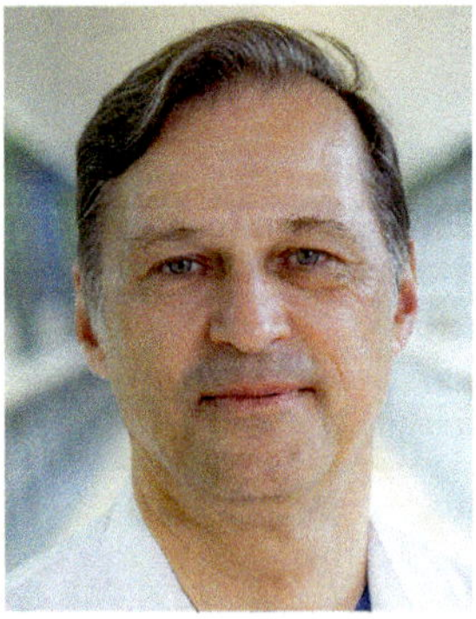

Marcus Blum, MD is Head of Department of Ophthalmology, Helios Klinikum Erfurt, Germany. He studied at the University of Heidelberg. He was resident in the Department of Ophthalmology at Heidelberg (Prof. H. E. Völcker) and fellow at the Department of Ophthalmology at Jena (Prof. J. Strobel). He was appointed Associate Professor at the University of Jena in 1999 and was involved in building up a technology network focusing on new technologies for Ophthalmology in Jena. Together with Walter Sekundo he pioneered using fs-lasers for lenticule extraction. In 2001, Prof. Blum became head of the Ophthalmology Department at the Helios Klinikum Erfurt. He has published 150 papers and book chapters and has given more than 300 presentations at national and international meetings. In 2024, he was elected as president of the German Society for Cataract and Refractive Surgery (DGII).

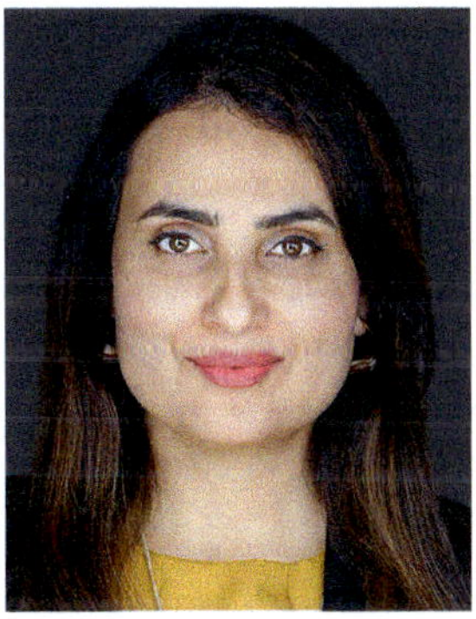

Sheetal Brar is Director, Cataract and Refractive surgery and Head of Research and academics at Brar Eye Hospital, Bathinda, Punjab. Trained > 200 trainees in phacoemulsification and complex cataract surgeries and > 100 surgeons in refractive surgery and participated in over 100 masterclasses and instructional courses and performed live surgeries of phacoemulsification and SMILE. 100+ publications in national and international peer-reviewed indexed journals. Sheetal Brar is Reviewer for *Journal of Refractive Surgery* (JRS), *Cornea*, *JCRS*, *BMC Ophthalmology*, *Open Journal of Ophthalmology*, and *IJO* journals. Sheetal Brar is Receiver of over 30 international film festival and best papers of session awards. 1st woman ophthalmologist from India to receive the prestigious APACRS Certified Educator (ACE) Award.

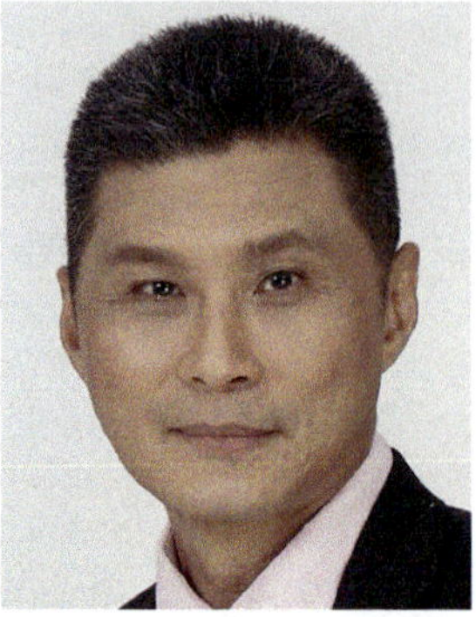

Ekktet Chansue is Medical Director of TRSC International LASIK Center in Bangkok, Thailand. Graduating from the Ramathibodi Hospital Faculty of Medicine, Mahidol University in Bangkok, Thailand in 1986, he went directly into Ophthalmology at the Department of Ophthalmology, Chiang Mai University. In 1989, he joined ORBIS International ("Project ORBIS" at that time) as a staff ophthalmologist and crew member, and later became the Field Medical Director. After his time on ORBIS, Dr. Chansue went to undertake a 2-year Cornea, External Disease, and Refractive Surgery fellowship at the Washington University in St. Louis, Missouri from 1991 to 1993. Returning to Thailand in 1993, he taught at the Ramathibodi Hospital Faculty of Medicine, Mahidol University, Bangkok, for several years. Dr. Chansue performed the first LASIK surgery in Thailand (and probably the first in South-East Asia) in 1994, and also performed the first SMILE in Thailand in 2010. In the same year, he designed the Chansue ReLEx Dissector, an instrument to aid in the separation and freeing of the lenticule during the SMILE procedure. The instrument has been widely adopted as a standard for the procedure worldwide. Dr. Chansue also helped develop the CIRCLE program for enhancement surgery after SMILE.

In his free time, he likes to play the guitar and has got into lutherie, making acoustic guitars from scratch. His interests include music and travels.

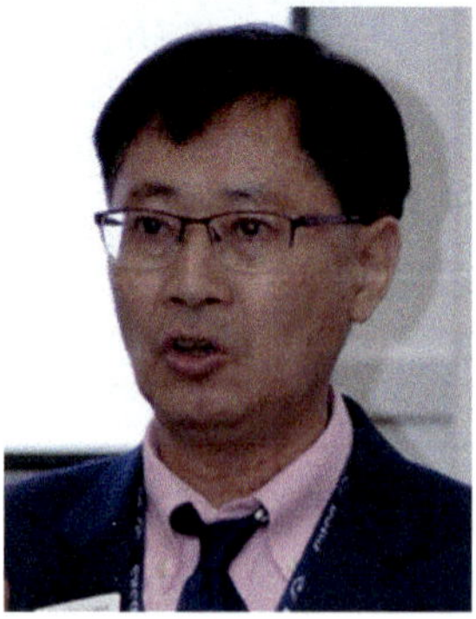

Hong Fu has been the principal inventor for ELITA Femtosecond Laser System and the industry first biconvex lenticule algorithm for corneal refractive surgery. He holds 40 patents or patent applications in laser related fields. He has been a primary contributing author on 25 peer-reviewed papers on laser, optics, and physics before joining industry. He has deep passion to apply mathematics and physics to improve the clinical outcome. Hong Fu is Research Fellow and Senior R&D Manager at Johnson-Johnson Vision in Silicon Valley, California, USA. Prior to Johnson-Johnson, he worked at various positions, including engineer, manager, director, VP for R&D and Engineering, and VP for manufacturing. Hong Fu earned Ph.D. in laser physics at University of Stuttgart, Germany; did graduate study at the Institute of Theoretical Physics of Chinese Academy of Sciences, Beijing; and earned BS degree in nuclear physics at Sichuan University, Chengdu, China. He pursued post-doctoral research at the Optical Sciences Center, University of Arizona, Tucson, USA.

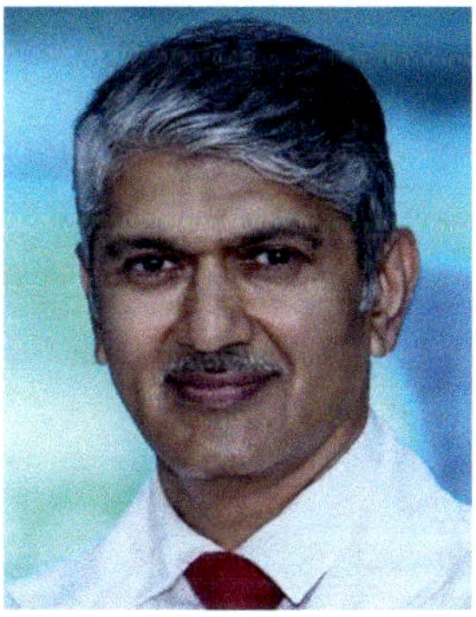

Sri Ganesh, MBBS, MS, DNB, DSC (Hon.), FRCS (Glasgow), FAICO, FWCRS, Founder of Nethradhama Hospitals Pvt. Ltd. and Shraddha Eye Care Trust. Dr. Sri Ganesh started his practice in 1994 and now runs 8 eye hospitals. He started his refractive surgery practice with RK in 1994, Lasik in 1997 and has been at the forefront of refractive surgery technologies. He has performed over 120,000 cataract surgeries and 75,000 refractive surgeries. He has over 60 peer-reviewed publications and has done some pioneering work on lenticule extraction techniques and using SMILE lenticules in tissue addition techniques for correction of hyperopia and keratoconus. He has contributed to 6 book chapters. He has trained over 200 national and international fellows in phaco and refractive surgeries. He was awarded the honorary doctorate from the Rajiv Gandhi University of Health Sciences in 2014 for his contributions to the field of Ophthalmology. He was awarded the honorary FRCS (Glasgow) in 2018. He has been awarded the Gold Medal oration at the AUSCRS in 2017 and the IIRSI Gold Medal in 2007 and BOA Gold Medal in 2011. He was awarded the prestigious Micheal Kritzinger award by ISRS at the AAO 2022 for contributions in refractive surgery and the Honorary FAICO in refractive surgery by All India Ophthalmological society. He is also a charter fellow of the WCRS. He has delivered numerous orations and lectures at various national and international conferences and conducted instruction courses and symposia. He has performed over 100 live surgical demonstrations in various national and international meetings. He is a member of several national and international ophthalmic societies including the "IIIC."

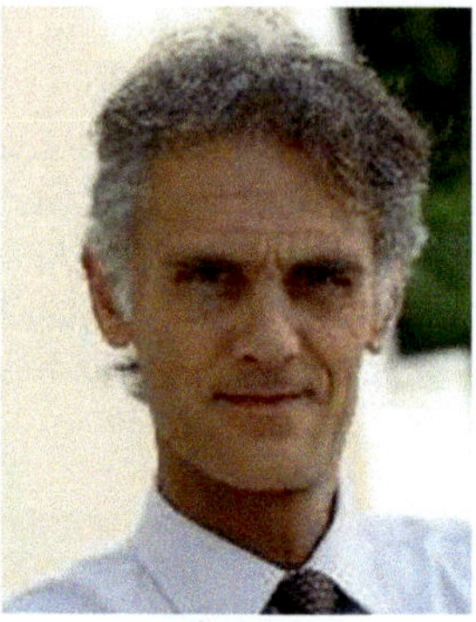

José L. Güell is dedicated to corneal transplant surgery, refractive surgery, and anterior segment reconstruction. He is an Associate Professor at the Autonoma University of Barcelona (Master at IMO) and coordinates the Department of Cornea and Refractive Surgery at IMO Miranza in Barcelona.

He has been President of the ESCRS and EuCornea and is still a director in both companies. He also coordinates the anterior segment modules at European School of Advanced Studies in Ophthalmology (ESASO) and is currently a Board Member of the Cornea Society in the United States and member of the Medical Council of the Veonet group.

Areas of interest are full and partial thickness corneal transplantation (Deep Anterior lamellar keratoplasty and endothelial keratoplasty), complex cataract and anterior segment reconstructive procedures including permanent keratoprothesis surgery (artificial cornea). Also, refractive surgery specially Excimer and femtosecond laser, Iris Claw style phakic IOL (Artisan-Artiflex) and Intracorneal Ring Segments have also been areas of interest. He has lectured since 1991 nationally and internationally on these topics. He has 700 conferences/talks in national and international meetings and 250 articles in peer-reviewed journals and several book chapters.

Main achieved Awards: Award Ramon Castroviejo 2020, Societat catalana d'Oftalmolgia. Lliurament Insignia al Soci d'Honor (per la seva trajectoria). Dr. Josep Ll.Güell. Barcelona. 24 Novembre 2018, Honorary Member. Societe Française d'Ophtalmologie. May 6th, 2018, Fyodorov Award:" Modern Approach for keratoconus patient" HSIOIRS Athens 2016, ISRS Land Award: AAO, Las Vegas 2015, Menezo Quintana Award: SECOIR Barcelona 2013, RolandSiccso Award: "DMEK complications." Annual SICSSO Meeting. Roma

2012, José Ignacio Barraquer Award: "How to enhance refractive outcomes." Videocattaratttarefractiva Milan 2010, ISRS Kritzinger Award. AAO 2008.

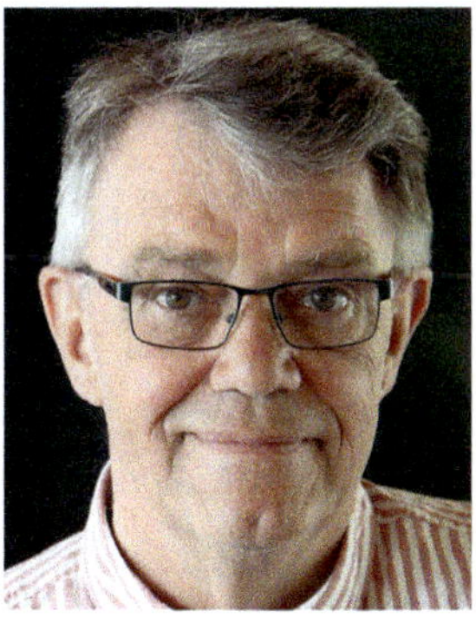

Jesper Hjortdal graduated from Aarhus University in 1988 and was clinically trained in Denmark and at Moorfields Eye Hospital, UK. In 1991–1992, he was Visiting Research Associate at Stanford University, working together with David Maurice. His research focus has mainly been in corneal optics, biomechanics, corneal transplantation, corneal banking, and refractive surgery, and he has published more than 250 papers/book-chapters. He became Senior Consultant at the Department of Ophthalmology, Aarhus University Hospital in 2001 and was appointed Clinical Professor in Corneal and Refractive Surgery at Aarhus University in 2009. In 2011, he was one of the first corneal surgeons to perform SMILE surgery in Europa and his group has published +20 papers on this technique. In 2009, Jesper Hjortdal also became Medical Director and Responsible Person for the Danish Cornea Bank located at Aarhus University Hospital. Jesper Hjortdal is past president of the Danish Ophthalmological Society, the European Eye Bank Association, and EuCornea. Currently he is Secretary of EU EYE, co-editor of Acta Ophthalmologica and Current Eye Research and head of the drafting group for Ocular Tissues in the *Guide to the quality and safety of tissues and cells for human application* published by the European Directorate for the Quality of Medicines and HealthCare (EDQM).

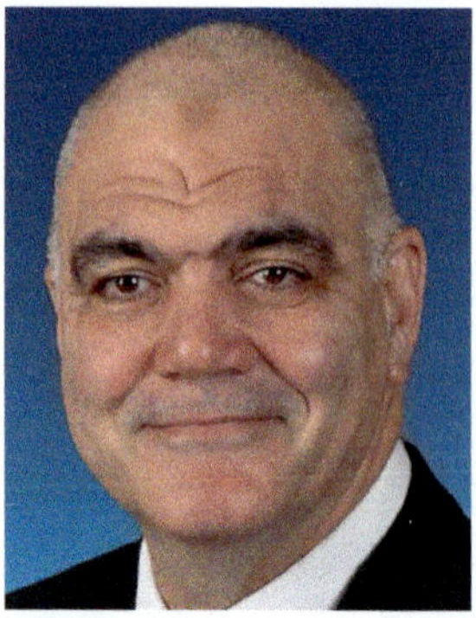

Osama Ibrahim Immediate Past President of Alexandria University and distinguished professor of Ophthalmology. He is the 23rd president of AU and the first elected president (December 2011). He completed Fellowship in Corneal and Refractive Surgery at Emory University, Atlanta, GA, USA between 1988 and 1990. During his 30 years of clinical practice and research development, he supervised and discussed more than 70 Master and Doctorate thesis both in Alexandria University and almost all other universities in Egypt.

Dr. Ibrahim has promoted Refractive Surgery all over the Arab world and Middle East and helped to establish many centers by educating, training and supervising many of his colleagues in the Arab world and operating in many countries. He is an active member of almost all prestigious Ophthalmic Societies in the world.

Dr. Ibrahim has been actively involved as a principal investigator and consultant for many clinical studies and research projects for most Excimer laser companies, Corneal topography, microkeratomes, and Femto second Laser systems and helped to develop many software programs and algorithms for their systems.

Professor Osama is the recipient of the MEACO Distinction Award for 2012, by the Middle East Africa Council of Ophthalmology (MEACO), and the Achievement Award for 2012, by the American Academy of Ophthalmology (AAO), and Casebeer Award for 2013, by the International Society of Refractive Surgery (ISRS).

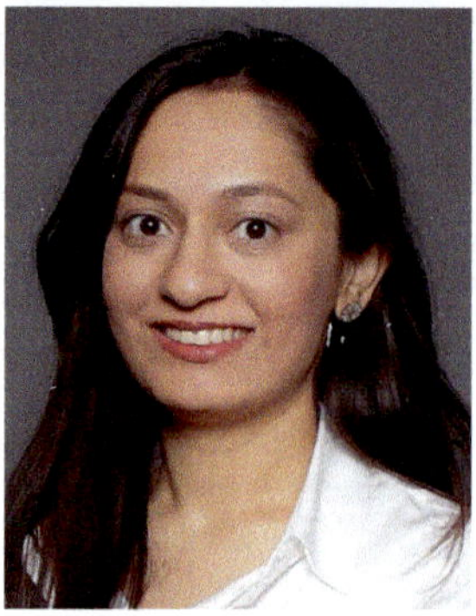

Pooja Khamar is a distinguished consultant in cataract and refractive services at Narayana Nethralaya Eye Institute. With extensive clinical and research experience, she has significantly advanced ophthalmology, particularly through her Ph.D. research on wound healing in refractive surgery at Maastricht University. Her specialized training includes a CORE fellowship at Narayana Nethralaya, Bengaluru, focusing on cataract and refractive surgery, dry eye, and keratoconus. Dr. Khamar is actively involved in translational research at the GROW and IBMS Lab, working on projects that benefit patients and the medical community. Recognized through numerous publications and as a faculty member at prestigious conferences, Dr. Khamar has been named one of the Top 10 Rising Stars of Ophthalmology and awarded the Troutman Award for her exceptional contributions to refractive surgery. Her work has been honored on both national and international platforms. With her extensive knowledge, clinical expertise, and research contributions, Dr. Khamar is a trusted authority in ophthalmology, dedicated to improving patient care and advancing scientific understanding.

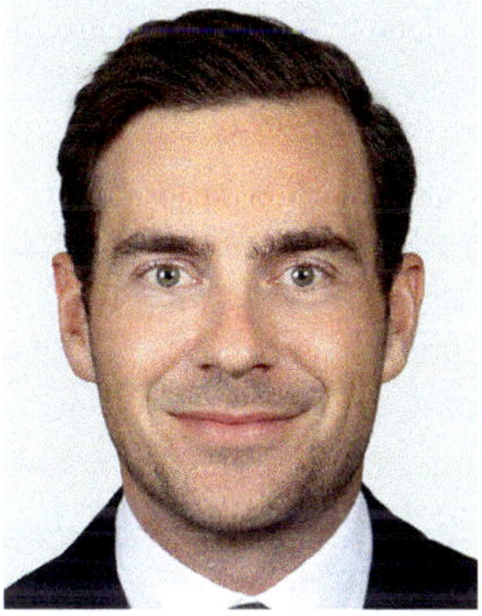

Nikolaus Luft, MD, Ph.D., FEBO, FWCRS, is a professor and consultant ophthalmologist at the Department of Ophthalmology, Ludwig-Maximilians-University in Munich, Germany. He began his scientific career with a research fellowship at the Vienna Institute for Research in Ocular Surgery (VIROS) after completing his medical degree at the Medical University of Vienna. Concurrently, he pursued a Ph.D. degree in Applied Medical Science at the same university, researching Laser Speckle Flowgraphy (LSFG), a novel non-invasive ocular perfusion quantification method. He was a resident at the Kepler University Clinic in Linz (Austria) and Ludwig-Maximilians-University in Munich. Dr. Luft was awarded the Highest Overall EBOD Score Award of 651 contestants from 28 countries at the 2018 European Board of Ophthalmology Diploma Examination in Paris (France). He acquired his venia docendi in 2020 focusing on optimizing the safety and efficiency of corneal refractive and lens surgery before being appointed Professor of Ophthalmology by the Ludwig-Maximilians-University in 2024. Dr. Luft has received several research awards, including the Best Poster Award from the American Academy of Ophthalmology. In 2022, he was elected to the board of the

Cornea Section of the German Ophthalmological Society (DOG), and in 2023, he was nominated as a fellow of the World College of Refractive Surgery and Visual Sciences (FWCRS) for his contributions to refractive surgery. Dr. Luft is a versatile ophthalmic surgeon covering therapeutic and refractive corneal surgery, corneal transplantation and complex lens surgery at the Ludwig-Maximilians-University and his private practices in Austria (Auge Laser Chirurgie, Linz and Vienna).

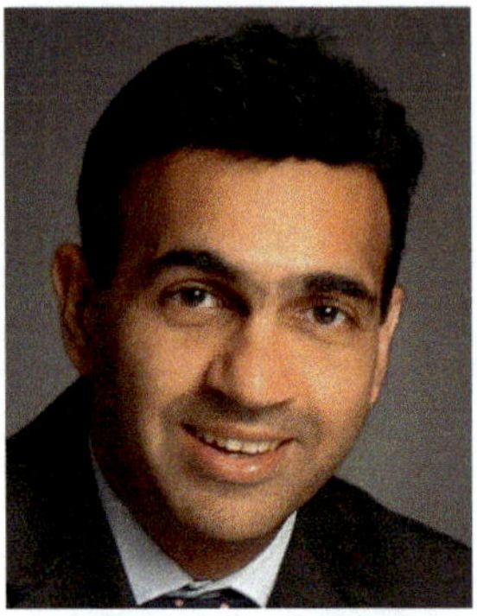

Jodhbir S. Mehta currently helms as the deputy medical director (Research), distinguished professor in Clinical Innovation in Ophthalmology, Singapore National Eye Centre (SNEC), and academic vice-chair (Research) with the SingHealth Duke-NUS Ophthalmology and Visual Science Academic Clinical Programme. He holds concurrent appointments as Executive Director of the Singapore Eye Research Institute (SERI) and heads the Tissue Engineering and Cell Therapy Research Group at SERI. He also serves as Senior Consultant and former Head of the Cornea and External Eye Disease Department at SNEC. Furthermore, he is a tenured professor at the Duke-NUS Medical School.

A highly accomplished Clinician Scientist, Prof. Mehta has been making instrumental contributions both internationally and in the Asia Pacific region. Clinically, he is one of the leading specialists in the world on corneal diseases and refractive surgical procedures; while academically he has demonstrated a remarkable track record in publications and securing funding among others. His research interests span outstandingly across all aspects of corneal external disease and refractive surgery, with corneal transplantation research as the key focus.

Directing a strong multi-disciplinary team and partnering a wide network of collaborators, Prof. Mehta has driven various research projects successfully, many of which have produced breakthroughs and patents with high translational potential.

Professor Mehta exhibits a prolific publication records, with over 520 peer-reviewed papers in acclaimed international journals and authored over 24 book chapters. He has earned a high H-index of 73 (with over 20,500 citations. He has published in *NEJM*, *Lancet*, *Lancet Respiratory Medicine*, *Nature Biomedical Engineering*, *Nature Review Disease Primers*, as well as high impact eye journals, e.g., *PRER*, *Ophthalmology*. He has filed 24 patents from his research work, of which

6 have been commercialized and licensed to companies. As a leader of one of the top research programs at SERI, he has received several competitive research grants, achieving over $15 million as Principal Investigator. As a further reflection of his high standing in the global ophthalmology community; he is currently ranked number 1 in the world for expertise in Cornea and number 2 for Refractive surgery on expertscape.com. He has given over 350 invited lectures and given 19 named lectures; and serves the editorial board of several ophthalmic and visual sciences journals.

Beyond research, Prof. Mehta is a committed educator. Apart from lecturing and teaching various local and international courses, he also supervises and mentors (Transition awards (NMRC), Foundation grant (Singhealth), NIG (NMRC), junior clinicians, fellows (over 30 local and international fellows), researchers (Ph.D. and M.Sc. students) and undergraduate students.

Professor Mehta has received many international awards for the excellent contributions and achievements from his research, clinical and educational endeavors. Some of his accolades include the Nakajima Award (Asia Pacific Academy for Ophthalmology, 2013), Senior Achievement Award (American Academy of Ophthalmology, 2017 and 2023), Doug Coster Lecture (Australia and New Zealand Cornea Society, 2018), Charles Tilett Lecture (Fuchs Society, USA, 2020), Casebeer Award (International Society of Refractive Surgery, AAO, 2020), and the Charles McGhee Medal (BSRS, Oxford UK, 2023), APAO Senior Achievement Award 2023, ACE Award APACRS 2023.

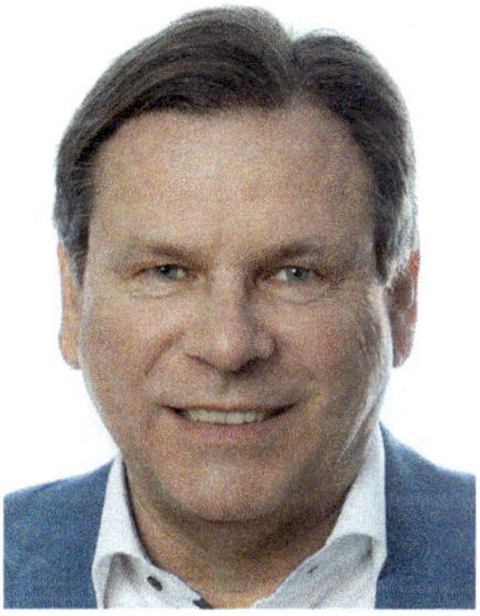

Bertram Meyer is a specialist in laser refractive surgery, with a career spanning over three decades since he began his practice in 1992. Notably, he has been performing SMILE (Small Incision Lenticule Extraction) procedures since 2010. Bertram Meyer offers his expertise in private clinics located in Cologne, Germany, and Dubai, UAE. His professional contributions extend beyond clinical practice. Bertram Meyer regularly shares his knowledge and advancements in the field through lectures and updates at prominent annual meetings, including those organized by the German Ophthalmological Society (DOG), the German Society of Cataract and Refractive Surgery (DOC), the German-speaking Society of Intraocular Lens Implantation (DGII), and the European Society of Cataract and Refractive Surgeons (ESCRS). These presentations primarily focus on Femto-Lasik and Laser-Assisted-Lenticule-Extraction, e.g., ReLEx®SMILE, reflecting his deep expertise and commitment to advancing laser refractive surgery.

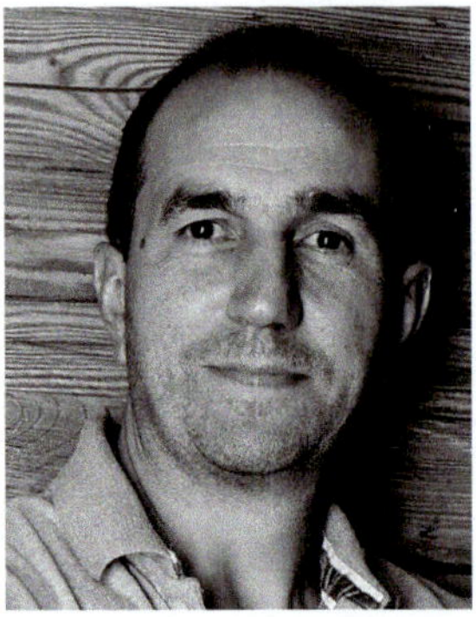

Samuel Arba Mosquera, Ph.D. is Senior Optical and Visual Scientist, Biomedical Engineering Office, SCHWIND eye-tech-solutions, Germany. He studied Physics in Santiago de Compostela (Spain). He further completed a Master's and Doctor's Degree in Sciences of Vision by the University of Valladolid in Spain. Dr. Arba Mosquera has published over 150 original papers, over 15 book chapters and is the inventor in over 100 patent applications. He gave countless presentations at national and international meetings. He is a reviewer for 21 Ophthalmic Journals. In the last 25 years, his research has been focused on corneal and refractive surgery.

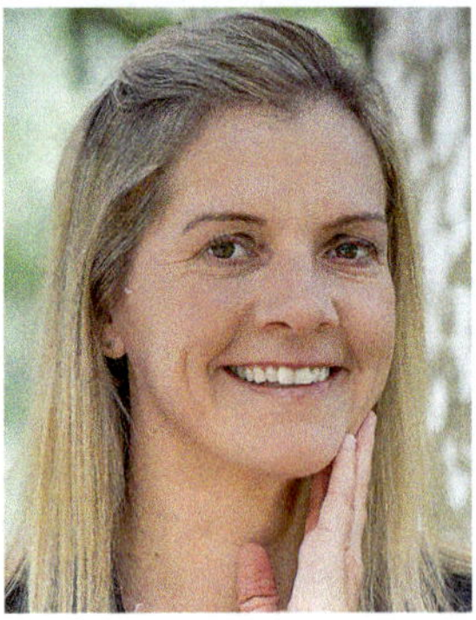

Stine Elkjær Nielsen is a consultant and assistant professor within the cornea and refractive section in the Department of Ophthalmology in Aarhus, Denmark. She received her Ph.D. in 2011. After this she started her ophthalmology residency training at the Department of Ophthalmology in Aarhus, Denmark, and finished training in 2016. She started performing SMILE procedures in 2016. Stine Elkjær

Nielsen has published 20 scientific papers. Her clinical, surgical, and research activity focuses on cataract, corneal refractive surgery, keratoplasty, keratoconus and corneal wound healing.

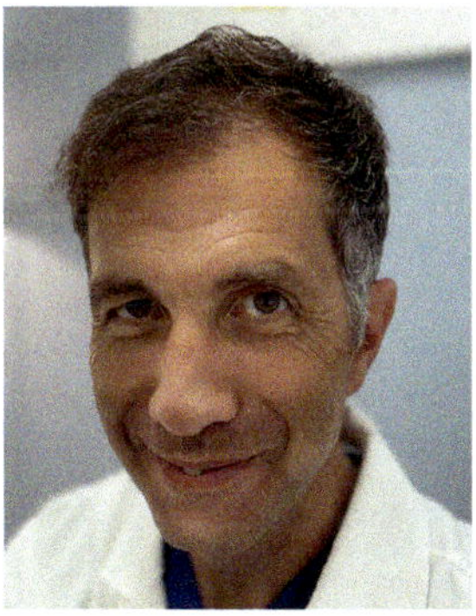

Mario Nubile is currently **Associate Professor in Ophthalmology and Director of the Cornea Service** of the University "G. d'Annunzio" of Chieti and Pescara—Italy. He completed his Residency Program in Ophthalmology in 2003 and his Ph.D. program in 2007. Since 2005, he has been appointed as *Assistant Professor in Ophthalmology* (Researcher) in service at the Ophthalmology Clinic, Center of Excellence in Ophthalmology, National High-Tech Eye Center, University of Chieti-Pescara, Italy. In *2017*, he received full qualification as *Associate Professor in Ophthalmology*, and in 2023 received the qualification for *Full Professor in Ophthalmology*.

He is Head of the "Cornea and Ocular Surface Service" of this University. Principle fields of interest include ocular surface diseases, corneal pathologies and surgery, keratoplasty, femtosecond laser refractive surgery, anterior segment imaging.

Dr. Nubile is Author of more than 160 scientific publications in ophthalmology, books and book chapters, of which 92 are published on international peer-reviewed journals with impact factor. (H-index 33; Citations: 2994)

Patent: EP20179055.7 (European Patent Office) New Drug Delivery System for Ophthalmic use (2020)

Teaching Activities: Teacher of Ophthalmology at the Medical School Program, Teacher of pathologies of the anterior segment and Anterior Segment surgery in the Residency program in Ophthalmology. Member of the Teacher Professors Collegium of the Ph.D. program in "Medical Biotechnology" of the University since 2013. Former External Examiner of International Ph.D. thesis in Europe (UK, Denmark, Spain).

He is Scientific Reviewer for several international scientific journals since 2005. He is member of the Executive Board of the EuCornea (European Society of the Cornea and Ocular Surface Specialists) with the function of Secretary General. He has been member of the ESCRS Research Committee (2016–2023) and he is currently Member of the ESCRS Program Committee (2024). He is Coordinator of the Anterior Segment Programs of the ESASO (European School for Advanced Studies in Ophthalmology).

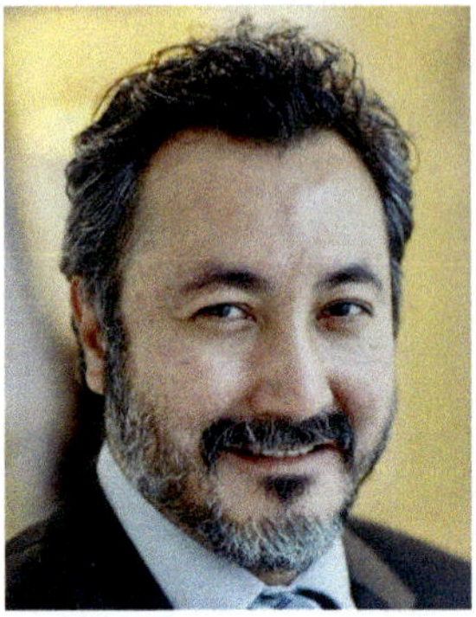

Dr. Kishore Raj Pradhan, born on 19 November 1973, is a highly skilled ophthalmologist and refractive surgery specialist based in Kathmandu, Nepal. After completing his MBBS in 1998 at Shyam Shah Medical College in Madhya Pradesh, India, he earned a Diploma in Ophthalmology (DOMS) from Kasturba Medical College, Karnataka, and an MD in Ophthalmology from the National Institute of Medical Sciences, Kathmandu. In 2010, he pursued advanced training in refractive surgery with Prof. Dan Z. Reinstein at the London Vision Clinic, England.

Dr. Pradhan began his career by dedicating four years (2001–2005) to charity eye camps in rural Nepal, providing cataract surgeries to underprivileged communities in partnership with Operation Eyesight Universal and Sight First International. Following this, he served as a Consultant Ophthalmologist and later specialized in refractive surgery at Tilganga Institute of Ophthalmology from 2008 to 2019, performing over 30,000 cataract surgeries and nearly 6,800 refractive procedures. His contributions to laser eye surgery include work with Schwind Laser Eye Tech in 2019/2020 on the Atos Femtosecond laser, awarded for scientific innovation in Germany.

Currently, Dr. Pradhan is the Medical Director and Proprietor of Matrika Eye Center in Kathmandu and the Matrika Eye Foundation in Birgunj, where he continues to support free eye surgeries for those in need. He has also served as the General Secretary of the Nepal Ophthalmic Society and is a global Key Opinion Leader for Carl Zeiss Meditech, Germany, influencing laser technology advancements. Dr. Pradhan's work is marked by his commitment to improving ophthalmic care in Nepal through clinical expertise and humanitarian outreach.

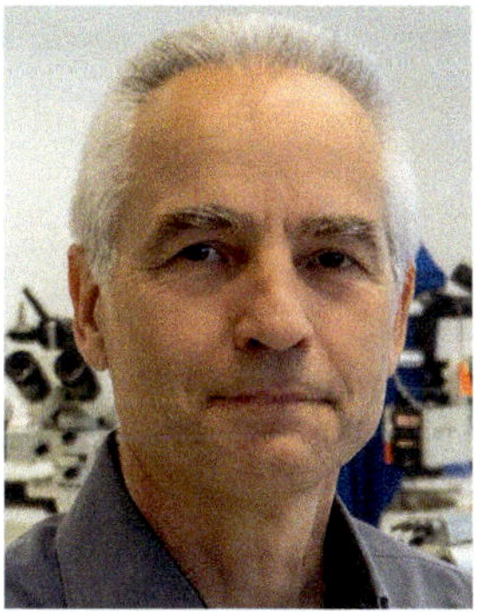

Christian Rathjen, Ph.D., is Vice President for Technology and Strategy at Ziemer Ophthalmic System, Port Switzerland. He is a femtosecond lasers expert with more than 20 years of experience. Previously, he worked at CERN, Geneva Switzerland, developing equipment for superconducting magnets and ultra-high vacuum for the LHC accelerator. He studied engineering at the University of Hannover, Germany, where he also served as a research assistant. In parallel to his professional work, Dr. Rathjen earned a Ph.D. in metrology, during which he invented and implemented a 3D scanning method for surface analysis. In addition to his academic role, he developed equipment to investigate the biomechanics of screw-bone connections, which led to the creation of automated surgical screwdrivers for the cervical spine. Dr. Rathjen's major contributions to ophthalmology include the invention of the Femto LDV Family of low energy femtosecond lasers and the Galilei Scheimpflug analyzer for anterior segment tomography and biometry. Recent contributions in which he plays a leading role include solid-state lasers for surface ablation and various femtosecond laser applications, such as lenticular extraction. His strong focus on innovation has resulted in over 350 granted patents.

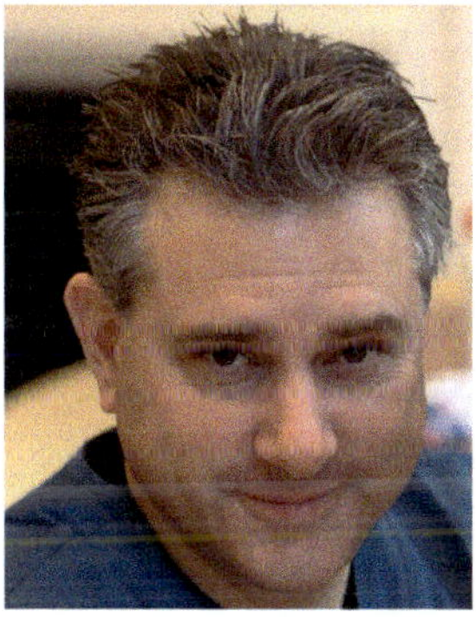

Dan Z. Reinstein, Founder and Medical Director of the London Vision Clinic and part of the EuroEyes Group, is a board-certified ophthalmologist in the USA and Canada, with professorships in the UK, New York, and Paris. Dedicated solely to Refractive Surgery since the 1990s, he has pioneered epithelium mapping and corneal 3D pachymetric imaging with VHF digital ultrasound and OCT. His extensive contributions include over 215 scientific papers, 1000+ lectures globally, and significant roles in Therapeutic Refractive Surgery and as Section Editor for the Journal of Refractive Surgery. He authored a definitive textbook on SMILE, contributed to 44 book chapters, and holds patents for VHF digital ultrasound technology, commercialized as the Insight 100 by ArcScan Inc., which is pivotal for the most accurate ICL sizing. Reinstein developed PRESBYOND Laser Blended Vision, now a part of the Carl Zeiss Meditec platform, and has been their Lead Refractive Surgery consultant since 2001. His achievements have earned him numerous awards, including the Waring Medal (2006), the Kritzinger Award (2013), the ISRS President's and AAO Senior Achievement Awards (2020), the Lifetime Achievement Award from UKISCRS (2023), and the Barraquer Award from AAO (2024). An accomplished saxophonist, he has maintained a monthly residency at the 606 Club in Chelsea for over 20 years.

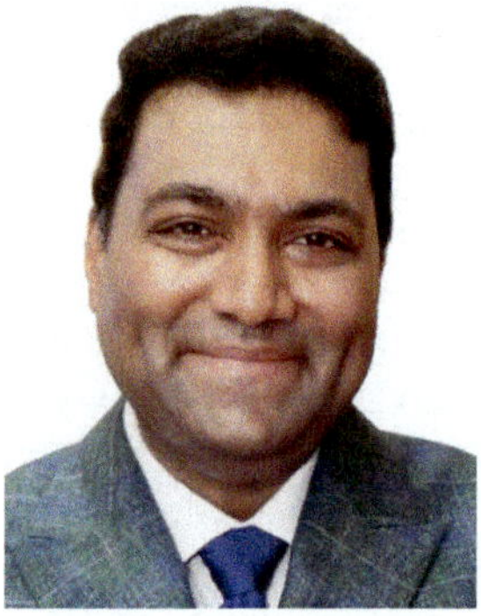

Prof. Dr. Rohit Shetty, DNB, FRCS, FWCRS, FACS, Ph.D. (Netherlands)
Chairman, Narayana Nethralaya, Bengaluru
Clinical and Translational Scientist, GROW Laboratories
Faculty, Department of Ophthalmology, Maastricht University

Professional Summary:

Dr. Rohit Shetty is a distinguished cornea-refractive surgeon and clinician-scientist with a profound interest in keratoconus and corneal ectatic disorders. With over 20 years of expertise in high-volume refractive surgery, Dr. Shetty has significantly contributed to the understanding of keratoconus as an inflammatory disorder and has been instrumental in pioneering novel therapeutic approaches aimed at mitigating inflammation and stabilizing the disease through medical management strategies.

His ground breaking research spans molecular biomarkers in various ocular conditions, including dry eye, keratoconus, retinal conditions, myopia, and glaucoma.

Driven by his passion for translational science, he has successfully translated these discoveries into practical applications, notably developing the "Bio M Pathfinder," the first point-of-care diagnostic kit for studying molecular biomarkers in clinical settings.

Furthermore, Dr. Shetty is actively involved in advancing gene therapy for corneal conditions such as keratoconus and other systemic and retinal dystrophies, cementing his status as a mentor par excellence in the field.

Education:

- Diplomate of the National Board (DNB) in Ophthalmology, St. Johns Medical College
- Fellow of the Royal College of Surgeons (FRCS), Glasgow, Scotland, UK
- Doctor of Philosophy (Ph.D.) in Ophthalmology (Netherlands)
- Fellow of the World College of Refractive Surgeons
- Fellow of the American College of Surgeons (FACS)

Professional Achievements:

- Chief Mentor for the Dual Academic Program (Ph.D. and Clinical Fellowship), Narayana Nethralaya Eye Institute, Bangalore, and Maastricht University
- Fellow of the American College of Surgeons (FACS)
- Recipient of the Casebeer Award for outstanding contribution to refractive surgery
- Awarded the Achievement Award by the American Academy of Ophthalmology and the Asia Pacific Academy of Ophthalmology for distinguished services and contributions to the field

Research Interests:

- One of the first to work on clinical applications on polarization sensitive OCT in clinical practice
- Keen interest in wound healing post-refractive surgery, with a special focus on lenticular-based procedures
- Biomarker discovery for various eye diseases to understand modern-day diseases and identify new drug targets

Publications and Research:

- Authored nearly 350 publications in peer-reviewed journals
- Dr. Shetty holds close to 25 patents in various areas in Ophthalmology.
- Reviewer for numerous indexed journals in ophthalmology
- Editorial board member of the *Journal of Refractive Surgery*

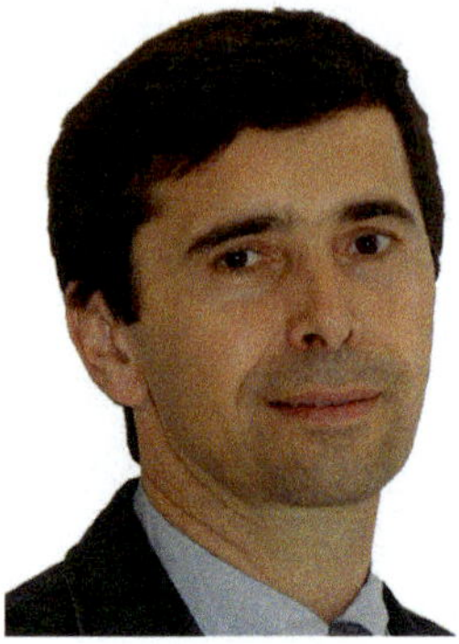

Pavel Stodulka Founder, chief surgeon and CEO of Gemini Eye Clinics in the Czech Republic and Vienna with 350 employees performing over 40,000 surgeries annually. In 2022 he founded corneal eye bank. AECOS Europe President (2024) and ESCRS council member (2017–2025). He teaches ophthalmology at Charles University in Prague and gave over 1000 presentations worldwide and holds several patents regarding ophthalmic devices. The world firsts: presbyopic diffractive phakic IOL implantation (2014). Co-inventor of CAPSULaser and performed world first CAPSULaser capsulotomy (2015) and received the 1st price in innovative category for CAPSULaser video at ESCRS meeting in Copenhagen (2016). World first hydrophobic trifocal FineVision IOL (2016) implantation and EDOF LuxSmart IOL (2021) implantation. He designed presbyopic bio-synthetic collagen corneal inlay and performed its world first implantation (2018). He performed the world first femtomatrix laser cataract surgery (2019) and the presbyopic SMILE (2023). Surgeon dedicated to innovations performed the first in his country lasik (1994), MICS (2001), femtolasik (2006), DMEK (2006), FLACS femtocataract (2012) and many other surgeries. High volume surgeon with over 50,000 surgeries. He received several honors including Emilio Campos Medal Lecture for innovations from Italian Ophthalmology Society (2022) and the reward from a president of the Czech Republic for services to the state (2022).

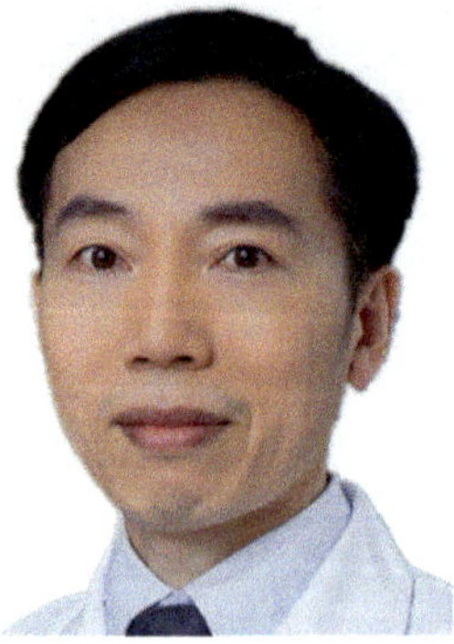

Prof. Xingtao Zhou, Ph.D. is a distinguished chief ophthalmologist, post-doctor of ophthalmology, Ph.D. supervisor, and professor of ophthalmology at EENT Hospital of Fudan University, China. He serves as the President of EENT Hospital and Director of the Shanghai Research Center of Ophthalmology and Optometry. He also holds the position of Deputy Head of the National Expert Group on Comprehensive Prevention and Control of Myopia in Children and Adolescents. Prof. Zhou is a section editor for *APJO* and a reviewer for prestigious journals such as *The Lancet*, *Ophthalmology*, *AJO*, *JRS*, *JCRS*, *IOVS*, *BJO*, etc. Renowned for his pioneering work in myopia prevention and laser treatment of refractive errors, Prof. Zhou has published over 200 SCI articles and holds more than 30 patents. He has been the principal investigator for 15 major research projects and edited 8 professional books. Notably, he performed the first SMILE procedure in China and has completed over 45,000 cases. He also performed the first case of TICL, epikeratophakia with SMILE lenticule. His innovative contributions to surgical equipment have earned him the National Invention Award and the National Science and Technology Progress Award. Prof. Zhou's dedication to public education is evident in his establishment of the Asian-Pacific ICL/TICL Education Center and the annual "Care for Myopia, Smile Symposium." His initiatives in myopia management span all age groups, from children to the elderly. His numerous accolades include the titles of Young and Middle-aged Experts with Outstanding Contributions to National Health, Outstanding Doctors of China, and Eye Health Hero, alongside multiple national and regional awards for science and technology progress.

Part I

Small Incision Lenticule Extraction (SMILE® and SMILE pro®): Basic Principles

Femtosecond Laser Keratomes for Refractive Lenticule Extraction

1

Mark Bischoff and Gregor Stobrawa

Abstract

This chapter looks at the technical fundamentals of refractive lens extraction. It covers the initial developments leading up to the SMILE procedure, which has become the preferred method of lens extraction. The chapter highlights the evolution of femtosecond laser-keratomes and their technical parameters; important differences among various femtosecond laser-keratomes available on the market are presented. The importance of accurate diagnosis, surgical planning, and the biomechanical effects of the treatment are briefly discussed.

Keywords

Femtosecond laser • Refractive lenticule extraction • Small incision lenticule extraction (SMILE) • Femtosecond lenticule extraction (FLEx) • Laser-assisted in situ keratomileusis (LASIK) • VISUMAX devices

The first refractive lenticule extraction in a human was done on May 4, 2006, at the eye clinic of the Helios Klinikum Erfurt, Germany, with a femtosecond laser keratome from ZEISS. This first treatment of an amblyopic patient already demonstrated the effectiveness of the new refractive correction method. However, in this first treatment, the lenticule was created along with a complete flap incision, not with a cap. This procedure, later known under the name FLEx, was revolutionary in terms of refractive lenticule generation and an exciting success for all those involved. But surgically it was somewhat easier than the SMILE lenticule extraction procedure commonly used today. The first SMILE treatment in humans was

M. Bischoff (✉) · G. Stobrawa
Carl Zeiss AG, Carl-Zeiss-Promenade 10, 07745 Jena, Germany
e-mail: mark.bischoff@zeiss.com

W. Sekundo and F. M. Wagner (eds.), *Femtosecond Laser Assisted Lenticule Extraction*,
https://doi.org/10.1007/978-3-031-60424-9_1

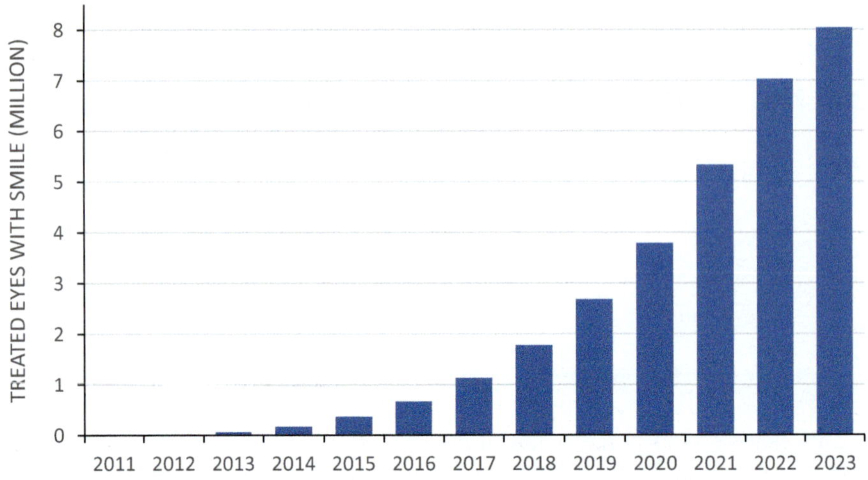

Fig. 1.1 Total number of lenticule extraction procedures performed with SMILE worldwide since market launch. Last considered status is August 2023

done on April 24, 2007, by Walter Sekundo. The SMILE lenticule extraction procedure convinced refractive surgeons worldwide and has now completely sidelined FLEx in clinical use. More than 16 years have passed since then with more than 8 million eyes having been treated with SMILE as of August 2023 (Fig. 1.1). The development history of this clinical procedure is described in detail in Chap. 4 by its pioneering clinicians, Marcus Blum and Walter Sekundo.

In terms of lenticule cutting geometry, there is no difference between the previous VisuMax instruments (500 kHz) and the new models VISUMAX 600 and VISUMAX 800 (2 MHz). Figure 1.2 shows the main features of the incisions created in SMILE for myopic corrections. The cap cut is always made parallel to the corneal surface and its thickness is defined by the surgeon. The refractive effect results from the interplay between the cap cut and the deeper lenticule cut. The latter is performed first by the laser keratome to avoid a shadowing effect of the laser beam due to bubbles in incisions above. Both incisions are connected to each other by the side cut at the edge of the lenticule, which is normally 10–15 μm in height. Today, most surgeons practicing the lenticule extraction procedure SMILE do so with just a single access incision of 2–4 mm width. Drawings of lenticules are almost always elongated in the direction of the optical axis (e.g., Fig. 1.2) in order to present various important characteristics. However, one should not get a false impression of the reality. Figure 1.3 illustrates the geometry of a typical lenticule using a uniform aspect ratio.

In addition to the spherical correction, the vision correction also often involves correction of astigmatism. This means that the lenticule thickness profile differs along different meridians. In SMILE, the lenticule cut has a toric geometry instead of a spherical geometry. Since VISUMAX devices scan the laser focus along contour lines of the curved cut surfaces, this results in elliptical instead of circular

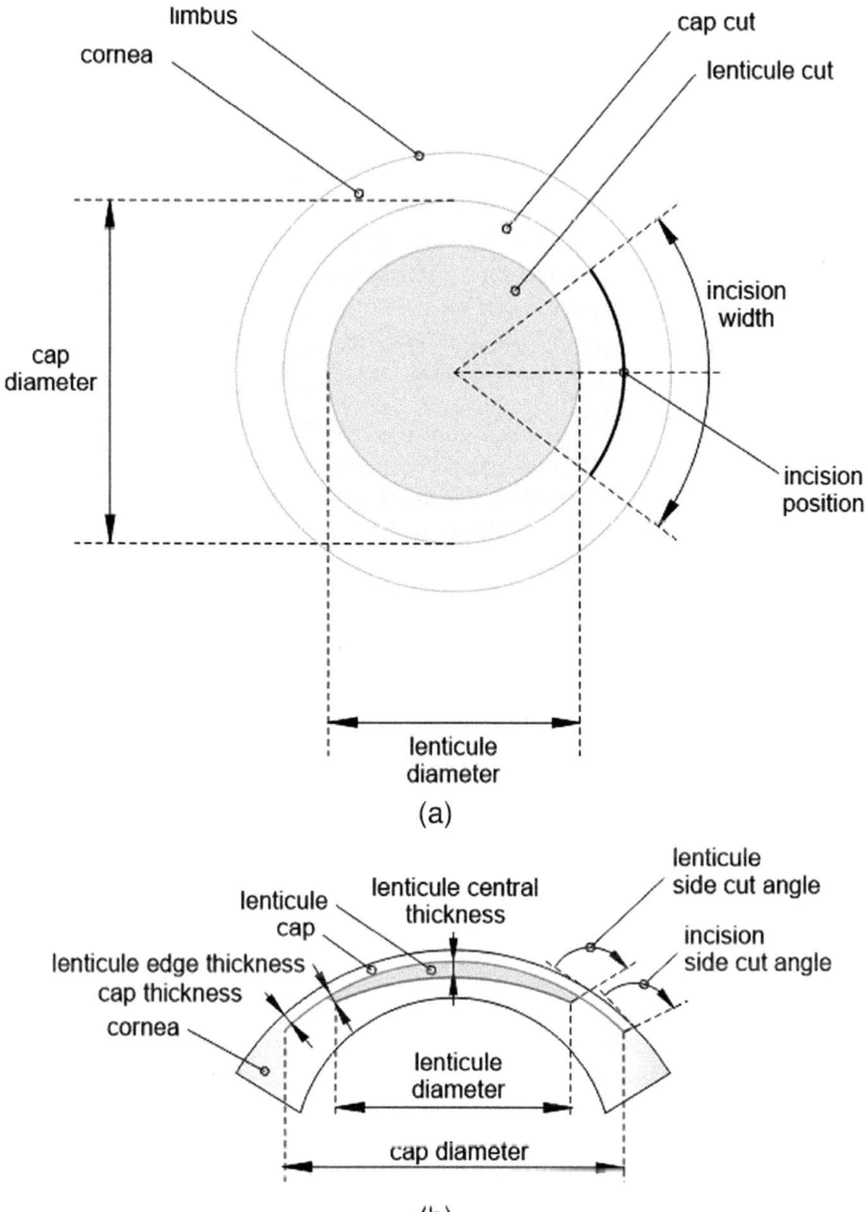

Fig. 1.2 Parameters associated with SMILE for myopia. Diagram at top (a) is a schematic view from above of a cornea with lenticule and cap already cut. The diagram at the bottom (b) is a side view of the same. Many parameters can be selected directly by the user, such as the opening incision width, the lenticule diameter, the cap thickness, the lenticule edge thickness, the cap diameter, and the cap and lenticule side cut angles. Other parameters such as the lenticule central thickness, the residual bed thickness, and the shape of the lenticule (not labeled) are calculated by the laser keratome based upon the manifest and target refraction values and preoperative corneal pachymetry entered by the user. (Note that the aspect ratio has been modified in this illustration.)

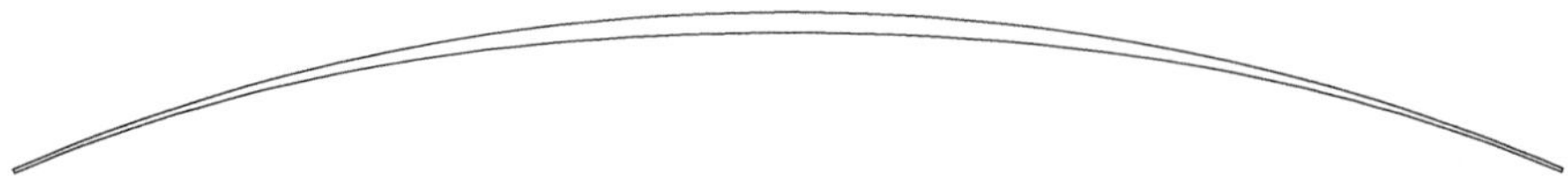

Fig. 1.3 Cross section of a typical lenticule for a correction of myopia, shown with a uniform aspect ratio for all axes and a scaling factor of approximately 25:1 (sphere = −5 diopters, cylinder = 0 diopters, diameter = 6 mm, minimum lenticule thickness = 15 μm, side cut angle = 90°)

scan trajectories for the lenticule cut. A narrow transition zone (0.1 mm width in Myopia SMILE) surrounds the elliptical cut surface and gives it a circular outer contour. Thanks to the VISUMAX' full-field objective, the surgeon can observe the complete cutting process and can even identify such fine details. A SMILE lenticule always has a precise circular outer contour with a defined thickness of 10–15 μm. Astigmatism correction is the subject of Chap. 8.

Ten years ago, when the first edition of this book was published, there was intense debate about the advantages and disadvantages of SMILE and LASIK. In the meantime, numerous high-quality clinical comparative studies have been published showing that the refractive results of the lenticule extraction with SMILE and LASIK are similar in clinical practice [1, 25, 34]. However, there are differences in the healing process, possible complications, and side effects. These are not due to the special interaction mechanism of femtosecond laser pulses with tissue, which is different from the interaction of excimer laser pulses with tissue. Rather, the differences result from the fact that, unlike in LASIK, no flap is cut in SMILE. Cap in SMILE instead of flap in LASIK results in preservation of integrity of the mechanical comparatively strong anterior layer of corneal stroma and its mainly intact innervation [3, 7, 32]. This has advantages for patients because it reduces some risks and thus reduces the extent and frequency of some side effects after LASIK [12, 33]. However, SMILE requires high technical effort in the laser system and surgical skill in the resection of the lenticule. The technique practiced today is based on the pioneering work of Sekundo and Blum [27] and was then gradually improved. Many outstanding refractive surgeons contributed to this, some of whom also appear in this book with their own contribution.

For VisuMax, VISUMAX 600, and VISUMAX 800, which all have a pulse length of approx. 300 fs and a focus diameter of just under 3 μm, the following sectioning parameters have proven to be well suited:

Pulse energy: 125–140 nJ.

Pulse density: 50.000–100.000 per mm^2.

One way to optimally adjust the parameters of a specific device is described in detail in Chap. 10 (Fig. 1.4).

When generating a lenticule, the size of the cut surfaces is primarily determined by the size of the optical zone. Since this is a patient-specific parameter, there is a typical diameter range of 6.5 to 7.5 mm. This results in a scan time of about 25 seconds for VisuMax with 500 kHz repetition rate and less than 10 seconds for devices of the new generation (VISUMAX 600/ VISUMAX 800), which use a laser pulse frequency of 2 MHz.

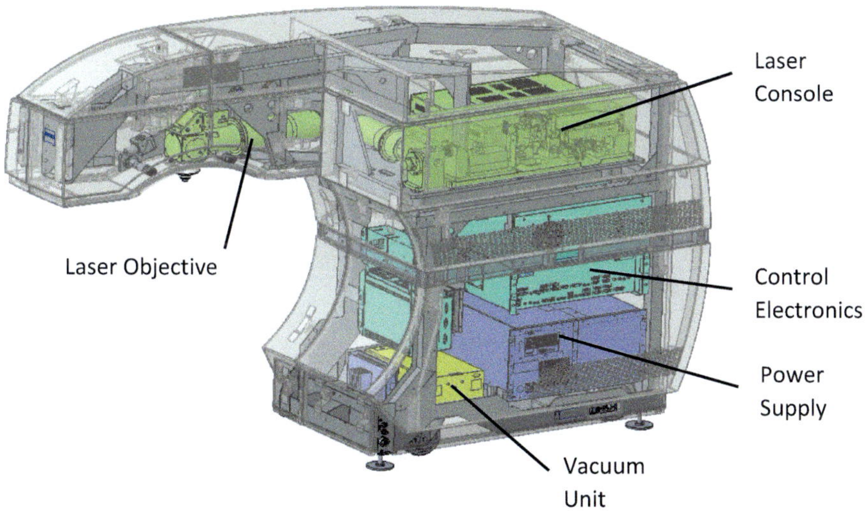

Fig. 1.4 Section through a VisuMax device (first generation) to illustrate the internal structure. Today, more than 1.500 devices of this type are in clinical use worldwide

When awarding the 2018 Nobel Prize in Physics for groundbreaking inventions in the field of laser physics to Donna Strickland and Gerard Mourou, the Nobel Committee cited SMILE as a vivid example of the practical significance of their method for generating intense ultrashort laser pulses [19]. The technology for optical amplification of ultrashort laser pulses, invented by these two outstanding physicists in 1985, was published under the name "chirped pulse amplification." It laid the laser physics groundwork for all of today's femtosecond laser keratomes. The lenticule extraction procedure developed by Carl Zeiss Meditec AG, as an "all-in-one femtosecond laser procedure" for vision correction, is an elegant technical application of this laser technology in ophthalmology. The ZEISS design combined the femtosecond laser with a high-performance optical system and extensive computer control. This medical device then creates the incisions in the cornea required for the separation of a lenticule with the accuracy required for vision correction according to the surgeon's specifications fast and automatically—one can certainly also say "robotically."

The first VisuMax was shown to the public in 2006 and was for many years the only system suitable for lenticule extraction. In the meantime, however, the first competing devices from other manufacturers have been introduced. They differ with regard to the details of the cutting geometry the laser parameters, the respective scan regime, and several other factors. All these systems are suitable for lenticule extraction in principle, but the exciting question is: Are there clinically relevant differences? Table 1.1 provides an overview of the key technical data of the systems currently on the market.

Table 1.1 Technical parameters of femtosecond laser keratomes for lenticule extraction procedures

Device	Manufacturer	Type of optical system	Typical pulse energy (nJ)	Max. pulse frequency (MHz)	Pulse density (#/mm^2)	Scanning time for lenticule (s)	Duration of eye suction (s)
VisuMax	ZEISS	Full field	100–150	0.5	40,000–160,000	25	30
VISUMAX 600 / VISUMAX 800	ZEISS	Full field	100–150	2	40,000–670,000	10	15
Z8	ZIEMER	Partial-field	< 100	< 10	ca. 1,000,000	35	~75
ATOS	Schwind	Partial-field	75–135	< 4	ca. 60,000–70,000	39	~95
ELITA	J&J	Partial-field	45–90	10	ca. 1,000,000	16	> 35

The scanning and suction times are derived from public videos. Other technical data are based on data published on FDA websites. *Source* [4, 6, 10, 15–17, 20, 21]

Today's femtosecond laser keratomes can be divided into two categories, distinguished by the optical systems they use. The first is the class of devices with full-field objective lenses, which include the ZEISS instruments. Such devices can address the full treatment field without moving their laser objective. Partial-field objectives were introduced by Ziemer (see Chap. 26). Devices of this second category can only address a small part of the actual treatment field without moving the objective. In the case of the full-field objective lenses, the high numerical aperture (large beam cone angle) is expensive and mechanically larger, which can present limitations when confronted with some patient's anatomy (nose, cheekbone). A partial-field objective lens is comparatively small and less costly to produce. The cost advantage of the manufacturer is offset by limitations and additional effort incurred when it comes to creating the cutting surfaces: Partial-field objective lens systems tend not to be the fastest at lenticule cutting.

From the patient's and surgeon's points of view, it is crucial that the laser treatment is safe and precise. The ease with which the lenticule can be dissected is an important prerequisite for a good lenticule extraction treatment. Deficiencies in this step would increase the manual challenges. Therefore, the use of proper surgical tools and a careful surgical approach to lenticule extraction are also important. The recommended standard procedure for SMILE taught by ZEISS in certified individual user training sessions is now performed by more than 2500 surgeons worldwide, and there are also numerous technical articles and books [23, 26] on all kinds of surgical challenges. The patient's perceived success of the treatment depends critically on careful diagnosis including accurate determination of refraction. It has been shown that clinics with a strict procedure for diagnosis and surgical planning are able to achieve the target refraction with an accuracy of ± 0.5 D for 90% or more of the treated eyes [8, 29]. The probability for the statistical event that neither of two treated eyes of a patient reaches the target refraction with this accuracy is then calculated as $0.1^2 = 0.01$. This means that less than 1% of (binocularly) treated patients have a refractive error of more than ± 0.5 D in both of their eyes. This fact and the proven low regression [8, 18] explain the usually low need for touch-up treatments. However, this is still one of the weaknesses of SMILE because the procedures currently used for touch-up usually convert SMILE to LASIK (using a CIRCLE procedure) or require a PRK treatment. The predictability of these procedures is high [30, 31] but they have some drawbacks compared to the lenticule extraction procedure SMILE (see Chap. 17).

One of the rare surgical challenges is that the very thin lenticule ruptures during resection, initially leaving a portion of the lenticule under the cap [2]. If this is initially unnoticed, follow-up treatment may be required. With a minimum thickness of the lenticule of typically 15 μm at its periphery, this complication is very rare in myopia correction because with a defined side cut thickness, an irregularity at the edge of the removed lenticule is easily recognizable for the surgeon [28]. As a consequence of this minimum peripheral thickness, the maximum thickness of the lenticule for a given diameter of the optical zone is somewhat larger than theoretically necessary. However, the side cut also ensures that the cut surfaces keep a minimum distance from each other. This is advantageous as a lenticule would create a poor optical quality of the correction if the cut surfaces were to be too close together. Even without a minimum thickness, one would be well advised to choose a sufficient distance of the cut surfaces across the entire optical zone. The SCHWIND ATOS® by SCHWIND eye-tech solutions GmbH solves this problem by surrounding the optical zone with a wide transition zone. For a 6.5 mm optical zone, such a lenticule then has an effective diameter of up to 7.8 mm [20] instead of 6.6 mm with VisuMax or VISUMAX 600/VISUMAX 800. With an equivalent correction, the removed corneal volume is thus approx. 0.1 mm^3 (approx. 5%) larger than with SMILE.

Correctly assessing the potential biomechanical effect of a treatment is one of the important medical tasks in treatment planning. In practice, the criterion of the residual stromal thickness (RST) limits has proven useful for PRK and LASIK. Its transfer to SMILE was logical and has also proven successful. There are several reasonable approaches to account for the largely preserved biomechanical potential of the cap [5, 22, 24]. Comparing the stromal volume removed by the treatment, a small advantage for SMILE over PRK is seen for higher corrections. For lower corrections, it is just the opposite (see Fig. 1.5). There is a tie (agreement) between the two procedures at about -3 dpt, depending on the rim thickness (minimum thickness) of the myopia SMILE lenticule. What does this mean for the biomechanical effect on the treated eye? The parameter Percent Volume Altered (PVA) provides an answer to this question. It is based on the calculation of the amount of corneal tissue removed or rendered biomechanically ineffective by the surgery. LASIK performs poorly in this comparison because the flap can no longer contribute to the biomechanical stability of the cornea—at least for quite some time after the procedure. Chapter 19 addresses this aspect in more detail.

A question that has been debated theoretically and also investigated clinically is that of the correct centration of the SMILE treatment. Chapter 15 is dedicated to this specific topic. Practically, it comes down to the question of whether the lenticule should be centered with respect to the pupil center or with respect to the vertex. Both variants are possible and provide good refractive results [9, 22, 24]. For eyes with small angle between pupillary axis and visual axis (angle kappa), it does not really matter, but this aspect is especially interesting for eyes with large angle kappa. From a theoretical point of view, one should remember that the position of a SMILE lenticule in the cornea depends on the positioning of the treatment, but not its shape (see Fig. 1.6). This is different for treatments with an excimer laser: In LASIK and PRK, the shape of the ablated tissue volume changes when the treatment is decentered with respect to the vertex because the ablation efficiency of the excimer laser pulses depends on their angle of incidence on the corneal surface.

The lenticule shape was designed by ZEISS with the intention of making the SMILE treatment as tolerant as possible to decentration. That is, the induction of higher-order aberrations should be as low as possible if a treatment is decentered. Clinical studies investigating the effect of decentration in myopia SMILE have confirmed the high tolerance of this procedure to decentration [9, 11, 13]. Furthermore, it seems that systematic vertex centration produces fewer aberrations even

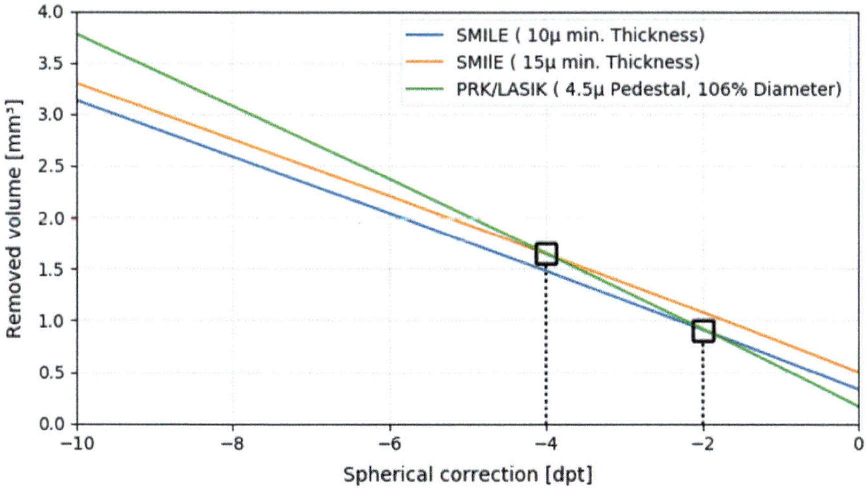

Fig. 1.5 Volume of the removed stromal tissue for a laser vision correction of pure myopia. Each graph represents a correction with a specified (negative) sphere value for an excimer laser treatment (green) and SMILE with a minimum thickness of 10 μm (blue) and 15 μm (orange). The two squares indicate data points where the volume of tissue removed during an excimer laser treatment matches the value of a SMILE treatment. PRK = photorefractive keratectomy; LASIK = laser in situ keratomileusis; dpt = diopters. *Source* Gatinel et al. [5]

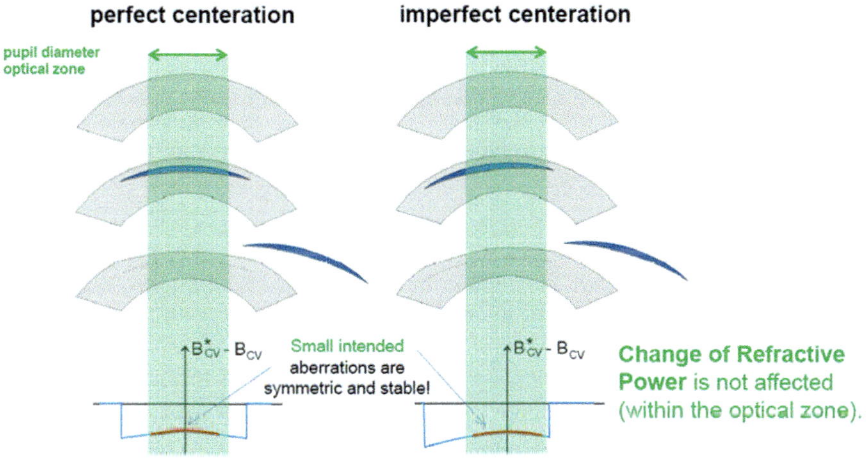

Fig. 1.6 Optical effect of a rotational decentration of the lenticule inside the stroma is similar to a shifting contact lens. This is due to the general method as well as the design of the SMILE lenticule. In the figure, the induced refractive power change (B_{CV}*-B_{CV}) is shown not to be sensitive for decentration of a SMILE treatment. The optical zone (green) and the corneal volume (gray) are shown in the preoperative state (top), with lenticule cut (middle) and with lenticule extracted (bottom). Perfect centration is shown on the left hand side and an example of decentration is shown on the right-hand side. Limitations of this simplified model are due to neglecting the induction of a small prism, biomechanical effects, and healing

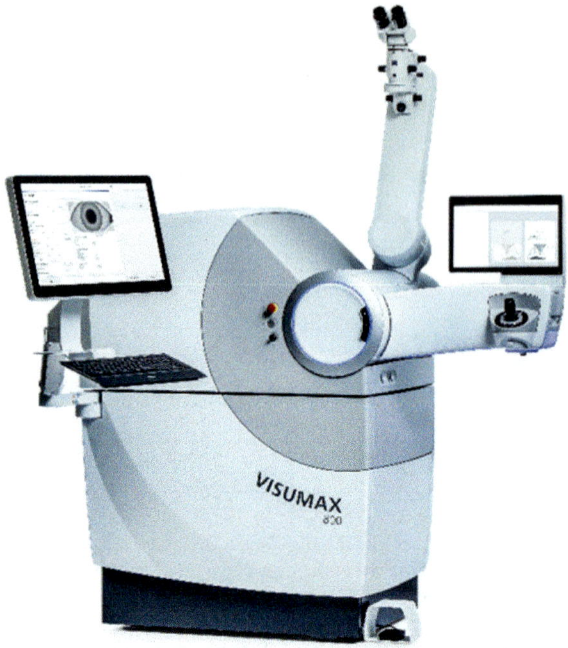

Fig. 1.7 VISUMAX 800 device is commercially available in the first markets since October 2021

with typical centration errors [14]. However, it should be considered that vertex centration requires a larger optical zone of the lenticule corresponding to the angle kappa (Fig. 1.7).

In lenticule extraction for Hyperopia, which is expected to be available in 2024 on VISUMAX 600/VISUMAX 800 with SMILE, there may be a greater dependence on centration. This is due not only to the typically larger angle kappa of hyperopic eyes, but also to the greater epithelial hyperplasia, which could lead to increased induction of postoperative aberrations (for details see Chap. 14). This emphasizes the practical relevance of the centration support introduced with the VISUMAX 600/VISUMAX 800. Future upgrades based on the new VISUMAX 600/VISUMAX 800 laser platform will provide even more support for surgeons in planning, performing, and analyzing their treatments. More than 16 years after the first SMILE treatment, these systems provide the technical basis to further increase the comfort, precision, safety, and efficacy of SMILE treatments.

References

1. Ang M, Farook M, Htoon HM, Mehta JS. Randomized clinical trial comparing femtosecond LASIK and small-incision lenticule extraction. Ophthalmology. 2020;724–30.
2. Asif MI, et al. Complications of small incision lenticule extraction. Indian J Ophthalmol. 2020;68(12):2711–22.
3. Bandeira F, Yusoff NZ, Yam GH-F, Mehta JS. Corneal re-innervation following refractive surgery treatments. Neural Regen Res. 2019;14(4):557–65.

4. Fuest M, Mehta JS. Advances in refractive corneal lenticule extraction. Taiwan J Ophthalmol. 2021;11(2):113–21.
5. Gatinel D, Weyhausen A, Bischoff M. The percent volume altered in correction of myopia and myopic astigmatism with PRK, LASIK, and SMILE. J Refract Surg. 2020;36(12):844–50.
6. Green JA. K223566 (ELITA™ femtosecond laser system, ELITA™ patient interface). Silver Spring: U.S. Food & Drug Administration; 2023.
7. Guo H, Hosseini-Moghaddam S, Hodge W. Corneal biomechanical properties after SMILE versus FLEX, LASIK, LASEK, or PRK: a systematic review and meta-analysis. BMC Ophthalmol. 2019;19(1).
8. Han T, et al. Four-year observation of predictability and stability of small incision lenticule extraction. BMC Ophthalmol. 2016;16(149):1–8.
9. Hjortdal JO, et al. Predictors for the outcome of small-incision lenticule extraction for Myopia. J Refract Surg. 2012;28(12):865–71.
10. Jain A. K213559 (FEMTO LDV Z8 femtosecond surgical laser). Silver Spring: U.S. Food & Drug Administration; 2022.
11. Kang DS, et al. Comparison of the distribution of lenticule decentration following SMILE by subjective patient fixation or triple marking centration. J Refract Surg. 2018;34(7):446–52.
12. Kobashi H, Kamiya K, Shimizu K. Dry eye after small incision lenticule extraction and femtosecond laser-assisted LASIK: meta-analysis. Cornea. 2016;36(1):85–91.
13. Li M, et al. Mild decentration measured by a scheimpflug camera andits its impact on visual quality following SMILE in the early learning curve. Cornea. 2014;55(6):3886–92.
14. Liu S, Zhang X, You Z, Zhou X. Comparison of the distribution of lenticule decentration following SMILE by pupil center or tear film mark centration. J Refract Surg. 2020;36(4):239–46.
15. Mehta JS. CLEAR for advanced refractive correction. CRST, Band new lenticule extraction platforms. 2021.
16. Nalley C. Refractive procedures in the pipeline. Rev Ophthalmol 2023.
17. Nanavaty MA, Naveed H, Ashena Z, Mukhija R. Ex-vivo study on the surface quality of corneal lenticule and stroma after low energy femtosecond laser lenticule extraction. Sci Rep. 2022;12(10034).
18. Papa-Vettorazzi MR, et al. Long-term efficacy and safety profiles following small incision lenticule extraction in eyes with ≥ 5-year follow-up. Eur J Ophthalmol. 2022;32(6):3333–9.
19. Physics TNCF. Groundbreaking inventions in laser physics. Stockholm: KUNGL. VETENSKAPS-AKADEMIEN; 2018.
20. Pradhan KR, Mosquera SA. SmartSight offers a twist. CRST, Band New Lenticule Extraction Platforms. 2021.
21. Pradhan KR, Mosquera SA. Twelve-month outcomes of a new refractive lenticular extraction procedure. J Optometry. 2023;16(1):30–41.
22. Reinstein DZ, Archer TJ, Randleman JB. Mathematical model to compare the relative tensile strength of the cornea after PRK, LASIK, and small incision lenticule extraction. J Refract Surg. 2013;29(7):454–60.
23. Reinstein DZ, Carp GI, Archer TJ. The surgeon's guide to smile: small incision lenticule extraction. 1 Hrsg. S.l.:SLACK; 2018.
24. Reinstein DZ, Gobbe M, Archer TJ. Coaxially sighted corneal light reflex versus entrance pupil center centration of moderate to high hyperopic corneal ablations in eyes with small and large angle kappa. J Refract Surg. 2013;29(5):518–25.
25. Schallhorn J, Seifert S, Schallhorn S. SMILE, topography-guided LASIK, and wavefront-guided LASIK: review of clinical outcomes in premarket approval FDA studies. J Refract Surg. 2019;35(11):690–8.
26. Sekundo W. Small incision lenticule extraction (SMILE). 1 Hrsg. Heidelberg: Springer; 2015.
27. Sekundo W, et al. First efficacy and safety study of femtosecond lenticule extraction for the correction of myopia: six-month results. J Cataract Refract Surg. 2008;34(9):1513–20.
28. Shah R. Complications after SMILE and its management including re-treatment. In: Sekundo W, editor. Small incision lenticule extraction (SMILE). Heidelberg: Springer; 2015. p. 97–105.

29. Sia RK et al. Visual outcomes after SMILE from the first-year experience at a U.S. military refractive surgery center and comparison with PRK and LASIK outcomes. J Cataract Refract Surg. 2020;46(7):995–1002.
30. Siedlecki J, et al. CIRCLE enhancement after myopic SMILE. J Refract Surg. 2018;34(5):304–9.
31. Siedlecki J, et al. Surface ablation versus CIRCLE for myopic enhancement after SMILE: a matched comparative study. Journal of Refract Surg. 2019;35(5):294–300.
32. Wei S, Wang Y. Comparison of corneal sensitivity between FS_LASIK and femtodesond lenticule extraction (ReLEx flex) or small-incision lenticule extraction (ReLEx smile) for myopic eyes. Graefes Arch Clin Exp Ophthalmol. 2013;251(6):1645–54.
33. Wong AHY, et al. Dry eye after SMILE. Asia Pac J Ophthalmol (Phila). 2019;8(5):397–405.
34. Xia L-K, et al. Three-year results of small incision lenticule extraction and wavefront-guided femtosecond laser-assisted laser in situ keratomileusis for correction of high myopia and myopic astigmatism. Int J Ophthalmol. 2018;11(3):470–7.

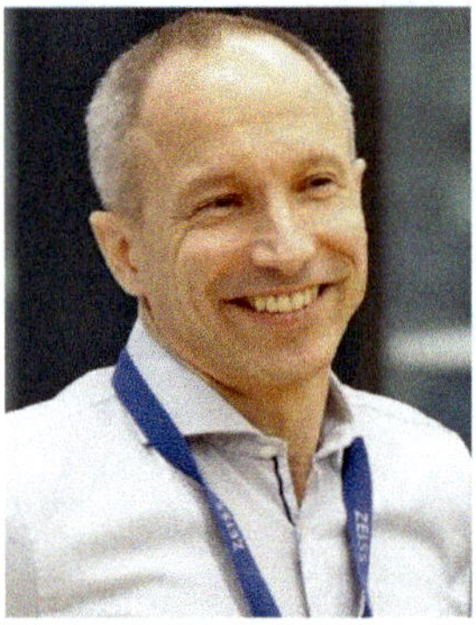

Mark Bischoff earned his Ph.D. in Physics from Friedrich-Schiller-University Jena in 2000. After working at IMRA America, Inc. from 2000 to 2001, he joined the EUV radiation source group at Friedrich-Schiller-University Jena. In 2002, he became a femtosecond laser specialist at Carl Zeiss Meditec's R&D department and was later appointed as the general project manager for the VISUMAX femtosecond laser device. He held various positions at Carl Zeiss Meditec AG, including Head of R&D Refractive Lasers. Currently, Mark is the Head of the Tissue Engineering Team at the Corporate Research and Technology Department of Carl Zeiss AG.

Wound Healing After Small Incision Lenticule Extraction (Relex® Smile) Surgery

2

Yu-Chi Liu and Jodhbir S. Mehta

Abstract

This chapter outlines the fundamental principles of femtosecond lasers, emphasizing wavelength, pulse duration, and their impact on tissue interaction. It also delves into corneal wound healing after lenticule extraction, exploring molecular and cellular aspects and comparing responses across different procedures. The clinical study section examines complications like corneal haze and diffuse lamellar keratitis (DLK), highlighting differences between small incision lenticule extraction (SMILE) and femtosecond laser-assisted in situ keratomileusis (FS-LASIK). The concluding section underscores the critical role of wound healing in postoperative outcomes, noting minimal inflammatory responses in the extracted lenticule plane and emphasizing the need for continued research, particularly in evolving lenticule extraction procedures.

Keywords

Femtosecond laser • ReLEx® • Small incision lenticule extraction (SMILE) • Corneal surgery • Lenticule extraction • Corneal complications • Diffuse lamellar keratitis (DLK)

Y.-C. Liu · J. S. Mehta (✉)
Department of Cornea and External Eye Diseases, Singapore National Eye Centre, Singapore, Singapore
e-mail: jodmehta@gmail.com

Cornea and Refractive Surgery Group, Singapore Eye Research Institute, Singapore, Singapore

Duke-NUS Graduate Medical School, Ophthalmology Academic Clinical Program, Singapore, Singapore

W. Sekundo and F. M. Wagner (eds.), *Femtosecond Laser Assisted Lenticule Extraction*,
https://doi.org/10.1007/978-3-031-60424-9_2

2.1 Basic Principles of Femtosecond Laser

The femtosecond laser consists of a solid-state laser source that emits impulses of wavelength close to the infrared spectrum and of duration measurable in femtoseconds [1]. The definition of a femtosecond is 10^{-15} seconds. Unlike photoablation generated by a 193 um wavelength of light from an argon fluoride excimer laser, the 1053 um wavelength of light used by the femtosecond laser produces a different tissue interaction, known as photodisruption. During the photodisruption process, plasma (free electrons and ions), an acoustic shockwave, thermal energy, and then a cavitation bubble are created (Fig. 2.1) [1]. This process of photodisruption, termed laser-induced optical breakdown, essentially vaporizes a small volume of tissue. The threshold for photodisruption is inversely related to the laser's intensity. The shorter the pulse's duration, the smaller the diameter of the laser spot and the lower the energy needed for photodisruption. The femtosecond laser permits the creation of corneal cuts of different shapes, at desired depths, but the fundamental requirement for this is corneal transparency, that allows precise focus of the laser spots [1]. The corneal surface is the reference plane for the laser. A lens with a higher numerical aperture will create a more focal laser spot in terms of its diameter and volume, which enhances the depth accuracy and overall precision of the lamellar cut. The VisuMax® laser systems (Carl Zeiss Meditec AG, Jena, Germany) use a larger numerical aperture lens, with a lower pulse energy and higher pulse frequency than conventional lasers (500 kHz with the VisuMax 500 and 2000 kHz with VisuMax 800) [2]. Lower pulse energy is generally associated with fewer unwanted side effects, such as an opaque bubble layer, collateral thermal damage, corneal inflammation, and diffuse lamellar keratitis as well as transient light sensitivity [3, 4].

2.2 Wound Healing After Keratorefractive Lenticule Extraction ReLEx SMILE®

Corneal wound healing has an important effect on the safety, efficacy, and stability of laser vision correction [5, 6]. Biological differences in wound healing responses are thought to be a major factor affecting the predictability of refractive surgery such as overcorrection, undercorrection, regression, and irregular astigmatism [5]. Corneal wound healing has also been reported to be associated with corneal haze, myopia regression, and non-infectious keratitis (diffuse lamellar keratitis) after femtosecond laser in situ keratomileusis (Fs-LASIK) [7–9].

Corneal wound healing involves a complex cascade of pathways. On the molecular and cellular level, cytokines and growth factors, such as interleukin (IL)-1, tumor necrosis factor (TNF)-α, epidermal growth factor, and platelet-derived growth factor, are released from the injured epithelium [10, 11]. This injury can take the form of an incision, femtosecond laser exposure, or other insults. The released cytokines and growth factors mediate stromal keratocytes apoptosis [12], followed by proliferation and migration of remaining stromal keratocytes within

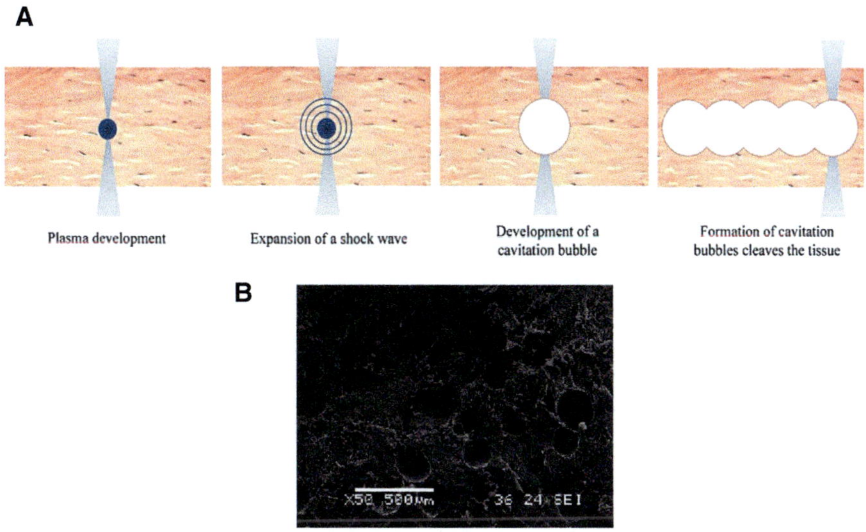

Fig. 2.1 Illustration of photodisruption process in corneal stroma (A). Scanning electron microscopic micrograph showing the cavitation bubbles generated during the photodisruption process

a few hours to restore stromal cellularity [12]. Within 24 h, inflammatory cells migrate to phagocytize the apoptotic cells and enhance the transformation of keratocytes to fibroblasts [6]. Transforming growth factor-β (TGF-β) and other cytokines then induce the differentiation of fibroblasts to myofibroblasts [13], and the appearance of myofibroblasts is the primary biological event associated with the development of corneal surface irregularity and corneal haze (Fig. 2.2) [14]. During the corneal wound healing response, the balance between myofibroblast precursor apoptosis and myofibroblast development is a critical determinant of whether corneal haze develops [14, 15]. Moreover, corneal avascularity, or the maintenance of a corneal "angiogenic privilege" state, is important for corneal transparency [16]. The maintenance of corneal avascularity depends on a fine balance between the production of angiogenic and anti-angiogenic factors [5].

2.2.1 Corneal Wound Healing and Inflammatory Response After ReLEx®: Animal Study

Our group has investigated and compared the early corneal wound repair and inflammatory responses after Femtosecond Lenticule Extraction (FLEx), a flap-based predecessor of SMILE and Fs-LASIK 1 day after surgery [17]. We demonstrated that (1) the expression of fibronectin, which is produced by activated keratocytes and plays an important role in cell adhesion, growth, migration, and differentiation during the corneal wound healing process, showed a less abundant expression around the incision line in the corneas that underwent FLEx than

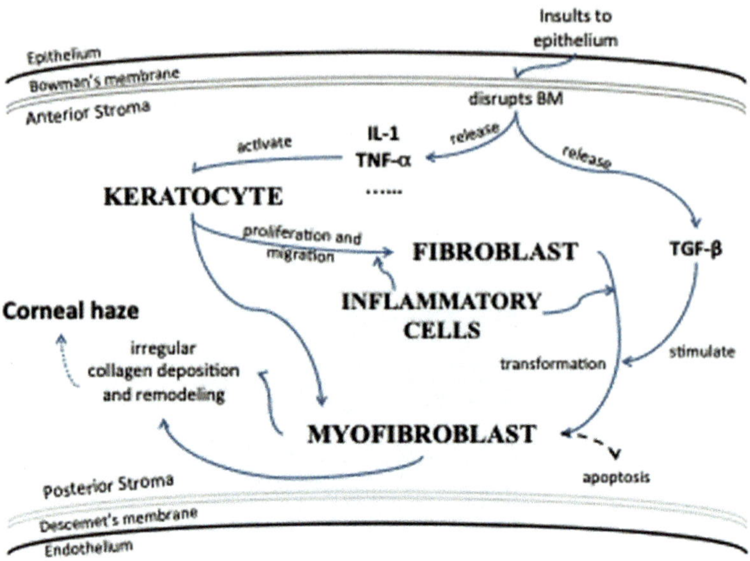

Fig. 2.2 Illustration of corneal wound healing cascade

Fs-LASIK. The differences became more marked as the power of correction was increased. This was because the higher energy of the excimer laser in Fs-LASIK caused an elevated intensity of fibronectin staining. Also in Fs-LASIK, a wider treatment zone including a 1.0-mm blend zone is performed (a conventional blend zone is not needed in ReLEx®). A similar trend was also seen in the number of CD11b-positive cells (a marker of monocytes), that play a role in inflammatory infiltration after injury. The results suggested that excimer laser treatment in Fs-LASIK stimulated a higher degree of inflammation. Furthermore, we found that there were no CD11b-positive cells seen along the laser vertical or lamellar cutting plane in the post-FLEx corneas when the lenticule was not removed. This indicated that the inflammatory response following ReLEx mainly comes from the surgical dissection, rather than the laser. (2) TUNEL-positive cells (indicating apoptotic cells) were detected in the corneal center and periphery of flap, suggesting femtosecond laser energy still induced keratocyte cell death in the absence of injured epithelium. There was no significant disparity in the number of apoptotic cells between Fs-LASIK group and ReLEx, although more apoptotic cells were observed in Fs-LASIK group. (3) Ki-67, a cell proliferation marker, was primarily present in the epithelial cells of the flap margin, rather than the epithelium of cornea center, for both groups. This indicated the proliferation activity was mainly seen in the areas where epithelium was damaged or displaced. No significant difference in the Ki-67 expression around the flap margin was observed between the two groups.

Dong et al. evaluated and compared the early corneal wound healing and inflammatory response after SMILE versus Fs-LASIK using a rabbit model [18].

The authors reported that (1) TUNEL-positive cells were detected at the lamellar interface after SMILE and Fs-LASIK procedures at postoperative 4 and 24 h. A statistically significantly fewer TUNEL-positive stromal cells were observed in the SMILE group than in the Fs-LASIK group at postoperative 4 and 24 h. (2) There were statistically significantly fewer Ki67-positive cells in the stroma in the SMILE group as compared to the fs-LASIK group, at day 3 and week 1 postoperatively, indicating that SMILE stimulated less stromal keratocyte proliferation. (3) The CD11b-positive cells were significantly less in the SMILE group at day 1, day 3, and week 1 postoperatively. The authors postulated this could be due to the following reasons: a small incision for SMILE produced fewer cytokines to attract inflammatory cells in the injury, the intrastromal dissection by a femtosecond laser contributed to less extent of tissue injury compared with the stromal ablation by an excimer laser, and there was less necrotic debris in the interface after SMILE.

It was reported that the recruitment of inflammatory cells begins as early as one hour after SMILE; hence, the authors suggested to start anti-inflammatory eye drops at a very early stage postoperatively [19]. Our group has also studied the early corneal wound healing inflammatory response following SMILE in a rabbit model. The small vertical incision and lamellar dissection wounds were observed on day 1 (Fig. 2.3A) but both of them almost healed at week 1 postoperatively (Fig. 2.3B). The CD11b-postive cells were apparent at 1 day postoperatively, more abundant around the vertical incision site (Fig. 2.4A) than the lamellar incision plane (Fig. 2.4B). This is understandable since the vertical incision cuts through the epithelium and basement membrane. In healthy and intact corneas, the basement membrane can function to bind cytokines [20], suggesting that it may act as a physical barrier for signaling molecules that are produced by the epithelial cells or tear fluid [20]. Thus, when the barrier is compromised, the underlying stroma is exposed to the signaling molecules, and the inflammatory cell infiltration is augmented. Moreover, the surgical manipulations around the incision, such as inserting instruments via the small incision to dissect the anterior and posterior surfaces of the lenticule, and to extract the lenticule, might elicit cytokines to attract inflammatory cells because of more disturbances on the basement membrane. It might also be due to some inadvertent minor epithelial abrasions or small tears at the incision site, which have been reported to be a common postoperative complication after SMILE [21]. At 1 week postoperatively, the CD11b expression was significantly reduced (Fig. 2.4C, D). This observation was different from what was reported by Dong et al. [18]. They showed an increase in CD11b-positive cells in the central cornea at 1 week compared to 1 day postoperatively. However, CD11b is an early inflammatory marker expressed on the surface of neutrophils. Monocytes, and macrophages, which have been reported to be attracted to the wound site within 24 h and be replaced by lymphocytes 3 days after the corneal insult [22]. Since we had previously shown that the expression of CD11b was related to the surgical trauma of lenticule extraction, the difference in the results between the two studies may be explained by differences in surgical technique in lenticule extraction. The expression of fibronectin appeared around the incision as well as along the anterior and posterior extracted lenticule planes at day 1 postoperatively (Fig. 2.5A, B), and the staining intensity in these two sites increased at week 1 postoperatively (Fig. 2.5C, D). Studies on rabbit wound healing models have shown that one day after an incision on the cornea, fibronectin appeared at the site of injury. During the following 1–2 weeks, the increased fibronectin provided a provisional matrix to support the migration of the remaining epithelial cells or keratocytes to cover the area of the defect [23]. After 2 weeks, the wound healing response was complete, and the expression of fibronectin began to decrease [24]. This explains why the expression of fibronectin appeared more distinct around both the small vertical incision and extracted lenticule plane at week 1 after SMILE. Heat shock protein 47 (HSP47) is a stress protein and functions as a collagen-specific molecular chaperon. It is induced in response to stress applied to cells [25]. Unlike the staining pattern of CD11b that mainly appeared in the vertical incision and resolved at 1 week following SMILE, the expression of HSP47 was observed throughout the whole cornea at day 1 postoperatively (Fig. 2.6A, B), suggesting that the laser-induced cell stress may affect the whole layer of cornea, as well as the small incision site. The HSP47-positive cells significantly reduced at 1 week postoperatively (Fig. 2.6C, D).

Corneal backscatter light intensity (LI) depth graphics (Z-scan), a feature of in vivo confocal microscopy (IVCM), has been reported to be used to evaluate corneal stromal reaction, keratocyte activation, and objective haze grading after refractive surgery [26]. Our group has also used IVCM to evaluate and compare the early corneal wound healing and inflammatory response after Fs-LASIK and FLEx in a rabbit model by semi-quantifying the reflectivity level using ImageJ software [17]. The difference in reflectivity level between the two groups was only significant at higher refractive corrections (> 6.0 D myopic correction), with higher reflectivity level in the Fs-LASIK group (Fig. 2.7). That was because greater levels of correction required more tissue to be ablated and longer exposure to the excimer, hence delivering more energy to the cornea. On the contrary, in the refractive lenticule extraction (ReLEx) procedure, either in FLEx or SMILE, the laser energy simply cuts a different shape of the lenticule with an energy of only about

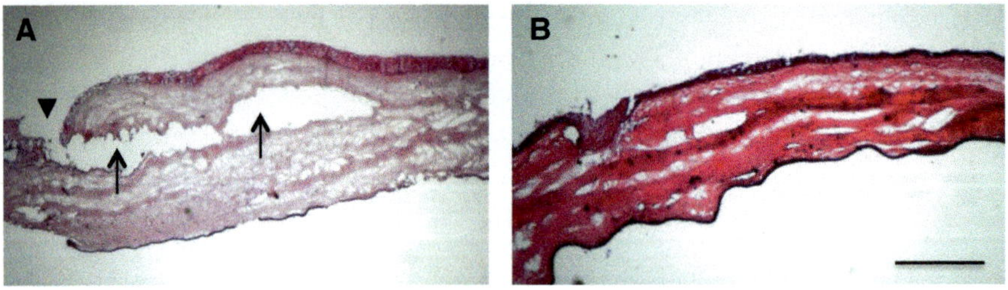

Fig. 2.3 Light microscopic cross-sectional histologic specimen in rabbit corneas stained by hematoxylin-eosin (H & E) stain showing the small incision (arrowhead) and lamellar dissection wound (arrows) were observed at day 1 postoperatively (A) but almost healed at week 1 postoperatively (B). Original magnification: 100x, scale bar 100 μm

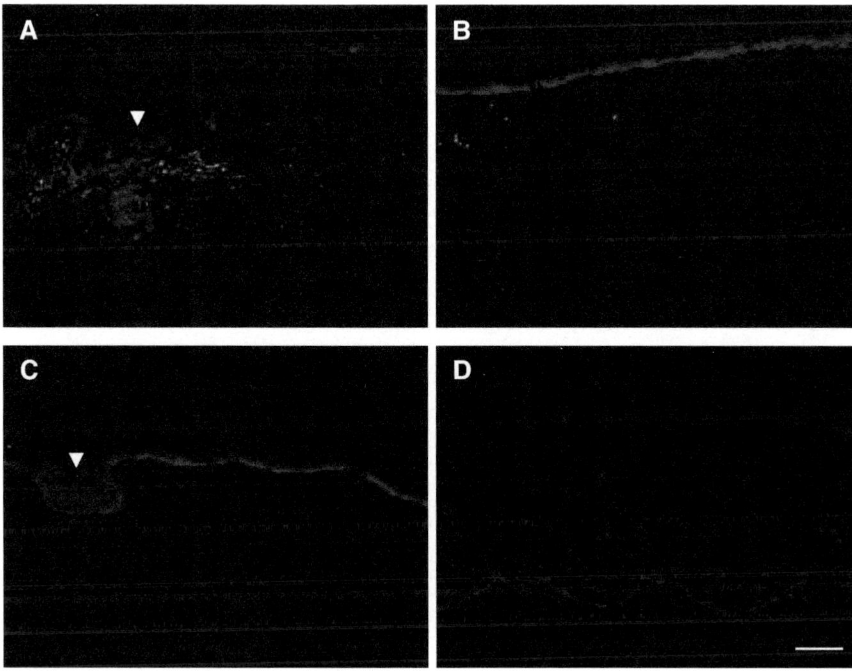

Fig. 2.4 Immunohistochemical staining showing the expression of CD11b in rabbit corneas 1 day (A, B) and 1 week (C, D) at the incision (A, C; arrowheads) and extracted lenticule plane (B, D) after −4.0 D SMILE. The CD11b-postive cells were apparent at 1 day, more abundant around the incision (A) than around the lamellar cutting plane (B) and significantly reduced at 1 week postoperatively (C, D). Original magnification: 200x, scale bar 100 μm

0.58 J (from Carl Zeiss Meditec), and the energy levels did not differ significantly between different attempted corrections [17].

There are other factors that also have an impact on the extent of corneal wound healing and inflammatory response after SMILE, including the laser cut energy level (laser cut energy index), spot size, spacing setting, surgical experience, and the refractive power corrected [27–29]. Although SMILE has been reported as a safe and efficient strategy to treat a wide range of myopia, and the energy levels to cut different-thickness lenticules do not differ significantly between different attempted corrections, the differences in the ease of dissection and lenticule extraction among different power of corrections may still have an impact on the postoperative wound healing and inflammatory response. In low myopic treatment, the delineation and dissection of the anterior surface of the lenticule may be difficult because the lenticule is thin. When the initial dissection undermines the posterior surface of the lenticule, the surgery may become difficult, as the lenticule sticks to the anterior corneal cap and is difficult to be extracted. Furthermore, it is more challenging to extract the lenticule when doing low myopic treatment because the lenticule is thin. These increased manipulations may lead to a greater

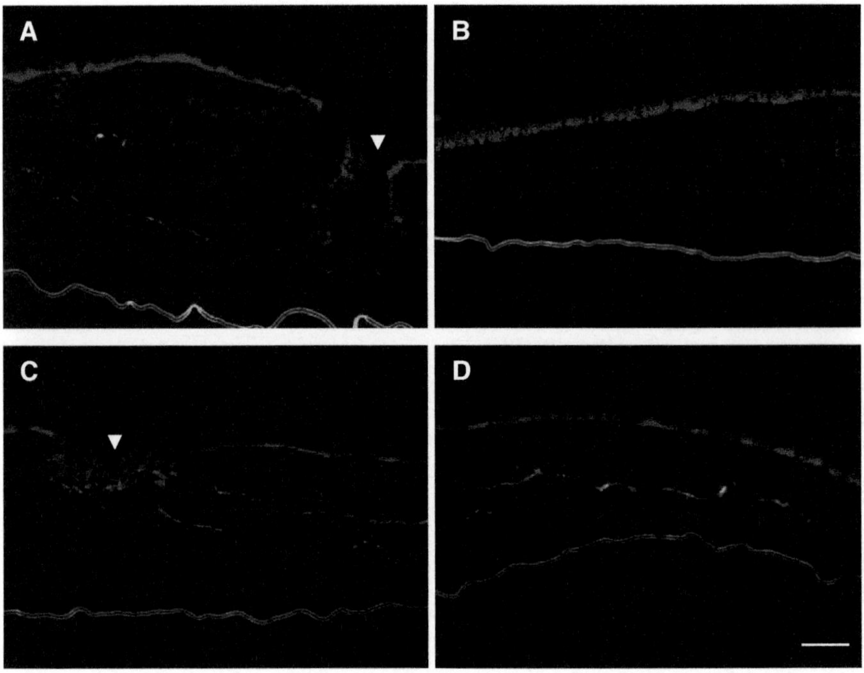

Fig. 2.5 Immunohistochemical staining showing the expression of fibronectin in rabbit corneas 1 day (A, B) and 1 week (C, D) at the incision (A, C; arrowheads) and extracted lenticule plane (B, D) after −4.0 D SMILE. The expression of fibronectin appeared around the incision as well as extracted lenticule plane at day 1 (A, B), and the staining intensity in these two sites became greater at week 1 postoperatively (C, D). Original magnification: 200x, scale bar 100 μm

extent of inflammatory process. Our group reported that less surgical experience resulted in an increased inflammatory response in low myopic corrections, while greater keratocyte response was seen in high myopic corrections irrespective of surgeon experience [27]. These parameters should be taken into account when interpreting the wound healing results among different studies.

The wound healing responses in different re-treatment options after SMILE have also been investigated. Our group examined the in-vivo tissue responses in (i) VisuMax Circle, followed by excimer ablation, (ii) secondary SMILE anterior to the primary procedure, and (iii) surface ablation. Enhancement with surface ablation induced a significantly greater extent of corneal haze, as well as more CD11b and TUNEL-positive cells in the corneal stroma [30]. Hence, the use mitomycin-C is suggested when using surface ablation as the enhancement procedure in order to reduce inflammation and modulate better wound healing.

As SMILE has been a well-established surgical technique for correcting myopia, there has been great interest in extending this treatment to the correction of hyperopia. A recent prospective multicenter trial including 374 eyes demonstrated its high level of efficacy, predictability, safety, and stability [31]. In terms

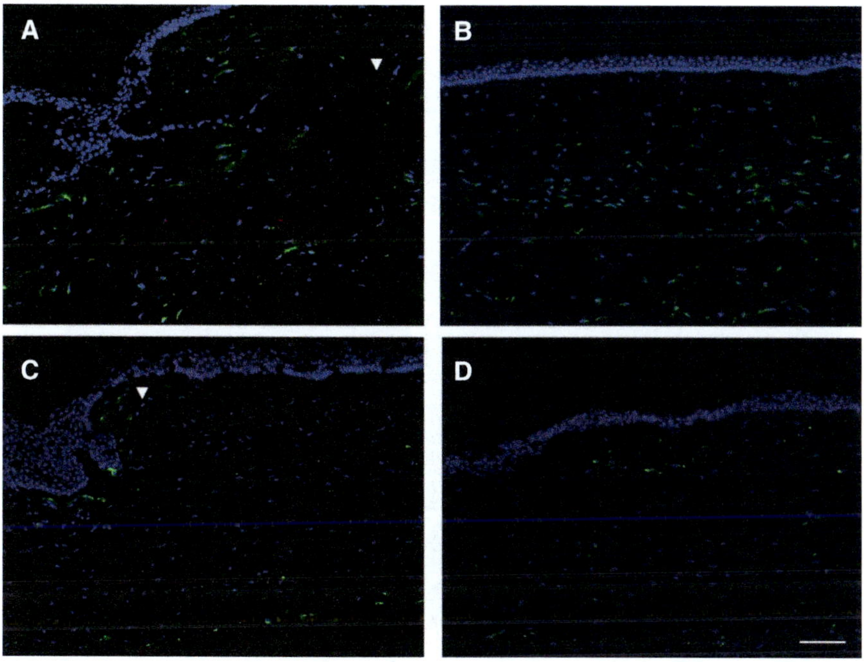

Fig. 2.6 Immunohistochemical staining showing the expression of HSP47 in rabbit corneas 1 day (A, B) and 1 week (C, D) at the incision (A, C; arrowheads) and extracted lenticule plane (B, D) after −4.0 D SMILE. HSP47-postive cells were observed throughout the whole cornea but significantly reduced at 1 week postoperatively. Original magnification: 200x, scale bar 100 μm

of the wound healing responses, our group compared its wound healing and inflammatory responses with those of hyperopic-LASIK, as well as myopic-SMILE, using a rabbit model. Our results showed that hyperopic-SMILE, compared to hyperopic-LASIK, had less postoperative wound healing response and stromal interface reaction, especially in higher refractive correction. However, compared to myopic-SMILE, hyperopic-SMILE resulted in more central deranged collagen fibrils. This might be because in myopic-SMILE, the anterior surface of the lenticule was cut from the center immediately after the completion of cutting the central posterior lenticule surface. In hyperopic-SMILE, there was a 6-second delay between the creation of the central posterior and anterior lenticule surfaces because of the creation of the transition zone. This might lead to increased displacement and distortion of the anterior stromal collagen lamellae to occur as a result of tissue edema and coalescence of cavitation bubbles at the central posterior lenticule surface, resulting in de-arrangements of collagen fibril [32].

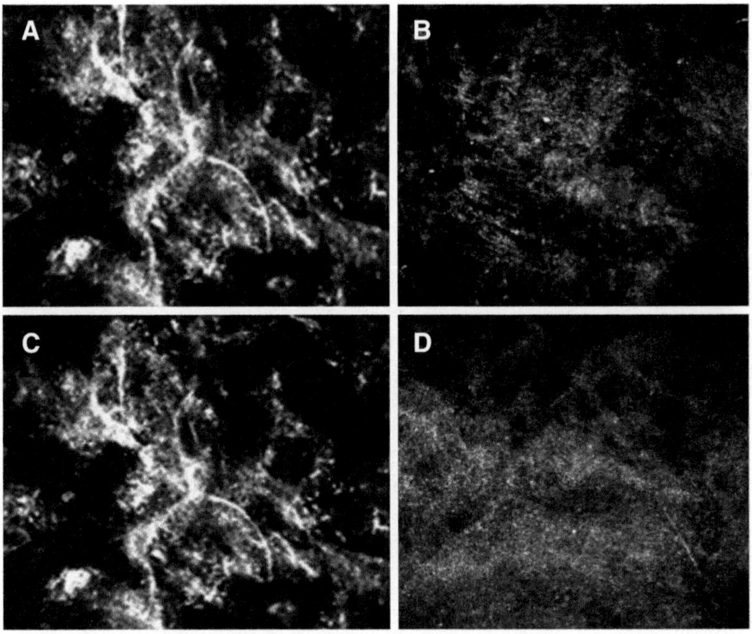

Fig. 2.7 In vivo confocal micrographs of the rabbit corneas 1 day after −3.0 D Fs-LASIK (A), −3.0 D SMILE (B), −9.0 D Fs-LASIK (C), and −9.0 D SMILE (D), at the flap interface (Fs-LASIK) or cap interface (SMILE). The interface site was acellular and light reflective. The difference in reflectivity level between the two groups was only significant at higher corrections (C, D), with higher reflectivity level in the Fs-LASIK group

2.2.2 Clinical Study

The sequelae of corneal wound healing in refractive surgery can lead to undesirable complications, such as corneal haze, diffuse lamellar keratitis (DLK), epithelial ingrowth, and regression [33, 34]. In a large study evaluating more than 1500 SMILE procedures [21], the authors reported that trace corneal haze (grade 0.5–1) was the most frequent postoperative complication noted 3 months after SMILE (127/1574 eyes, 8.1%). Among these 127 eyes that had corneal haze, ten of them had notes of perioperative complications, with six cases of difficult lenticule extraction and four minor tears at the incision. These perioperative complications may trigger greater extent of inflammatory cytokines release, leading to corneal haze. In five cases (0.3%), the patients presented with one or more interface infiltrates 1 week after surgery. Samples were taken for microbiological investigation, but specific pathogens could not be identified. Four eyes (0.3%) experienced interface inflammation during the first week after surgery and were successfully treated with dexamethasone eye drops. DLK occurs in approximately 1.6–2.2% of SMILE surgery [35, 36], with the majority of patients (94%) at stage 1 or 2. Thinner lenticule thickness has been identified as a risk factor associated with DLK. One explanation is that with thinner lenticules, the accumulation of gas bubbles might induce a more intensive inflammatory response at the interface because the anterior and posterior planes of the lenticule would be pressed together more tightly under the compressive force. Another reason might be that thinner lenticules resulted in more wound healing responses due to more technically difficult lenticule separation or extraction [35]. In another large-scaled retrospective review of 4000 eyes, the incidence of DLK was 0.45%. Topical steroid therapy resolved the DLK in all cases with no sequelae and no adverse effect on refractive or visual outcome at one-year postoperatively [37].

Agca et al. [38] conducted a randomized clinical trial enrolling 30 patients who underwent SMILE in one eye and Fs-LASIK in the fellow eye and reported that the mean backscattered LI at all measured depths were significantly higher in the SMILE group than the Fs-LASIK group at all postoperative visits from 1 week to 3 months. The authors stated that this increased corneal backscatter in the early postoperative period in the SMILE group did not necessarily result in decreased vision, increased incidence of complications, or increased inflammation, but it reflected a different healing response after SMILE, and whether this difference has any positive or negative clinical consequences is still unknown (see Chap. 17 for details).

Kamiya et al. [39] also reported that transient interface haze was the most common adverse complication in SMILE, although it was mild and resolved with time. The authors also stated that this mild degree of interface haze may account for the tendency for a slight delay of visual recovery in the early postoperative period (especially 1 week postoperatively) in SMILE or FLEx compared to Fs-LASIK.

After refractive surgery, corneal epithelium remodels by altering its thickness in response to underlying stromal irregularities in an attempt to establish a smooth optical surface [40]. This epithelial remodeling has been shown to be responsible for the postoperative regression after PRK and LASIK [41, 42]. A comparative study reported that the topographic epithelial remodeling patterns differ following Fs-LASIK or SMILE, and the epithelial remodeling appears to stabilize more rapidly following SMILE than Fs-LASIK [43]. Ganesh et al. also demonstrated a statistically significant epithelial thickness increase was observed in the central zone in all post-SMILE eyes (6.83% increase for low myopia, 9.26% increase for moderate myopia, and 12.7% increase for high myopia). This epithelial thickness increase was correlated positively with the degree of myopia corrected [40]. Another prospective study found that postoperative epithelial modulation exerted a significant impact on corneal HOA alterations in SMILE [44].

On a molecular level, results from a randomized controlled trial with paired-eye design demonstrated that there was significant up-regulation in leukocyte migration and wound healing at 1 week, humoral immune response and apoptosis at 1 month, negative regulation of endopeptidase activity at 3–6 months, and extracellular structure organization at 1 year in the post-LASIK eyes, in comparison with post-SMILE eyes [45].

Topical steroid treatment has been used in limiting corneal haze and myopic regression in highly myopic patients after photorefractive keratectomy (PRK) and

LASIK [46, 47]. It was reported that SMILE and Fs-LASIK had a similar risk of myopic regression for low to moderate myopia. Similar to the study results in LASIK [48], a higher preoperative sphere increased myopic regression, while a larger optical zone was a protector against regression [49]. There is no standard protocol for topical steroid use following SMILE. Most of the institutes, including our institute, use a regimen of topical steroids four times a day for 1 week with a tapering dose for the following week. Some institutes use postoperative steroids for even a shorter period [50]. However, in cases of difficult lenticule extractions, higher dose steroids maybe required if extensive manipulations occur at the incision site.

A second-generation VisuMax femtosecond laser, the VisuMax 800, was introduced in 2022. Compared to Visumax 500, it has an increased pulse frequency of 2000 kHz, reducing the lenticule delineation time from approximately 30 s to less than 10 s [51]. The impact of this higher pulse frequency on the tissue responses remains uncertain. In terms of corneal epithelial remodeling, as the lenticule profile and geometry of the Visumax 800 are identical to that of the VisuMax 500, the epithelial remodeling process is expected to be identical between 2 laser systems [51].

2.3 Conclusions

Corneal wound healing process has a major impact on the postoperative visual outcomes, complications, and corneal biomechanical changes after ReLEx®SMILE. Based on rabbit SMILE models, SMILE leaves a small epithelial incision that heals within 1 week. The extracted lenticule plane itself and the remaining stromal bed undergo little inflammatory response, and the inflammatory response seems to primarily result from surgical manipulation to extract the lenticule, rather than laser itself. The postoperative complications resulting from impaired wound healing or inflammatory response, such as corneal haze or DLK, are reported to be low and were mainly associated with perioperative complications, such as difficult lenticule extraction. Corneal epithelial remodeling is related to postoperative regression. Further research is required to investigate the wound healing responses in the newer generation of lenticule extraction procedures.

References

1. Sugar A. Ultrafast (femtosecond) laser refractive surgery. Curr Opin Ophthalmol. 2002;13(4):246–9.
2. Lubatschowski H. Overview of commercially available femtosecond lasers in refractive surgery. J Refract Surg. 2008;24(1):S102-107.
3. Santhiago MR, Wilson SE. Cellular effects after laser in situ keratomileusis flap formation with femtosecond lasers: a review. Cornea. 2012;31(2):198–205.

4. de Paula FH, Khairallah CG, Niziol LM, Musch DC, Shtein RM. Diffuse lamellar keratitis after laser in situ keratomileusis with femtosecond laser flap creation. J Cataract Refract Surg. 2012;38(6):1014–9.
5. Azar DT, Chang JH, Han KY. Wound healing after keratorefractive surgery: review of biological and optical considerations. Cornea. 2012;31(Suppl 1):S9–19.
6. Dupps WJ Jr, Wilson SE. Biomechanics and wound healing in the cornea. Exp Eye Res. 2006;83(4):709–20.
7. Vaddavalli PK, Hurmeric V, Wang J, Yoo SH. Corneal haze following disruption of epithelial basement membrane on ultra-high-resolution OCT following femtosecond LASIK. J Refract Surg. 2012;28(1):72–4.
8. Kanellopoulos AJ, Asimellis G. Epithelial remodeling after femtosecond laser-assisted high myopic LASIK: comparison of stand-alone with LASIK combined with prophylactic high-fluence cross-linking. Cornea. 2014;33(5):463–9.
9. Mohan RR, Mohan RR, Kim WJ, Wilson SE. Modulation of TNF-alpha-induced apoptosis in corneal fibroblasts by transcription factor NF-kappaB. Invest Ophthalmol Vis Sci. 2000;41(6):1327–36.
10. Yang LWY, Mehta JS, Liu YC. Corneal neuromediator profiles following laser refractive surgery. Neural Regen Res. 2021;16(11):2177–83.
11. Tuominen IS, Tervo TM, Teppo AM, Valle TU, Gronhagen-Riska C, Vesaluoma MH. Human tear fluid PDGF-BB, TNF-alpha and TGF beta1 vs corneal haze and regeneration of corneal epithelium and subbasal nerve plexus after PRK. Exp Eye Res. 2001;72(6):631–41.
12. Jester JV, Petroll WM, Cavanagh HD. Corneal stromal wound healing in refractive surgery: the role of myofibroblasts. Prog Retin Eye Res. 1999;18(3):311–56.
13. Netto MV, Mohan RR, Sinha S, Sharma A, Dupps W, Wilson SE. Stromal haze, myofibroblasts, and surface irregularity after PRK. Exp Eye Res. 2006;82(5):788–97.
14. Ambati BK, Nozaki M, Singh N, et al. Corneal avascularity is due to soluble VEGF receptor-1. Nature. 2006;443(7114):993–7.
15. Lim RR, Tan A, Liu YC, et al. ITF2357 transactivates Id3 and regulate TGFbeta/BMP7 signaling pathways to attenuate corneal fibrosis. Sci Rep. 2016;6:20841.
16. Chang JH, Gabison EE, Kato T, Azar DT. Corneal neovascularization. Curr Opin Ophthalmol. 2001;12(4):242–9.
17. Riau AK, Angunawela RI, Chaurasia SS, Lee WS, Tan DT, Mehta JS. Early corneal wound healing and inflammatory responses after refractive lenticule extraction (ReLEx). Invest Ophthalmol Vis Sci. 2011;52(9):6213–21.
18. Dong Z, Zhou X, Wu J, et al. Small incision lenticule extraction (SMILE) and femtosecond laser LASIK: comparison of corneal wound healing and inflammation. Br J Ophthalmol. 2014;98(2):263–9.
19. Sun Y, Zhang T, Liu M, et al. Early corneal wound healing response after small incision lenticule extraction. Cornea. 2019;38(12):1582–8.
20. Zieske JD, Mason VS, Wasson ME, et al. Basement membrane assembly and differentiation of cultured corneal cells: importance of culture environment and endothelial cell interaction. Exp Cell Res. 1994;214(2):621–33.
21. Ivarsen A, Asp S, Hjortdal J. Safety and complications of more than 1500 small-incision lenticule extraction procedures. Ophthalmology. 2014;121(4):822–8.
22. Nakamura M, Sato N, Chikama T, Hasegawa Y, Nishida T. Fibronectin facilitates corneal epithelial wound healing in diabetic rats. Exp Eye Res. 1997;64(3):355–9.
23. Tervo K, van Setten GB, Beuerman RW, Virtanen I, Tarkkanen A, Tervo T. Expression of tenascin and cellular fibronectin in the rabbit cornea after anterior keratectomy. Immunohistochemical study of wound healing dynamics. Invest Ophthalmol Vis Sci. 1991;32(11):2912–8.
24. Nishida T. The role of fibronectin in corneal wound healing explored by a physician-scientist. Jpn J Ophthalmol. 2012;56(5):417–31.
25. Nagata K. Expression and function of heat shock protein 47: a collagen-specific molecular chaperone in the endoplasmic reticulum. Matrix Biol. 1998;16(7):379–86.

26. Moller-Pedersen T, Vogel M, Li HF, Petroll WM, Cavanagh HD, Jester JV. Quantification of stromal thinning, epithelial thickness, and corneal haze after photorefractive keratectomy using in vivo confocal microscopy. Ophthalmology. 1997;104(3):360–8.
27. Liu YC, Teo EP, Lwin NC, Yam GH, Mehta JS. Early Corneal wound healing and inflammatory responses after SMILE: comparison of the effects of different refractive corrections and surgical experiences. J Refract Surg. 2016;32(5):346–53.
28. Shah R, Shah S, Sengupta S. Results of small incision lenticule extraction: all-in-one femtosecond laser refractive surgery. J Cataract Refract Surg. 2011;37(1):127–37.
29. Hu MY, McCulley JP, Cavanagh HD, et al. Comparison of the corneal response to laser in situ keratomileusis with flap creation using the FS15 and FS30 femtosecond lasers: clinical and confocal microscopy findings. J Cataract Refract Surg. 2007;33(4):673–81.
30. Riau AK, Liu YC, Lim CHL, et al. Retreatment strategies following small incision lenticule extraction (SMILE): in vivo tissue responses. PLoS ONE. 2017;12(7): e0180941.
31. Reinstein DZ, Sekundo W, Archer TJ, et al. SMILE for hyperopia with and without astigmatism: results of a prospective multicenter 12-month study. J Refract Surg. 2022;38(12):760–9.
32. Liu YC, Ang HP, Teo EP, Lwin NC, Yam GH, Mehta JS. Wound healing profiles of hyperopic-small incision lenticule extraction (SMILE). Sci Rep. 2016;6:29802.
33. YC Liu, AK Riau, Mehta J. Cornea, vol. 4. Philadelphia: Elsevier Mosby; 2016.
34. Liu YC, Pujara T, Mehta JS. New instruments for lenticule extraction in small incision lenticule extraction (SMILE). PLoS ONE. 2014;9(12): e113774.
35. Zhao J, He L, Yao P, et al. Diffuse lamellar keratitis after small-incision lenticule extraction. J Cataract Refract Surg. 2015;41(2):400–7.
36. Wang Y, Ma J, Zhang L, et al. Postoperative corneal complications in small incision lenticule extraction: long-term study. J Refract Surg. 2019;35(3):146–52.
37. Reinstein DZ, Stuart AJ, Vida RS, Archer TJ, Carp GI. Incidence and outcomes of sterile multifocal inflammatory keratitis and diffuse lamellar keratitis after SMILE. J Refract Surg. 2018;34(11):751–9.
38. Agca A, Ozgurhan EB, Yildirim Y, et al. Corneal backscatter analysis by in vivo confocal microscopy: fellow eye comparison of small incision lenticule extraction and femtosecond laser-assisted LASIK. J Ophthalmol. 2014;2014: 265012.
39. Kamiya K, Shimizu K, Igarashi A, Kobashi H. Visual and refractive outcomes of femtosecond lenticule extraction and small-incision lenticule extraction for myopia. Am J Ophthalmol. 2014;157(1):128–34e122.
40. Ganesh S, Brar S, Relekar KJ. Epithelial thickness profile changes following small incision refractive lenticule extraction (SMILE) for myopia and myopic astigmatism. J Refract Surg. 2016;32(7):473–82.
41. Lohmann CP, Reischl U, Marshall J. Regression and epithelial hyperplasia after myopic photorefractive keratectomy in a human cornea. J Cataract Refract Surg. 1999;25(5):712–5.
42. Spadea L, Fasciani R, Necozione S, Balestrazzi E. Role of the corneal epithelium in refractive changes following laser in situ keratomileusis for high myopia. J Refract Surg. 2000;16(2):133–9.
43. Ryu IH, Kim BJ, Lee JH, Kim SW. Comparison of corneal epithelial remodeling after femtosecond laser-assisted LASIK and small incision lenticule extraction (SMILE). J Refract Surg. 2017;33(4):250–6.
44. Liu M, Jin C, Lu L, et al. The impact of corneal epithelial thickening and inhomogeneity on corneal aberrations after small incision lenticule extraction. J Refract Surg. 2023;39(1):23–32.
45. Liu YC, Yam GH, Lin MT, et al. Comparison of tear proteomic and neuromediator profiles changes between small incision lenticule extraction (SMILE) and femtosecond laser-assisted in-situ keratomileusis (LASIK). J Adv Res. 2021;29:67–81.
46. Vetrugno M, Maino A, Quaranta GM, Cardia L. The effect of early steroid treatment after PRK on clinical and refractive outcomes. Acta Ophthalmol Scand. 2001;79(1):23–7.
47. Price FW Jr., Willes L, Price M, Lyng A, Ries J. A prospective, randomized comparison of the use versus non-use of topical corticosteroids after laser in situ keratomileusis. Ophthalmology. 2001;108(7):1236–44; discussion 1244–5.

48. Zhou J, Gao Y, Li S, Gu W, Wu L, Guo X. Predictors of myopic regression for laser-assisted subepithelial keratomileusis and laser-assisted in situ keratomileusis flap creation with mechanical microkeratome and femtosecond laser in low and moderate myopia. Ophthalmic Epidemiol. 2020;27(3):177–85.
49. Zhou J, Gu W, Gao Y, Wang W, Zhang F. Survival analysis of myopic regression after small incision lenticule extraction and femtosecond laser-assisted laser in situ keratomileusis for low to moderate myopia. Eye Vis (London). 2022;9(1):28.
50. Sekundo W, Kunert KS, Blum M. Small incision corneal refractive surgery using the small incision lenticule extraction (SMILE) procedure for the correction of myopia and myopic astigmatism: results of a 6 month prospective study. Br J Ophthalmol. 2011;95(3):335–9.
51. Reinstein DZ, Archer TJ, Potter JG, Gupta R, Wiltfang R. Refractive and visual outcomes of SMILE for compound myopic astigmatism with the VISUMAX 800. J Refract Surg. 2023;39(5):294–301.

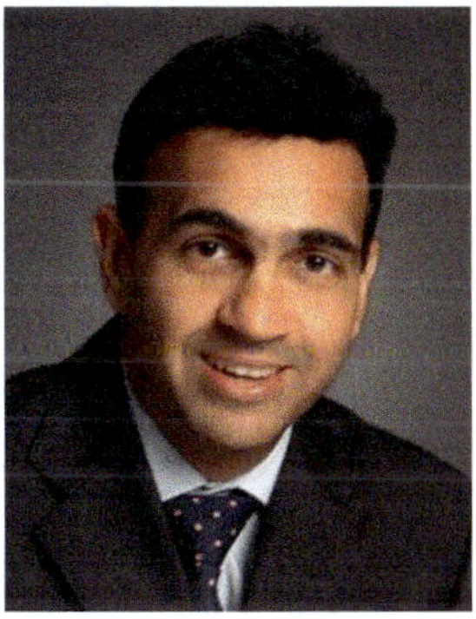

Jodhbir S. Mehta currently helms as the Deputy Medical Director (Research), Distinguished Professor in Clinical Innovation in Ophthalmology, Singapore National Eye Centre (SNEC) and Academic Vice-Chair (Research) with the SingHealth Duke-NUS Ophthalmology and Visual Science Academic Clinical Programme . He holds concurrent appointments as Executive Director of the Singapore Eye Research Institute (SERI) and heads the Tissue Engineering and Cell Therapy Research Group at SERI. He also serves as Senior Consultant and former Head of the Cornea and External Eye Disease Department at SNEC. Furthermore, he is a tenured Professor at the Duke-NUS Medical School.

A highly accomplished Clinician Scientist, Prof Mehta has been making instrumental contributions both internationally and in the Asia Pacific region. Clinically, he is one of the leading specialist in the world on corneal diseases and refractive surgical procedures; while academically he has demonstrated a remarkable track record in publications and securing funding among others. His research interests span outstandingly across all aspects of corneal external disease and refractive surgery, with corneal transplantation research as the key focus.

Directing a strong multi-disciplinary team and partnering a wide network of collaborators, Prof Mehta has driven various research projects successfully, many of which have produced breakthroughs and patents with high translational potential.

Prof Mehta exhibits a prolific publication records, with over 520 peer-reviewed papers in acclaimed international journals and authored over 24 book chapters. He has earned a high H-index of 73 (with over 20,500 citations. He has published in NEJM, Lancet, Lancet Resp Medicine, Nature Biomedical Engineering, Nature Review Disease Primers, as well as high impact eye journals e.g. PRER, Ophthalmology. He has filed 24 patents from his research work, of which 6 have been commercialised and licensed to companies. As a leader of one of the top research programmes at SERI, he has received several competitive research grants, achieving over $15 million as Principal Investigator. As a further reflection of his high standing in the global ophthalmology community; he is currently ranked number 1 in the world for expertise in Cornea and number 2 for Refractive surgery on expertscape.com. He has given over 350 invited lectures and given 19 named lectures; and serves the editorial board of several ophthalmic and visual sciences journals.

Beyond research, Prof Mehta is a committed educator. Apart from lecturing and teaching various local and international courses, he also supervises and mentors (Transition awards (NMRC), Foundation grant (Singhealth), NIG (NMRC), junior clinicians, fellows (over 30 local and international fellows), researchers (PhD and MSc students) and undergraduate students.

Prof Mehta has received many international awards for the excellent contributions and achievements from his research, clinical and educational endeavours. Some of his accolades include the Nakajima Award (Asia Pacific Academy for Ophthalmology, 2013), Senior Achievement Award (American Academy of Ophthalmology, 2017 and 2023), Doug Coster Lecture (Australia and New Zealand Cornea Society, 2018), Charles Tilett Lecture (Fuchs Society, USA, 2020), Casebeer Award (International Society of Refractive Surgery, AAO, 2020), and the Charles McGhee Medal (BSRS, Oxford UK, 2023), APAO Senior Achievement Award 2023, ACE Award APACRS 2023.

Corneal Nerve and Keratocyte Response to SMILE® Surgery

3

Leonardo Mastropasqua and Mario Nubile

Abstract

Any kind of laser corneal refractive surgery has an impact on the ocular surface and corneal innervation and, therefore, on the postoperative symptoms and quality of life of patients. Minimizing the aforementioned rare, but possible, side effects, represents one of the main goals of modern laser surgery. It is claimed that small incision lenticule extraction (SMILE) induces less dry eye and wound healing phenomena as compared with laser-assisted in situ keratomileusis (LASIK) and other excimer laser-based techniques. In this chapter, the fundamentals and updates on corneal neural and keratocytes response to femtosecond lenticule extraction surgery are presented.

Keywords

Laser corneal refractive surgery • Small incision lenticule extraction (SMILE) • Laser-assisted in situ keratomileusis (LASIK) • Excimer laser • Corneal innervation • Corneal nerve fibers • Corneal sensitivity • Dry eye • Corneal epitheliopathy

3.1 Introduction

Any kind of laser corneal refractive surgery has an impact on the ocular surface and corneal innervation and, therefore, on the postoperative symptoms and quality of life of patients. Minimizing the aforementioned rare, but possible, side effects, represents one of the main goals of modern laser surgery. It is claimed that SMILE induces less dry eye and wound healing phenomena as compared with LASIK and

L. Mastropasqua · M. Nubile (✉)
National High-Tech Eye Center, University of Chieti, Pescara, Italy
e-mail: m.nubile@unich.it

W. Sekundo and F. M. Wagner (eds.), *Femtosecond Laser Assisted Lenticule Extraction*,
https://doi.org/10.1007/978-3-031-60424-9_3

other excimer laser-based techniques. In this chapter, the fundamentals and updates on corneal neural and keratocytes response to femtosecond lenticule extraction surgery are presented.

Corneal laser refractive surgery gained popularity among ophthalmologists since the beginning of the nineties of the last century and rapidly substituted the old manual incisional surgery such as radial and astigmatic keratotomies [1–3]. In fact, excimer laser surgical procedures for the treatment of ametropias changed completely the approach to refractive corrections, basing the modification of the corneal shape on the mechanism of the so called laser "photoablation" of the corneal stroma, which makes possible to sculpt the cornea with microscopic accuracy [4]. Laser in situ keratomileusis (LASIK), photorefractive keratectomy (PRK), and, among the surface ablation procedures, the variations called laser-assisted sub-epithelial keratectomy (LASEK) and Epi-LASIK represented the most exploited, successfully used and evolving corneal laser surgical interventions for the correction of myopia and other ametropias [5, 6].

Despite the great precision of corneal refractive excimer laser ablations, and the recent improvement of the techniques, drawbacks intrinsic to the procedures still persist unsolved, including surgical-induced nerve damages, triggering of stromal wound healing and keratocytes changes [7]. These post-surgical corneal alterations are generally transient but in some cases may be persistent and often can lead to undesirable side effects and symptoms in treated patients. Damage to the corneal nerve plexus is frequent cause of corneal neurotrophic epitheliopathy, with related dry eye symptoms and altered tear film dynamics, while keratocyte apoptosis, stromal inflammation, and wound healing can be responsible for regression of the achieved corrections and loss of corneal transparency (haze) [7].

Recent investigations suggest that ReLEx techniques, due to the photodisruption mechanism and the flap-less approach (for SMILE), may exert different effects on corneal nerve fibers and keratocytes after myopic and astigmatic refractive correction as compared to the traditional excimer laser-based surface ablation and LASIK techniques.

3.2 Surgical Anatomy of the Corneal Nerves and Stromal Keratocytes

3.2.1 Nerve Fibers

The cornea is a highly sensitive structure and is innervated by the ophthalmic division of the trigeminal nerve. Superficial corneal nerve density is estimated to be approximately 300–600 times that of skin and 20 times that of tooth pulp [8]. The human cornea receives most of its sensory innervation from the two long ciliary nerves that enter the posterior globe adjacent to the optic nerve and course forward in the suprachoroidal space at the nasal and temporal meridians [9]. Prior to reaching the corneoscleral limbus, the nerves branch into smaller bundles and anastomose repetitively with branches of the short ciliary nerves that approach the limbus radially from all directions. The nerves that enter the cornea can be considered as mixed sensory and autonomic nerves. Recent investigations redefined the knowledge of the neural architecture and distribution of the corneal nerves [10–12].

Approximately, 30–60-thick nerve bundles enter the human cornea in a relatively equal distribution around the circumference of the limbus and thereafter run toward the central cornea, dividing into several branches in the peripheral area. In the stroma, nerves organize in parallel to collagen lamellae, branch into smaller fascicles as they become more superficial and form interconnections (anterior stromal plexus). It is evident that nerve density increases while nerve diameter thins moving anteriorly toward the superficial stroma. It is remarkable to note that a small number of stromal nerves terminate as free endings while some fibers directly innervate keratocytes [13]. After passing through the Bowman's zone, the original stromal fibers terminate into "bulb-like thickenings" from which multiple sub-basal nerves arise [10]. The stromal nerves penetrate the Bowman's layer (perforation sites) mainly in the mid-peripheral cornea with relatively fewer perforation sites in the central or peripheral cornea (See Fig. 3.1). Approximately, 25–30 perforation sites were observed in the human central cornea versus 125–160 perforation sites in the mid-peripheral cornea [10]. After the perforation, nerve fibers branch and divide further and then run below the epithelium to originate the sub-basal plexus.

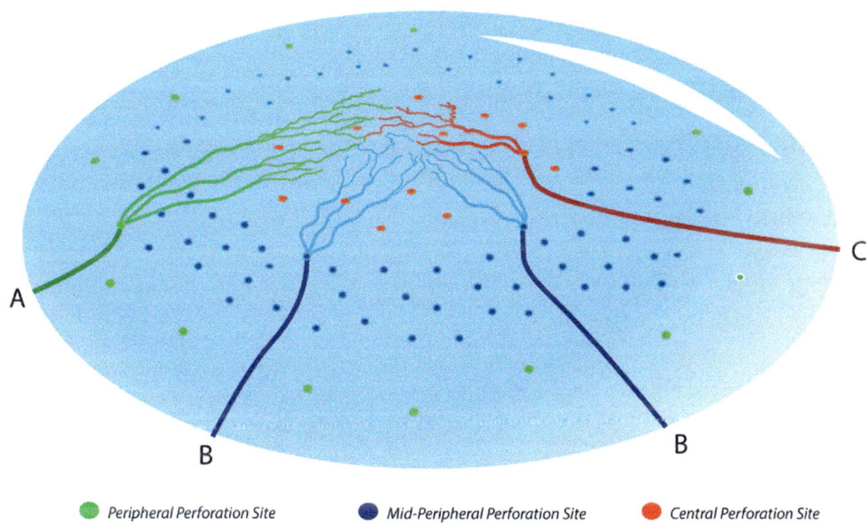

Fig. 3.1 Schematic representation of the anatomy of corneal nerves. Nerve fibers enter the cornea at the limbal region and then run radially toward the center as stromal fibers. These fibers tend to reach the stromal superficial layers and perforate the Bowman's layer at different topographical locations (different colors). The sites of Bowman's membrane perforation are depicted by colored dots. After gaining the superficial location, they give origin to the sub-basal fibers

It is of interest to consider that when surface refractive ablations (i.e. PRK) are performed, the epithelial removal and the superficial ablation remove the central Bowman's layer and anterior stroma, therefore eliminating the epithelial, sub-basal, and most anterior stromal nerve fibers. In case of LASIK surgery, although the epithelium, Bowman's zone, and very anterior stroma are preserved from ablation in the flap, the nerve fibers are resected peripherally due to the flap circumferential side cut, while deeper stromal fibers are damaged by the ablation under the flap. When a femtosecond refractive lenticule is dissected and removed, in the SMILE technique, stromal nerve fibers within the lenticule are resected but the absence of surface damage and of the flap creation represent the anatomical basis for a different pattern of corneal nerve damage that will be discussed further in this chapter.

3.2.2 Stromal Keratocytes

Corneal keratocytes (corneal fibroblasts) are specialized fibroblast cells residing in the stroma. These cells are interspersed within the structure of the stroma that is built up from highly regular orthogonally arranged collagenous lamellae and extracellular matrix components. Keratocytes play a key role in maintaining the stromal structure and transparency of the cornea, being the source of stromal collagen and proteoglycans. They also mediate corneal wound healing and tissue repair and are capable of undergoing phenotypic transformations in wounds due to the influence of growth factors and cytokines. These specialized cells are therefore involved in healing corneal wounds and synthesizing its components. In the unperturbed cornea, keratocytes are normally quiescent, but they can rapidly respond and change into repair phenotypes following injury [14, 15]. Stromal keratocyte density has been evaluated both ex-vivo and in vivo, and it is known to be higher in the anterior third of the stroma, while it progressively decreases in the mid and rear stroma (Fig. 3.2).

In excimer laser surface ablation techniques, the very anterior keratocytes (depending on the ablation depth) are damaged and apoptosis mechanisms, with subsequent wound healing cascade, are triggered in the most keratocyte-populated area of the stroma. In LASIK technique, the keratocyte and stromal healing phenomena occur at a deeper level (in the residual stromal bed under the flap stroma and the ablated tissue), where the keratocyte density is lower. In SMILE and to some extent in FLEx techniques, the unique use of femtosecond laser dissection with no photoablation induces a different pattern, of keratocyte changes and wound healing (in the anterior-mid stroma), characterized by less apoptosis and inflammation, as already discussed in the previous chapter.

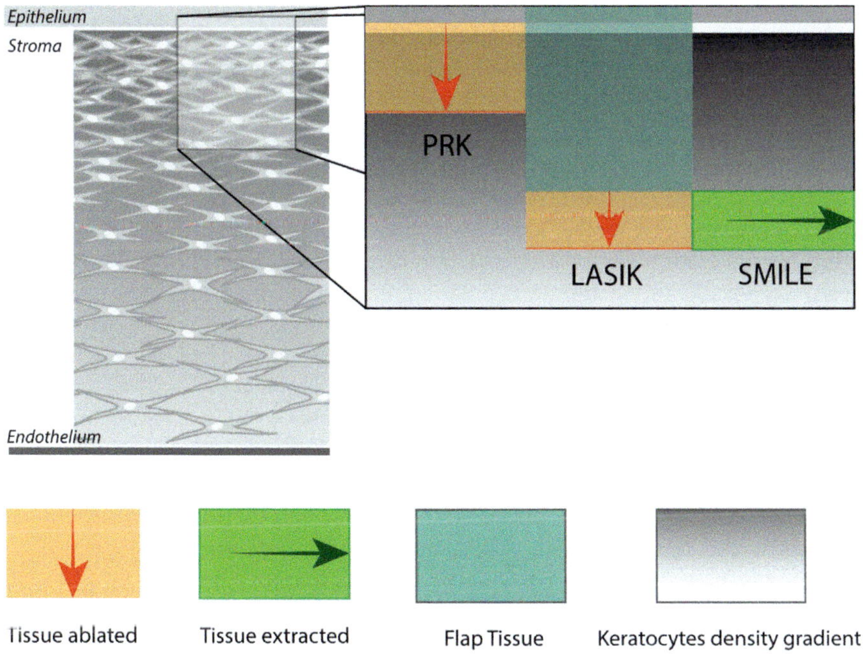

Fig. 3.2 Schematic representation illustrating the keratocyte distribution within the corneal stroma and the surgical anatomy of three different corneal refractive surgical techniques: PRK, LASIK, and SMILE (section)

3.2.3 In Vivo Confocal Microscopy of the Cornea: An Imaging Technique for Nerves and Keratocytes

In vivo confocal microscopy (IVCM) has gained a notable popularity and consensus as a powerful imaging tool among cornea specialists in the last 2 decades. It is a non-invasive diagnostic imaging system that allows viewing of tissues, in particular the cornea at its microscopic details, one depth level at a time [16–18]. This kind of microscope is designed for non-invasive, real-time, in vivo examination of tissues without the need of stains or dyes but does require operator-dependent expertise and skill in optimizing the quality of the obtained images and their interpretation. Currently, two different confocal technologies are available for clinical use: the laser scanning and the white-light scanning confocal microscopy. These two confocal systems clearly differ in the capacity of ocular tissue imaging depending on the type of light source used [18]. White-light confocal microscopy offers a detailed view of the corneal layers, provides an optical pachymetry of the entire cornea or of selected sublayers, and allows for automatic cell counts (i.e., keratocytes and endothelial cell density), but the imaging quality is affected by tissue transparency and stromal edema more than laser scanning confocal systems. Due to the fact that the cornea is generally a nearly transparent tissue, with minimal light absorption, the increase in axial resolution allows confocal microscopy to scan optical sections of the entire corneal thickness producing high magnification (between 600 and 1000 X) "en face images" of the cornea (maintaining lateral and axial resolution within values comprised between 1 and 3 μm and 5 up to 10 μm, respectively). Almost all anatomical corneal layers are clearly imaged by confocal microscopy: superficial epithelium, basal epithelium, Bowman's membrane, sub-epithelial nerve plexus, corneal stroma with resident keratocytes, deep nerve fibers, Descemet's membrane, and endothelium. Figure 3.3 presents a composition of images illustrating confocal microscopic anatomy of the central human corneal layers. As visible in the figure, in vivo confocal images are oriented parallel to the microscope objective and to the corneal surface, differently than histological specimens, which are sectioned perpendicular to the surface of the cornea, and thus, the observer has to become familiar with the imaging in the coronal plane.

On IVCM evaluation, patients undergoing refractive surgery generally present a decrease in corneal nerve density, diameter, and total length, as well as an increase in corneal tortuosity, branching, and beading. Hence, it is important to identify reliable and reproducible quantitative tools to measure the extent of corneal denervation and subsequent nerve regeneration following refractive surgery [19].

Computer-based software for standardizing the reproducibility of nerve metric evaluation became recently available, and their use can help for better correlation

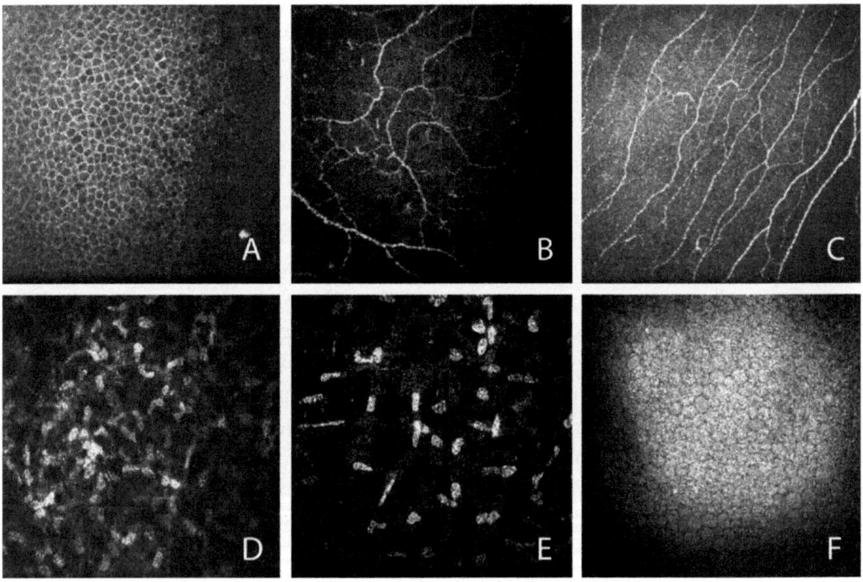

Fig. 3.3 Composition of images illustrating confocal microscopic anatomy of the central human corneal layers, with emphasis on visualizing nerve fibers and keratocytes. A) Basal epithelium. B-C) Different pattern of sub-epithelial nerve plexus. D) High density of anterior stromal keratocytes. E) Mid-stromal keratocytes present a lower density. F) Normal endothelial cell mosaic

of corneal nerve analysis by IVCM images to clinical outcomes and postoperative symptoms such as transient dry eye or ocular surface neurotrophic disease.

3.3 Nerve Fibers Change After ReLEx Refractive Surgery: Morphology and Pathophysiology

3.3.1 Nerve Fibers and Tear Film Alterations After Excimer Laser Surgery

Any kind of subtractive laser refractive surgery has the disadvantages of inducing a variable degree of damage to the corneal nerve fibers. It is well known that the integrity of nerve fibers is fundamental for the physiological maintenance of the ocular surface tear film dynamics and corneal epithelial homeostasis. Tear secretion is regulated through a neural reflex initiated by trigeminal primary afferent neurons innervating the corneal epithelium. Dry eye phenomena may be induced by a dysfunction in the tear-secreting glands or in the neuronal circuit regulating these glands [20].

Patients' complain of dry eye symptoms and related epitheliopathy commonly occur after traditional refractive surgery techniques. The most frequently reported manifestations are ocular dryness, that takes place in almost 40% of laser-assisted in situ keratomileusis (LASIK) and photorefractive keratectomy (PRK) treated eyes, but also non-specific ocular surface discomfort associated with mild corneal epitheliopathy and reduced lubrication may occur [21]. At the present time, LASIK (either performed with microkeratomes or with Fs-Laser) is considered as one of the gold standard refractive procedures, supported by numerous investigations, for its visual outcomes and rapid postoperative recovery. The LASIK technique induces morphological and functional effects on the corneal surface. Changes in corneal shape, tear film dynamic, and sub-epithelial innervation after surgery exert a significant influence in ocular discomfort syndrome onset. The impact of these factors produces detrimental effects to visual results including fluctuation of vision quality, decrease of contrast sensitivity and, in some cases, of best spectacle-corrected visual acuity [22]. One of the key points to consider in the occurrence of these phenomena is the fact that different patients may present a variable spectrum of symptoms to identical surgical stimuli, and that pre-existing dry eye before surgery can be a risk factor for severe ocular discomfort after refractive surgery.

As explained, excimer laser-based procedures (either LASIK or surface ablation techniques such as PRK) result in a sudden central corneal nerve fiber damage related to the flap cut, in LASIK, and to the excimer photoablation of the anterior stroma containing nerve fibers, that takes time to recover, often only partially. The wound healing of central corneal sub-epithelial nerves fibers has been reported to be only slightly different between LASIK and similar flap-based procedures, regarding the time to recovery and the morphological appearance of the regenerated nerve plexus. At one month after surgery, the central cornea appears devoid of nerve fibers in conventional LASIK procedure, Sub-Bowman's keratomileusis

(SBK), and femtosecond laser-assisted-LASIK (Fs-LASIK) [23]. The process of re-innervation begins in the early period after surgery in the peripheral flap region with the formation of thin non-branching fibers crossing the side cut. Nerve morphology changes rapidly across the following months reaching the central 3 mm area at 6 months [23]. In spite of this nerve regrowth, the density and the nerve morphology remain altered for years after surgery, representing the basis for some clinical conditions of dryness and recurrent superficial epithelial punctate erosions. Surface excimer laser ablations showed a faster recovery time, with two years of mean time-to-restoration against five years of the flap-based procedures [24].

Along with the corneal neural impairment, patients show an altered corneal sensitivity that follows a similar pattern by decreasing significantly immediately after, persisting reduced in the first three months, and returning to normal values at six months after surgery [25]. Previous investigations reported a persistent non-complete normalization at one year and more [26].

The risk of developing "Dry Eye Syndrome" appears to be correlated with the degree of preoperative myopia and the depth of laser ablation/stromal dissection; moreover, in dry eye-affected patients, the risk of myopic regression is increased [27, 28]. The status of the ocular surface and tear film before and after refractive surgery can adversely affect the outcomes in terms of complications, refractive results, optical quality, patient satisfaction, and the severity and duration of dry eye after LASIK [29].

The switching from microkeratome-based to Fs-Laser flap making in the clinical use in corneal refractive surgery favored significant improvements in the reliability of LASIK procedures by increasing flap precision (thickness, shape, diameter), setting up planar configuration of the flap cut geometry, and giving more predictable depth of dissection and reduction of intraoperative complications incidence [30]. Despite these advantages with Fs-Laser-created flaps, corneal nerve plexus presents the above-described modification and remains affected by severe damage for a long time. In fact, the flap creation implies the transection of all nerve fibers at the lamellar border. In spite of the better alignment of flap margins achieved with Fs-LASIK, the re-innervation process emerges to be similar to the well-known microkeratome-LASIK procedures. Central nerve fibers density reduction and slow progressive recovery turned out to be comparable in both techniques as long as three years after surgery [30]. Similarly, the incidence of dry eye symptoms after surgery is similar in both procedures. Therefore, the planar configuration of thin Fs-LASIK flaps is not associated with faster re-innervation compared with the microkeratome flaps and does not provide clinically significant advantages in terms of induced neurotrophic epitheliopathy. Patients complaining of post-refractive surgery dry eye symptoms are generally treated by frequent instillations of lubricant eye drops and occasionally local steroids and/or topical cyclosporin A for weeks to months after surgery; however, there is no recognized and definite treatment for such condition.

3.3.2 Corneal Nerve Fibers After ReLEx: Anatomical Bases and Scientific Evidence

Femtosecond laser refractive surgery received a notable advancement with the introduction of "all-femto" SMILE technique. The capacity of the femtosecond laser of designing intrastromal dissection planes with three-dimensional cut complex geometry helps the surgeons to remove corneal tissue without a flap by creating a lenticule and a small incision to extract it. The first dissection plane designs the backside face of the lenticule, while the second one creates its anterior face and extends further to form a spaced intrastromal pocket to facilitate the extraction maneuvers (edge of the so called "cap"). The complete procedure happens without affecting the superficial tissue, fashioning an intrastromal "disk" that can be easily extracted through the 40–50 arc degrees single superficial incision.

The basis that explains the pattern of nerve fiber resection induced by SMILE (similarly to other refractive surgical procedure) relies in the anatomy of the intracorneal distribution of the fibers that give origin to the sub-basal nerve plexus and of the topography of emerging fibers that penetrate the Bowman's layer (BL) running, thereafter, superficially. As explained previously in this chapter, the stromal nerves, coming from the suprachoroidal space through the limbal region, course toward the center in a radial manner and penetrate the Bowman's layer at different locations, mostly situated in the mid-peripheral zone (outside the central 6 mm), creating, thereafter the sub-basal plexus. A schematic representation illustrating the nerve fiber pathway that runs centripetally is presented in Figs. 3.1 and 3.4A. When a flap-based technique (LASIK, Fs-LASIK, or FLEx) is performed, all nerve fibers that are running across the flap side cut circumference are resected (the majority of the central and paracentral stromal fibers). The excimer laser ablation on the stromal bed further vaporizes remaining deeper stromal fibers. Only the fibers that run in the region of the flap hinge (few fibers) may course undisturbed within the lifted flap as sub-basal fibers (see Fig. 3.4B). This supposed mechanism is in agreement with the described clinical and confocal observations that reported a remarkable reduction of corneal sensitivity and of the central sub-basal corneal nerve plexus after LASIK.

On the other hand, when a SMILE procedure is performed, it is presumed that a different pattern of nerve resection occurs.

1. A certain amount of fibers running centripetally in the superficial stroma and in the sub-epithelial zone are resected due to the side cut where the incision is placed.
2. Other stromal fibers that run toward the surface perforating the Bowman's zone inside the refractive lenticule and cap area might be interrupted by the lenticule/cap planar dissection itself.
3. Conversely, fibers that gained the superficial sub-epithelial location after perforating the BL in areas located outside the lenticule—cap area may run untouched (inside the stromal and epithelial component of the cap) over

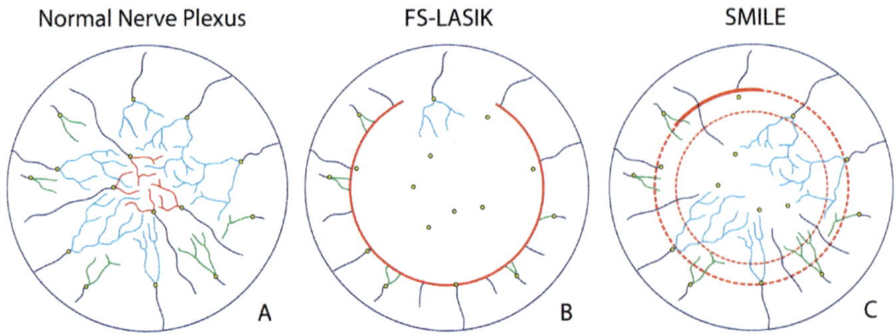

Fig. 3.4 **A)** Stromal nerve fibers bundles run centripetally and toward the surface perforating the Bowman's layer (spots indicated by yellow circles). Once the fibers penetrate the BL, the sub-basal nerve plexus is originated. Different colors illustrate the sub-basal fibers originating from central (red), paracentral (light blu), and peripheral (green) perforating stromal fibers, respectively. **B)** In the LASIK procedure, all fibers are cut throughout the extension of the 300–310° degree of arc flap side cut; moreover, all deeper fibers are disrupted within the photoablation area. **C)** With the SMILE procedure, in the absence of a full flap side cut, peripheral nerve fibers are resected only where the 50° arc of the incision is placed (thick red line). Moreover, fibers are resected if rising superficially to perforate the BL within the area of the created and extracted refractive lenticule. The other fibers that had penetrated the BL outside the lenticule area may run undisturbed as sub-basal nerve plexus. (For simplicity central sub-basal surviving fibers are not depicted in the central zone)

the refractive zone without interruption with the exception of the mentioned peripheral incision (see Fig. 3.4C).

Some recent investigations have evaluated the corneal innervation and corneal sensitivity after ReLEx surgery. Authors that investigated changes in corneal sensitivity reported it to be significantly better after SMILE than after LASIK in every corneal area. Interestingly, corneal sensitivity values were found to reach preoperative levels as soon as 3 months after SMILE surgery, therefore suggesting that long-lasting changes, typical after LASIK procedures, should not occur after flap-less ReLEx SMILE surgery [31]. Vestergaard et al. evaluated corneal sensitivity and used confocal microscopy to study the sub-basal nerve plexus morphology comparing two groups of femtosecond laser refractive surgery treated patients: the SMILE procedure as compared to the FLEx technique (the original approach to all-femto refractive myopic lenticule extraction, based on a complete flap lifting) [32]. The authors observed a better corneal sensitivity and a significantly higher density of central corneal nerve fibers as observed by confocal microscopy in the SMILE group with respect to the FLEx group at six months follow-up time. This study highlighted the importance of a flap-less procedure to favor a rapid nerve restoration; however, it does not take into account the early postoperative phase, and the LASIK technique was not investigated. Another investigation used in vivo confocal microscopy to evaluate changes of corneal innervation following SMILE surgery as compared to Fs-LASIK treated eyes [33]. It reported a decrease in sub-basal nerve fiber density less severe after SMILE in comparison to Fs-LASIK in the early postoperative phase (1 week to three months) while nerve density reached similar values at six months following both procedures. Nerve density values were found to correlate well with corneal aesthesiometry.

As demonstrated, by the means of laser scanning in vivo confocal microscopy (IVCM) remarkable differences in the induced sub-basal nerve fiber changes and subsequent nerve regeneration patterns can be found between flap-based refractive procedures and SMILE for similar myopic corrections.

When studying the peripheral nerve fiber integrity (in the areas corresponding to the flap side cut in the LASIK, and the lenticule-cap area in the SMILE group, respectively), all fibers running centripetally are resected by the presence of the side cut. This concept is illustrated in Fig. 3.4B, and confocal images are presented in Fig. 3.5. In flap-based procedures (Fs-LASIK or FLEx), the fibers are circumferentially interrupted by the flap side cut at the time of surgery. The following stromal excimer ablation (or lenticule removal in FLEx) further contributes to damage deeper fibers (Fig. 3.5A). In the SMILE procedure, peripheral fibers may be observed running centripetally, non-resected, in the area overlying the edge of the lenticular lamellar cut as shown in Fig. 3.5B. As it happens in LASIK, the superficial radial nerve fibers are resected where the SMILE incision is placed (Fig. 3.5C).

In LASIK treatments, the inferred mechanisms responsible for corneal nerve damage include:

1. The peripheral transection of the nerve superficial nerve fibers that perforated the BL outside the flap area (flap side cut)
2. Resection of stromal nerve fibers crossing at any level the planar dissection of the flap
3. Further damage to deeper stromal fibers by the excimer photoablation.

These features may explain the fact that, soon after surgery, the central nerve fibers density is markedly reduced in the LASIK treatments (Fig. 3.6A). The drop in central nerve fiber density produced by LASIK surgery is considered to be as high as 80 to 95% [22–24, 30, 33, 34]. A partial recovery of the fiber density takes months to occur.

Conversely, in the SMILE technique, the reduction of the nerve fiber density was found to be significantly lower with faster central re-innervation than LASIK. Approximately, 20 to 40% of the central fibers are spared by SMILE surgery [31–34]. The reasons for partial nerve sparing in SMILE are:

1. Absence of the side cut that transects all edge-crossing fibers
2. Smaller area of the lenticule planar cut (6.5 mm in average plus the small pocket dissection) that is approximately 30% smaller than LASIK flap cut) [35].

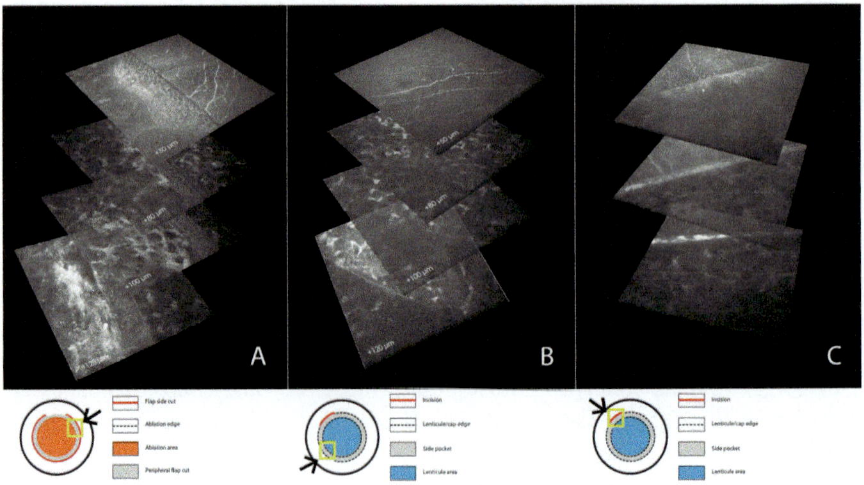

Fig. 3.5 Side cut IVCM stack reconstruction. FS-LASIK (A), SMILE periphery (lenticule edge) (B), and SMILE incision (C). A) In FSL-LASIK, all fibers are resected throughout the extension (approximately 300°) of side cut of the flap (top panel shows resected fibers at the flap border one week after surgery; underlying panels show deeper stromal layers). B) In SMILE, non-damaged superficial fibers can be observed (top panel). They typically run over the lenticule stromal edge (bottom panel), toward the center, as they perforated the BL outside the lenticule-cap dissection. C) "Small incision" represents a zone of superficial nerve fiber resection in the SMILE technique (top panel)

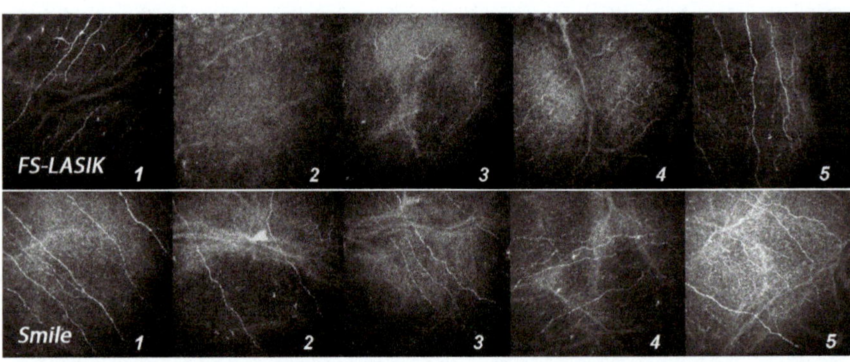

Fig. 3.6 In vivo confocal microscopy images of the central sub-basal nerve plexus before and after FS-LASIK (top line) and SMILE (bottom line). 1 = preoperative, 2 = 1 week; 3 = 1 month; 4 = 3 months; 5 = 6 months. Note that distinct sub-basal fibers are visible at one week and one month after SMILE surgery; recovery of nerve fiber density takes a longer time after LASIK

3. Preservation of the integrity of the crossing fibers that reached the superficial sub-basal location outside the lenticule-cap area (probably 20–30%), as shown in Fig. 3.5B.
4. Absence of excimer laser collateral stromal damage (further discussed in the last paragraph of this chapter)

These features probably play an important role in maintaining a partial corneal innervation in the early postoperative period and may be also responsible for the faster nerve regrowth observed in the first months after surgery with respect to LASIK, as presented in Fig. 3.6. Central nerve fibers are detectable at one week and after SMILE (Fig. 3.6), and a rapid gain of central nerve fiber density can be observed by IVCM.

It is commonly believed that the corrected refractive power is correlated with the extent of postoperative corneal nerve depletion and restoration. However, only recently the corneal denervation and refractive power after LASIK and SMILE have been analyzed in a comparative fashion. Interestingly, the extent of corneal denervation and impairment of TBUT increases with the increase of laser refractive correction, and LASIK was associated with a significant greater damage on corneal nerves than SMILE, given the same corrected refractive power [36].

Another important concept that influences the degree of surgical denervation in corneal refractive surgery is the uneven distribution of the corneal nerve density, which is higher in the periphery and lower at the center, and the different profiles of tissue subtraction in hyperopic versus myopic corrections. Hyperopic patients will undergo subtraction of peripheral tissue with greater impact on nerves, since corneal nerve density is higher at the site where tissue removal is most intense. Whereas in myopic surgical profiles, the tissue removal, mostly focused on the central part, will harm less nerves than hyperopic treatments [37].

Similarly, larger optical zones and cap diameter in SMILE (as well as flap diameter in LASIK) are correlated with a more pronounced nerve damage [34].

In a recent meta-analysis, it was shown that the overall corneal nerve injury in FS-LASIK is worse than that in SMILE, being the nerve regeneration and recovery from neurotrophic symptoms faster in a flap-less technique. However, in the long-term period, from 6 to 24 months after surgery, the difference between the two techniques seems to be less evident [38].

Another reason for less nerve fiber damage in SMILE in comparison to LASIK may correlate to the higher level of collateral damage and decellularization of keratocytes induced by the excimer laser [34, 39]. It is not clear yet whether viable keratocytes are needed to sustain corneal nerve function or vice versa, but prolonged keratocyte apoptosis and acellularity have been observed after excimer laser-based techniques in which an extended period of postoperative denervation is common [34, 40]. As mentioned earlier, some stromal nerves fibers directly innervate stromal keratocytes [13]. Both structures probably mediate the complex wound healing pattern occurring after keratorefractive laser procedures and are likely to be involved in the delicate system aimed to restore the corneal integrity, transparency, and epithelial dynamics after surgery.

3.4 Keratocyte Changes After SMILE® Refractive Surgery: In Vivo Evaluation and Wound Healing Patterns

The immediate postoperative stromal modification of LASIK or surface ablation is dominated by the laser-tissue interaction and the keratocyte-mediated wound healing cascade. These events are known to actively influence the refractive outcome and optical transparency of the cornea particularly in surface ablation procedures. There is a specific type of inflammation and wound healing [41] with a central role of keratocyte apoptosis in activation of the wound healing cascade effecting corneal nerves, lacrimal glands, and tear film [7].

Keratocyte activation stimulated by LASIK has a short duration compared with that reported after surface ablation techniques. Regardless of the method used for flap creation, the stromal tissue presents early morphological changes in keratocytes located below the flap, at the edge of the photoablation [41] (see also Fig. 3.2). However, the presence of this new virtual space—"the surgical interface"—allows the collection of liquid or particles as well as the spread of inflammatory cells.

IVCM morphology of the stromal interface (either in LASIK and SMILE) is characterized by the discontinuity of the stromal cellular architecture. Examples of microscopic characteristics of SMILE® stromal interfaces are shown in Fig. 3.7.

The interface is generally imaged microscopically as a poorly cellulated layer within the anterior stroma, with variable amount of reflective debris and particles clearly distinguishable from the other corneal layers [42]. A typical feature at the interface, which has been confirmed by IVCM, is the lower cellular activity and stromal remodeling. It has been shown that "acellular zones" are present on both sides of the interface [43] and appear thicker when investigated in the first days

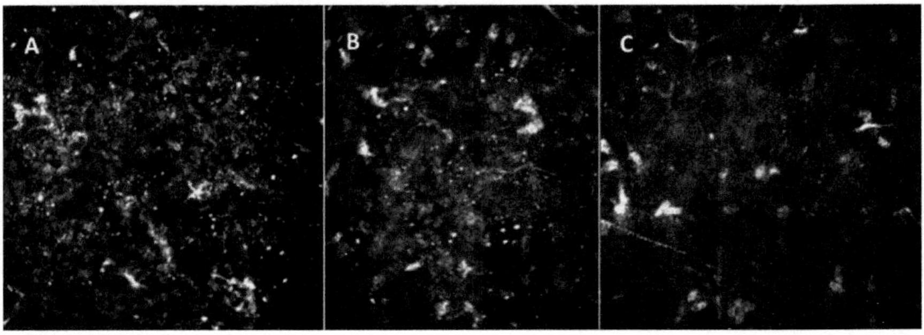

Fig. 3.7 IVCM images of SMILE lamellar interface at different intervals after surgery. A) Stroma interface one week after SMILE shows increased matrix reflectivity, apoptotic keratocytes, bright reflective particles, and mild edema. B) One month after surgery viable keratocyte nuclei are visible along with improved reflectivity. C) At six months after surgery, the interface appears stable, with rare keratocytes interspersed and linear structure of a regenerating nerve fiber. Keratocyte density is always reduced at the interface

after surgery, whereas keratocyte is visible closer to the interface in the following weeks [44]. The keratocyte-free layers probably represent zone undergoing apoptosis or necrosis, an assumption supported by histological investigation [45].

IVCM analysis of SMILE interface and stromal keratocyte changes over time are presented in Fig. 3.8.

In SMILE® surgery, keratocyte apoptosis is mostly confined in the stromal sub-layer adjacent to the extracted lenticules, and surrounding tissue is generally affected by minimal apoptotic/necrotic effect and inflammation, in the early postoperative period. If surgical excessive manipulation and irrigation of the interface are performed during surgery, a certain degree of stromal edema, with packed keratocytes within fluid cystic spaces, can be observed by IVCM in the first days after procedure. This feature may not be clearly evident at slit lamp examination and can be responsible for delayed visual recovery, often observed in the first week (Fig. 3.9A). The interface and the adjacent layers generally become transparent few days after surgery, and keratocytes response generally persists mild to moderate, as compared with excimer laser ablations (Fig. 3.8). Fs-LASIK also exerts an excimer ablation effect in addition to the femtosecond laser dissection compared with SMILE, and this is probably related to the greater keratocytes activation observed for a few weeks after surgery (Fig. 3.8). Keratocyte stability probably equals that of SMILE at three months (unpublished data). The occurrence of persistent keratocytes activation, which may be responsible for abnormal collagen deposition and optical degradation of the interface quality in SMILE, is a rare phenomenon and generally can be reversed by prolonged use of steroid eye drops similarly to excimer laser surgery (Fig. 3.9B).

Recently, a new-generation femtosecond laser system has been introduced in the clinical use, which is characterized by higher laser pulse frequency of 2,000 kHz. This allows a significant reduction in the lenticule delineation time (from approximately 30 s to less than 10 s), without effecting the quality of visual outcome or ease of lenticule separation [46]. In vivo imaging after lenticule extraction in patients treated with the 2 MHz system is presented in Fig. 3.10, as compared to the standard laser, and preliminary results showed that no significantly different wound healing pattern is triggered in the corneal stroma after lenticule separation and extraction with the newer laser pulse frequency.

3.5 Summary

In vivo findings suggest that surgical denervation is significantly less in SMILE as compared to other laser refractive procedures. Also a faster nerve regeneration is likely to occur after SMILE. These advantages are thought to be related to the neuro-anatomy of the cornea and to the particular flap-less procedure of the SMILE technique. However, also in SMILE, nerve fibers intersecting the lenticule/cap plane become transected by the femtosecond laser cut and degenerate thereafter, reducing the overall central corneal nerve fibers density. This damage appears

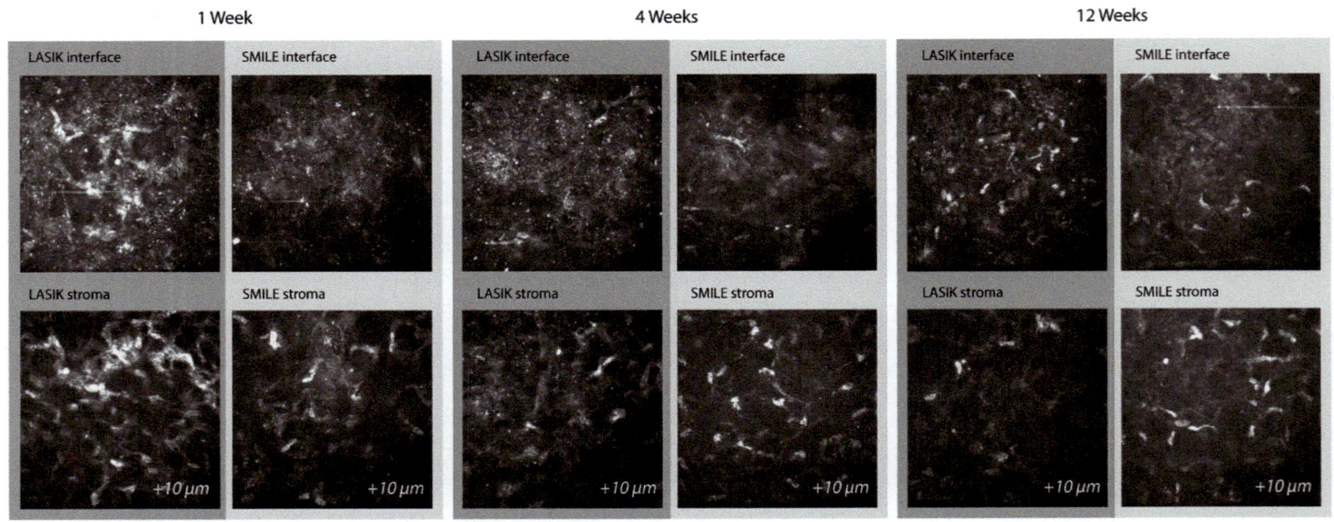

Fig. 3.8 IVCM images showing the interface and stromal keratocyte characteristics after SMILE and Fs-LASIK. In the first row, confocal images of the lamellar interface comparing LASIK and SMILE at different time courses are presented. SMILE interfaces generally show lower degree of bright particles and present visible keratocyte nuclei, indicating lower apoptosis. The second row presents images of the stromal layers immediately below the interface (+ 10 microns), showing greater keratocytes activation in the first weeks after surgery (probably related to the excimer ablation effects in addition to the femtosecond laser dissection). Keratocytes distribution tends to equal three months after surgery

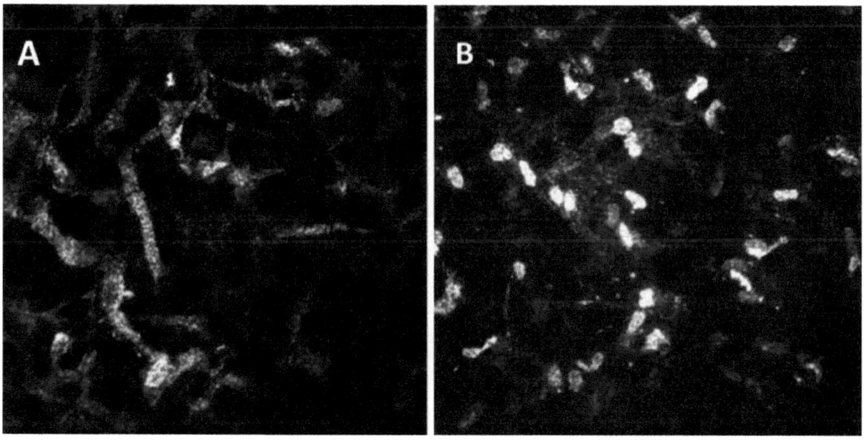

Fig. 3.9 The A) Stromal postoperative edema with cystic extracellular spaces (honeycomb pattern) and packed keratocytes with increased reflectivity. B) Activated keratocytes in the anterior stroma characterized by bright nuclei and visible cytoplasmic processes

significantly less as compared to flap-based and surface ablation techniques, in which the fiber resection is almost total.

After SMILE, some of the spared stromal fibers run over the lenticule plane, in the mid-periphery, piercing the BL outside the treatment area and therefore remain intact and contributing to the sub-basal central plexus. Based on these observations, SMILE surgery favors a better preservation of the corneal neural architecture and a greater postoperative corneal sensitivity leading to a lower incidence and course of the neurotrophic epitheliopathy. Dry eye symptoms are less pronounced after SMILE to those occurring with LASIK, and time to recovery is generally faster.

Keratocytes apoptosis, stromal inflammation, and secondary keratocyte activation are seen as mild to moderate, without substantial differences in any intrastromal refractive techniques. Thus, an abnormal healing compromising the optical quality of the lamellar interface and remaining stroma is unlikely to occur. Newer laser systems will probably improve the overall quality of corneal wound healing, minimizing the intraoperative collateral tissue damaging, while maintaining the advantages of faster procedure and high precision and predictability.

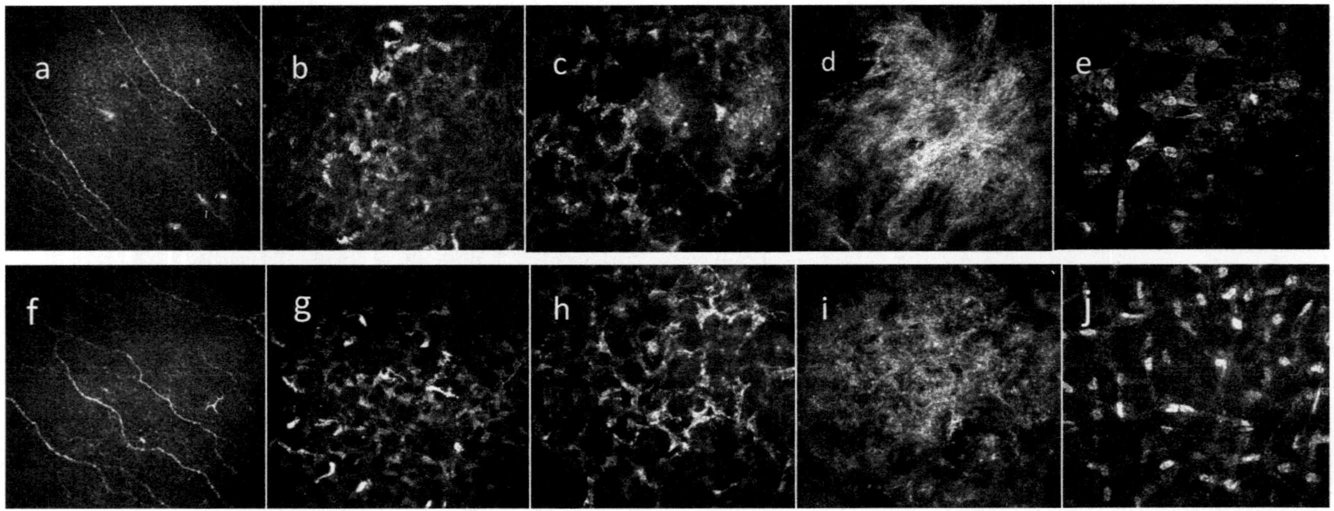

Fig. 3.10 IVCM images showing different corneal anterior layers after myopic SMILE with two different laser systems at one month after surgery. First row (a-e), central cornea after 500 kHz FSL lenticule extraction (VisuMax 500, Carl Zeiss Meditec, Germany). Bottom row (f-j) shows the same corneal layers after new-generation 2000 kHz FSL lenticule extraction (VisuMax 800, Carl Zeiss Meditec, Germany). Panels a, f: sub-basal nerve fibers; b, g: anterior stromal keratocytes in the cap stroma; c, h: anterior stroma activated keratocytes adjacent to the interface; d, i: interface devoid of cells with increased reflectivity due to new collagen deposition; e, j: activated stromal keratocytes adjacent to the interface in the residual stromal bed

References

1. Sutton GL, Kim P. Laser in situ keratomileusis in 2010—a review. Clin Experiment Ophthalmol. 2010;38(2):192–210.
2. Reynolds A, Moore JE, Naroo SA, Moore CB, Shah S. Excimer laser surface ablation—a review. Clin Exp Ophthalmol. 2010;38(2):168–82.
3. Ang EK, Couper T, Dirani M, Vajpayee RB, Baird PN. Outcomes of laser refractive surgery for myopia. J Cataract Refract Surg. 2009;35(5):921–33.
4. Arba-Mosquera S, Klinner T. Improving the ablation efficiency of excimer laser systems with higher repetition rates through enhanced debris removal and optimized spot pattern. J Cataract Refract Surg. 2014;40(3):477–84.
5. Sakimoto T, Rosenblatt MI, Azar DT. Laser eye surgery for refractive errors. Lancet. 2006;367(9520):1432–47.
6. O'Brart DP. Excimer laser surface ablation: a review of recent literature. Clin Exp Optom. 2014;97(1):12–7.
7. Dupps WJ Jr, Wilson SE. Biomechanics and wound healing in the cornea. Exp Eye Res. 2006;83(4):709–20.
8. Rózsa AJ, Beuerman RW. Density and organization of free nerve endings in the corneal epithelium of the rabbit. Pain. 1982;14(2):105–20.
9. Müller LJ, Marfurt CF, Kruse F, Tervo TM. Corneal nerves: structure, contents and function. Exp Eye Res. 2003;76(5):521–42.
10. Al-Aqaba MA, Fares U, Suleman H, Lowe J, Dua HS. Architecture and distribution of human corneal nerves. Br J Ophthalmol. 2010;94(6):784–9.
11. Shaheen BS, Bakir M, Jain S. Corneal nerves in health and disease. Surv Ophthalmol. 2014;59(3):263–85.
12. He J, Bazan NG, Bazan HE. Mapping the entire human corneal nerve architecture. Exp Eye Res. 2010;91(4):513–23.
13. Müller LJ, Pels L, Vrensen GF. Ultrastructural organization of human corneal nerves. Invest Ophthalmol Vis Sci. 1996;37(4):476–88.
14. Wilson SE, Chaurasia SS, Medeiros FW. Apoptosis in the initiation, modulation and termination of the corneal wound healing response. Exp Eye Res. 2007;85(3):305–11.
15. West-Mays JA, Dwivedi DJ. The keratocyte: corneal stromal cell with variable repair phenotypes. Int J Biochem Cell Biol. 2006;38(10):1625–31.
16. Chiou AG, Kaufman SC, Kaufman HE, et al. Clinical corneal confocal microscopy. Surv Ophthalmol. 2006;51:482–500.
17. Dhaliwal JS, Kaufman SC, Chiou AG. Current applications of clinical confocal microscopy. Curr Opin Ophthalmol. 2007;18:300–7.
18. Nubile M, Mastropasqua L. In vivo confocal microscopy of the ocular surface: where are we now? Br J Ophthalmol. 2009;93(7):850–2.
19. Chin JY, Yang LWY, Ji AJS, Nubile M, Mastropasqua L, Allen JC, Mehta JS, Liu YC. Validation of the use of automated and manual quantitative analysis of corneal nerve plexus following refractive surgery. Diagnostics (Basel). 2020;10(7):493.
20. Meng ID, Kurose M. The role of corneal afferent neurons in regulating tears under normal and dry eye conditions. Exp Eye Res. 2013;117:79–87.
21. Hovanesian JA, Shah SS, Maloney RK. Symptoms of dry eye and recurrent erosion syndrome after refractive surgery. J Cataract Refract Surg. 2001;27(4):577–84.
22. Ambrósio R Jr, Tervo T, Wilson SE. LASIK-associated dry eye and neurotrophic epitheliopathy: pathophysiology and strategies for prevention and treatment. J Refract Surg. 2008;24(4):396–407.
23. Zhang F, Deng S, Guo N, Wang M, Sun X. Confocal comparison of corneal nerve regeneration and keratocyte reaction between FS-LASIK, OUP-SBK, and conventional LASIK. Invest Ophthalmol Vis Sci. 2012;53(9):5536–44.

24. Erie JC, McLaren JW, Hodge DO, Bourne WM. Recovery of corneal subbasal nerve density after PRK and LASIK. Am J Ophthalmol. 2005;140(6):1059–64.
25. Pérez-Santonja JJ, Sakla HF, Cardona C, Chipont E, Alió JL. Corneal sensitivity after photorefractive keratectomy and laser in situ keratomileusis for low myopia. Am J Ophthalmol. 1999;127(5):497–504.
26. Murphy PJ, Corbett MC, O'Brart DP, Verma S, Patel S, Marshall J. Loss and recovery of corneal sensitivity following photorefractive keratectomy for myopia. J Refract Surg. 1999;15(1):38–45.
27. De Paiva CS, Chen Z, Koch DD, Hamill MB, Manuel FK, Hassan SS, Wilhelmus KR, Pflugfelder SC. The incidence and risk factors for developing dry eye after myopic LASIK. Am J Ophthalmol. 2006;141(3):438–45.
28. Albietz JM, Lenton LM, McLennan SG. Chronic dry eye and regression after laser in situ keratomileusis for myopia. J Cataract Refract Surg. 2004;30(3):675–84.
29. Albietz JM, Lenton LM. Management of the ocular surface and tear film before, during, and after laser in situ keratomileusis. J Refract Surg. 2004;20(1):62–71.
30. Patel SV, McLaren JW, Kittleson KM, Bourne WM. Subbasal nerve density and corneal sensitivity after laser in situ keratomileusis: femtosecond laser vs mechanical microkeratome. Arch Ophthalmol. 2010;128(11):1413–9.
31. Wei S, Wang Y. Comparison of corneal sensitivity between Fs-LASIK and femtosecond lenticule extraction (ReLEx FLEx) or small-incision lenticule extraction (ReLEx SMILE) for myopic eyes. Graefes Arch Clin Exp Ophthalmol. 2013;251(6):1645–54.
32. Vestergaard AH, Grønbech KT, Grauslund J, Ivarsen AR, Hjortdal JØ. Subbasal nerve morphology, corneal sensation, and tear film evaluation after refractive femtosecond laser lenticule extraction. Graefes Arch Clin Exp Ophthalmol. 2013;251(11):2591–600.
33. Li M, Niu L, Qin B, Zhou Z, Ni K, Le Q, Xiang J, Wei A, Ma W, Zhou X. Confocal comparison of corneal reinnervation after small incision lenticule extraction (SMILE) and femtosecond laser in situ keratomileusis (Fs-LASIK). PLoS ONE. 2013; 9;8(12):e81435.
34. Mohamed-Noriega K, Riau AK, Lwin NC, Chaurasia SS, Tan DT, Mehta JS. Early corneal nerve damage and recovery following small incision lenticule extraction (SMILE) and laser in situ keratomileusis (LASIK). Invest Ophthalmol Vis Sci. 2014;55(3):1823–34.
35. Reinstein DZ, Archer TJ, Randleman JB. Mathematical model to compare the relative tensile strength of the cornea after PRK, LASIK, and small incision lenticule extraction. J Refract Surg. 2013;29:454–60.
36. Liu C, Lin MT, Lee IXY, Mehta JS, Liu YC. Impact of corrected refractive power on the corneal denervation and ocular surface in small-incision lenticule extraction and LASIK. J Cataract Refract Surg. 2023;49(11):1106–13.
37. Bandeira F, Yusoff NZ, Yam GH, Mehta JS. Corneal re-innervation following refractive surgery treatments. Neural Regen Res. 2019;14(4):557–65.
38. Jiang X, Wang Y, Yuan H, Li Y, Wang H, An Z, Li X. Influences of SMILE and FS-LASIK on corneal sub-basal nerves: a systematic review and network meta-analysis. J Refract Surg. 2022;38(4):277–84.
39. Riau AK, Angunawela RI, Chaurasia SS, Lee WS, Tan DT, Mehta JS. Early corneal wound healing and inflammatory responses after refractive lenticule extraction (ReLEx). Invest Ophthalmol Vis Sci. 2011;52:6213–21.
40. Erie JC, Patel SV, McLaren JW, Hodge DO, Bourne WM. Corneal keratocyte deficits after photorefractive keratectomy and laser in situ keratomileusis. Am J Ophthalmol. 2006;141:799–809.
41. Alio JL, Javaloy J. Corneal inflammation following corneal photoablative refractive surgery with excimer laser. Surv Ophthalmol. 2013;58(1):11–25.
42. Vesaluoma M, Pérez-Santonja J, Petroll WM, et al. Corneal stromal changes induced by myopic LASIK. Invest Ophthalmol Vis Sci. 2000;41:369–76.
43. Erie JC, Nau CB, McLaren JW, et al. Long-term keratocyte deficits in the corneal stroma after LASIK. Ophthalmology. 2004;111:1356–61.

44. MH, Petroll WM, Perez-Santonja JJ, et al. Laser in situ keratomileusis flap margin: wound healing and complications imaged by in vivo confocal microscopy. Am J Ophthalmol. 2000;130:564–73.
45. Dong Z, Zhou X, Wu J, Zhang Z, Li T, Zhou Z, Zhang S, Li G. Small incision lenticule extraction (SMILE) and femtosecond laser LASIK: comparison of corneal wound healing and inflammation. Br J Ophthalmol. 2014;98(2):263–9.
46. Reinstein DZ, Archer TJ, Potter JG, Gupta R, Wiltfang R. Refractive and visual outcomes of SMILE for compound myopic astigmatism with the VISUMAX 800. J Refract Surg. 2023;39(5):294–301.

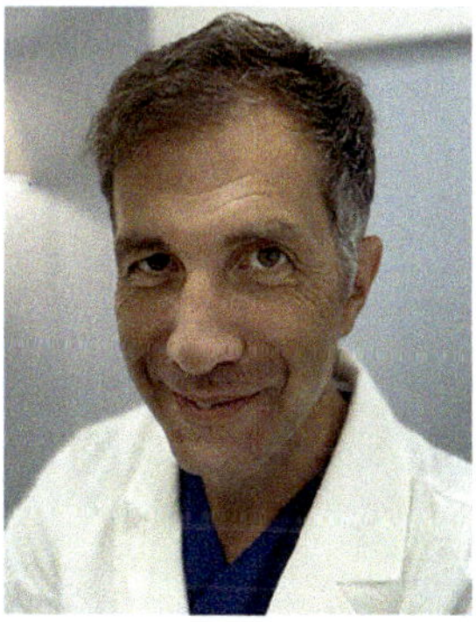

Mario Nubile is currently **Associate Professor in Ophthalmology and Director of the Cornea Service** of the University "G. d'Annunzio" of Chieti and Pescara – Italy. He completed his Residency Program in Ophthalmology in 2003 and his PhD program in 2007. Since 2005, he has been appointed as *Assistant Professor in Ophthalmology* (Researcher) in service at the Ophthalmology Clinic, Center of Excellence in Ophthalmology, National High-Tech Eye Center, University of Chieti-Pescara, Italy . In *2017* he received full qualification as *Associate Professor in Ophthalmology,* and in 2023 received the qualification for *Full Professor in Ophthalmology.*

He is the Head of the "Cornea and Ocular Surface Service" of this University. Principle fields of interest include ocular surface diseases, corneal pathologies and surgery, keratoplasty, femtosecond laser refractive surgery, anterior segment imaging.

Dr. Nubile is Author of more than 160 scientific publications in ophthalmology, books and book chapters, of which 92 are published on international peer reviewed journals with impact factor. (H-index 33; Citations: 2994)

Patent:EP20179055.7 (European Patent Office) New Drug Delivery System for Ophthalmic use (2020)

Teaching Activities: Teacher of Ophthalmology at the Medical School Program, Teacher of pathologies of the anterior segment and Anterior Segment surgery in the Residency program in Ophthalmology. Member of the Teacher Professors Collegium of the PhD program in "Medical Biotechnology" of the University since 2013. Former External Examiner of International PhD thesis in Europe (UK, Denmark, Spain).

He is Scientific Reviewer for several international scientific journals since 2005. He is member of the Executive Board of the EuCornea (European Society of the Cornea and Ocular Surface Specialists) with the function of Secretary General. He has been member of the ESCRS Research Committee (2016-2023) and he is currently Member of the ESCRS Program Committee (2024). He is Coordinator of the Anterior Segment Programs of the ESASO (European School for Advanced Studies in Ophthalmology).

Part II

Small Incision Lenticule Extraction (SMILE® and SMILE pro®): Clinical Development and Current Techniques

Historical Overview of the Clinical Development of Laser-Assisted Lenticule Extraction

4

Marcus Blum and Walter Sekundo

Abstract

This chapter provides a historical overview of laser-assisted lenticule corneal resection for myopia correction, tracing the evolution from early mechanical devices to the development of advanced femtosecond laser systems like VisuMax. It highlights the transition from femtosecond lenticule extraction (FLEx) to small incision lenticule extraction (SMILE), emphasizing the global acceptance of SMILE as a minimally invasive procedure for myopia and myopic astigmatism. Additionally, the chapter explores lenticule extraction for hyperopia, detailing modifications for improved outcomes, and recognizes collaborative efforts between surgeons and laser manufacturers, shaping the present and future of femtosecond laser surgery.

Keywords

Laser-assisted lenticule surgery • Corneal resectional refractive procedures • In Situ keratomileusis • Femtosecond laser systems • VisuMax • Femtosecond lenticule extraction (FLEx) • Small incision lenticule extraction (SMILE) • Myopia • Myopic astigmatism correction

Corneal resectional refractive procedures for the correction of myopia were pioneered by Barraquer and Ruiz [1]. They removed a layer of intrastromal tissue

M. Blum (✉)
Department of Ophthalmology, Helios Hospital Erfurt, Erfurt, Germany
e-mail: marcus.blum@helios-gesundheit.de

W. Sekundo
Department of Ophthalmology, Philipps University of Marburg, Marburg, Germany

W. Sekundo and F. M. Wagner (eds.), *Femtosecond Laser Assisted Lenticule Extraction*,
https://doi.org/10.1007/978-3-031-60424-9_4

utilizing a microkeratome and called this procedure "in situ keratomileusis." However, the results of the procedure performed with mechanical devices were not entirely satisfactory [2, 3].

A few years later, lasers entered the field of refractive surgery, and in 1989, Stern reported the use of lasers to ablate the cornea [4]. The first use of a laser instead of a microkeratome to achieve an intrastromal lenticule was described in 1996 [5]. Using a picosecond laser, an intrastromal lenticule was generated and was then removed manually after lifting the flap. In two highly myopic eyes, a fair amount of manual dissection was required resulting in an irregular surface [6]. Its use was therefore limited to animal studies [7, 8]. It is noteworthy that in the early 1990s of the last century, the idea of full femtosecond laser system-based refractive correction had already been born.

First clinical results with a laser-induced extraction of a refractive lenticule were reported with 5 blind or amblyopic eyes in 2003 [9]. Unfortunately, these first studies lack a sufficient number of eyes and a detailed analysis of the achieved refractive data. The studies have not been continued with a representative study cohort.

For several years, the advanced femtolaser systems were restricted to the creation of flaps as a replacement for mechanical microkeratomes, while the actual refractive procedure remained the domain of the 193 nm-ArF-excimer laser [10]. With regard to the quality of the surgical outcome, femtosecond laser microkeratomes have advantages over mechanical devices [11–13].

After several years, intensive laboratory research around the turn of the century a prototype femtosecond laser system—now known as VisuMax®—was developed by Carl Zeiss Meditec AG, Jena, Germany. In order to enable intraoperative target fixation by the patient, an illuminated and curved treatment interface (so-called contact glass) that does not elevate the intraocular pressure above the diastolic blood pressure was developed and tested beforehand on animals (Fig. 4.1) and in human volunteers in 2005. Mainly because the suction is applied at the cornea rather than at the sclera (as with other fs-lasers), the IOP raises to only 70–80 mmHg [14, 15]. This enables patients to see the blinking target and results in a good centration preventing clinically relevant induction of high order aberrations (HOA) [16] even with a laser without iris registration and centration assistance, such as VisuMax 500. Furthermore, the concept with its low suction and a continuous fixation target may reduce potential risks for the posterior segment [17]. To prove the function of the VisuMax fs-laser as a femto microkeratome, a study combining the fs-flap cut with the MEL 80 Excimer laser ablation was performed parallel to the further development of the FLEx procedure described below [18].

During this period of time in 2005 and 2006, a series of studies by Blum and Sekundo (unpublished data) on animals, blind and amblyopic eyes underwent a new refractive procedure, which no longer required an excimer laser (Fig. 4.2). The procedure was called femtosecond lenticule extraction (FLEx) in order to distinguish it from other known refractive procedures. In autumn of 2006, during the American Academy of Ophthalmology Meeting in Las Vegas/USA, Sekundo and Blum presented the very first ten cases of corneal refractive correction using

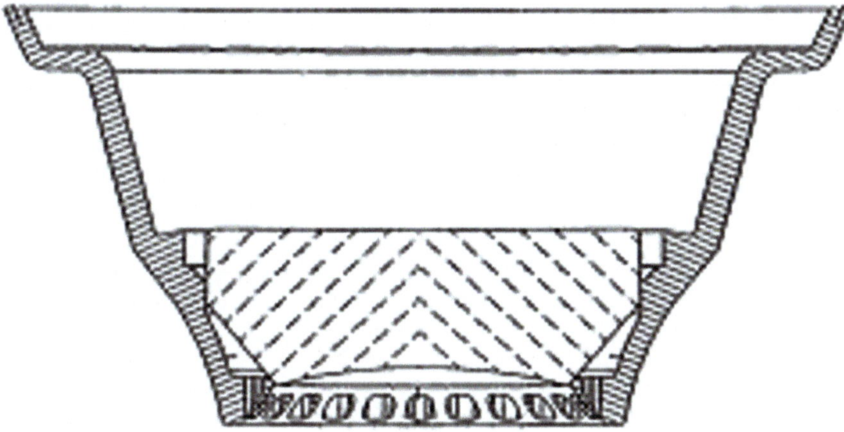

Fig. 4.1 Treatment pack

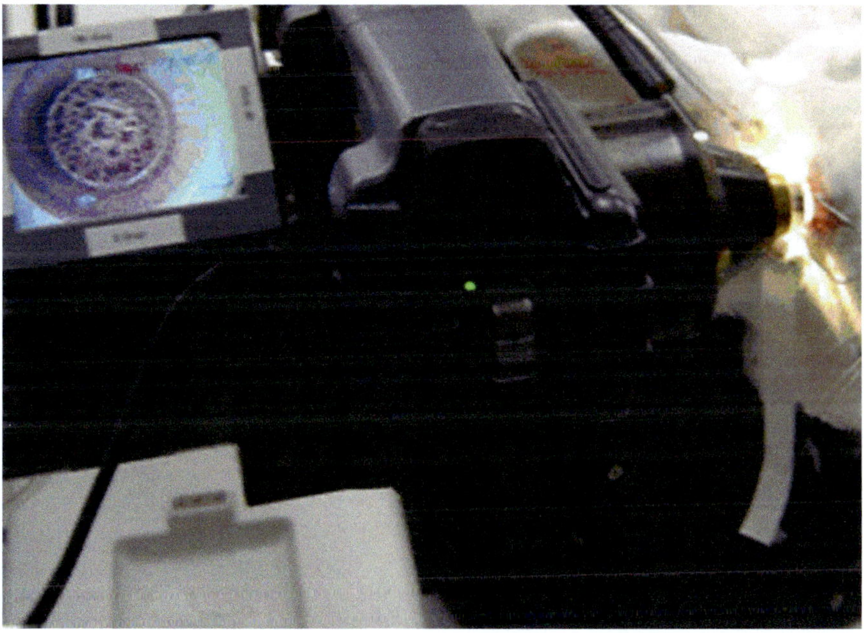

Fig. 4.2 Photograph from the first animal experiments testing femtosecond lenticule extraction

a prototype of the VisuMax femtosecond laser. The first peer-reviewed article was published by Sekundo et al. [19]. Animation images of the procedure reproduced from the first award-winning surgical video shown by Sekundo and Blum at the 2008 ASCRS Meeting in Chicago are summarized in Fig. 4.3.

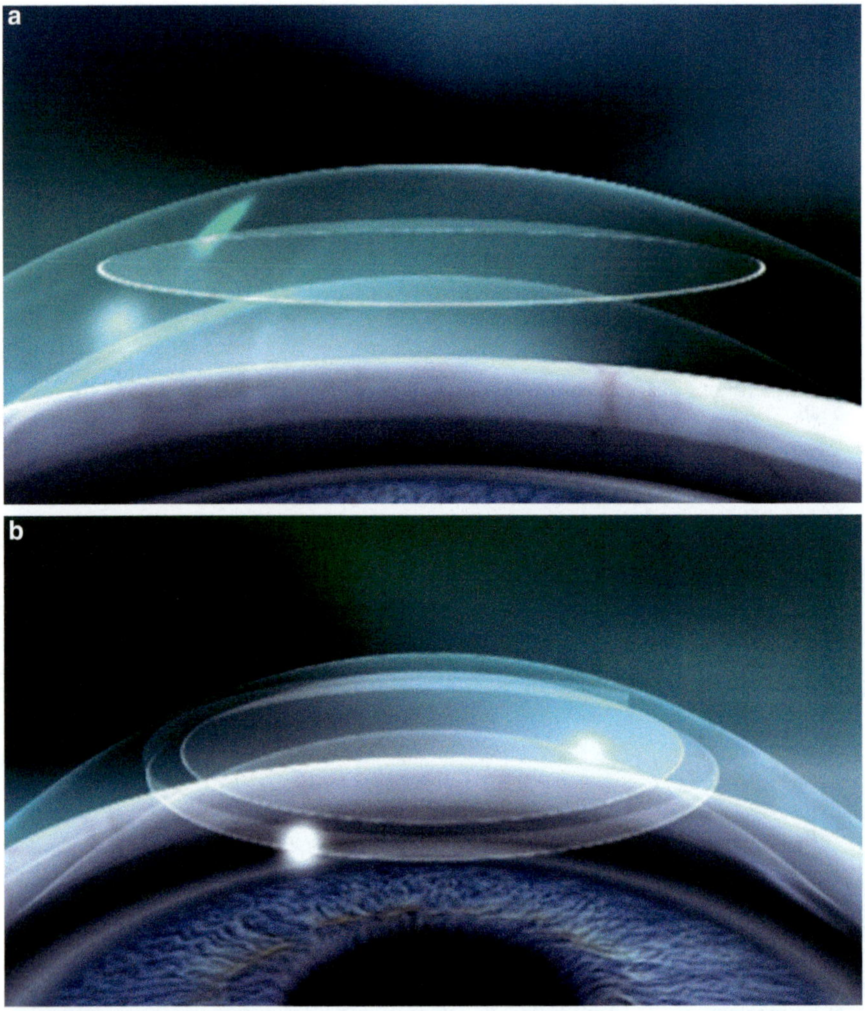

Fig. 4.3 Schematic drawing of the FLEx procedure. The VisuMax® femtosecond laser system cuts the back of the refractive lenticule followed by its front surface incision followed by a vertical incision leaving an arc of 50° untouched (hinge). The final step is performed manually, with the flap being lifted with the spatula and the lenticule removed manually using forceps. The flap is then repositioned

A cohort of fully seeing eyes treated for myopia and myopic astigmatism followed this very first report. A total of 108 eyes had been recruited and treated from 56 patients with spherical myopia between −2 and −8.5 D and myopic astigmatism up to −6 D cyl. These eyes were followed up for 6 months and—on a voluntary basis—for 12 months [20, 21]. Meanwhile, the ten-year results of this initial cohort have been published [22].

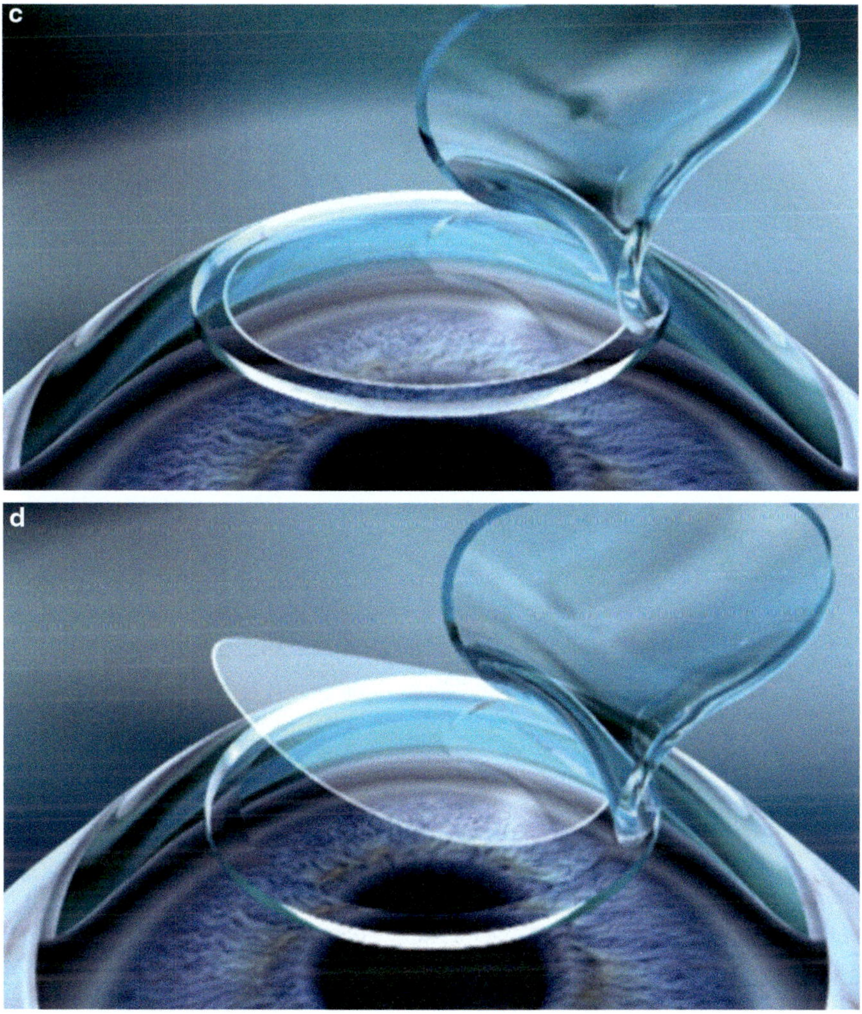

Fig. 4.3 (continued)

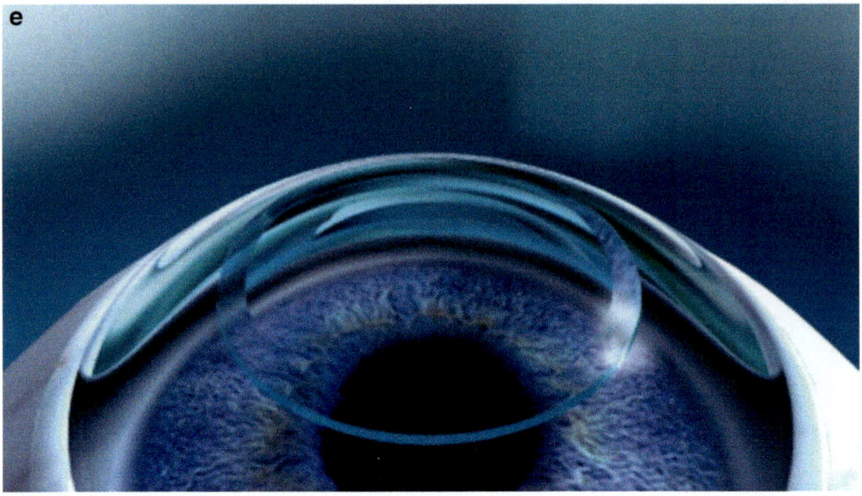

Fig. 4.3 (continued)

In this first larger series, the intended flap thickness varied between 110 and 160 μm; the flap diameter was chosen between 7.0 and 8.5 mm. In all 108 cases, a superior hinge, 50° in chord length, was left. The lenticule diameter varied between 6.0 and 7.3 mm according to patient's scotopic pupil diameter. No nomograms were available at the beginning, and a special equation (Patent No. DE 102006053120 A1) based on Mannerlyn's formula was used to calculate the geometry and the thickness of the refractive lenticule. The postoperative regimen consisted of preservative free antibiotic, steroid, and hyaluronic acid lubricating drops four times per day each for 1 week. Keeping in mind that this first prospective clinical study started without a nomogram, the results of 98.1% of eyes within 1 D of refractive target were satisfactory and exceeded the expectations.

Rupal Shah was the third surgeon in the world who took up the refractive lenticule extraction (ReLEx) technique (as it was called those days) and significantly contributed to its development in the early phase of this procedure. Her main achievement was not only to optimize laser settings for the 200 kHz machine used at this stage of development in a substantial number of patients, but also to realize that also the laser scan (or cut) direction matters [23].

Following the successful implementation of FLEx, the next aim was to further develop a surgical procedure in which a flap no longer was necessary. This procedure was named small incision lenticule extraction (SMILE): by passing a dissector through a small 2–3 mm incision the anterior and posterior lenticular interfaces are separated and the lenticule is than removed through the incision (Fig. 4.4). This eliminates the need to create a flap and the cornea above the upper interface of the lenticule is now referred to as the cap. The first surgical video of SMILE was shown during the Cataratta refractiva in Milano in 2009. However, it took another three years till peer-reviewed publications appeared in the scientific literature [24, 25]. The first larger series of eyes operated with the SMILE technique was published by Sekundo, Blum et al. and, unlike in today's SMILE, were carried out through two opposite entering incisions, 4 mm each [24]. A total of 91 eyes clearly demonstrated the "prove of principle," and the encouraging results motivated a number of researchers to test the new surgical technique [25, 26]. This resulted in a variety of smaller changes in surgical technique, but the main elements remained unchanged: The laser first created the lower interface, followed by the upper interface of the lenticule either using an out-to-in direction or using an in-to-out direction. Shah was the first surgeon to use a single entering incision [25], and it was also her who systematically worked toward very small incision used today.

Although the refractive results were good in the first study (very close to those observed in LASIK), visual recovery time was slightly longer. The effect of different scanning patterns, optimization of energy parameters, and spot spacing settings led to much improved visual recovery times [23, 26, 28, 29]. Furthermore, a 500-kHz-Laser was released, and the precision of lenticule creation was improved [30, 31]. In terms of safety and complications, SMILE has also been shown to be quite outstanding [32].

This minimally invasive procedure has meanwhile become internationally established for the treatment of myopia and myopic astigmatism, and both data from large patient cohorts and long-term results are available. Similarly to the development of SMILE for myopia and astigmatism, hyperopia was initially approached by a flap-based femtosecond lenticule extraction (FLEx), but the early results were discouraging, as systematic regression worsened the outcome [33]. Modification of the lenticule geometry and enlargement of the optical zone led to significantly better results [34, 35] (Fig. 4.5). The influence of the diameter of the optical zone and the optimal centration of the hyperopic lenticule were studied by a research group in Nepal [36, 37], and the same group also tested the new femtolaser profiles resulting in improved outcomes [38]. After these smaller studies, a prospective, multicentre, international study conducted at seven sites demonstrated that lenticule extraction shows equally good results as hyperopic fs-LASIK [39].

After 2010–2011, the technique of lenticule extraction became increasingly popular and many outstanding surgeons joined the "SMILE community" improving the quality of this procedure step by step. While Carl Zeiss Meditec AG used this time to develop a new VisuMax 800 laser requiring 9–10 s for the full laser scan in myopic and 12 s in hyperopic treatments and enriching it with centration and cyclotorsion assisting systems, other laser manufactures have either developed or modified their laser systems for lenticule extraction. They introduced different applanation, cutting, and lenticule shape strategies as well as centration assistance. Because of the proprietary reasons, these procedures have a different branding, such as SmartSight® (Schwind), CLEAR® (Ziemer) and SILK® (Johnson & Johnson).

It is a pleasure to see several companies and many of the surgeons working on the improvement of fs-laser lenticule extraction as co-authors of this book, sharing their view of the present and the future of "all-in-one" femtosecond laser surgery.

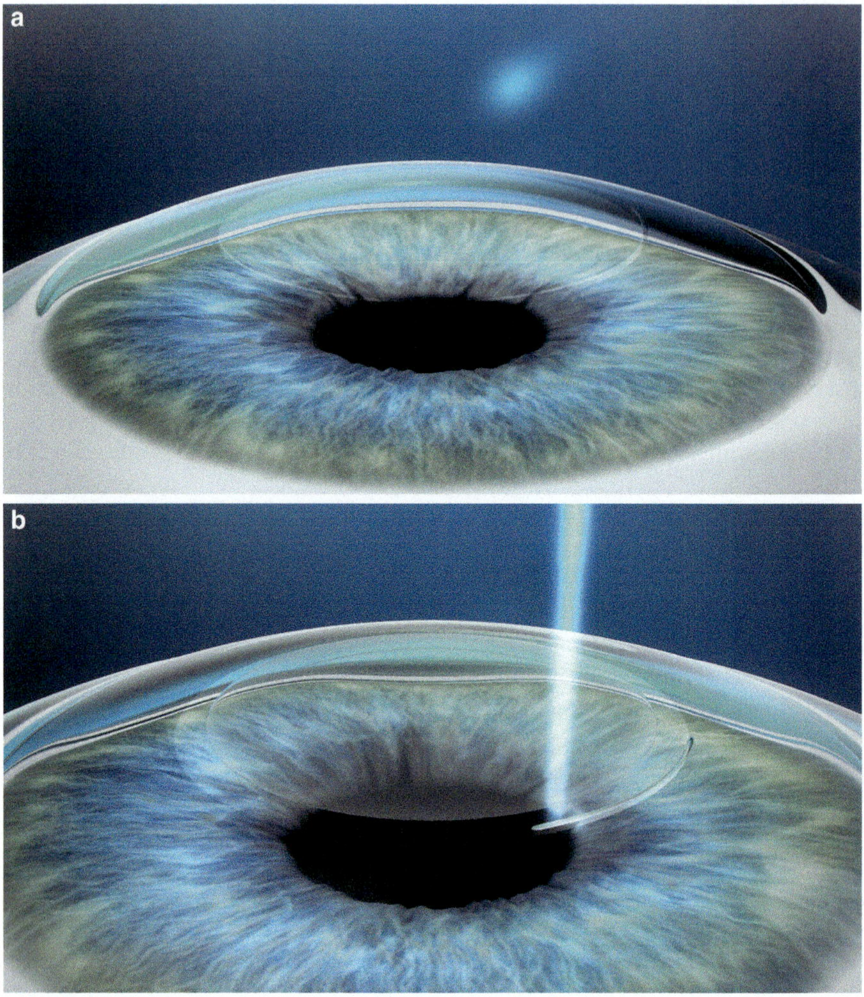

Fig. 4.4 Schematic drawing of the SMILE procedure

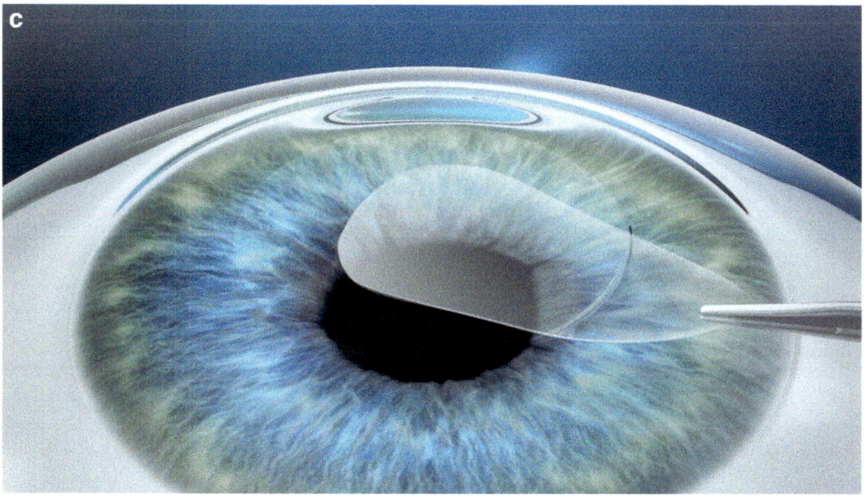

Fig. 4.4 (continued)

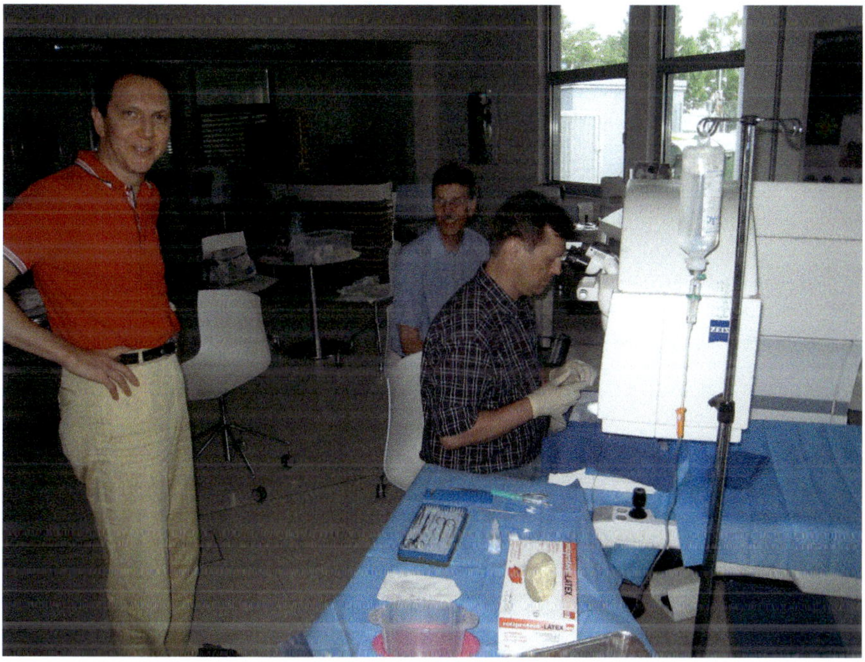

Fig. 4.5 Marcus Blum, Walter Sekundo, and Matthias Wottke (Carl Zeiss Meditec Ag) in the wetlab in Jena testing first modern profiles for hyperopic lenticule extraction on porcine eyes

References

1. Barraquer JI. The history and evolution of keratomileusis. Int Ophthalmol Clin. 1996;36:1–7.
2. Ibrahim O, Waring GO, Salah T, El Maghraby A. Automated in situ Keratomileusis for myopia. J Refract Surg. 1995;11:431–41.
3. Wiegand W, Krusenberg B, Kroll P. Keratomileusis in situ bei hochgradiger Myopie. Erste Ergebnisse. Ophthalmologe. 1995;92:402–9.
4. Stern D, Schoenlein RW, Puliafito CA. Corneal ablation by nanosecond, picoseconds, and femtosecond lasers at 532 and 625 nm. Arch Ophthalmol. 1989;107:567–92.
5. Ito M, Quantock AJ, Malhan S, Schanzlin DJ, Krueger RR. Picosecond laser in situ keratomileusis with a 1053-nm Nd: YFL laser. J Refract Surg. 1996;12:721–8.
6. Krueger RR, Juhasz T, Gualano A, Marchi V. The picosecond laser for nonmechanical laser in situ keratomileusis. J Refract Surg. 1998;14:467–9.
7. Kurtz RM, Horvath C, Liu HH, Krueger RR, Juhasz T. Lamellar refractive surgery with scanned intrastromal picoseconds and femtosecond laser pulses in animal eyes. J Refract Surg. 1998;14:541–8.
8. Heisterkamp A, Mamon T, Kermani O, Drommer W, Welling H, Ertmer W, Lubatschowski H. Intrastromal refractive surgery with ultrashort laser pulses: in vivo study on the rabbit eye. Graefes Arch Clin Exp Ophthalmol. 2003;241:511–7.
9. Ratkay-Traub I, Ferincz IE, Juhasz T, Kurtz RM, Krueger RR. First clinical results with the femtosecond neodymium-glass laser in refractive surgery. J Refract Surg. 2003;19:94–103.
10. Nordan LT, Slade SG, Baker RN. Femtosecond laser flap creation for laser in situ keratomileusis: six-months follow-up of the initial US clinical series. J Refract Surg. 2003;19:8–14.
11. Kezirian GM, Stonecipher KG. Comparison of the IntraLase femtosecond laser and mechanical microkeratome for laser in situ Keratomileusis. J Cataract Refract Surg. 2004;30:26–32.
12. Durrie DS, Kezirian GM. Femtosecond laser versus mechanical keratome flaps in wavefront-guided laser in situ keratomileusis: prospective contralateral eye study. J Cataract Refract Surg. 2005;31:120–6.
13. Tran DB, Sarayba MA, Bor Z, et al. Randomized prospective clinical study comparing induced aberrations with IntraLase and Hansatome flap creation in fellow eyes: potential impact on wavefront-guided laser in situ keratomileusis. J Cataract Refract Surg. 2005;31:97–105.
14. Vetter JM, Holzer MP, Teping C, Weingartner WE, Gericke A, Stoffelns B, Pfeiffer N, Sekundo W. Intraocular pressure during corneal flap preparation: comparison among four femtosecond lasers in porcine eyes. J Refract Surg. 2011;27:427–33.
15. Vetter JM, Faust M, Gericke A, Pfeiffer N, Weingärtner WE, Sekundo W. Intraocular pressure measurements during flap preparation using 2 femtosecond lasers and 1 microkeratome in human donor eyes. J Cataract Refract Surg. 2012;38:2011–8.
16. Sekundo W, Gertnere J, Bertelmann T, Solomatin I. One-year refractive results, contrast sensitivity, high-order aberrations and complications after myopic small-incision lenticule extraction (ReLEx SMILE). Graefes Arch Clin Exp Ophthalmol. 2014.
17. Reviglio VE, Kuo IC, Gramajo L, et al. Acute rhegmatogenous retinal detachment immediately following laser in situ keratomileusis. J Cataract Refract Surg. 2007;33:536–9.
18. Blum M, Kunert K, Gille A, Sekundo W. First experience in Femtosecond LASIK with the Zeiss VISUMAX® laser. J Refract Surg. 2009;25:350–6.
19. Sekundo W, Kunert K, Russmann Ch, Gille A, Bissmann W, Strobrawa G, Stickler M, Bischoff M, Blum M. First efficacy and safty study of femtosecond lenticule extraction for the correction of myopia. J Cataract Refract Surg. 2008;34:1513–20.
20. Blum M, Kunert K, Schröder M, Sekundo W. Femtosecond lenticule extraction (FLEX) for the correction of myopia: 6 months results. Graefes Arch Clin Exp Ophthalmol. 2010;248:1019–27.
21. Blum M, Kunert KS, Engelbrecht Ch, Dawczynski J. Sekundo W Femtosekunden-Lentikel-Extraktion (FLEX) – Ergebnisse nach 12 Monaten bei myopem Astigmatismus. Klin Monatsbl Augenheilkd. 2010;227:961–5.

22. Blum M, Lauer AS, Kunert KS, Sekundo W. 10-year results of small incision lenticule extraction. J Refract Surg. 2019;35:618–23.
23. Shah R, Shah S. Effect of scanning patterns on the results of femtosecond laser lenticule extraction refractive surgery. J Cataract Refract Surg. 2011;37:1636–47.
24. Sekundo W, Kunert K, Blum M. Small incision femtosecond lenticule extraction (SMILE) for the correction of myopia and myopic astigmatism: results of a 6 months prospective study. Br J Ophthalmol. 2011;95:335–9.
25. Shah R, Shah S, Segupta S. Results of small incision lenticule extraction: all-in-one femtosecond laser refractive surgery. J Cataract Refract Surg. 2011;37:127–37.
26. Hjortdal JO, Vestergaard AH, Ivarsen A, Ragunathan S, Asp S. Predictors for the outcome of small-incision lenticule extraction for Myopia. J Refract Surg. 2012;28:865–71.
27. Kamiya K, Shimizu K, Igarashi A, Kobashi H. Visual and refractive outcomes of femtosecond lenticule extraction and small-incision lenticule extraction for myopia. Am J Ophthalmol. 2014;157:128–34.
28. Kunert KS, Blum M, Duncker GIW, Sietmann R, Heichel J. Surface quality of human corneal lenticules after femtosecond laser surgery for myopia comparing different laser parameters. Graefes Arch Clin Exp Ophthalmol. 2011; 249:1417–24.
29. Heichelt J, Blum M, Duncker GIW, Sietmann R, Kunert KS. Surface quality of porcine corneal lenticules after femtosecond lenticule extraction. Ophthalmic Res. 2011;46:107–12.
30. Reinstein DZ, Archer TJ, Gobbe M. Accuracy and reproducibility of cap thickness in small incision lenticule extraction. J Refract Surg. 2013;29:810–5.
31. Ozgurhan EB, Agca A, Bozkurt E, Gencer B, Celik U, Cankaya KI, DEmirok A, Yilmaz OF. Accuracy and precision of cap thickness in small incision lenticule extraction. Clin Ophthalmol. 2013;7:923–6.
32. Ivarsen A, Asp S, Hjortdal J. Safty and complications of more than 1500 small incision lenticule extraction procedures. Ophthalmology. 2014;121:822–82.
33. Blum M, Kunert KS, Vossmerbaeumer U, Sekundo W. Femtosecond lenticule extraction (ReLEx®) for correction of hyperopia—first results. Graefes Arch Clin Exp Ophthalmol. 2013;251:349–55.
34. Sekundo W, Reinstein DZ, Blum M. Improved lenticule shape for hyperopic femtosecond lenticule extraction (ReLEx FLEx): a pilot study. Lasers Med Sci. 2016;31:659–64.
35. Sekundo W, Messerschmidt-Roth A, Reinstein DZ, Archer TJ, Blum M. Femtosecond lenticule extraction (FLEx) für spherocylindrical hyperopia using new profiles. J Refract Surg. 2018;34:6–10.
36. Reinstein DZ, Pradhan KR, Carp GI, Archer TJ, Gobbe M, Sekundo W, Khan R, Citron K, Dhungana P. Small incision lenticule extraction (SMILE) for hyperopia: optical zone centration. J Refract Surg. 2017;33:150–6.
37. Reinstein DZ, Pradhan KR, Carp GI, Archer TJ, Gobbe M, Sekundo W, Khan R, Citron K. Dhungana P (2017) Small incision lenticule extraction (SMILE) for hyperopia: optical zone diameter and spherical aberration induction. J Refract Surg. 2017;33:370–6.
38. Pradhan KR, Reinstein DZ, Carp GI, Archer TJ, Dhungana R. Small incision lenticule extraction (SMILE) for hyperopia: 12-month refractive and visual outcomes. J RefractSurg. 2019;35:442–50.
39. Reinstein DZ, Sekundo W, Archer TJ, Stodulka P, Ganesh S, Cochener B, Blum M, Wang Y, Zhou X. SMILE for hyperopia with and without astigmatism: Results of a prospective multicenter 12-month study. J Refract Surg. 2022;38:760–9.

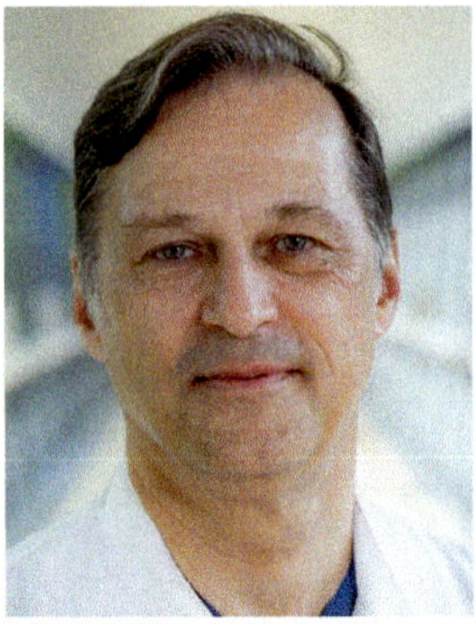

Marcus Blum MD is Head of Department of Ophthalmology, Helios Klinikum Erfurt, Germany. He studied at the University of Heidelberg. He was resident in the Department of Ophthalmology at Heidelberg (Prof. H.E. Völcker) and fellow at the Department of Ophthalmology at Jena (Prof. J. Strobel). He was appointed Associate Professor at the University of Jena in 1999 and was involved in building up a technology network focussing on new technologies for Ophthalmology in Jena. Together with Walter Sekundo he pioneered using fs-lasers for lenticule extraction. In 2001 Prof. Blum became head of the Ophthalmology Department at the Helios Klinikum Erfurt. He has published 150 papers and book chapters and has given more than 300 presentations at national and international meetings. In 2024 he was elected as president of the German Society for Cataract and Refractive Surgery (DGII).

Current Technique and Instrumentation for SMILE

5

Ekktet Chansue and Walter Sekundo

The ReLEx® SMILE procedure is typically performed under topical anesthesia and can be divided into two steps: the femtosecond laser application and the manual removal of the lenticule. The femtosecond laser cuts are intrastromal, without any external corneal wound, and subsequently can be performed in a "clean" fashion, i.e., no disinfection needed. The second step requires sterility of the field.

Bilateral Surgery

The procedure can be performed bilaterally provided that the patient has been properly counseled and has gone through proper informed consent process. For bilateral ReLEx SMILE, the procedure can be performed either as two sequential unilateral procedures (complete laser cuts and lenticule extraction in one eye, then the same in the other) or as a stepwise bilateral operation (sequential laser cuts in both eyes, followed by sequential lenticule extraction in both eyes). The advantages of completing the whole procedure one eye at a time are:

- More conventional feel.
- Simpler setup of the operating room. Less manpower needed.

Supplementary Information The online version contains supplementary material available at https://doi.org/10.1007/978-3-031-60424-9_5.

E. Chansue (✉)
Bangkok, Thailand
e-mail: echansue@gmail.com

W. Sekundo
Department of Ophthalmology, Phillipps University of Marburg, Marburg, Germany

W. Sekundo and F. M. Wagner (eds.), *Femtosecond Laser Assisted Lenticule Extraction*,
https://doi.org/10.1007/978-3-031-60424-9_5

The advantages of doing each step bilaterally are:

- This clearly separates the "clean" and the "sterile" parts of the procedure, making contaminations less likely.
- The dissection and extraction of the lenticules can be performed with another microscope, perhaps one the individual surgeon prefers over that of the laser. This will also free the laser bed for the preparation of the next patient. This is especially useful in high-flow practices, with adequate manpower in the operating room.
- The laser applications occur in rapid succession, decreasing the risks of overdehydration of the surface of the second eye, which may lead to slow visual recovery and possibly variations in refractive results.
- Uneventful completion of femtosecond laser cuts in both eyes helps ensure that lenticule extraction can be successfully performed in both eyes. Should there be any problem in the laser part of the procedure in either eye, the surgeon and the patient have the options of proceeding or aborting the procedure.

5.1 Femtosecond Laser Application

Much like the setting of the excimer laser in LASIK, the surgeon is ultimately responsible in setting up parameters of the laser to get optimum results. The details of the femtosecond laser settings are discussed elsewhere in this textbook (see Chap. 10).

The procedure involving the docking and the application of the laser cuts are similar to that in FemtoLASIK flap creation. The difference is that FemtoLASIK flap cuts only involve two cuts (the planar cut and the edge cut), whereas ReLEx® SMILE involves four cuts: (a) the posterior (Lenticule-Bed, LB) plane cut, (b) the lenticule edge cut, (c) the anterior (Cap-Lenticule, CL) plane cut, and (d) the entrance incision cut (Fig. 5.1). Consequently, it takes roughly twice the duration to complete the ReLEx cuts, compared to flap cuts.

This is the most critical part of the procedure refractively because it is where the femtosecond laser defines the anterior and posterior plane between which the lenticule will be created. The dimension and shape of the lenticule determine the amount of spherical and cylindrical correction and the effective optical zone of treatment.

The smoothness of the cuts affects the smoothness of the corneal surface once the lenticule has been extracted. The smoothness of the surface is further affected by the postoperative epithelial remodeling (see Chap. 13), but the initial smoothness immediately after the procedure has significant effects on the early visual quality and recovery.

In bilateral cases, while the first eye is receiving the laser treatment, the second eye should be held shut with an adhesive strip, to prevent uneven dehydration of the epithelium that may lead to temporary roughness of the surface, in turn affecting the smoothness of the laser cuts and the visual recovery time (Fig. 5.2).

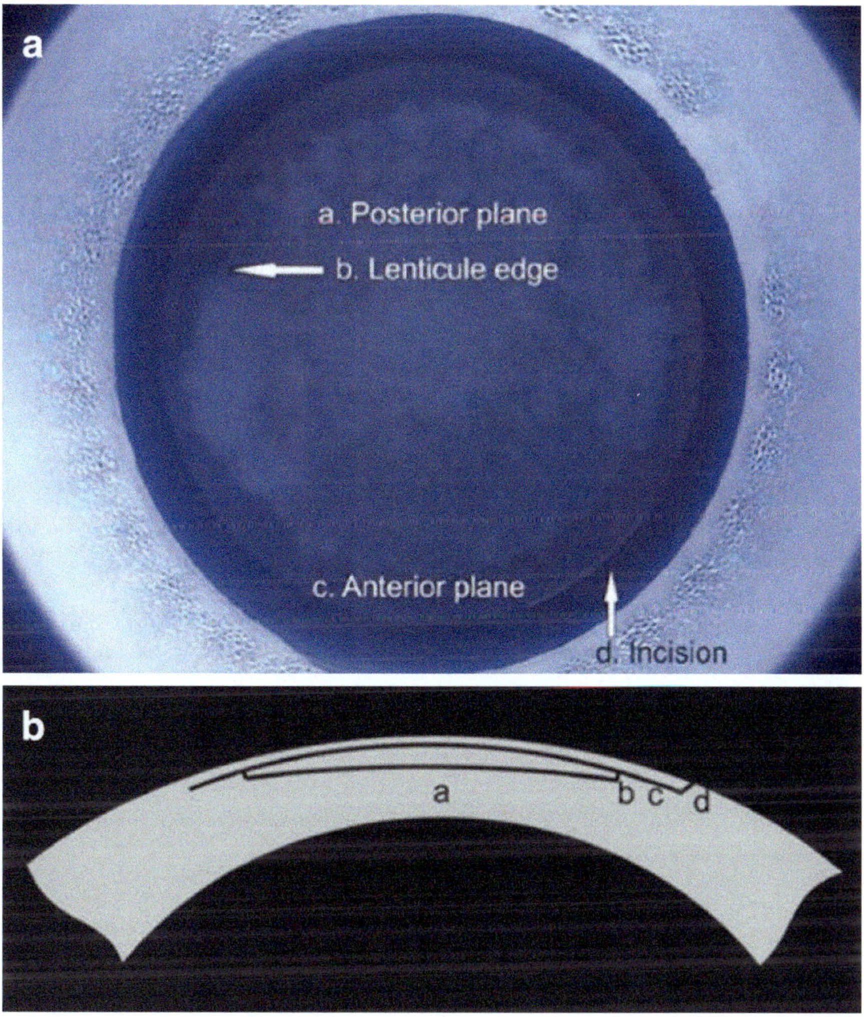

Fig. 5.1 Femtosecond laser ReLEx® cuts: (1a) frontal, and (1b) cross-sectional views. a) Posterior (Lenticule-Bed: LB) plane; b) lenticule edge cut; c) anterior (Cap-Lenticule: CL) plane; d) incision cut

5.2 Lenticule Extraction

Immediately after the femtosecond laser cuts are completed, the lenticule is still not freely retrievable, as there are still micro-bridges between the interfaces. The surgeon breaks those micro-bridges by bluntly dissecting in the plane between the lenticule and the stromal cap and that between the lenticule and the stromal bed, to free the lenticule from its surroundings. The lenticule is then retrieved and removed from the pocket.

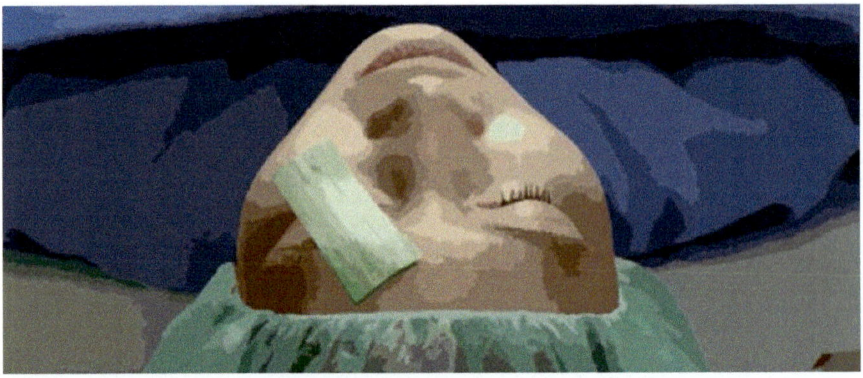

Fig. 5.2 Second eye is taped shut before the laser application to the first eye

Instrumentation

The lenticule extraction part of ReLEx® SMILE requires minimal instrumentation. This includes:

Basic Instruments: Eyelid speculum, absorbent surgical spears, sterile balanced-salt solution (15 cc bottle), blunt irrigating cannula, and Kelman-McPherson-type forceps.

An Eyelid Speculum: A solid-bladed, self-retaining speculum. Here, pediatric-sized specula are preferred, as the shorter blades create more vertical space resulting in a roughly hexagonal, rather than rectangular, exposure. This is especially useful in the eyes with shorter palpebral fissures (Fig. 5.6).

Specific Instruments: Lenticule dissector for freeing the lenticule and microforceps for retrieving the freed lenticule.

Lenticule Dissectors

The Chansue ReLEx® Dissector

When I started performing ReLEx® in 2010, the standard instrument recommended by the laser manufacturer for dissecting the lenticule was the Seibel flap lifter or a simple phako spatula and the Blum modified McPherson forceps. As the name implies, Seibel flap lifter was designed to be used for flap lifting in FemtoLASIK. It worked quite well as a dissector for ReLEx® FLEX, as the flap and the lenticule were lifted in the same manner as the flap in FemtoLASIK. However, the instrument lent itself poorly to lenticule dissection when a small incision was intended, as it was too straight and too long. Consequently, I designed an instrument specifically for ReLEx® lenticule dissection later that year. It has a curved tapering circular shaft which ends in a conical semi-blunt dissecting tip. The curvature of the dissecting shaft conforms with the average corneal curvature, to minimize distortion and stress to the anterior stromal cap during the dissection

(Fig. 5.3a). The other end of the dissector bears a Sinskey-style hook in the same fashion as does the Seibel Flap Lifter but is slightly longer to facilitate the delineation of both the Cap-Lenticule (CL) and the Lenticule-Bed (LB) planes. The instrument is called the Chansue ReLEx® Dissector (CRD). Since then, the CRD has been widely adopted and is available from various instrument manufacturers. However, when the commercially available CRD's were examined, it was found that they tended to differ and deviate from the original design. Most notably, the length of the dissecting shaft was usually too long, which reduces the surgeon's control of the tip. The shaft being too long also made the action of sweeping the dissecting shaft (while trying not to tear the entrance incision) more complex. Another notable deviation was the tip usually being too sharp, which made it easier for the instrument to create false planes and to perforate the cap.

(As a side note, there is even an "Advanced" CRD available which I was not involved in designing.)

The Chansue ReLEx® Dissector 2

A few years later, I made a modification to the CRD's tip to facilitate locating and entering both the CL and the LB planes without the help of the hook.

Starting near the tip, the instrument tapers down from a circular cross-section into a flat tip, in a shape similar to a duck's bill, its semi-circular leading edge still semi-blunt (Fig. 5.3e).

Using this new design, one can make the entrance incision, find the CL plane, locate the lenticule edge, and enter the LB plane using the dissector side only. The hook end of the instrument still persists (for the rare cases in which the lenticule edge is difficult to locate) but is rarely used anymore. This modified CRD is called the Chansue ReLEx® Dissector 2 (CRD2).

Meanwhile, some further modifications of different instruments were made by other surgeons in co-operation with other ophthalmic instruments manufacturers, but they are generally speaking one of these designs:

1. Spatulas resembling the CRD, but with different lengths and diameter (e.g., Kostin spatula/Medin-Ural/Russia, Fig. 5.3b) or
2. Dissectors featuring a combination of the CRD and Blum spoon (e.g., Tan dissector/ASICO/USA, Güell dissector/Geuder/ Germany, Reinstein single-use dissector/Malosa/UK, Sekundo spade dissector for forward and backward cutting/Titan Surgical/Russia). See also Fig. 5.3c, d, f.
3. More recently, an instrument has been in development by Dr. Dishler (Denver, CO, USA) which has a modified tip design that vibrates in a specific way at relatively low frequency and moves only about 10–15 microns. There is feedback as to resistance encountered that controls instantly the amount of force of the movement, thus making it a "smart device. (Fig. 5.3g)

Time will tell whether assisted dissection tools will replace manual dissectors and spatulas.

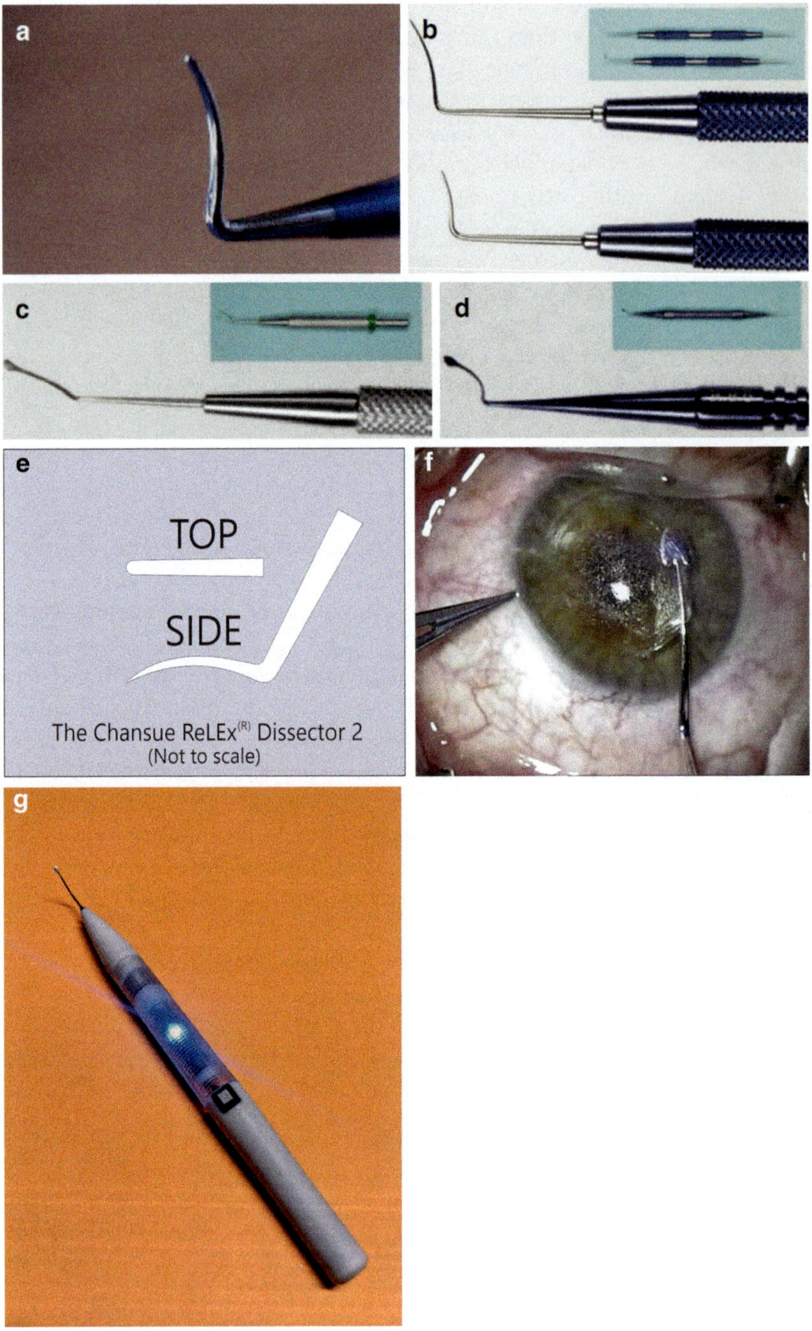
a
b
c
d
e
TOP
SIDE
The Chansue ReLEx(R) Dissector 2
(Not to scale)
f
g

◂**Fig. 5.3** (a) Original Chansue ReLEx® Dissector (CRD). (b) Kostin spatulas (Medin-Ural/Russia) are slightly slender compared to the original Chansue dissector and are produced in two different lengths. (c) The original Blum "spoon" (Geuder GmbH/Germany) designed at the early stage of ReLEx® development features a semi-sharp ending similar to a hockey knife. (d) and (e) Due to a better laser cut quality of the VisuMax® 500 and 800, Blum spoon was replaced by several similar instruments featuring a blunt, rounded, and polished head as shown in this "advanced" Chansue dissector. (f) "Spade" spatula was designed by Sekundo to address the backward cutting of the lenticule edge particularly juxtaincisionaly as shown on this screenshot (g) Recently introduced Dishler's (Denver, CO, USA) instrument has a modified tip design that vibrates in a specific way at relatively low frequency and moves only about 10–15 microns

Lenticule-Retrieving Microforceps

Marcus Blum's modified McPherson forceps with serrated jaws (Fig. 5.4a) was the first lenticule retrieving instrument designed for ReLEx® procedure. However, when the entering incision becomes smaller than 2.5 mm, microforceps are recommended. The standard microforceps instrument is the Advanced Lenticule forceps, which is a modification of the Shah Lenticule forceps, designed by Dr. Rupal Shah in 2011 (Fig. 5.4b).

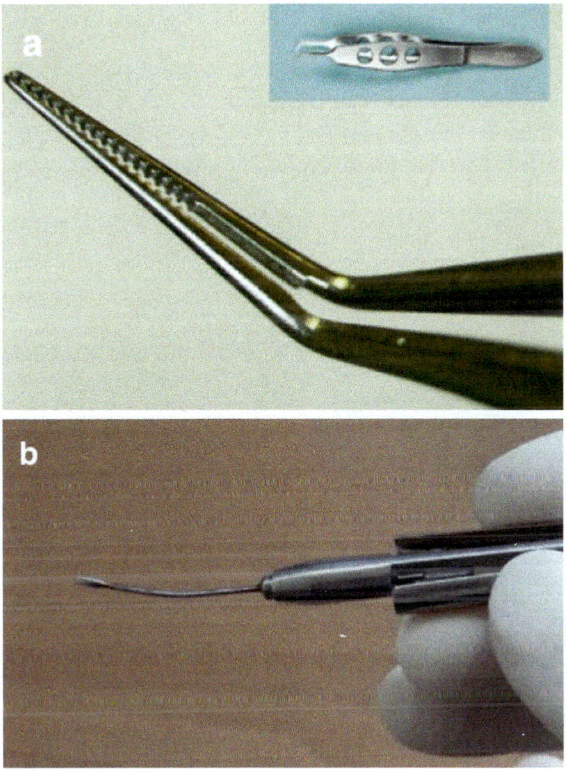

Fig. 5.4 (a) McPherson serrated forceps (Geuder GmbH, Germany) modified by Blum is a simple forceps for lenticule extraction for entering incisions of 2.5 mm or longer. (b) Advanced Lenticule forceps

5.3 Globe Stabilization

The dissection can be performed with the patient self-fixating on the microscope illuminator, and usually no additional physical fixation is needed. However, immediately after the femtosecond laser application, the central cornea becomes cloudy because of the microbubbles created by the laser energy. This makes fixation difficult for the patient. To partially clear the central cornea of these microbubbles, pointed pressure can be applied on the central corneal epithelial surface with a smooth instrument. The heel part of the CRD can be used to do this, as it provides a small pressure point and the shiny smoothness of its surface minimizes epithelial disturbances. This allows some of the microscope light to get through the central cornea and helps the patient fixate (Fig. 5.6). Fixation on the microscope light not only distracts the patient away from their anxiety, but also helps the surgeon with the dissection, as it creates opposing force to that caused by the dissector separating the planes.

Some surgeons feel more comfortable to manually stabilize the globe with the nondominant hand using either a micro-spear sponge or Fine-Thornton's fixating ring for contra-pressure or a pair of toothed forceps to hold the globe (see Fig. 5.7).

5.4 Dissecting Efficiency

The dissector has the highest dissecting power at the tip. The quality of the femtosecond laser cuts in the previous step determines how effectively the dissector separates the interfaces. In some eyes, the dissector can only advance a few millimeters with each sweep of the dissecting tip, whereas in others, just one sweep will separate the whole expanse of the pocket.

5.5 Surgical Steps

Standard lenticule extraction using the original CRD:

1. Sterile field with routine disinfection and draping of the upper half of the face. Some surgeons also prefer to drape the eyelids and the eyelashes.
2. Placement of eyelid speculum (Fig. 5.5).
3. Pointed pressure in the center of the cornea, just enough to create a relatively clear stroma through which the patient can see the microscope light and fixate. The patient is instructed to fixate on the light at all times (Fig. 5.6).
4. The hook end of the CRD is used to break the entrance incision open (Fig. 5.8).
5. A small pocket (1×2 mm) is made with the hook. While doing the planar dissection of this pocket, care should be taken to keep the most distal part of the hook parallel to the corneal surface (or pointed slightly up and away from the eye) to ensure that this pocket is in the CL plane (Fig. 5.9).

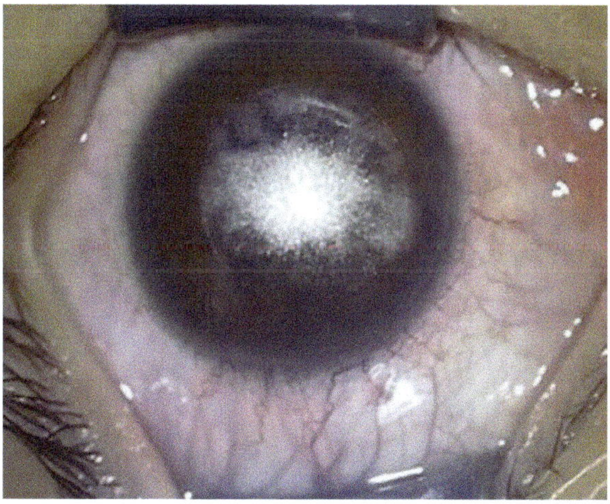

Fig. 5.5 Short blades of the pediatric eyelid speculum create hexagonal exposure

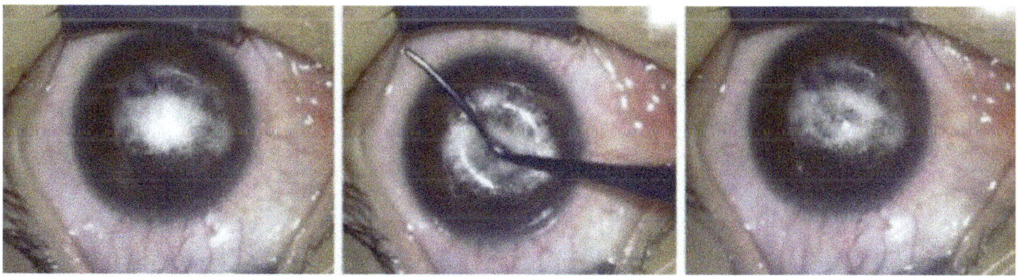

Fig. 5.6 Central microbubbles are pushed away by pointed pressure on the epithelial surface, creating a relatively clear area though which the patient can fixate at the microscope illuminator

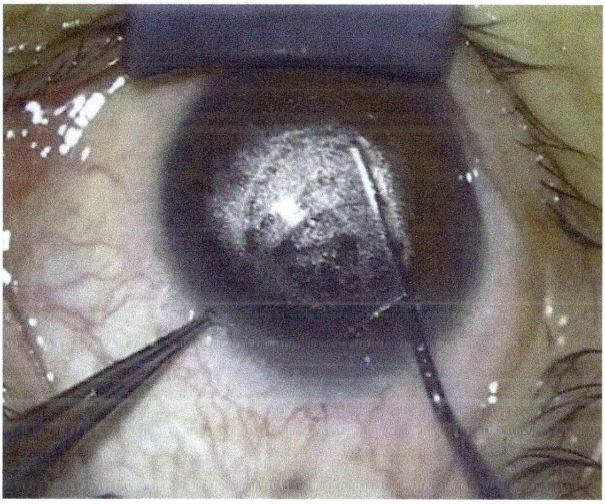

Fig. 5.7 Manual globe fixation with 0.12 toothed forceps

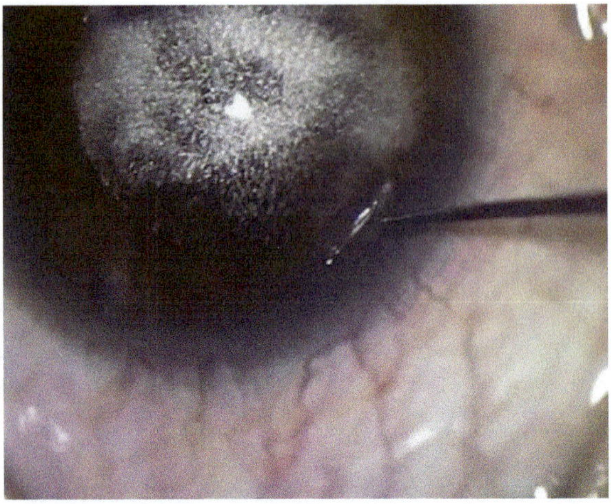

Fig. 5.8 Creating the incision

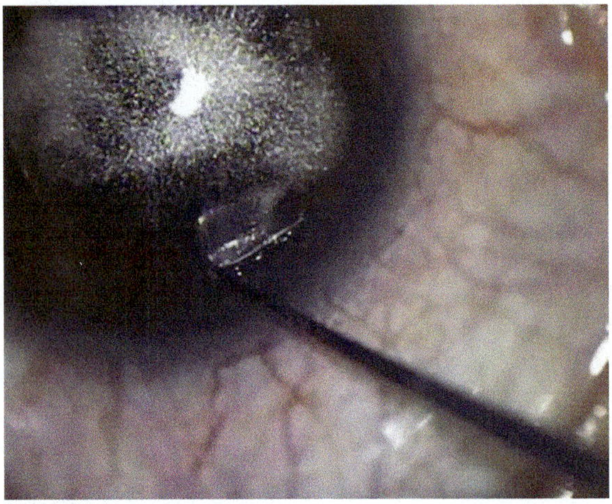

Fig. 5.9 Small pocket is created with the hook. The tip of the hook is pointed upward in an attempt to stay in the plane anterior to the lenticule

6. The CRD is then rotated around its handle so that the tip of the hook is pointed down toward the center of the eyeball. The tip is then pressed down and pushed across centripetally in a tangential direction. This action helps the tip find the edge of the lenticule. Only 1 mm-long separation is sufficient to serve as a marker for the lenticule edge. This step ensures that the instrument is correctly in the CL plane before the dissection is started (Fig. 5.10).
7. Once the lenticule edge has been located, the dissecting end of the CRD is used to separate CL plane (Fig. 5.11).
8. Going under the lenticule edge identified in step 6, the CRD is then used to dissect the LB plane to free the lenticule from its stromal bed (Fig. 5.12).
9. The patient is then instructed to look down and the lenticule forceps are used to remove the freed lenticule from the stromal pocket (Fig. 5.13).

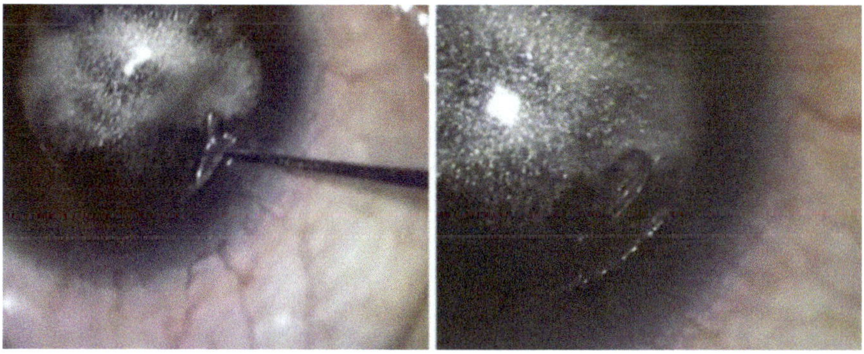

Fig. 5.10 Left: Locating the edge of the lenticule ensures that the two planes are positively identified. Right: Partially separated edge of the lenticule is visible under the cap

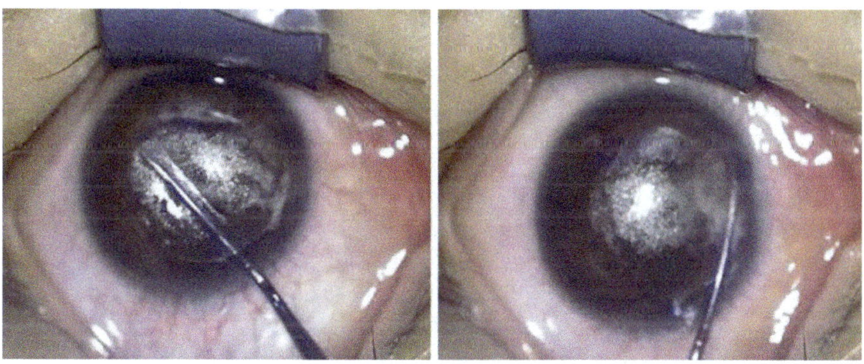

Fig. 5.11 Sweeping motion of the dissector is created by the rotation of the handle. The surgeon moves his/her hand position back and forth to maintain pivot at the small incision

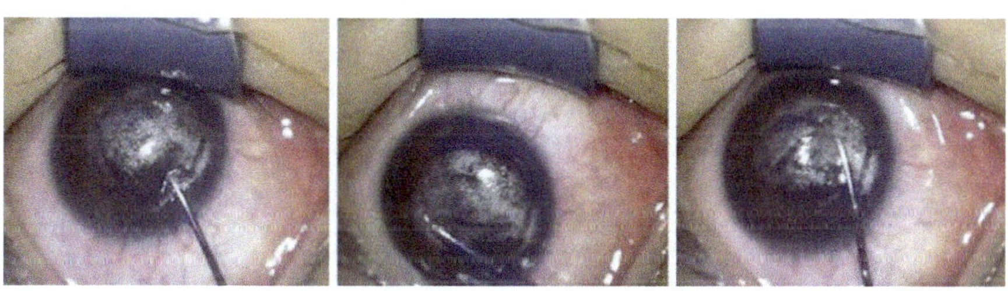

Fig. 5.12 Posterior plane dissection to free the lenticule

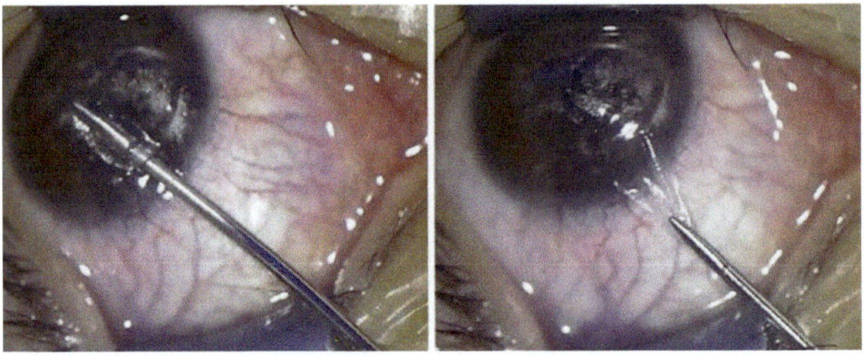

Fig. 5.13 Lenticule is removed from the pocket with a pair of microforceps

10. Optionally the pocket may be irrigated to wash out debris or foreign bodies such as epithelial cells. This also floats up the cap and lets it drape evenly back to the stromal bed, minimizing irregularity in the cap (Fig. 5.14).

Strategic Prioritization of the Dissection Area

To aid in the dissection of the LB plane, strategic placements of undissected edge areas of 1 to 2 mm can stabilize the about-to-be-freed lenticule (Fig. 5.15).

Similarly, in cases where one anticipates difficulties in dissection, such as when there is a presence of dark spots or Opaque Bubble Layer (OBL) in some areas, it is advisable to dissect those difficult areas first, utilizing the benefits of stabilization of the lenticule by the undissected (but easier to dissect) areas around them.

Fig. 5.14 Irrigating the pocket

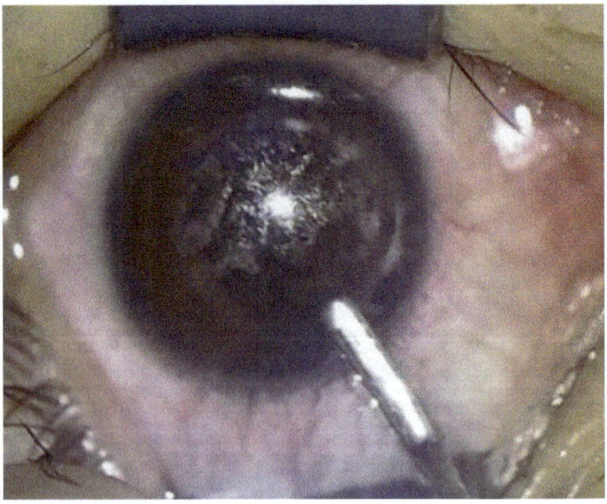

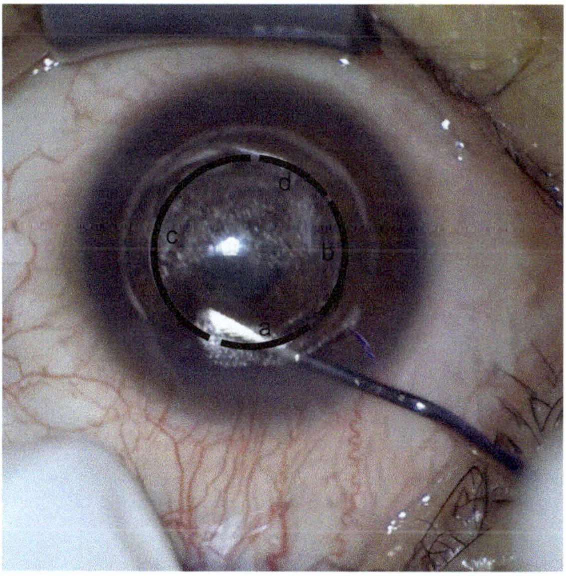

Fig. 5.15 Example of the order of dissecting the lenticule edge

Intraoperative Communication with the Patient
As the procedure is performed under topical anesthesia, patient co-operation is of high importance. I feel it useful to use verbal communications all through the procedure. This helps relax the patient, increases their level of co-operation, and actually makes the procedure easier and safer.

Intraoperative communications are mostly one-way, with the surgeon speaking to the patient constantly. Messages should include:

1. Instructions to concentrate on the fixation light.
2. Feedback and praise for good co-operation by the patient ("That is great; you're doing a great job," etc.).
3. Warning of any anticipated change in patient's perception ("The white light is going to move back and forth, follow it please," "Now you're going to feel a little cool fluid," etc.).

What not to say: The one thing to avoid is to describe to the patient real-time what the surgeon is actually doing ("Now I'm entering the wound and going to separate the layers"), as it can put scary images in the patient's mind, making them more anxious, and distract the patient from concentrating on the fixation light.

5.6 Variations in Instrumentation and Technique

No-Hook Lenticule Extraction with the CRD2

The CRD2's dissector tip can be used to find and separate the edges of femto cuts in place of the hook's pointed end. This enables the surgeon to separate the entrance incision, find and separate the CL plane, locate and separate the lenticule edge, and separate the LB plane all with only one end of the instrument and without having to turn the instrument around (Fig. 5.16).

This reduces the number of times the surgeon needs to enter and exit the pocket in order to free the lenticule to just one.

The Deep-Dive Dissection (3D) Technique

The 3D technique was devised based on the observation that in cases where the lenticules are on the thin side and there happened to be a lenticule tear, most or the tears occur roughly between 5 to 7 o'clock. The 3D technique attempts to address this problem by the surgeon dissecting the tear-prone area first, before the cap is completely separated. The adhesion between the lenticule and the cap makes the edges less likely to be torn by the dissector.

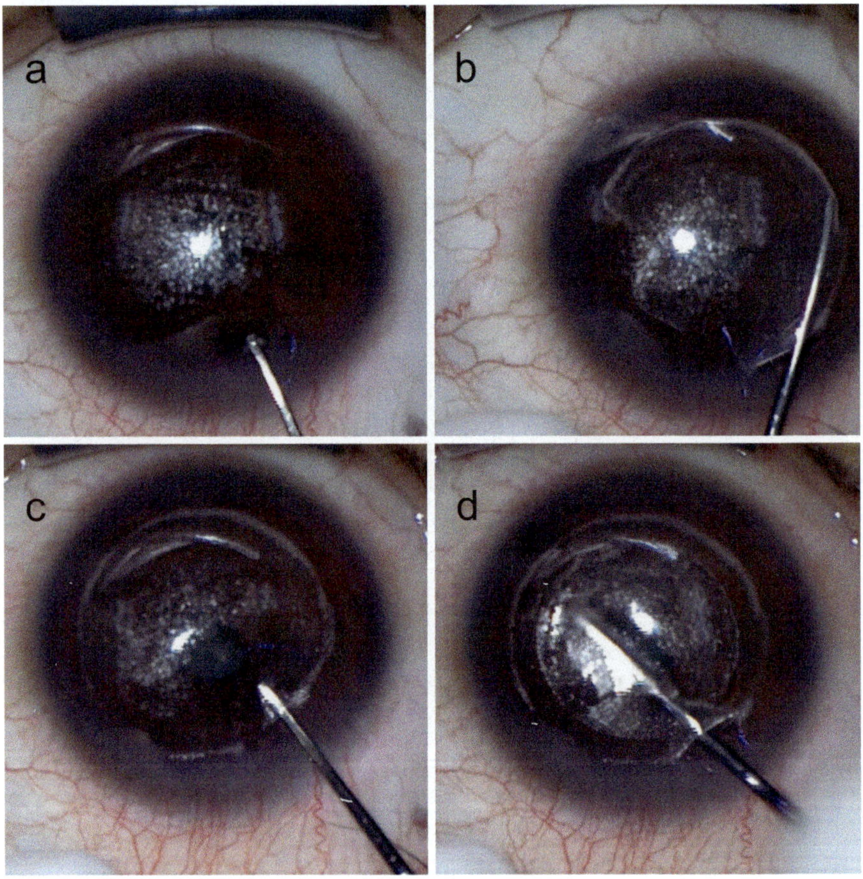

Fig. 5.16 No-hook dissection. a) Entrance incision, b) CL plane dissection, c) locating edge of lenticule, and d) LB plane dissection

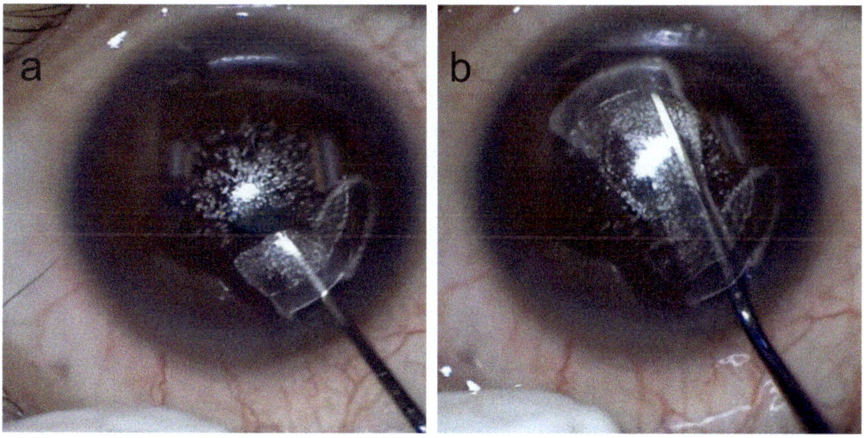

Fig. 5.17 Deep-dive dissection (3D): (a) Locating the entrance incision and the CL plane, (b) locating and separating the LB plane to free (approximately) 5 to 7 o'clock edge of the lenticule

After the CL plane in the para-incision area has been separated, before the entire plane is dissected, the CRD2 is used to find the anterior edge of the lenticule, and width-limited dissection of the LB plane is performed so that the 5 to 7 o'clock lenticule edge gets separated from the stromal bed (Fig. 5.17). Subsequently, the rest of the dissection is performed in the above-mentioned, routine fashion.

Hydroexpression of the Lenticule

After the lenticule has been extracted, the surgeon has the choice of whether or not to irrigate the pocket. There are advantages and disadvantages of either choice, which are not discussed here. For those who routinely irrigate the pocket, however, hydroexpression of the lenticule appears to be a sensible way to combine the retrieval of the lenticule and the irrigation, doing away with the microforceps altogether.

After the lenticule has been completely freed from the cap and the bed, usually by visual confirmation, it can be extracted from the pocket with a push of balanced-salt solution (BSS). Most of the time the lenticule is cleanly pushed out. This involves using a 15 ml bottle of the balanced-salt solution (BSS) attached to a blunt-tip, flat, angulated cannula. The tip of the cannula is inserted into the pocket with the surgeon maintaining a slight positive pressure by lightly squeezing the BSS bottle. The tip of the cannula is then used to push the lenticule inferiorly so that most of it is in the lower one-third of the pocket. The tip of the canula is then directed posteriorly to the lenticule and inferiorly toward the bottom of the pocket. The surgeon then expresses the lenticule by squeezing on the BSS bottle (Fig. 5.18).

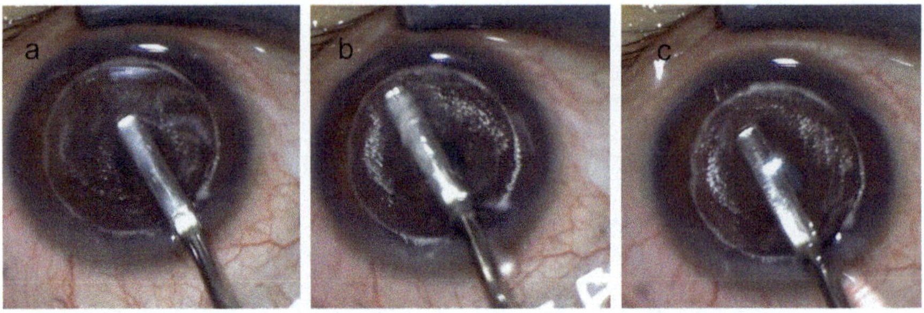

Fig. 5.18 Hydroexpression of the lenticule: a) Pushing down the lenticule, b) reaching behind and below the lenticule, c) pushing out the lenticule with BSS pressure

Caveats:

- The surgeon must maintain slight positive pressure all the time that the cannula tip is in the pocket, lest external fluids be drawn into the pocket and cause inflammation or infection.
- The expressed lenticule mostly stays in the upper fornix after exiting the pocket through the incision. However, it may also float directly down into the fluid-collecting bag of the drape. So, if one needs to examine the lenticule, or if the patient wants their lenticules for souvenir (which is not rare), it is preferable to retrieve it with microforceps.

Using the no-hook technique with the CRD2 and hydroexpression, the surgeon enters and exits the pocket only twice during the whole procedure.

Although ReLEx® SMILE has already gained much popularity, as more surgeons perform this procedure, there are bound to be variations both in the instrumentation and the surgical technique. The following are only a few examples of the presently performed variations.

Double entrance. Some surgeons advocate the use of two entrance incision cuts about 90° apart. An extra entrance can act as a “safety net” in case of difficulties at the other entrance incision. It can also act as an exit incision to push the freed lenticule through and obviate the need of lenticule forceps.

Liquid infiltration method. Some surgeons find that using balanced-salt solution to wet the interface makes for easier dissection.

There are also other methods and dissector designs being used effectively by various surgeons around the world, and the reader is referred to the surgical video library enclosed with this book.

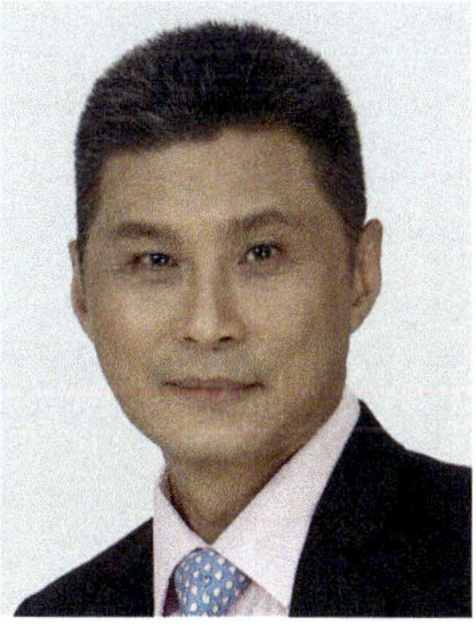

Ekktet Chansue is the Medical Director of TRSC International LASIK Center in Bangkok, Thailand. Graduating from the Ramathibodi Hospital Faculty of Medicine, Mahidol University in Bangkok, Thailand in 1986, he went directly into Ophthalmology at the Department of Ophthalmology, Chiang Mai University. In 1989 he joined ORBIS International ("Project ORBIS" at that time) as a staff ophthalmologist and crew member, and later became the Field Medical Director. After his time on ORBIS, Dr. Chansue went to undertake a 2-year Cornea, External Disease, and Refractive Surgery fellowship at the Washington University in St. Louis, Missouri from 1991 to 1993. Returning to Thailand in 1993, he taught at the Ramathibodi Hospital Faculty of Medicine, Mahidol University, Bangkok for several years. Dr. Chansue performed the first LASIK surgery in Thailand (and probably the first in South-East Asia) in 1994, and also performed the first SMILE in Thailand in 2010. In the same year, he designed the Chansue ReLEx Dissector, an instrument to aid in the separation and freeing of the lenticule during the SMILE procedure. The instrument has been widely adopted as a standard for the procedure worldwide. Dr. Chansue also helped develop the CIRCLE program for enhancement surgery after SMILE.

In his free time he likes to play the guitar and has got into lutherie, making acoustic guitars from scratch. His interests include music and travels.

From VisuMax 500 to VisuMax 800 Refining Results with SMILE: Tips and Tricks

6

Sri Ganesh

Corneal refractive procedures for the correction of myopia were pioneered by Barraquer and Ruiz [1]. They removed a layer of intrastromal tissue utilizing a microkeratome and called this procedure "in situ keratomileusis". Few years later, lasers entered the field of refractive surgery, and in 1989, Stern reported the use of lasers to ablate the cornea [2]. Surgeons experimented with femtosecond lasers in refractive surgery in the 1990s, and since then there has been an exceptional amount of development in this arena, with today's platforms having wavelengths in the near-infrared range, allowing surgeons to cut the clear cornea with minimal side effects.

Following the successful implementation of femtosecond lenticule extraction (FLEX), the procedure was advanced to small incision lenticule extraction (SMILE or ReLEx-SMILE). In SMILE, a dissector is passed through a small 2–5-mm incision to separate the lenticular interfaces and allows the lenticule to be removed, without the need to create a flap [3]. In 2011, Carl Zeiss received European conformity approval (Conformité Européenne, CE) for SMILE with VisuMax (200 kHz shortly thereafter upgraded to 500 kHz), which was then approved by the US Food and Drug Administration (FDA) for the treatment of myopia in 2016. In 2018, astigmatism correction was added, so that the current SMILE FDA approval is for myopia of −1.0 to −10.0 D and astigmatism of −0.75 to −3.0 D with a

Supplementary Information The online version contains supplementary material available at https://doi.org/10.1007/978-3-031-60424-9_6.

S. Ganesh (✉)
Bangalore, India
e-mail: chairman@nethradhama.org

W. Sekundo and F. M. Wagner (eds.), *Femtosecond Laser Assisted Lenticule Extraction*,
https://doi.org/10.1007/978-3-031-60424-9_6

maximum spherical equivalent (myopia plus half of the astigmatism) correction of no more than −10.0 D [4].

With laser refractive surgery already achieving excellent clinical visual outcomes, it is often difficult to demonstrate that newer procedures are superior to the established techniques.

Lenticule extraction with SMILE has become an established procedure in the refractive surgery community with over 8 million patients treated since its launch in 2011 [5]. Considering the benefits and excellent outcomes, SMILE now accounts for nearly 90% of the myopic refractive laser surgeries, redefining refractive surgery as we know it [6]. ZEISS is at the forefront of this minimally invasive laser vision correction. ZEISS SMILE runs on the ZEISS VisuMax Femtosecond Laser System (Carl Zeiss Meditec AG, Jena, Germany) which allows surgeons to perform precise and safe procedures with remarkable details as the basis for excellent, highly individualized treatment process.

6.1 The Environment

The laser room environment is critical for excimer laser surgery, and both temperature and humidity should be maintained at optimal levels. The VisuMax femtosecond laser is more robust and less sensitive to changes in humidity and temperature, but I have found that maintaining a temperature of around 22 °C and humidity of 50% is optimal and gives the best tissue dissection. A lower temperature affects the fluence and the bubble pattern with the VisuMax 500 in particular, which may make dissection of the tissue planes more difficult.

6.2 VisuMax 500®

As mentioned above, the VisuMax 500 has been a working horse for far over the decade and with its installation base worldwide of nearly 2000 devices the mostly frequent laser used for lenticule extraction. Many of us, who also had the privilege to purchase the VisuMax 800 at the very early stage, still have the VisuMax 500 as a robust back-up machine. Moreover, the VisuMax 800 has not been approved in all markets as of 2023, and many colleagues will rely on this device for several more years to come. Hence, the important tips and tricks for the “older” machine are presented briefly.

6.3 Optimal Fluence (Laser Energy)

The laser energy is of utmost importance to get a good bubble pattern and greatly influences the ease of dissection and surgical time. Whilst the energy adjustment is discussed in detail in Chap. 10, let me concentrate on the opaque bubble layer (OBL) which is much more common with VisuMax 500 compared to 800. There is a general tendency to increase the laser energy when dissection is difficult, but this may be counterproductive and give rise to more OBL.

It is important to carefully observe the OBL pattern and make necessary changes in the fluence levels to get an optimal bubble layer. If you notice a fast OBL—the OBL occurs preceding or during the spiral pattern of the laser wave, the energy is high and needs to be reduced (Fig. 6.1). A slow OBL, which occurs after the laser dissection is seen if the fluence is lower and indicates that the energy may have to be, increased (Fig. 6.2). A perfect bubble layer is observed at optimal laser energy with no OBL and a uniform density of the bubble layer (Fig. 6.3). Generally, this is obtained for most VisuMax 500 lasers between fluence levels of 26–32 (130–150 nJ) at a 4.5 μm spacing.

Fig. 6.1 Fast OBL (opaque bubble layer)

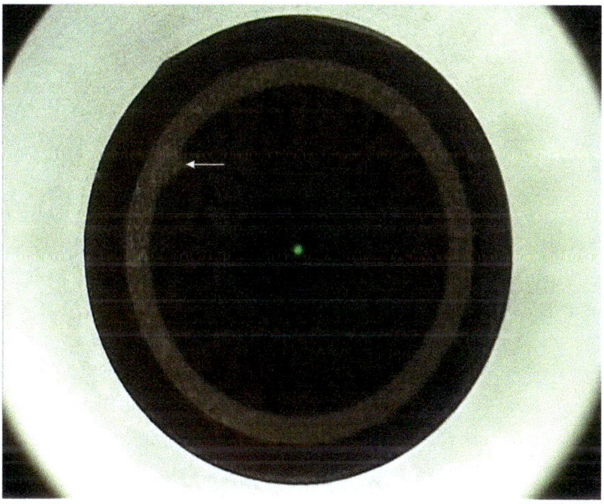

Fig. 6.2 Slow OBL

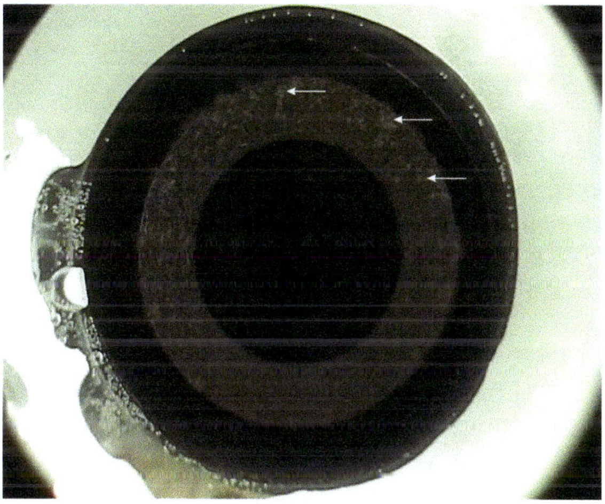

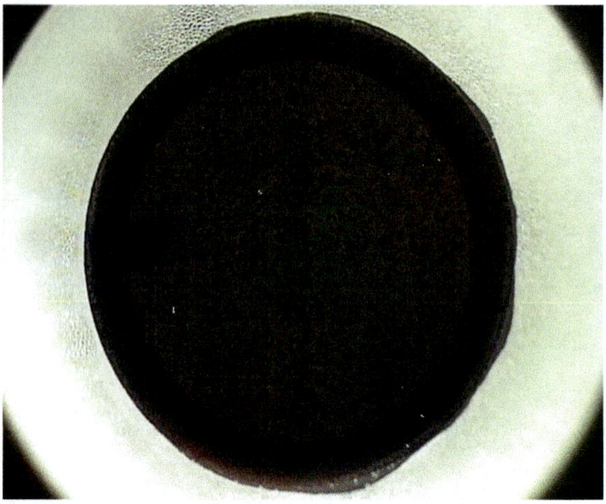

Fig. 6.3 Normal bubble pattern

6.4 Nomogram Adjustment

Results vary with every laser and every surgeon, and it is imperative that all surgeons develop a nomogram adjustment to refine their results. Ideally, one should use a dedicated software (e.g. Datagraph/Pieger Engineering GmbH, Germany or VISULYZE/Carl Zeiss Meditec, Germany) to get the best possible refractive results. However, if you just start your first surgeries with the VisuMax 500, I would recommend to add 10% to myopic astigmatic treatments in patients who are between 20 and 30 years and if scotopic pupil size is larger than 6 mm.

Other tips such as cyclorotation adjustment, patient's positioning and corneal surface management prior and during the applanation are discussed in detail in Chaps. 5 and 8.

6.5 VisuMax 800

In September 2021, ZEISS introduced its new evolution a second-generation femtosecond laser, the VisuMax 800, following the knowledgeable input and learnings from 10 years of experience with several improvements on the existing VisuMax (500 kHz) design, to optimize the performance of the new laser. The result is an updated and upgraded system that brings benefits for surgeons, surgical staff and patients [6].

The VisuMax 800 includes a faster 2-MHz frequency laser, a centration aid (CentraLign), a cyclotorsion aid (OcuLign), separate laser and microscope arms, and heads-up docking.

The VisuMax 800 is physically a completely new device: it is compact and mobile, having separate laser and microscope arms, with moving parts integrated into the laser arms, with no attached bed; speaking a language of design meets functionality. Thus, taking up less space in the operating theatre and allows for what we believe is a wider, more comfortable environment for patients. Additionally, it has a user-friendly graphic interface which is integrated into the refractive workflow, hence helping in planning and verifying the treatment for the surgeon prior to the surgery.

6.6 Reduced Time

Although the laser head and optical pathway of the VisuMax 800 are identical to the VisuMax (500 kHz), the main hardware difference is in the driving of the femtosecond laser head at an increased pulse frequency of 2000 kHz. The VisuMax operates at 500 kHz, with which flap creation takes under 20 seconds and a lenticule creation takes under 30 s. With the VisuMax 800, flaps are created in under 7 seconds and a lenticule delineation takes less than 10 seconds [7].

The VisuMax (500 kHz) was already associated with less intraocular pressure (IOP) increase, less patient fear, pain and subconjunctival haemorrhage compared to other femtosecond laser systems [8–10], because of its curved soft patient interface, docking merely to the cornea. The faster speed with VisuMax 800 further reduces the risk of the above-mentioned complication which brings benefits for surgeons and patients and is one of the most striking enhancements.

The difference in the time for lenticule creation with VisuMax 800 is especially noteworthy because docking time is probably the most critical and stressful time for both patients and surgeons during a procedure, as almost all patients are nervous undergoing a laser vision correction procedure.

Thus, the faster cutting time with VisuMax 800 lessens the discomfort the patient might experience from increased intraocular pressure (IOP) during docking, hence helping them feel more satisfied with their entire surgical experience.

Nevertheless, faster creation of the lenticule with the VisuMax 800 might even help shortening the learning curve in terms of suction stability management for surgeons starting with SMILE.

Additionally, the separate swivelling laser and microscope arms of the VisuMax 800 allowed us to device a different workflow at our centre: bilateral sequential docking followed by bilateral lenticule dissection which was possible due to the advancement in the body of the VisuMax 800.This in addition to the reduced docking and lenticule creation time, supported to efficiently reduce the overall surgical time and hence levering in an enhanced workflow without compromising on the safety quotient (see Chap. 7 for details of the study) [11].

6.7 Easier Lenticule Extraction

The VisuMax 800 is a fantastic piece of engineering, with high-frequency laser of 2 MHz; this makes the laser produce more efficient and easier tissue cutting. The lenticule extraction was also very good with the VisuMax (500 kHz), but this seems even more easier with the VisuMax 800, attributing to its near elimination of opaque bubble layer formation due to an optimized energy per area and a faster laser source.

6.8 Centration Guide with CentraLign

The current treatment protocol for the VisuMax (500 kHz) optimizes centration by the use of printed reference images for the expected position of the corneal reflex in relation to the pupil (e.g. the topography eye image and/or the Hirschberg test) [12] whereas in VisuMax 800, a computer-assisted centration aid is included: "CentraLign". This feature gives surgeons full control of centration during the docking phase, allowing the (x, y) location of the corneal vertex to be manually entered into the software, and the surgeon is guided by real-time visual overlays on the treatment monitor to align the eye to corneal vertex accurately [13].

6.9 OcuLign for Cyclotorsion

With the VisuMax (500 kHz), cyclotorsion can be achieved by using corneal marks and manually rotating the contact glass to align the marks after applying suction [12, 14, 15].

The VisuMax 800 allows for quick cyclotorsion alignment through digital rotation of the laser pattern, which is important for astigmatism correction and a very helpful feature for beginner surgeons. The OcuLign is the cyclotorsion compensatory aid which gets activated after docking. The treatment monitor displays a reticule guideline overlay representing the horizontal axis of the contact glass. The surgeon can align the treatment to the previously marked 0–180 markings manually by rotating joystick or can have an automatic cyclotorsion with the help of iris images which are imported from IOL master [13].

The optics and laser delivery systems of the VisuMax 800 are identical to those of the VisuMax (500 kHz). The optimal operating spot spacing and energy levels will be specific to each VisuMax 800 unit. These optimal settings are reached by the Standard VisuMax Optimisation Protocol [12], which enables us to determine on first installation the required energy and spot/track spacing settings in the same way as has been done during the past 10 years for the VisuMax (500 kHz).

6.10 Visual Efficacy

At our centre, we conducted a prospective study to assess the clinical outcome of small incision lenticule extraction using the VisuMax 800 in 1000 eyes of 502 patients, under 45 years of age with CDVA of 20/20 or greater. All the surgeries were performed by a single experienced surgeon using a standard technique. The patients were followed up on post-operative days 1 and 15 and at 3 months.

Uncorrected (UDVA) and corrected visual acuity (CDVA), manifest refraction, slit lamp examination, topography, tomography, aberrometry and objective scatter index (OSI) were all evaluated. The results of our study showed the mean pre-operative spherical equivalent of -4.24 ± 1.91 D and mean pre-operative cylinder of -1 ± 0.53D. The spherical equivalent (SE) at 3-month follow-up in 99% of the eyes was seen to be within ± 0.5 D. The mean pre-operative CDVA was found to be -0.052 $\pm$ 0.05 LogMAR, which was almost similar to the mean post-operative CDVA of -0.084 ± 0.067 LogMAR at 3-month follow-up (Fig. 6.4).

The study also showed a significant improvement in the quality of vision measured by OSI. The study showed 3-month post-operative follow-up to demonstrate

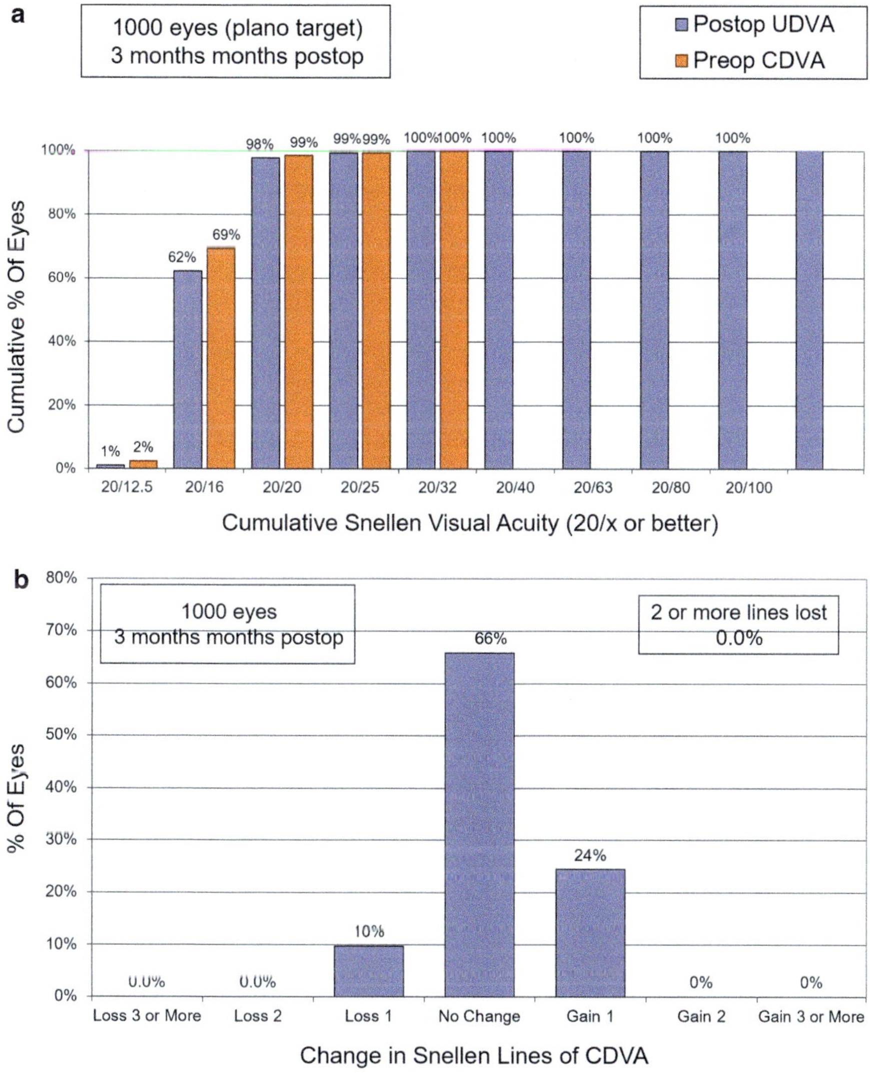

Fig. 6.4 Standard 9 charts graph of the results of 1000 eyes treated with VisuMax 800

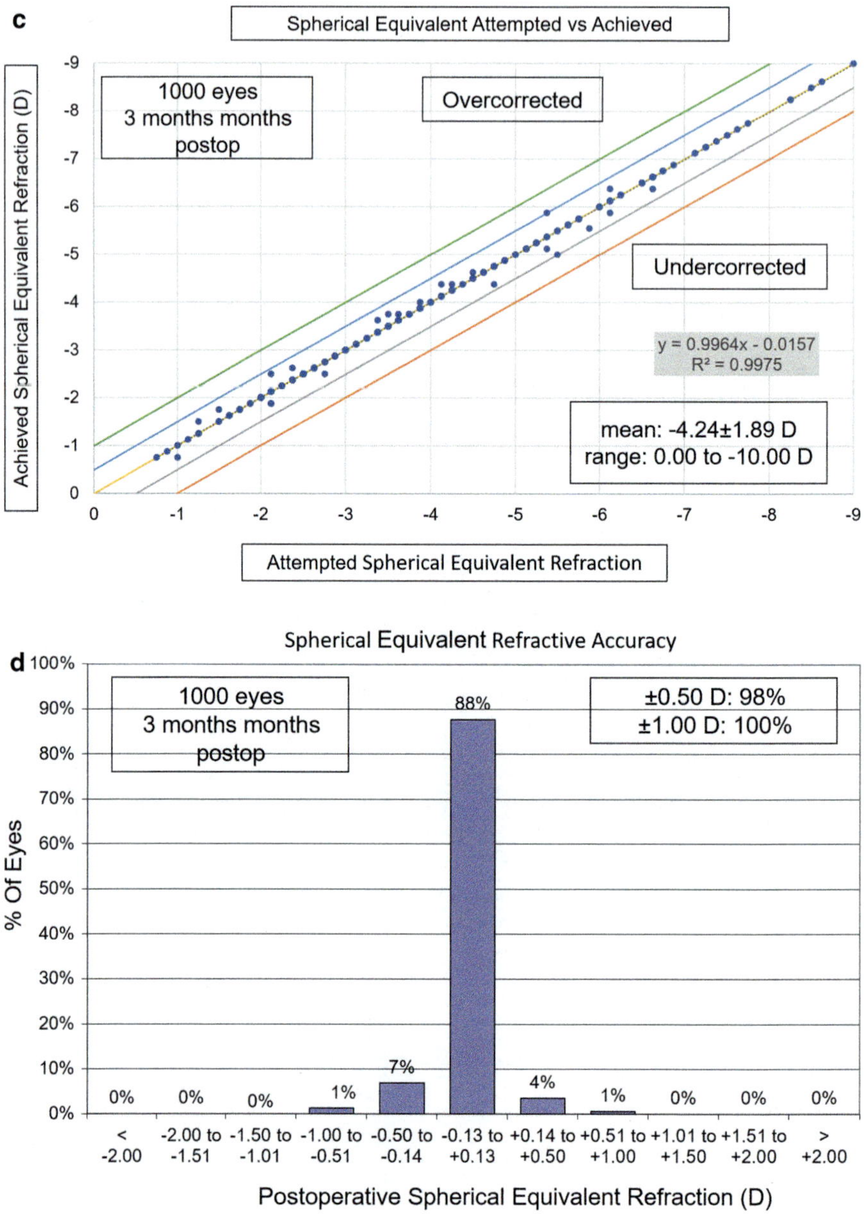

Fig. 6.4 (continued)

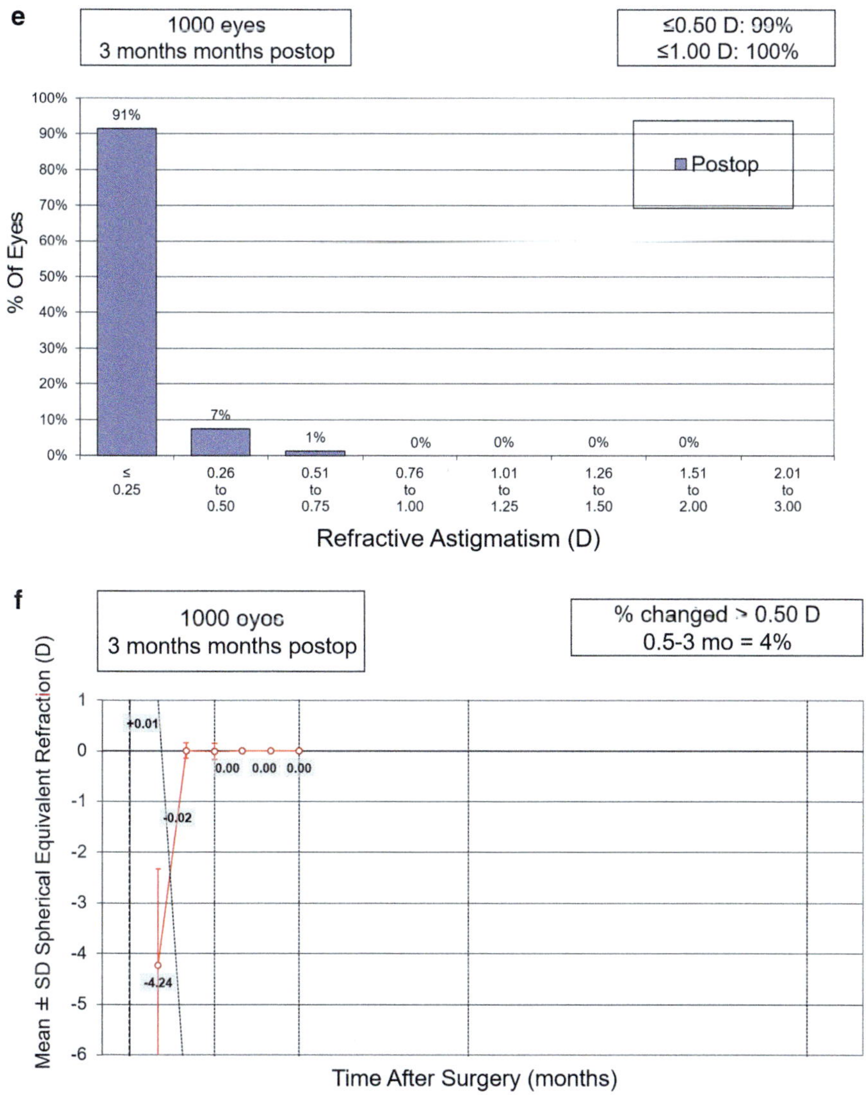

Fig. 6.1 (continued)

excellent correction and visual outcomes with no patients showing loss of two lines. The efficacy and safety index were seen to be 1.23 and 1.08 per cent, respectively, quantifying to the safety and efficacy of the procedure. The initial studies done using this laser have had smaller sample sizes. Our study compromises a data of 1000 eyes, which being a large sample set, and further reinforces upon the reliability and safety of the outcomes reported.

Table 6.1 Comparison table of results at post-operative day 15 between SMILE and SMILE Pro

POD 15	SMILE	SMILE Pro	P-Value
UDVA	−0.03 ± 0.059	−0.01 ± 0.069	0.20
Sphere	0	−0.01 ± 0.055	0.16
Cylinder	−0.01 ± 0.26	−0.03 ± 0.32	0.40
Spherical Equivalent	−0.03 ± 0.32	0	0.30
CDVA	−0.04 ± 0.05	−0.02 ± 0.05	0.24
OSI	1.02 ± 0.45	1.16 ± 0.52	0.20

6.11 Safety and Patient Satisfaction

We have another ongoing contralateral eye study at our centre to assess the patient experience, visual and refractive outcomes of patients treated with VisuMax 500 in one eye and VisuMax 800 in the contralateral eye. The new VisuMax has several advancements over its predecessor; thus, it would be interesting to see whether the new laser in addition to improving the workflow also contributes to improved clinical outcomes. This study was approved by the institutional review board of Nethradhama Superspeciality Eye Hospital, Bangalore. By the end of 2023, a total of 20 patients have undergone bilateral SMILE procedure. Both eyes of each patient have been randomized (using computer-generated numbers) to receive treatment with VisuMax 800 in one eye and with VisuMax 500 femtosecond laser in contralateral eye for correction of myopia and myopic astigmatism. Patients were appropriately counselled regarding the nature of the study, and both oral and written consents were obtained. At present, 20 patients have completed their follow-ups up to post-operative day 15. The mean UDVA, CDVA and OSI in both the groups at the post-operative days 1 and 15 did not show any statistical significance (Table 6.1). This may be attributed to our small sample size and short follow-up time.

The patient experience was recorded by means of a questionnaire in our study. It was found that out of the 20 patients, 17 recorded no difference in their experience between both the eyes, with three patients recorded a better experience in the eye operated with VisuMax 800 femtosecond laser. There were no intraoperative or post-operative complications noted. Intraoperatively, the opaque bubble layer (OBL) was found to be < 25% in 17 patients in both the eyes, two patients showed it to be between 25 and 50% in both the eyes; however, one patient showed it to be better (<25%) in the eye which underwent SMILE with VisuMax 800 in comparison with (25–50%) the eye undergone SMILE with VisuMax 500.The ease of separation in majority of our 15 patients was found to be very easy in both the eyes. Thus, our results reflect the safety of SMILE with VisuMax 800 due to the near elimination of the OBL and the ease of separation due to an optimized and faster energy laser, especially advantageous for newer surgeons, with no complications reported per se.

6.12 Conclusion

Technology like art is a soaring exercise of human imagination. The VisuMax 800 laser is equipped with a number of new capabilities that makes it a state-of-the art platform, raising SMILE to a new level.

Like they say "If there is a way to do it better, find it". Likewise, for refractive surgery now and into the future, VisuMax with the addition of the automated centration and cyclotorsion control tools: CentraLign and OcuLign, holds to improve the workflow with greater consistency in results amongst surgeons, thus providing a comprehensive, safe and effective refractive solution.

Abbreviations

FLEX	Femtosecond lenticule extraction
SMILE	Small incision lenticule extraction
FDA	Food and Drug Administration
UDVA	Uncorrected distance visual acuity
CDVA	Corrected distance visual acuity
OSI	Objective scatter index
POD	Post-operative day

References

1. Barraquer JI. The history and evolution of keratomileusis. Int Ophthalmol Clin. 1996;36. https://doi.org/10.1097/00004397-199603640-00003
2. Stern D, Schoenlein RW, Puliafito CA. Corneal ablation by nanosecond, picosecond, and femtosecond lasers at 532 and 625 nm. Arch Ophthalmol. (1989);107. https://doi.org/10.1001/ARCHOPHT.1989.01070010601038
3. Sekundo W, Kunert KS, Blum M. Small incision corneal refractive surgery using the small incision lenticule extraction (SMILE) procedure for the correction of myopia and myopic astigmatism: results of a 6 month prospective study. Br J Ophthalmol. 2011;95. https://doi.org/10.1136/BJO.2009.174284
4. Fuest M, Mehta JS. Advances in refractive corneal lenticule extraction. Taiwan J Ophthalmol. 2021;11. https://doi.org/10.4103/TJO.TJO_12_21
5. Breyer DRH. VISUMAX 800—why speed matters. 2014;3:423–9.
6. Wiltfang R. Smile for correcting myopia with astigmatism enhancing the premium refractive procedure with the VISUMAX 800, the new evolution femtosecond laser. Accessed Nov 2023
7. Zeiss visumax 800 brochure en-int-34–010–0027ii.pdf [Internet] [cited 2023 Aug 12]. Available from: https://www.zeiss.com/content/dam/z/med/reference-master/product-portfolio/refractivelasers/femtosecondlasersolution/visumax-800/downloads/zeiss-visumax-800-brochure-en-int-34-010-0027ii.pdf
8. Vetter JM, Faust M, Gericke A, Pfeiffer N, Weingärtner WE, Sekundo W. Intraocular pressure measurements during flap preparation using 2 femtosecond lasers and 1 microkeratome in human donor eyes. Journal of Cataract and Refractive Surgery 2012;38:. https://doi.org/10.1016/J.JCRS.2012.05.042
9. Strohmaier C, Runge C, Seyeddain O. Profiles of intraocular pressure in human donor eyes during femtosecond laser procedures--a comparative study. Invest. Ophthalmol. Vis. Sci. 2013;54. https://doi.org/10.1167/IOVS.12-11155

10. Hall RC, Rosman M, Chan C. Patient and surgeon experience during laser in situ keratomileusis using 2 femtosecond laser systems. J Cataract Refract Surg 2014;40. https://doi.org/10.1016/J.JCRS.2013.08.056
11. Brar S, Ganesh S, Bhargav S. Comparison of intraoperative time taken for docking, lenticule dissection, and overall workflow for SMILE performed with the VisuMax 800 versus the VisuMax 500 femtosecond laser. J Refract Surg. 2023;9:648.
12. Reinstein D, Archer T, Carp G. The surgeon's guide to small incision lenticule extraction (SMILE). (2018).
13. Reinstein DZ, Archer TJ, Potter JG. Refractive and visual outcomes of SMILE for compound myopic astigmatism with the VISUMAX 800. J Refract Surg. 2023;39(5). https://doi.org/10.3928/1081597X-20230301-02
14. Ganesh S, Brar S, Pawar A. Results of intraoperative manual cyclotorsion compensation for myopic astigmatism in patients undergoing small incision lenticule extraction (SMILE). J Refract Surg 2017;33. https://doi.org/10.3928/1081597X-20170328-01
15. Kang DSY, Lee H, Lee H. Comparison of the distribution of lenticule decentration following SMILE by subjective patient fixation or triple marking centration. J Refract Surg. 2018;34. https://doi.org/10.3928/1081597X-20180517-02

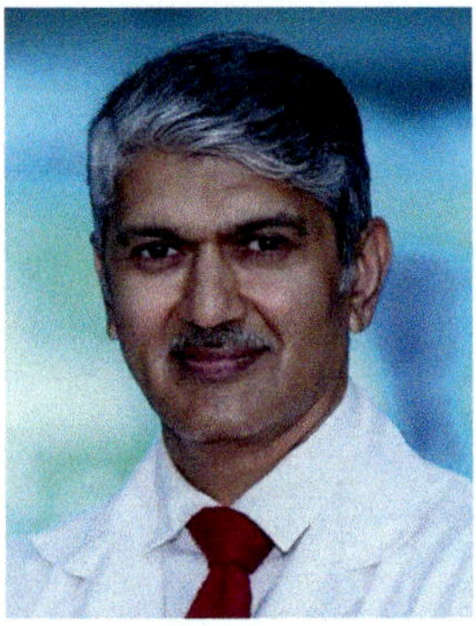

Sri Ganesh MBBS, MS, DNB, DSC(Hon.), FRCS (Glasgow), FAICO, FWCRS, Founder of Nethradhama Hospitals Pvt Ltd and Shraddha Eye Care Trust . Dr. Sri Ganesh started his practice in 1994 and now runs 8 eye hospitals. He started his refractive surgery practice with RK in 1994, Lasik in 1997 and has been at the forefront of refractive surgery technologies. He has performed over 120,000 cataract surgeries and 75,000 refractive surgeries. He has over 60 peer reviewed publications and has done some pioneering work on lenticule extraction techniques and using SMILE lenticules in tissue addition techniques for correction of hyperopia and keratoconus. He has contributed to 6 book chapters. He has trained over 200 national and international fellows in phaco and refractive surgeries. He was awarded the honorary doctorate from the Rajiv Gandhi University of Health Sciences in 2014 for his contributions to the field of Ophthalmology. He was awarded the honorary FRCS (Glasgow) in 2018. He has been awarded the Gold Medal oration at the AUSCRS in 2017 and the IIRSI Gold Medal in 2007 and BOA Gold Medal in 2011. He was awarded the prestigious Micheal Kritzinger award by ISRS at the AAO 2022 for contributions in refractive surgery and the Honorary FAICO in refractive surgery by All India Ophthalmological society. He is also a charter fellow of the WCRS. He has delivered numerous orations and lectures at various national and international conferences and conducted instruction courses and symposia. He has performed over 100 live surgical demonstrations in various national and international meetings. He is a member of several national and international ophthalmic societies including the "IIIC".

Main Features of VisuMax 800, Programming and Workflow

7

Sheetal Brar and Sri Ganesh

Abstract

This chapter delves into the main features of the VisuMax 800 femtosecond laser, contrasting it with its predecessor, the VisuMax 500. Highlighting a smaller footprint and improved functionality, the VisuMax 800 boasts enhanced mobility, comfort for patients, and reduced treatment times for flap and lenticule creation. Distinctive features include CentraLign for precise centration and OcuLign for cyclotorsion control. The chapter further explores the programming and workflow, emphasizing the integrated computer, touch user interfaces, and data management capabilities with VISULYZE. The innovative bilateral sequential docking and lenticule extraction workflow of VisuMax 800 is discussed, revealing significantly shorter surgical times compared to the conventional VisuMax 500, without compromising safety or postoperative outcomes.

Keywords

VisuMax 800 • Femtosecond laser • Surgical workflow • Bilateral sequential docking • Lenticule extraction • CentraLign • OcuLign

7.1 Main Features of VisuMax 800

The VisuMax 800 (see Chap. 1, Fig. 7) is a new device in terms of the physical presentation, appearance, and functionality, compared to its predecessor VisuMax 500. The main differentiating features being: a smaller footprint, thus requiring less space in the operating room, which makes it mobile and easy to relocate within the OR. The bed is immobile for better patients comfort and the moving parts,

S. Brar (✉) · S. Ganesh
Bangalore, India
e-mail: brar_sheetal@yahoo.co.in

W. Sekundo and F. M. Wagner (eds.), *Femtosecond Laser Assisted Lenticule Extraction*,
https://doi.org/10.1007/978-3-031-60424-9_7

i.e., the laser and microscope are separated and presented as two swivel arms, the LM for laser and OM for operating microscope, both of which are controlled by a joystick. Additionally, a foot pedal has been provided, which is attached with the operating microscope for fine focusing. The laser is equipped with a slit lamp and two screens. The large screen is used for data management and. It can also be used by the OR assistant to observe the surgery, while the other screen provides comprehensive visualization throughout the surgery and thereby ensures ergonomic comfort for the surgeon. It also encompasses two cameras for positioning and docking (top and side view) [1].

Although the laser head and optical pathway of the VisuMax 800 are identical to the VisuMax (500 kHz), the main hardware difference is in the driving of the femtosecond laser head at an increased pulse frequency of 2000 kHz. This obviously translates into faster treatment times for both flap and lenticule creation. The VisuMax operates at 500 kHz, with which flap creation takes under 20 s and a lenticule creation takes under 30 s. With the VisuMax 800, flaps are created in under 7 s and a lenticule delineation takes less than 10 s. The reduction in lenticule creation time using the VisuMax 800 is noteworthy considering that movement of the head, eye, and eyelids during this step can result in loss of suction [2]. Furthermore, the incidence of IOP increase, patient discomfort, and subconjunctival hemorrhage compared to other femtosecond laser systems has further reduced, resulting in better confidence among surgeons while treating otherwise nervous/anxious patients.

Apart from the above differences, there are two other unique features in VisuMax 800 that differentiates it from its predecessor.

7.2 Centration Guide (CentraLign)

The current method of centration in VisuMax (500 kHz) involves an active patient controlled centration or the use of printed reference images for the expected position of the corneal reflex in relation to the pupil (e.g., the topography eye image and/or the Hirschberg test). Whereas in VisuMax 800, a computer-assisted centration aid is included: CentraLign, this feature gives surgeons full control of centration during the docking phase, allowing the (x,y) location of the corneal vertex to be manually entered into the software and the surgeon is guided by real-time visual overlays on the treatment monitor to align the eye to corneal vertex accurately (see Chap. 15, Fig. 7a and 7b and video in Chap. 6).

7.3 Cyclotorsion Control (OcuLign)

In high cylinders, with the VisuMax (500 kHz), compensation of the static cyclotorsion was shown to be achieved by using corneal marking in 0–180 degrees, followed by manually rotation of the contact glass to align the marks with eye

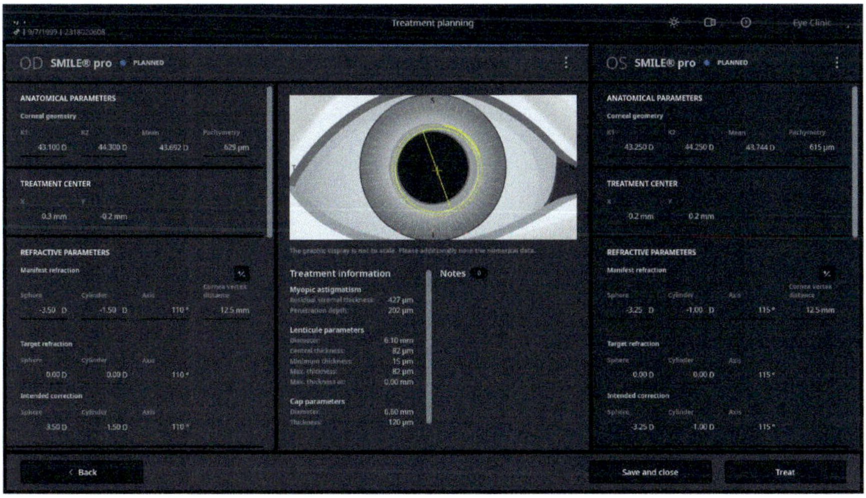

Fig. 7.1 Appearance of the main screen of the VisuMax 800 with simultaneous data of both eyes and a sketch of the centration according to the x–y data

piece reticule after application of the suction [5]. This maneuver could potentially result in suction loss, especially in higher degrees of cyclorotation.

On the other hand, the VisuMax 800 is equipped with OcuLign features that allows for cyclotorsion alignment through digital rotation of the laser pattern, instead of manual rotation of the contact glass. The OcuLign is activated after docking, wherein the treatment monitor displays a reticule guideline overlay representing the horizontal axis of the contact glass, (see Chap. 8, Fig. 7.1). The surgeon can then align the treatment to the previously marked 0–180 markings by rotating the joystick or can use an automatic cyclotorsion compensation with the help of iris images imported from the IOL master.

7.4 Programming and Workflow

The integrated computer with special software and corresponding touch user interfaces enables comfortable operation of the device and saves treatment data; more computers control and monitor the internal processes. The monitors or touch screens are used to plan the treatment, give instructions to the user, and display the progress of the treatment.

The laser source is in the device head. The laser beam exits the laser source and passes through the beam control assembly. There the characteristics of the laser radiation are adjusted to the planned application.

The deflection unit, treatment optics, and contact glass allow the laser radiation to be focused into the cornea of the patient's eye and spatially guided there when the laser arm is in treatment position.

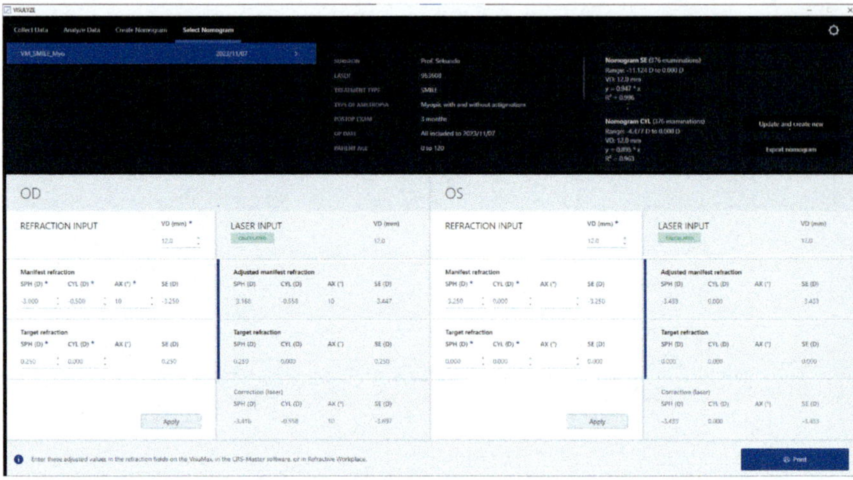

Fig. 7.2 Preparation of nomogram-corrected refractive data using VISULYZE software. The nomogram-corrected data can be instantly imported into the VisuMax 800 laser

Before planning the surgery, selection, and size of treatment pack, the effective white-to-white diameter is done. After switching on the device, the patient and treatment data are entered under the "Patient management" and checked.

Treatment planning can be done either at the laser or remotely on a dedicated software called the Refractive Workplace. Unlike VisuMax, wherein one eye is planned at a time, in VisuMax 800, both eyes can be planned simultaneously using an intuitive graphic user interface (GUI) (Fig. 7.1). The VisuMax 800 is fully integrated into the refractive workflow, wherein it is connected via FORUM with other devices and with software platforms. Data management and treatment planning are hence centralized to one place. It has a user-friendly graphic interface, thus allowing the treatment planning to be verified and done outside the OR prior and sent via a click to the FORUM and from there to the particular laser.

Data management capabilities with VISULYZE (Carl Zeiss Meditec AG; Jena, Germany) provide surgeons an excellent tool for refining and personalizing their nomograms so that the nomograms match the surgeon's unique surgical environment and techniques. This customization has great potential to further optimize the outcomes (Fig. 7.2).

7.5 Importing Externally Planned Treatments

Treatments planned with external planning software are available in the FORUM. The device is connected to a network and configured for FORUM integration. The treatment is planned and completed in the following steps:

1. After switching on the main switch, the treatment software is started, and the login window appears on the treatment screen.
   After logging in, enter the patient list by pressing [Patient management] button.
2. Use the filter to select only patients for whom a treatment has been planned.
3. Set further filter criteria if required (e.g., name).
4. Tap the [Find] button.
5. Select single, multiple, or all patients displayed.
6. The selected patient and planning data are imported, and patient and planning data already stored in the device are updated.
7. The planning data on the device are in the "not validated" state.
8. Check the correctness of displayed data.
9. Press the [Save] button in the planning dialog to confirm.
10. The data are checked and can be used for treatment.
11. Check the correct alignment of the patient supporting system relative to the device.
12. Bring the patient into the treatment room.
13. Lay the patient on the patient supporting system and position him/her for treatment in dorsal position.
14. Ensure that the patient is in a correct and comfortable position.
15. Check the patient data (select the eye to be treated on the treatment screen (OD/OS), verify personal data, treatment parameters, and eye to be treated, e.g., by talking to the patient or by using the Surgical Safety Checklist on the treatment screen). Then, confirm your verification.
16. Start the treatment procedure on the planning screen of the device.
17. Check the identity of the patient again using the master data.
18. Activate the laser mode.
19. Use the side-view camera video and the corresponding overlay on the planning screen to check the correct position of the patient head.
20. If necessary, correct the position of the head using the patient supporting system or by moving the device head via entries on the planning screen.
21. Use the laser arm joystick to position the laser arm over the eye to be treated.
22. Ensure that the eye to be treated is approximately in the middle of the live image display of the treatment screen.
23. Ask the patient to fixate upon the green fixation light and use the live image display of the treatment screen to inspect the patient's eye.
24. Make sure that no parts of the body, except the eye, come into contact with the contact glass or device. To avoid accidental nose contact with the laser objective, tilt the patient head. Make sure that the limbus is not covered by the eyelid retractor, outer eyelid angle, or tear film meniscus.
25. Use the laser arm joystick to position the laser arm. Observe all movements of the laser arm and constantly check the position of the patient's eye in relation to the contact glass on the treatment screen.

26. Position the laser arm so that the visual axis of the eye to be treated is exactly in the center of the contact glass as soon as the eye meets the contact glass. When approaching, the treatment illumination reflex should be in the center of the live image display of the treatment screen.
27. Bring the cornea into contact with the contact glass, using the live image display on the treatment screen and the centering assistant (overlay) to center on the planned treatment center.
28. Switch on the vacuum suction and allow the eye to be suctioned.
29. The suction pressure can be observed on the vacuum display on the treatment screen.
30. When the suction pressure has reached the required range, the "Laser ready" status is displayed on the treatment screen, followed by which the laser is fired.
31. After the laser delivery, the laser arm ascends, and the microscope arm descends.
32. The refractive treatment can then be completed by manual treatment steps using the integrated surgical microscope when the OPMI arm is in the observation position.

For the contralateral eye treatment, steps 15–32 are repeated in the same order. The above signifies a conventional workflow, wherein one eye is treated (from docking to lenticule extraction) at one time.

However, the unique feature of the swiveling separate laser and microscope arms prompted us to explore a different workflow involving bilateral sequential docking when the laser arm was brought down for docking followed by bilateral sequential lenticule dissection when the microscope arm was brought down for surgical extraction of the lenticule. Video 1 in Chap. 6 (available in the online version) demonstrates the sequence of steps of the new workflow followed while performing a bilateral SMILE procedure using the VisuMax 800 [3]. The purpose of the study was to compare the overall surgical workflow of performing a bilateral small incision lenticule extraction (SMILE) procedure with the VisuMax 800 femtosecond laser (Carl Zeiss Meditec AG) [1] using a new workflow versus the VisuMax 500 femtosecond laser (Carl Zeiss Meditec AG) using the conventional workflow [3].

This study included a total of 60 patients undergoing bilateral SMILE for myopia or myopic astigmatism between -1.00 and -10.00 diopters (D). Patients with spherical equivalent and manifest cylinder of less than 1.50 D (not requiring limbal marking) were randomly divided to receive treatment with the VisuMax 800 ($n = 30$) or VisuMax 500 ($n = 30$) femtosecond laser. A new workflow was followed for the VisuMax 800 group (bilateral sequential docking and lenticule extraction, i.e., laser–laser followed by extraction–extraction) versus the conventional workflow (operating on one eye at a time, i.e., laser extraction, laser extraction) in the VisuMax 500 group.

The docking time and overall surgical time in the VisuMax 800 group were 133.63 ± 38.88 s and 6.96 ± 1.67 min, respectively. This was significantly shorter when compared to the VisuMax 500 group (194.11 ± 47.59 s and 9.52 ± 1.72 min, respectively) ($P < 0.001$). The mean combined lenticule dissection time was comparable between groups (VisuMax 800 group = 99.06 ± 20.19 s, VisuMax 500 group = 115.40 ± 45.03 s) ($P = 0.07$). The mean overall surgical time for performing one bilateral procedure with the VisuMax 800 was 6.96 ± 1.67 min compared to 9.52 ± 1.72 min with the VisuMax 500. These results were statistically significant ($P < 0.001$). There were no significant differences in the one-day and two-week postoperative uncorrected distance visual acuity, objective scatter index, or patient's subjective intraoperative experience between the groups ($P > 0.05$ for all parameters). No complications, especially suction loss, occurred in either group.

The reduced docking and lenticule creation time, in addition to the time saved by performing immediate sequential bilateral docking followed by lenticule extraction in the same manner, played a major role in decreasing the overall surgical time in the VisuMax 800 group.

Thus, the new VisuMax 800 laser appears to support the enhanced efficiency in workflow in SMILE procedure without compromising the safety, which could be attributed to the technological advancements incorporated in the new laser.

References

1. Carl Zeiss Meditec. Zeiss VisuMax 800. https://www.zeiss.com/content/dam/z/med/reference-master/product-portfolio/refractivelasers/femtosecondlasersolution/visumax-800/downloads/zeiss-visumax-800-brochure-en-int-34-010-0027ii.Pdf.
2. Huang TZ, Shen L, Yu XN, Jin HY. Risk factors and incidence of suction loss during small incision lenticule extraction (SMILE) in 8493 eyes. BMC Ophthalmol. 2020;20(1):412.
3. Brar S, Ganesh S, Bhargav S. Comparison of intraoperative time taken for docking, lenticule dissection, and overall workflow for SMILE performed with the visumax 800 versus the visumax 500 femtosecond laser. J Refract Surg. 2023;39(9):648. https://doi.org/10.3928/1081597X-20230726-03. Epub 2023 Sep 1. PMID: 37675905.

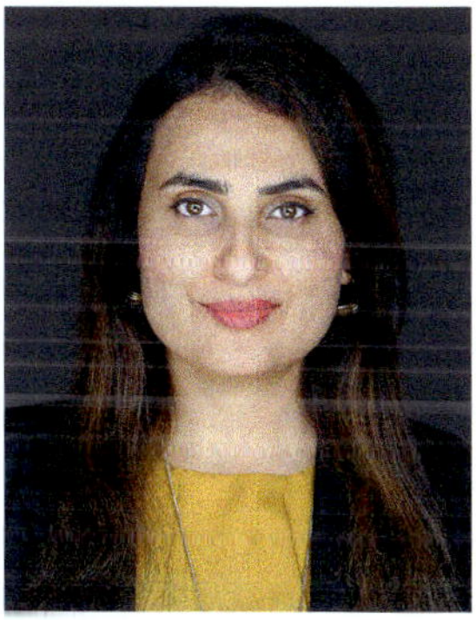

Sheetal Brar Director Cataract and Refractive surgery & Head of Research and academics at Brar Eye Hospital, Bathinda, Punjab. Trained > 200 trainees in phacoemulsification and complex cataract surgeries and > 100 surgeons in refractive surgery. Participated in over 100 masterclasses & instructional courses and performed live surgeries of phacoemulsification and SMILE. 100 + publications in national and international peer reviewed indexed journals. Reviewer for Journal of Refractive Surgery(JRS), Cornea, JCRS, BMC Ophthalmology, Open Journal of Ophthalmology, and IJO journals. Receiver of over 30 international film festival and best papers of session awards. 1st woman ophthalmologist from India to receive the prestigious APACRS Certified Educator (ACE) Award.

Astigmatism Correction

8

Marcus Blum and Walter Sekundo

Abstract

This chapter explores the types and dynamics of astigmatism, focusing on surgical treatments, including incisional techniques, excimer laser-based methods, and lenticule extraction. The authors evaluate the efficacy of all-femto lenticule extraction for correcting myopic astigmatism using vector analysis. Manual treatment cone adjustment is a popular technique with the VisuMax 500 laser. The chapter also highlights the role of the VisuMax 800 laser with built-in software-based rotation adjustment in improving astigmatic outcomes.

Keywords

Astigmatism • Astigmatic keratotomy (AK) • Limbal relaxing incisions (LRI) • VisuMax 800 • Excimer laser • Lenticule extraction • Callisto eye image-guiding software • ATOS laser

8.1 Introduction

The dome shape of the cornea is spherical if all the meridians have the same curvature. In astigmatism, the refractive power of the cornea varies in its vertical and horizontal meridians, and therefore, a point image of a point object cannot be formed. The meridians of maximum and minimum curvature are called the principal meridians, and in regular astigmatism, these are at 90° to each other. From the curvature of the cornea, the mean corneal power and the cylinder power

M. Blum (✉)
Department of Ophthalmology, Helios Hospital Erfurt, Erfurt, Germany
e-mail: marcus.blum@helios-gesundheit.de

W. Sekundo
Department of Ophthalmology, Philipps University of Marburg, Marburg, Germany

W. Sekundo and F. M. Wagner (eds.), *Femtosecond Laser Assisted Lenticule Extraction*,
https://doi.org/10.1007/978-3-031-60424-9_8

can be calculated, and clinically, this is described by the axis of the cylinder and its power in diopters (D) [1].

Depending on the orientation of the principal meridians, different types of astigmatism can be distinguished:

- *With-the-rule Astigmatism*: The vertical meridian has higher refractive power (90° ± 15°).
- *Against-the-rule Astigmatism* (so-called because it occurs less frequently): The horizontal meridian has higher refractive power (0° ± 15° or 180° ± 15°).
- *Oblique Astigmatism:* The principal meridians are tilted by an angle between 15° and 75° (or 105° and 165°) but are still perpendicular to each other.

It is a well-known fact that refractive error is not static throughout life. The highest incidence of astigmatism (up to 65%) is reported in the first year of life [2]. The decrease in astigmatism demonstrated over the first years in life appears to be a result of the increase in eye size and flattening of the cornea [3]. By adulthood, this high incidence of astigmatism has disappeared. The incidence of astigmatism greater than 1.0 D in adults is reported in up to 8% of patients [4].

8.2 Surgical Treatment of Astigmatism

8.2.1 Incisional and Excimer Laser-Based Techniques

Several surgical concepts have been tested for the therapy of astigmatism. Astigmatic keratotomy (AK) and limbal relaxing incisions (LRI) became popular as these procedures can be used in combination with cataract surgery [5]. Recent generations of excimer lasers provide an effective surgical technique to correct astigmatism with satisfactory results. However, the excimer laser treatment of spherical myopia has been shown to be more predictable than the correction of myopic astigmatism [6].

One study reported surgically induced astigmatism by corneal flap making. Huang et al. found an average of 0.12 D with-the-rule astigmatism induced after LASIK with a superior hinge [7]. The conclusion was that the astigmatic shift is an effect of the circular keratotomy and the absence of the keratotomy at the site of the superior hinge. The superior hinge causes a steepening of the astigmatism on the 90° axis, whilst the circular keratotomy causes a reduction of corneal astigmatism overall. However, other authors could not find this evidence.

8.2.2 Astigmatic Correction by Lenticule Extraction Techniques

Within a short period of time, continuous improvements of the lenticule extraction technique led to comparable results regarding safety and stability of the refractive results [8–12]. The first detailed report on the treatment of astigmatism analysing the results using vector analysis was given by Kunert and co-authors in 2013 [13]. A vector analysis was done with the refractive data, which mainly followed the definitions and formulas given by Eydelman and co-workers [14]. It should be stressed that in this study, the very first 200 kHz VisuMax® femtosecond laser was used for all procedures and all eyes had the flap lifted for the removal of the lenticule.

Her study evaluated the efficacy, predictability, and safety of the all-femto lenticule extraction procedure for correction of myopic astigmatism. A complete set of refractive data of 182 treatments (87 left and 95 right eyes) for the follow-up periods of 1 week and 1, 3, and 6 months is reported. The study consisted of 182 eyes of 113 patients with spherical myopia between 0 D and −8.75 D (MV − 4.10 D, SD = 1.51 D) and myopic astigmatism between −0.25 D to and −6.0 D (MV 0.96 D, SD ± 0.87 D). The dataset encompassed treatments of sphere and astigmatism. Vector analysis was performed to study the astigmatic results at each follow-up visit. The data allowed a quantitative analysis of under- and overcorrection of astigmatism in a very early stage of the 200 kHz laser. The slope of the linear regression lines expressed the factor of over- and undercorrection. All over the four follow-up periods of 1 week and 1, 3 and 6 months, the factors amount to 0.96, 0.89, 0.91, and 0.88, respectively. These data correspond to undercorrections of 4, 11, 9, and 12%, respectively.

The undercorrections seemed to develop until 1 month and showed negligible variation at 1 month and thereafter. Looking at the data in more detail, there was a slight overcorrection in the low astigmatism group (0.5D) and a undercorrection in higher astigmatism. In the range 1–3 D, the correction index was 0.87 and 0.93.

After this first study by Kunert and co-workers, a number of changes took place—the 500 kHz VisuMax® femtosecond laser was on the market, and according to the results with the 200 kHz laser, an adjustment of the nomogram was added to the software. Furthermore, the flapless SMILE replaced lenticule extraction by FLEx, and therefore, the lifting of the flap was no longer an issue. However, corneal flap making has been reported to induce astigmatism [7], and the presence (in FLEx) or absence (in SMILE) of a flap could affect astigmatic outcomes after surgery. Kobashi et al. compared the two techniques and found no statistically significant differences, suggesting that the lifting or non-lifting of the flap does not significantly affect astigmatic outcomes [15]. The Huang study was published in 2000 and used microkeratome-created flaps. With today's femtosecond technology, it is possible to create thinner and more uniform flaps, and this might have resolved the astigmatism induction issue.

Several of studies reported the outcomes of astigmatism correction with the SMILE technique using vector analysis. Ivarsen published results of SMILE treatments reporting an undercorrection with increased errors in treatment in higher astigmatism [16]. Zhang and co-workers came to a similar conclusion [17], and Chan, in direct comparison with femto-assisted LASIK, found less favourable outcomes even in low and moderate astigmatism [18]. One possible reason for the observed undercorrection could be cyclotorsion. Prakash et al. reported that iris registration with eye tracking in LASIK gave better astigmatic results [19]. In the 500 kHz VisuMax fs laser, iris registration was not available for the lenticule extraction procedure. Khalifa discussed that the difference might be the result of the absence of a cyclotorsion control [20]. A compensation method by marking the horizontal axis on the cornea preoperatively in a sitting position and re-adjust the treatment pack by manual rotation was reported [21] and is shown in Fig. 15.5. Whilst this manoeuvre improved the astigmatic outcomes in the first Indian study as well as a later study by Chen et al. [22] and also corresponds to the experience of the authors of this chapter, it did not become evident in the study by Xu et al. [23] or Sachdev et al. [24] Ivarsen found less undercorrection occurring in against-the-rule astigmatism than in with-the-rule astigmatism and excluded the influence of the back surface curvature of the cornea [25]. Improved nomograms, meticulous patient positioning as well as higher accuracy in axis determination improved the outcomes of astigmatic correction in small incision lenticule extraction [26]. In fact, in our experience, the bridge of the patient's nose can influence the cyclorotation. In patients with the high nose bridge, the head has to be tilted to the side in order to obtain good applanation leading to an increased cyclotorsion. Hence, we apply this technique in patients with a prominent nose bridge (more common in men) and cylindrical power of 1.5 D cyl or more.

Whilst the manual treatment cone adjustment is a surrogate technique used with the VisuMax 500 laser, the new VisuMax 800 laser is already equipped with an official built-in software-based rotation adjustment using joystick, the so-called OcuLign tool (Fig. 8.1; also see Chap. 15.3.2).

At the time of writing this chapter, only the ink mark-based cyclotorsion adjustment is available. However, automatic adjustment based on IOL Master 700 (Carl Zeiss Meditec) iris image shell follow in due course and will hopefully further improve the astigmatic outcomes. In fact, in a setting of Callisto eye image-guiding software (Carl Zeiss Meditec) connected to the VisuMax 500 microscope, Köse

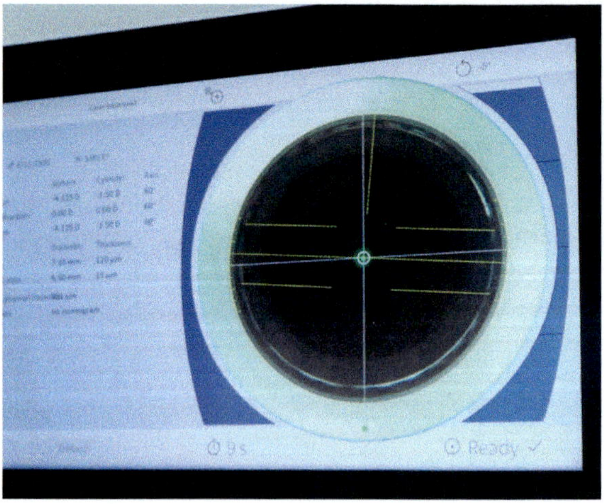

Fig. 8.1 OcuLign cyclotorsion adjustment is executed by rotating a reticule guideline with the joystick to match the preplaced corneal ink marks

showed the reduction of axis misalignment from 3.76° to 1.18° corresponding to the reduction of the mean astigmatism from -0.45 ± 0.38 D cyl (range: -1.50 to 0.00 D) to -0.19 ± 0.17 D cyl (range: -0.50 to 0.00 D) [27]. In the first publication on VisuMax 800 results, Reinstein et al. reported a similar astigmatic outcome as with the manual axis adjustment with VisuMax 500 [28] confirming that both techniques work. However, there is no doubt that iris registration can be transferred to lenticule extraction surgery as already implemented in the ATOS laser (Schwind) (see Chap. 25).

References

1. Olsen T. On the calculation of power from the curvature of the cornea. Br J Ophthalmol. 1986;70:152–4.
2. Howland HC, Sayles N. Photorefractive measurements of astigmatism in infants and young children. Invest Ophthalmol Vis Sci. 1984;25:93–102.
3. Abrahamsson M, Fabian G, Sjorstrand J. Changes in astigmatism between the ages of 1 and 4 years: a longitudinal study. Br J Ophthalmol. 1988;72:145–9.
4. Saunders KJ. Early refractive development in humans. Surv Ophthalmol. 1995;40:207–16.
5. Thornton SP. Astigmatic keratotomy: a review of basic concepts with case reports. J Cataract Refract Surg. 1990;16:430–5.
6. Bailey MD, Zadnik K. Outcomes of LASIK for myopia with FDA-approved lasers. Cornea. 2007;26:246–54.
7. Huang D, Sur S, Seffo F, Meisler DM, Krueger RR. Surgically induced astigmatism after laser in situ keratomoleusis for spherical myopia. J Refract Surg. 2000;16:515–8.
8. Blum M, Kunert K, Schröder M, Sekundo W. Femtosecond lenticule extraction for the correction of myopia: preliminary 6-month results. Graefes Arch Clin Exp Ophthalmol. 2010;248:1019–27.
9. Blum M, Kunert KS, Engelbrecht C, Dawczynski J, Sekundo W. Femtosecond lenticule extraction (FLEx)—results after 12 months in myopic astigmatism. Klin Monbl Augenheilkd. 2010;227:961–5.
10. Sekundo W, Kunert KS, Blum M. Small incision corneal refractive surgery using the small incision lenticule extraction (SMILE) procedure for the correction of myopia and myopic astigmatism: results of a 6 month prospective study. Br J Ophthalmol. 2011;95:335–9.
11. Shah R, Shah S. Effect of scanning patterns on the results of femtosecond laser lenticule extraction refractive surgery. J Cataract Refract Surg. 2011;37:1636–47.
12. Blum M, Flach A, Kunert KS, Sekundo W. Five-year results of refractive lenticule extraction. J Cataract Refract Surg. 2014;40:1425–9.
13. Kunert KS, Russmann CH, Blum M, SluytermanvanLangenweyde G. Vector analysis of myopic astigmatism corrected by femtosecond refractive lenticule extraction. J Cataract Refract Surg. 2013;39:759–69.
14. Eydelman MB, Drum B, Holladay J, Hilmantel G, Kezirian G, Durrie D, Stulting RD, Sanders D, Wong B. Standardized analyses of correction of astigmatism by laser systems that reshape the cornea. J Refract Surg. 2006;22:81–95.
15. Kobashi H, Kamiya K, Ali MA, Igarashi A, Elewa MEM, Shimizu K. Comparison of astigmatic correction after femtosecond lenticule extraction and small incision lenticule extraction for myopic astigmatism. PLoS ONE. 2015;10(4): e0123408. https://doi.org/10.1371/journal.pone.0123408.
16. Ivarsen A, Hjortdal J. Correction of myopic astigmatism with small lenticule extraction. J Refract Surg. 2014;30:240–7.

17. Zhang J, Wang Y, Wu W, Xu L, Li X. Dou R (2015) Vector analysis of low and moderate astigmatism with small incision lenticule extraction (SMILE): results of a 1-year follow-up. BMC Ophthalmol. 2015;15:8.
18. Chan TCY, Ng ALK, Cheng GPM, Wang Z, Ye C, Woo VCP, Tham CCY, Jhanji V. Vector analysis of astigmatic correction after small incision lenticule extraction and femtosecond-assisted LASIK for low to moderate myopic astigmatism. Br J Ophthamol. 2016;100:553–9.
19. Prakash G, Agrawal A, Ashok Kumar D, Jacob S, Agrawal A. Comparison of laser in situ keratomileusis for astigmatism without iris registration, with iris registration, and with iris registration-assisted dynamic eye tracking. J Cataract Refract Surg. 2011;37:574–81.
20. Kahlifa MA, Ghoneim AM, Shaheen MS, Pinero DP. Vector analysis of astigmatic changes after small incision lenticule extraction and wavefront-guided laser in situ keratomileusis. J Cataract Refract Surg. 2017;43:819–24.
21. Ganesh S, Brar S, Pawar A. Results of intraoperative manual cyclotorsion compensation for myopic astigmatism in patients undergoing small incision lenticule extraction (SMILE). J Refract Surg. 2017;33:506–12.
22. Chen P, Ye Y, Zhang X, et al. Comparison of SMILE surgery with and without cyclotorsion error correction for patients with astigmatism. Cornea. 2019;38:723–9.
23. Xu J, Liu F, Yang X, et al. Effect of cyclotorsion compensation with a novel technique on SMILE for the correction of myopic astigmatism. J Refarct Surg. 2019;35:301–8.
24. Sachdev GS, Patekar KB, Ramamurthy S. Comparative analysis of visual outcomes following SMILE with or without cyclotorsion compensation in eyes with high astigmatism: contralateral eye study. Indian J Ophthalmol. 2023;71:476–80.
25. Ivarsen A, Gyldenkerne A, Hjortdal J. Correction of astigmatism with small incision lenticule extraction: impact of against the-rule and with-the-rule astigmatism. J Cataract Refract Surg. 2018;44:1066–72.
26. Chan TCY, Wang Y, Ng ALK, Zhang J, Yu MCY, Jhanji V, Cheng GPM. Vector analysis of high (≥3 diopters) astigmatism correction using small incision lenticule extraction and laser in situ keratomileusis. J Cataract Refract Surg. 2018;44:802–10.
27. Köse B. Detection of and compensation for static cyclotorsion with an image-guided system in SMILE. J Refract Surg. 2020;36:142–9.
28. Reinstein DZ, Potter ATI, Gupta R, Wiltfang R. Refractive and visual outcomes of SMILE for compound myopic astigmatism with the VisuMax 800. J Refract Surg. 2023;39:294–301.

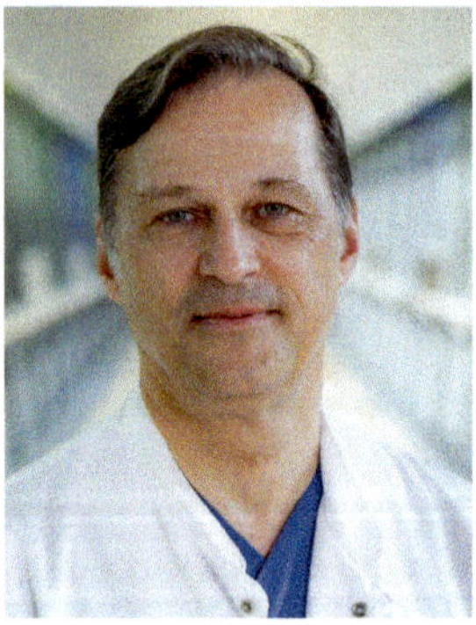

Marcus Blum is Head of Department of Ophthalmology, Helios Klinikum Erfurt, Germany. He studied at the University of Heidelberg. He was resident in the Department of Ophthalmology at Heidelberg (Prof. H.E. Völcker) and fellow at the Department of Ophthalmology at Jena (Prof. J. Strobel). He was appointed Associate Professor at the University of Jena in 1999 and was involved in building up a technology network focussing on new technologies for Ophthalmology in Jena. Together with Walter Sekundo he pioneered using fs-lasers for lenticule extraction. In 2001 Prof. Blum became head of the Ophthalmology Department at the Helios Klinikum Erfurt. He has published 150 papers and book chapters and has given more than 300 presentations at national and international meetings. In 2024 he was elected as president of the German Society for Cataract and Refractive Surgery (DGII).

Hyperopic Correction by SMILE

9

Dan Z. Reinstein, Walter Sekundo, Kishore Raj Pradhan, Timothy J. Archer, Ruchi Gupta, and Marcus Blum

Abstract

This chapter reviews the evolution of hyperopic correction through small incision lenticule extraction (SMILE). Initial challenges with femtosecond lenticule extraction (FLEx) prompted modifications, including increased pulse frequency and lenticule shape enhancements leading to the current outcomes being at least as good as those of modern Femto-LASIK.

Keywords

Hyperopic correction • Small incision lenticule extraction (SMILE) • Refractive lenticule extraction (ReLEx) • Femtosecond lenticule extraction (FLEx) • VisuMax 800

D. Z. Reinstein (✉) · T. J. Archer · R. Gupta
London Vision Clinic, 138 Harley Street, London W1G 7LA, UK
e-mail: dzr@londonvisionclinic.com

D. Z. Reinstein
Columbia University Medical Center, New York, NY, USA

W. Sekundo
Department of Ophthalmology, Philipps University of Marburg, Marburg, Germany

K. R. Pradhan
KRP Matrika Eye Center, Kathmandu, Nepal

M. Blum
Department of Ophthalmology, Helios Hospital Erfurt, Erfurt, Germany

W. Sekundo and F. M. Wagner (eds.), *Femtosecond Laser Assisted Lenticule Extraction*,
https://doi.org/10.1007/978-3-031-60424-9_9

9.1 Hyperopic Correction by ReLEx FLEx

Despite an increasing popularity of the ReLEx procedure, it still has some drawbacks. One of them is the absence of software for the VisuMax 500 laser to treat hyperopia. Indeed, the idea of "all-in-one surgery" can only become a true femtosecond-laser-alone procedure if all refractive errors can be treated without excimer laser.

9.1.1 The First Study

Our group published the first paper on this topic in 2013 [1]. In this study, we performed FLEx in 47 hyperopic eyes of 26 patients utilizing the 200 kHz VisuMax® femtosecond laser system. Forty-two out of 47 hyperopic eyes of the treatment group completed the final 9-month follow-up. The patients' mean age was 42.3 (±9.0) years. Their preoperative mean spherical equivalent (SE) was +2.80 ± 1.3 D (range: +0.25 to +5.38 D). The authors (W.S., M.B.) performed all surgeries. Intended flap thickness was 120 μm. Because of the longer treatment time with the 200 kHz laser as compared to today's 500 kHz laser, we used the S "contact glass" in the vast majority of treated eyes. Thus, the flap diameter was chosen between 7.0 and 8.5 mm depending on the lenticule diameter. In all cases, a superior hinge, 50° in chord length, was left. The lenticule diameter varied between 6.2 and 7.6 mm according to patient's mesopic pupil diameter and white-to-white distance. The lenticule's minimal thickness varied between 20 and 25 μm. In this first study, we used a pseudo-transition zone created by an oblique (slope-like) angle of the lenticule edge. Nine months postoperatively, 64% of eyes treated were within ±1.00 D, and 38% of eyes within ±0.50 D of intended correction. One eye out of 47 (2.1%) lost more than two Snellen lines, but none of the eyes had UCVA less than 20/40. While we could show that hyperopic treatment was feasible and that good centration was not an issue, the rate of refractive regression (Fig. 9.1) was unacceptable in comparison with modern excimer laser correction of low to moderate hyperopia [Reinstein]. Thus, several patients have received excimer laser enhancement. Moreover, we had one serious complication with a lenticule remnant in the center of the optical zone, due to a buttonhole through the lenticule, leading to a "central island" appearance.

9.1.2 The Second Hyperopic FLEx Study

An improved lenticule shape was developed (Fig. 9.2) that had identical optical properties within the optical zone as in the original study, but with a number of differences mainly relating to the creation of a dedicated transition zone. The key features of the larger transition zone were based on the positive long-term experience with hyperopic ablation profiles of the MEL 80 excimer laser [Reinstein]. The transition zone was selected for each case individually, according to

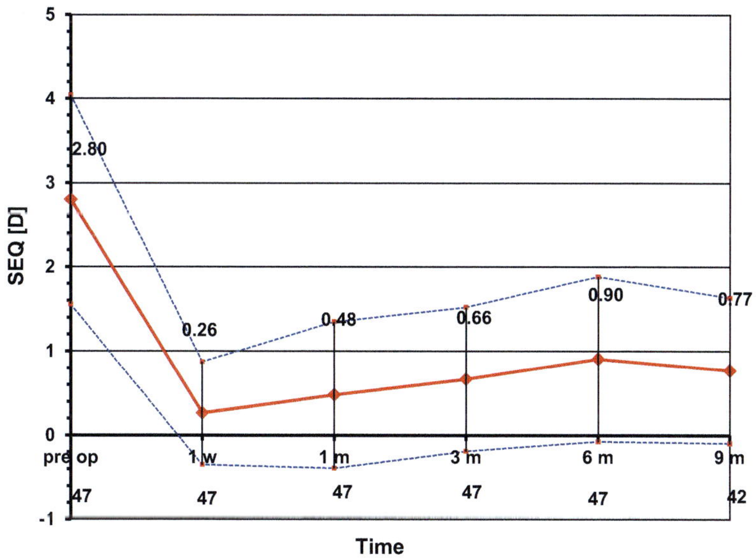

Fig. 9.1 Stability of refractive outcome over the 9-month follow-up period in the initial hyperopic study (reprinted from Blum et al. [1])

the corneal curvature, lenticule optical zone diameter, and the dioptric power of treatment (Fig. 9.2).

However, the total extent of the optical zone and transition zone is limited by the size of the VisuMax® contact glass being used, as the contact glass is applied to the cornea for suction. Therefore, in order to maximize the total lenticule diameter,

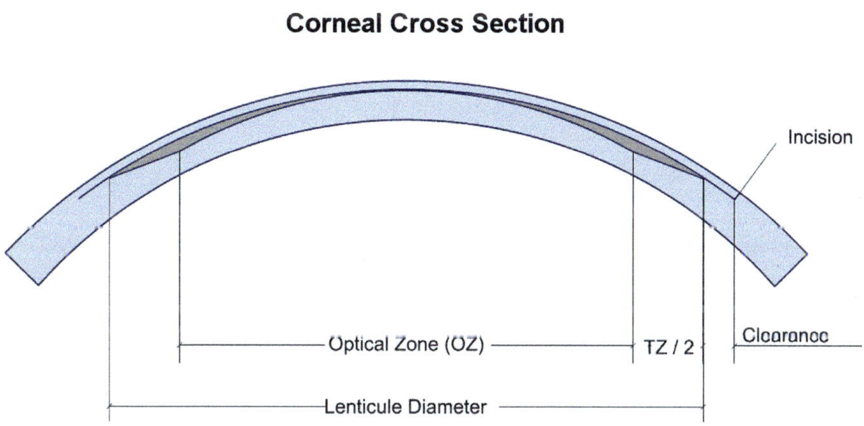

Fig. 9.2 Diagram of the improved lenticule shape used in the hyperopic FLEx study. *Note* a large transition zone and the minimal lenticule thickness at the edge and in the center

we used a medium (M) size contact glass in all cases rather than a small (S) size contact glass as in the majority of eyes in the previous study (similarly to myopic treatments). In order to obtain treatment zones as large as possible, the clearance between the edge of the lenticule and the edge of the flap was reduced to as low as 0.5 mm, compared to the 1 mm clearance that was used in the first study. When planning the lenticule and flap dimensions, the corneal diameter was also considered; as the treatments were centered on the corneal vertex, the flap diameter was confirmed to be within the diameter of the cornea in cases with an angle kappa, where the center of the treatment would not be aligned with the center of the cornea.

The other change between the two studies was that the pulse frequency of the VisuMax® had been increased from 200 to 500 kHz. This increase in pulse frequency meant that the new lenticule shape (with increased optical zone, transition zone, and flap diameters) could be performed without increasing the total treatment time, and therefore did not affect safety in relation to the risk of suction loss.

Because of the above-mentioned complication in the first study, where one eye developed a central buttonhole in the lenticule, we paid a lot of attention to the question of the central minimum lenticule thickness. After extensive ex vivo experiments with pig eyes and human corneas not eligible for corneal transplantation, this value was set at 25 μm in all eyes without any exception, rather than sometimes using 20 μm in the first study.

The Ethics Committees recommended that the study be divided into a pilot study with 10 eyes (initial spherical cohort) to be followed by a larger study of 40 eyes (second, spherocylindrical cohort) only after the 9-month data had been reported for the first treatment group.

The results of the initial spherical cohort reporting the results of nine eyes from five patients were published in 2016 [2]. Patients' average age at the time of surgery was 55.5 (range: 46 to 63) years. The mean preoperative manifest spherical equivalent refraction (SE) was $+1.82 \pm 0.56$ D (range: $+1.25$ to $+2.75$ D). As all patients were of presbyopic age, an overcorrection was intended in all cases and the mean target SE was -0.86 ± 0.41D (range -1.25 to 0.00 D).

The mean flap diameter was 8.46 ± 0.09 mm (range: 8.4 to 8.6 mm), the optical zone was 5.75 mm for all eyes, and the mean transition zone was 2.02 ± 0.14 mm (range: 1.78 to 2.29 mm). The femtosecond laser energy was adjusted between 180 and 160 nJ during the study with a fixed laser spot and track distance of 4.5 μm.

At one month, 3, 6, and 9 months, 33, 67, 22, and 22% of eyes were within 0.50 D of intended correction and 78% of eyes were within 1.00 D of target refraction. The analysis of attempted versus achieved refraction over time shows a regression between month 3 and month 9 of approximately 0.50 D in all but two eyes which were overcorrected. There were neither decentrations nor any other adverse effects (Fig. 9.3). Despite a mean refractive undercorrection of approximately 0.17 D, all patients were happy with the achieved results, simply because we purposely aimed at low myopia and in this way managed to bring all eyes into a comfortable zone for the presbyopic age (Fig. 9.4).

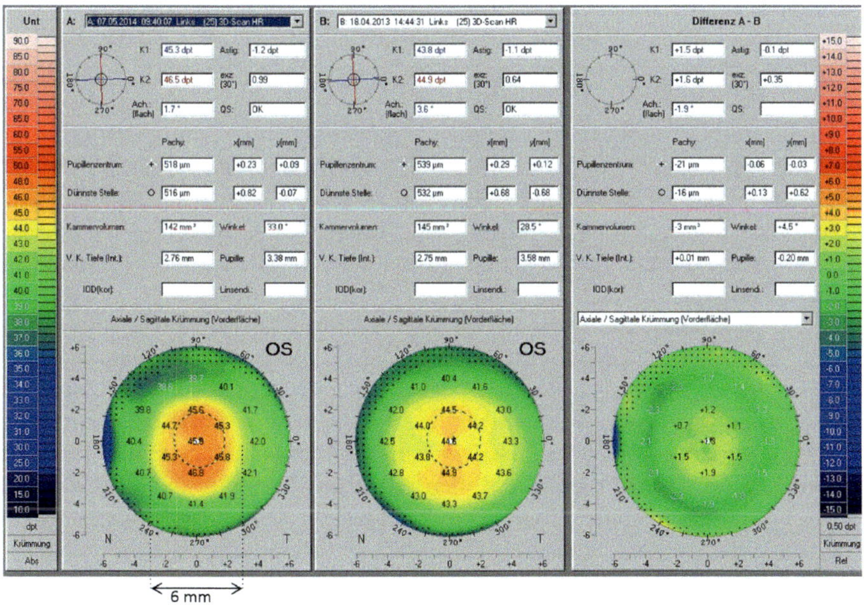

Fig. 9.3 Example of the pre- and post-op topography with steepened and well-centered central cornea (A: pre-op, B: 9 months, C: 3 months, D: 6 months after surgery). Also note that the differential map B-D shows minute changes only while the optical zone measures 6 mm on Pentacam's scale

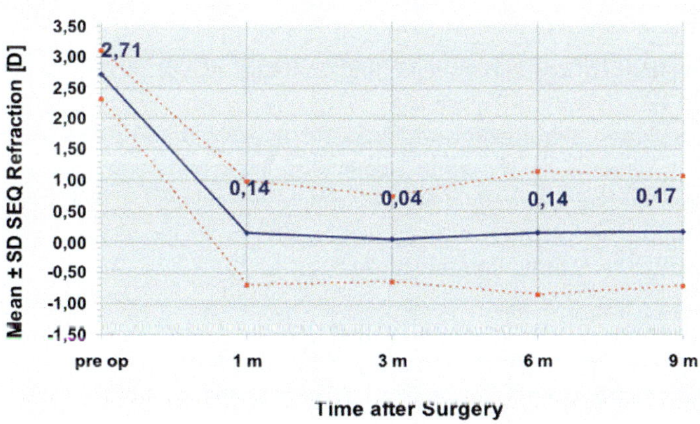

Fig. 9.4 Stability of the manifest refraction shown as change in spherical equivalent over time

As planned, the second phase of the study included a larger cohort of 39 eyes from 22 patients and the results were published in 2018 [3]. The second phase of the study introduced an updated femtosecond laser cutting sequence to decrease the laser treatment time. Patients' average age at the time of surgery was 49 (range: 27 to 56) years. The mean preoperative manifest spherical equivalent refraction (SE) was $+1.96 \pm 1.04$ D (range: + 0.63 to + 4.50 D) with mean preoperative sphere of + 2.24 ± 1.09 D (range: +0.75 to + 4.75 D) and mean astigmatism of -0.56 ± 0.45 D (range: 0 to -1.75 D). Of these 39 eyes, 16 eyes were targeted for emmetropia, whereas a myopic target was used for the other 23 eyes to induce micro-monovision.

In the pilot study, the femtosecond laser cutting sequence was to first create the lenticule interface from out-to-in, followed by the transition zone starting at the diameter of the optical zone and then scanning peripherally. For phase II, this sequence was changed to combine the optical zone and transition zone into a single continuous scan. Thus, the femtosecond laser cutting started at the outer diameter of the transition zone and then proceeded smoothly onto the lenticule interface within the optical zone. This modification shortened the overall laser treatment time by approximately 6 s, lasting on average 32 s. In addition, the initial experience of an undercorrection in the phase I study was compensated by applying a nomogram adjustment, adding +0.50 D to the intended correction.

The efficacy was calculated for the 16 eyes with a plano target, and the uncorrected distance visual acuity (UDVA) was 20/32 in 88% of eyes, 20/25 in 38%, and 20/20 in 6%. However, only 50% of these eyes had a preoperative CDVA of 20/20. At the final 9-month follow-up visit, the mean spherical equivalent was -0.40 ± 0.61 D (range: -1.50 to + 0.75 D), with 69% of eyes treated within ± 0.50 D and 90% of eyes within $\pm$ 1.00 D of intended correction. As expected for hyperopic treatments, there was a regression of $+0.35 \pm 0.51$ D until the end of the study (9 months). However, between 6 and 9 months, the refraction changed by + 0.03 D only.

This prospective investigation of FLEx for hyperopia and hyperopic astigmatism using a lenticule design with a dedicated large transition zone adjusted to both the optical zone and magnitude of correction produced visual and refractive outcomes similar to excimer laser correction of low to moderate hyperopia and had no visually threatening complications.

9.2 Hyperopic Correction by SMILE: Optical Zone Diameter and Spherical Aberration Induction

Pradhan and Reinstein presented the first results of hyperopic SMILE using two 2 mm incisions at the APAC Meeting 2014. They designed a multiphase study starting with four blind eyes, followed by six densely amblyopic eyes and 10 mildly amblyopic eyes, and published the results in 2017 [4, 5]. The lenticule shape was partially reminiscent to the one mentioned above, but the optical zone

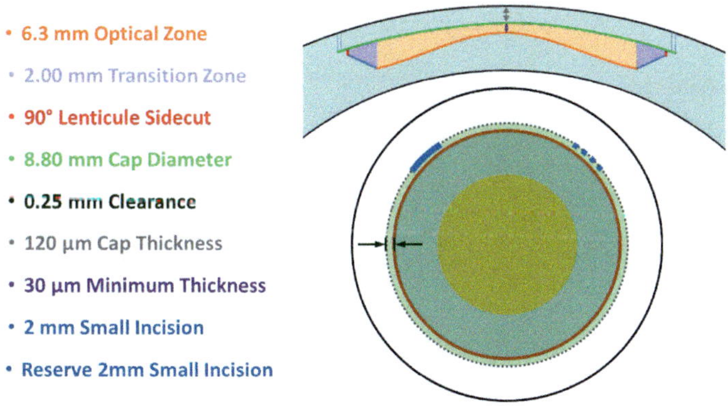

Fig. 9.5 Schematic diagram of hyperopic SMILE lenticule geometry used in Pradhan and Reinstein's study

of 6.3 mm was much larger, a transition zone of 2 mm was used for all eyes, and the minimal thickness was set to 30 μm (Fig. 9.5).

Study inclusion criteria were a maximum intended sphere up to + 7.00 D with astigmatism up to 6.00 D, age ≥ 21 years, CDVA 20/100 or worse. Retinoscopic refraction and Atlas topography were obtained before and 1 month after surgery. Twenty eyes were included and 1-month data were available in 11 eyes at the time of writing. MEL80 corneal vertex centered LASIK eyes matched for sphere and cylinder (±0.50 D) were randomly mined from our database to make two control groups: optical zone 6.50 mm or 7.00 mm (both with a 2 mm transition zone diameter). Mean SEQ was + 4.68 ± 1.30 D (range: +3.00 to +6.42 D). Mean refractive astigmatism was 1.09 ± 0.65 D (range: 0.50 to 2.75 D).

Mean post-op SEQ was +0.10 ± 0.91 D (range: −1.16 to + 1.50 D) with 27% of eyes within ± 0.50 D and 82% within ± 1.00 D of the target SEQ (N.B. these were retinoscopy refractions in blind or densely amblyopic eyes). Mean spherical aberration change was −0.49 μm in the 6.3 mm SMILE group, which was found to be equivalent to the 7 mm LASIK group (−0.47 μm, $p = 0.916$), but less than the 6.5 mm LASIK group (−0.79 μm, $p = 0.002$).

Optical zone centration was analyzed using the difference map of the Atlas tangential curvature to measure the distance between the center of the optical zone and the corneal vertex (the intended treatment center). Mean optical zone offset was equal for all groups ($p > 0.73$), being 0.30 ± 0.18 mm in the 6.3 mm SMILE group, 0.34 ± 0.26 mm in the 7 mm LASIK group, and 0.29 ± 0.15 mm in the 6.5 mm LASIK group. This demonstrated that the centration in SMILE was equivalent to LASIK despite the fact that SMILE does not use an eye tracker.

Mean achieved optical zone diameter was 5.55 ± 0.35 mm in the 6.3 mm SMILE group, which was found to be larger than the 6.5 mm LASIK group (4.65 ± 0.18 mm, $p < 0.001$) and the 7 mm LASIK group (4.93 ± 0.32 mm, $p < 0.001$). Figure 9.6 shows three example postoperative topographies from this hyperopic SMILE population alongside the topography of a matched LASIK case.

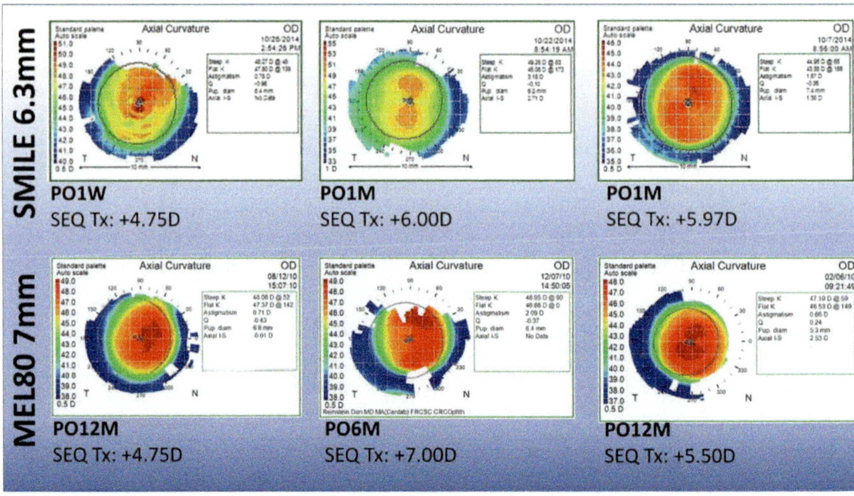

Fig. 9.6 Comparison of achieved optical zones with 6.3 mm lenticule diameter and 7 mm ablation zone showing a slight superiority of SMILE treated eyes

These examples visually demonstrate the encouraging optical zone diameter and centration results for SMILE.

In summary, optical zone centration was equivalent between vertex centered hyperopic SMILE and LASIK. Less spherical aberration was induced by 6.3 mm SMILE than 6.5 mm LASIK and was equivalent to 7 mm LASIK. Achieved topographic optical zone diameter was larger for 6.3 mm SMILE than 6.5 and 7 mm LASIK. Refraction change by retinoscopy appeared relatively accurate although longer-term sighted eye studies will be required to refine nomograms and balance these with observed regression.

9.3 Hyperopic Correction by SMILE: Refractive and Visual Outcomes

A prospective multiphase study was designed by Pradhan and Reinstein, to report the refractive and visual outcomes for hyperopic SMILE, which was published in 2019 [6]. The initial phases were designed as a feasibility study in poorly sighted eyes to optimize energy settings and demonstrate topographic safety before proceeding to investigate visual and refractive outcomes in sighted eyes.

Study inclusion criteria were attempted correction in the maximum hyperopic meridian between +1.00 and +7.00 diopters (D), astigmatism up to 6.00 D and medically suitable for SMILE. A complete ophthalmologic examination was performed prior to surgery by an in-house optometrist, as has been described previously [7]. Inclusion criteria included corrected distance visual acuity (CDVA) of 20/200 or worse for phase I, 20/100 and 20/200 for phase II, 20/40 and 20/80 for phase III, and 20/40 or better for phase IV of the study. Phases were advanced once safety had been demonstrated for the previous group.

All SMILE treatments were performed using the 500-kHz VisuMax femtosecond laser. In all eyes, two incisions were created: a 2-mm incision superonasally and a 2-mm incision superotemporally. Intended cap thickness was 120 μm in all eyes. Cap diameter used was 8.8 mm in all eyes, using a medium (M) contact glass. Optical treatment zone diameter was between 6.3 and 6.7 mm, with a 2 mm transition zone. The minimum lenticule thickness was 30 μm in all eyes. The spot and track distance were 4.6 μm for the cap and lenticule interfaces, 1.5 μm for the lenticule side cut, and 2 μm for the small incision. The energy level was set to 34 (170 nJ) in the VisuMax software.

A total of 93 eyes of 63 patients underwent hyperopic SMILE, and 12-month data were available in 72 eyes (71%). Mean SEQ was $+5.61 \pm 1.21$ D (range: +1.00 to +6.90 D). Mean refractive astigmatism was 0.90 ± 0.67 (range: 0.00 to 3.50 D). At 12 months after hyperopic SMILE, UDVA was 20/32 or better in 62% of eyes, relative to 62% with preoperative CDVA of 20/32 or better. Spherical equivalent refraction was within ± 0.50 D in 53% and within ± 1.00 D in 76% of eyes. There was one line loss CDVA in 16% of eyes, and no eyes lost two or more lines (Fig. 9.7). The results were similar to those for LASIK and refractive lens exchange for high hyperopia, as demonstrated in a previous literature review [8].

Refractive and visual outcomes including stability 12 months after SMILE for hyperopia were promising, given the high degree of hyperopia corrected and relatively reduced CDVA in this population. The authors concluded further follow-up is required to document refractive stability over 2 years and over the long term. Over the course of this prospective study for hyperopic SMILE, it was demonstrated that topographic centration, achieved topographic optical zone, induced higher-order aberrations, refractive and visual outcomes, and refractive and topographic stability are similar to the results of modern, large optical zone hyperopic LASIK.

9.4 Hyperopic Correction by SMILE: Prospective Multicenter 12-Month Study

Following the early studies, a large scale, multicenter, international, prospective study was conducted for hyperopic SMILE and published in 2022 [9]. Study inclusion criteria were age ≥ 18 years, hyperopic sphere up to +6.00 D, subjective astigmatism up to +5.00 D, maximum hyperopic meridian of + 7.00 D, and calculated postoperative residual stromal thickness of 250 μm or greater. A complete ophthalmologic examination was performed prior to surgery by an in-house optometrist, as has been described previously [7].

A total of 374 eyes of 199 patients underwent SMILE for hyperopia, data were available at 12 months in 323 eyes (86.4%). Follow-up percentages were slightly lower than projected due to the coronavirus disease 2019 (COVID-19) pandemic.

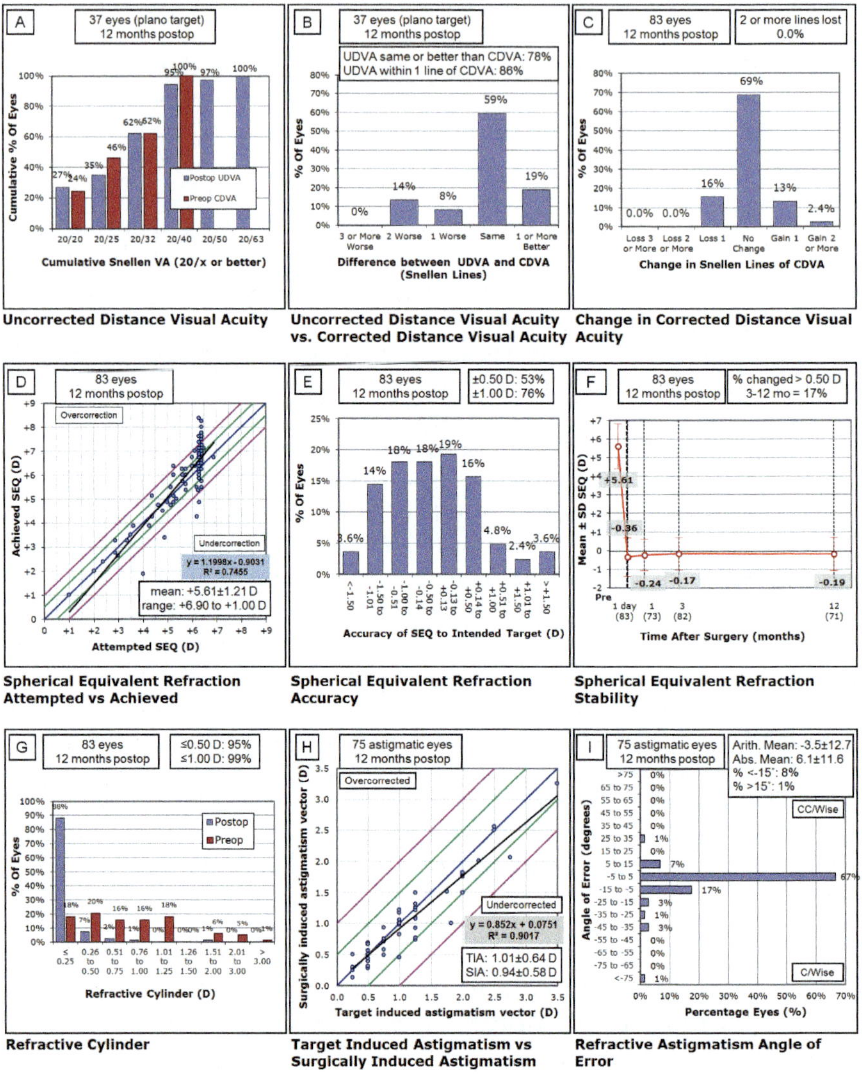

Fig. 9.7 Nine standard graphs for reporting refractive surgery showing the visual and refractive outcomes for 83 eyes 12 months after hyperopic SMILE. UDVA = uncorrected distance visual acuity; CDVA = corrected distance visual acuity; D = diopters; Post-op = postoperative; Pre-op = preoperative; SEQ = spherical equivalent refraction; TIA = target-induced astigmatism; SIA = surgically induced astigmatism

Mean SEQ was + 3.20 ± 1.48 D (range: 0.25 to +6.50 D). Mean refractive astigmatism was 0.88 ± 0.87 (range: 0.00 to 4.75 D). At 12 months after hyperopic SMILE, UDVA was 20/20 or better in 68% of eyes, relative to 85% with preoperative CDVA of 20/20 or better. UDVA was 20/16 or better in 28% and was 20/40 or better in all eyes. SEQ predictability was within ±0.50 D in 81% and within ±1.00 D in 93% of eyes at the 12-month visit. There was a gain of one line of CDVA in 10% of eyes, whereas there was one line loss in 11% and two or more lines loss in 1.2% at the 12-month visit (Fig. 9.8).

Intraoperative complications that occurred during this study were all previously described and at rates observed for routine myopic SMILE with the only exception being that the suction loss rate was higher at 1.34%. We attributed this to the larger treatment pack (size "M") and suction times reaching up to 35 s. In addition, hyperopic eyes are often those with a smaller white-to-white diameter. The least anticipated postoperative complication was interface haze, seen more frequently than expected for myopic SMILE. Interface haze occurred with a peak of 17% at the 6-month follow-up visit and decreased to 6.5% at the 12-month visit. Interface haze is known to be related to the degree of interface dissection trauma which is related to the optimization of the SMILE energy setting parameters, Haze prevention by use of topical corticosteroids for longer than the standard of 1 week as used in myopic SMILE, and energy setting optimization is the subject of future investigation in hyperopic SMILE.

SMILE was found to be an effective treatment method for the correction of compound hyperopic astigmatism, demonstrating a high level of efficacy, predictability, safety, and stability. The multicenter study revealed that hyperopic SMILE performed in a broader refractive surgical community achieved refractive results comparable to modern hyperopic corneal refractive surgery outcomes.

9.5 Discussion

While the first study demonstrated the feasibility of hyperopic correction by femtosecond laser alone, the more recently published studies deliver results comparable to the current state-of-the art excimer laser correction. Three major issues appear to be satisfactorily answered by these investigations:

(1) The patient's "self-centration" appears to work well in hyperopic eyes, where the centration issue is more crucial compared to myopic treatments
(2) The results achieved are stable and can be used for nomogram development.
(3) Lenticule parameters as described above appear to satisfy the requirements to safely dissect and remove a lenticule.

Apart from the advantages known from myopic SMILE, treatment of hyperopia using SMILE definitely eliminates any excimer laser fluence projection and truncation (exposed stromal bed smaller than ablation zone) errors. It is anticipated that the introduction of the VisuMax 800 laser for hyperopia will further improve

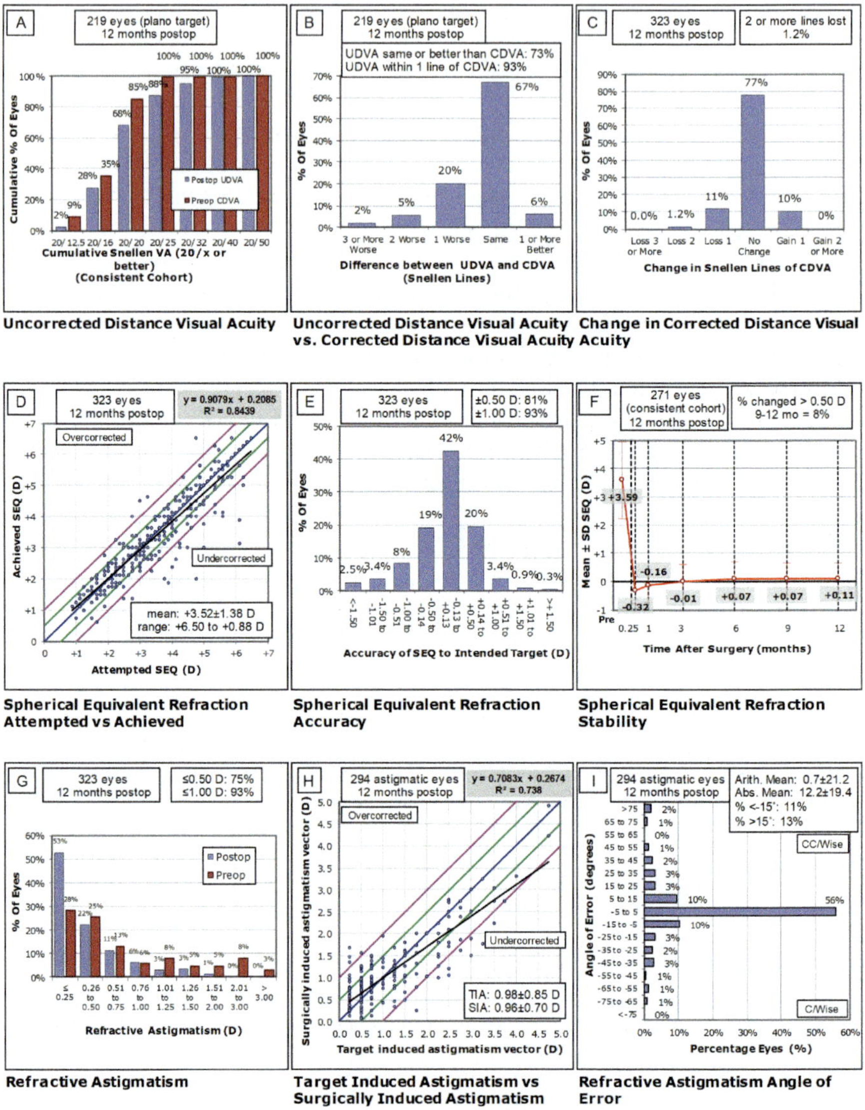

Fig. 9.8 Nine standard graphs for reporting refractive surgery showing the visual and refractive outcomes 12 months after hyperopic SMILE using the VisuMax femtosecond laser (Carl Zeiss Meditec, Jena, Germany). UDVA = uncorrected distance visual acuity; CDVA = corrected distance visual acuity; D = diopters; Post-op = postoperative; Pre-op = preoperative; SEQ = spherical equivalent refraction; TIA = target-induced astigmatism; SIA = surgically induced astigmatism

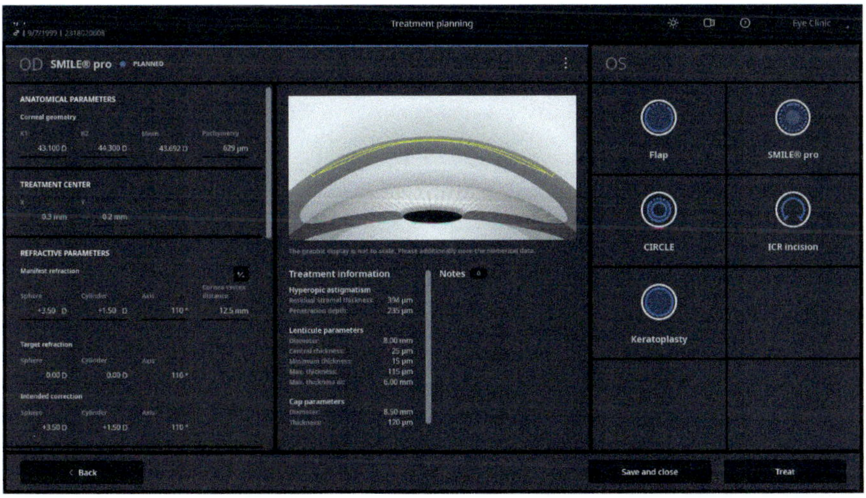

Fig. 9.9 VisuMax 800 data entry display for hyperopia and hyperopic astigmatism

safety and outcomes. The centration and cyclotorsion software should be of particular benefit in hyperopic patients who tend to have larger angle kappa. The femtosecond cutting speed is three times faster with the VisuMax 800 enabling a hyperopic treatment to be completed in 12 s, which should reduce the incidence of suction loss. The authors are therefore convinced that hyperopic SMILE, which will become available in 2024 with the VISUMAX 800, will enrich the refractive correction choice in the foreseeable future. Figure 9.9 shows the data entry screen for hyperopic SMILE.

We will also see the limits of hyperopic corneal surgery based on tissue extraction as opposed to tissue addition (see Chap. 22 for details).

References

1. Blum M, Kunert KS, Vossmerbaumer U, Sekundo W. Femtosecond lenticule extraction (ReLEx) for correction of hyperopia—first results. Graefes Arch Clin Exp Ophthalmol. 2013;251:349–55.
2. Sekundo W, Reinstein DZ, Blum M. Improved lenticule shape for hyperopic femtosecond lenticule extraction (ReLEx® FLEx): a pilot study. Lasers Med Sci. 2016;31:659–64.
3. Sekundo W, Messerschmidt-Roth A, Reinstein DZ, Archer TJ, Blum M. Femtosecond lenticule extraction (FLEx) for spherocylindrical hyperopia using new profiles. J Refract Surg. 2018;34:6–10.
4. Reinstein DZ, Pradhan KR, Carp GI, Archer TJ, Gobbe M, Sekundo W, Khan R, Dhungana P. Small incision lenticule extraction (SMILE) for hyperopia: optical zone diameter and spherical aberration induction. J Refract Surg. 2017;33:370–6.
5. Reinstein DZ, Pradhan KR, Carp GI, Archer TJ, Gobbe M, Sekundo W, Khan R, Citron K, Dhungana P. Small incision lenticule extraction (SMILE) for hyperopia: optical zone centration. J Refract Surg. 2017;33:150–6.

6. Pradhan KR, Reinstein DZ, Carp GI, Archer TJ, Dhungana P. Small incision lenticule extraction (SMILE) for hyperopia: 12-month refractive and visual outcomes. J Refract Surg. 2019;35:442–50.
7. Reinstein DZ, Yap TE, Carp GI, Archer TJ, Gobbe M. Reproducibility of manifest refraction between surgeons and optometrists in a clinical refractive surgery practice. J Cataract Refract Surg. 2014;40:450–9.
8. Reinstein DZ, Pradhan KR, Carp GI, Archer TJ, Day AC, Sekundo W, Dhungana P. Small incision lenticule extraction for hyperopia: 3-month refractive and visual outcomes. J Refract Surg. 2019;35:24–30.
9. Reinstein DZ, Sekundo W, Archer TJ, Stodulka P, Ganesh S, Cochener B, Blum M, Wang Y, Zhou X. SMILE for hyperopia with and without astigmatism: results of a prospective multicenter 12-month study. J Refract Surg. 2022;38:760–9.

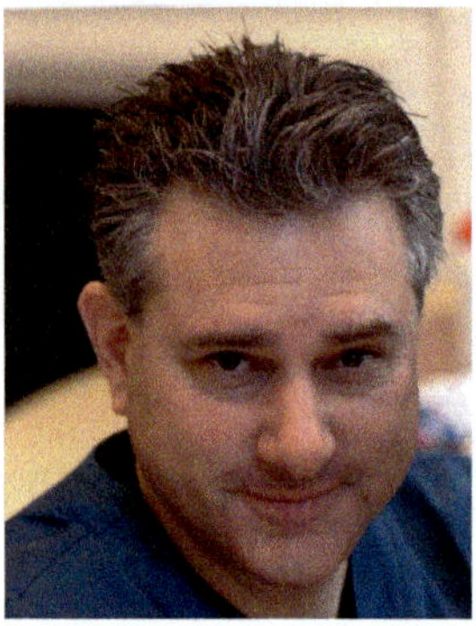

Dan Z. Reinstein, Founder and Medical Director of the London Vision Clinic and part of the EuroEyes Group, is a board-certified ophthalmologist in the US and Canada, with professorships in the UK, New York, and Paris. Dedicated solely to Refractive Surgery since the 1990s, he has pioneered epithelium mapping and corneal 3D pachymetric imaging with VHF digital ultrasound and OCT. His extensive contributions include over 215 scientific papers, 1000 + lectures globally, and significant roles in Therapeutic Refractive Surgery and as the Section Editor for the Journal of Refractive Surgery. He authored a definitive textbook on SMILE, contributed to 44 book chapters, and holds patents for VHF digital ultrasound technology, commercialized as the Insight 100 by ArcScan Inc., which is pivotal for the most accurate ICL sizing. Reinstein developed PRESBYOND Laser Blended Vision, now a part of the Carl Zeiss Meditec platform, and has been their Lead Refractive Surgery consultant since 2001. His achievements have earned him numerous awards, including the Waring Medal (2006), the Kritzinger Award (2013), the ISRS President's and AAO Senior Achievement Awards (2020), the Lifetime Achievement Award from UKISCRS (2023), and the Barraquer Award from AAO (2024). An accomplished saxophonist, he has maintained a monthly residency at the 606 Club in Chelsea for over 20 years.

Management of Laser Settings for Better SMILE Surgery

10

Bertram Meyer, Rainer Wiltfang, Rupal Shah, and Sri Ganesh

Abstract

This chapter focuses on optimizing laser parameters, particularly for the VisuMax 500, to enhance the outcomes of small incision lenticule extraction (SMILE) surgery. It delves into the critical interplay between energy levels, spot size, and track distance, addressing challenges such as delayed visual recovery and tissue distortion. The authors explore the introduction of the high-speed VisuMax 800, highlighting its benefits in shortened treatment times, reduced spot and tracking distances, and lower energy per spot, ultimately contributing to advancements in refractive surgery settings.

Keywords

Small incision lenticule extraction surgery (SMILE) • VisuMax 500 • Refractive surgery

B. Meyer (✉)
Eye Center Cologne, Cologne, Germany
e-mail: Meyer@augencentrumkoeln.de

R. Wiltfang
Smile-Eyes Center, Munich, Germany

S. Ganesh
Bengaluru, India

R. Shah
New Vision Laser Centers-Centre for Sight, Mumbai, India

W. Sekundo and F. M. Wagner (eds.), *Femtosecond Laser Assisted Lenticule Extraction*,
https://doi.org/10.1007/978-3-031-60424-9_10

10.1 Introduction

SMILE® has some compelling advantages presented by this refractive procedure as it has demonstrated notable safety and efficacy and proved to be much less independent of environmental conditions and corneal hydration as compared to excimer laser-based procedures. However, in comparison with the excimer laser, the femtosecond laser parameters adjustments are paramount for an excellent visual outcome.

During the early stages of implementing SMILE, we encountered several challenges, including delayed visual recovery in the initial postoperative days, determining the optimal approach for enhancement, and defining the long-term treatment range. This chapter elucidates our efforts to optimize clinical settings and enhance the overall clinical outcome of the treatment, when VisuMax 500 was introduced to the market. It will provide the reader with the understanding of laser energy–corneal tissue interaction and encourage the surgeon to get actively involved in optimizing of laser settings in his/her device.

10.2 Basic Understanding of Laser–Tissue Interaction

All VisuMax® lasers on the market provide surgeons with the ability for laser settings adjustments. In the VisuMax 500, the mode is called "expert mode" while the VisuMax 800 gives one opportunity to adjust the setting on the small screen (see Chap. 7). This brief chapter aims to elucidate the interplay between energy, spot size, and track distance.

Our primary focus was on identifying parameters influencing delayed visual recovery, leading us to three potential factors:

1. Energy Level

   Elevated energy levels may induce the development of gas bubbles, intensifying tissue compression and resulting in an irregular surface characterized by abnormal topography.
2. Optimized Spot and Track Spacing

   Fine-tuning these parameters holds the promise of reducing the roughness of the residual stroma and lenticule surface.
3. Speed of the Laser Cut

   Slower laser cut speed allows more time for gas bubbles formation resulting in opaque bubble layer (OBL).

The precision of tissue preparation prior and during the cut is crucial for achieving accurate refractive outcomes. Preventing tissue distortion is of essential importance.

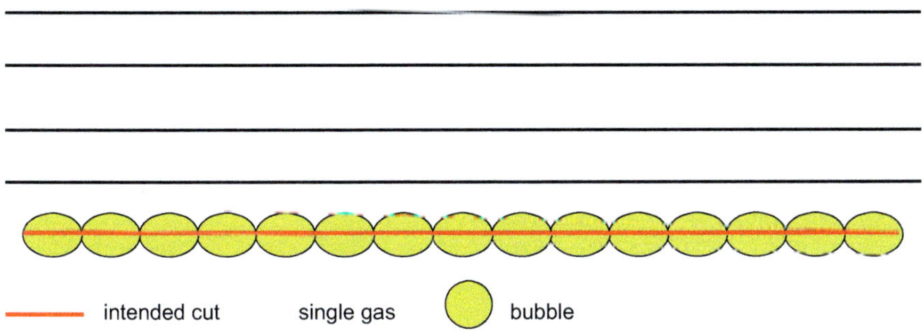

Fig. 10.1 .

To minimize tissue distortion before the cut, we took advantage of a curved patient's interface (also called "treatment pack" or "contact glass") and preferred a low corneal suction pressure, causing minimal applanation in the central cornea.

In contrast to flap cutting, where only one plane is produced by the laser, the interaction between the two adjacent planes (refractive and non-refractive cuts) is crucial in SMILE. Therefore, our second goal was to achieve a smooth bubble layer during the first deeper cut to prevent tissue distortion while performing the second cut.

The generation of optical breakdown induces plasma, leading to the formation of gas bubbles. This intricate process underscores the importance of understanding and managing the interaction between laser energy and tissue dynamics for optimal outcomes (Fig. 10.1).

As a physiological principle, the coalescence of individual gas bubbles into larger entities occurs when they are in close proximity. These enlarged bubbles have the potential to deform the surrounding tissue (Fig. 10.2).

As a result, the upper cut is generated within this distorted tissue (Fig. 10.3).

Following tissue relaxation and the absorption of gas bubbles, the intended layer of the cut may deviate from the actual cut. Extracting such a "deformed" lenticule

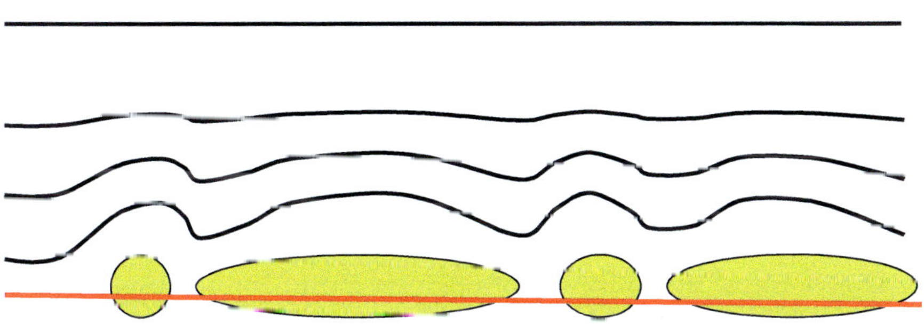

Fig. 10.2 .

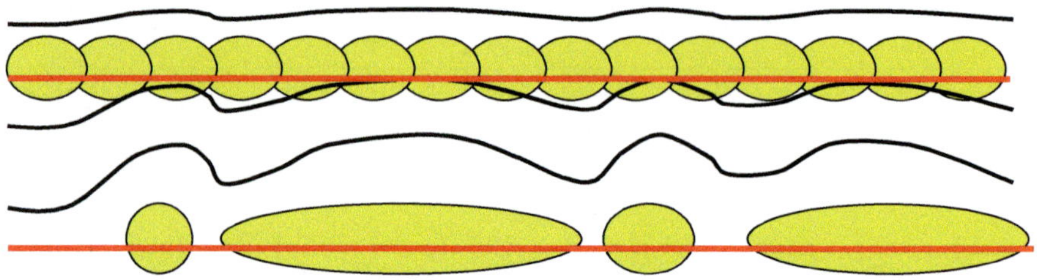

Fig. 10.3 .

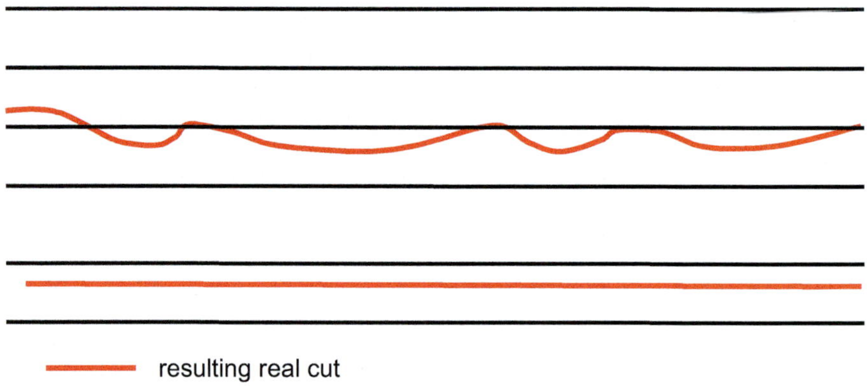

Fig. 10.4 .

would lead to substantial iatrogenic aberrations and a diminished quality of visual outcomes (Fig. 10.4).

To mitigate these challenges, it is imperative to minimize the volume of gas bubbles, ensuring that the distance between individual bubbles is both sufficiently small for effective separation and large enough to prevent tight junctions.

The initial effort to reduce the time between the laser cuts at the two interfaces—the "bottom" and the "roof"—within the central cornea (the optical zone) was successfully implemented by Shah through altering the cut direction. This is the rationale behind the current "spiral-in" followed by "spiral-out" approach [1].

10.3 First Study Comparing Energy Levels and Spot/Track Distances

To advance our understanding and optimize the SMILE® procedure, we aimed to identify the optimal combination of energy levels, spot distances, and tracking distances to improve cut quality and facilitate tissue separation.

10.3.1 Methods

To achieve precision in laser settings, we embarked on a foundational phase of basic research. Initial trials were conducted on porcine eyes to explore the limits of energy and spot distances: Table 10.1 illustrates the determination of the outer limits for the three specified variables.

Note: VisuMax laser uses an "index" for laser energy settings. For simplicity, we maintain this "index" as a unit familiar to VisuMax users. However, it is essential to know that one index unit is equivalent to 5 nJ (Table 10.1).

At high energy levels (index 60) and small spot and tracking distances (2.0 or 3.5 μ), we observed the formation of stromal ring-shaped structures. Conversely, at low energy levels (index 22) and large spot and tracking distances (5.0 μ), achieving controlled tissue separation became unattainable.

Through systematic analyses, we identified the optimal combination of energy level, spot size, and tracking distance for enhanced cut quality and ease of tissue separation. This optimal combination fell within two distinct ranges (Table 10.2).

Subsequently, we did adjustments by reducing the energy from index 28 to index 24 while maintaining the recommended spot and tracking distances. This alteration resulted in a slightly improved uncorrected distance visual acuity (UDVA) on the first day after treatment, although the improvement was not statistically significant.

Additionally, we analyzed the impact of enlarging the recommended spot and tracking distances while keeping the energy level consistent (index 24/26), expanding from 3.0 to 3.8 μ. This modification resulted in a statistically significant improvement in UDVA on the first day postoperatively.

Table 10.1 .

ID	Sphere/lenticule thickness	Flap energy/lenticule energy	Track distance/spot distance
5	−5D/96 μm	Index* 60	2.0/2.0 μm
6	−10D/166 μm	Index 60	2.0/2.0 μm
11	−5D/96 μm	Index 60	3.5/3.5 μm
12	−10D/166 μm	Index 60	3.5/3.5 μm
13	−5D/96 μm	Index 22	5.0/5.0 μm
14	−10D/166 μm	Index 22	5.0/5.0 μm

Table 10.2 .

ID	Sphere/lenticule thickness	Flap energy/lenticule energy	Track distance/spot distance
7	−5D/96 μm	Index 22	3.5/3.5 μm
8	−10D/166 μm	Index 22	3.5/3.5 μm
15	−5D/96 μm	Index 40	5.0/5.0 μm
16	−10D/166 μm	Index 40	5.0/5.0 μm

Consequently, our inference was that a decrease in energy per unit area might be the key to optimized settings. This can be achieved either by adjusting the energy level itself or by enlarging the spot/track distances. We decided on the second option and reduced the energy level per area from 4.1 μ/index 36 to 4.5 μ/index 36.

10.3.2 Results

Our key findings were as follows:

- Facilitated lenticule extraction with increased spot and tracking distance.
- Absence of critically low energy levels that might lead to uncontrolled tissue separation.
- Enhanced adjustability due to higher energy levels.
- Statistically significant improvements in UDVA on the first day post-op.
- Reduced treatment time with a reduced risk of suction loss.

The comprehensive results are summarized and presented in Figs. 10.5 and 10.6.

10.3.3 Discussion

Based on the outcomes of our extensive testing, we concluded: The application of a 4.5 μ spot and tracking distance, combined with an energy level of 180 nJ per spot, achieved an optimized low energy density. This configuration minimizes tissue distortion and facilitates easy lenticule extraction, particularly with the 500 kHz VisuMax laser. These refined settings have been successfully integrated into the VisuMax 500 femtosecond laser system by Carl Zeiss Meditec as early as 2014.

Our initial work benefited patients and surgeons alike because of:

- Shorter Treatment Time: Up to a 30% reduction, accompanied by a decreased risk of suction loss.
- Faster Visual Recovery: Especially evident in uncorrected distance visual acuity (UDVA) on the first day postoperatively.
- More Precise Refraction: Improved accuracy observed on the first day postoperatively.
- Reduced Tissue Affection: Immediate postoperative effects such as edema and stromal disorder are minimized.

Our initial work gave a rise to many studies related to the energy settings, quality of the cut surface, which in turn relates to the light scatter and ultimately the best corrected visual acuity. However, the concept of low energy also has its limits. While Donate and Thaëron claimed that reducing the energy just above plasma

a

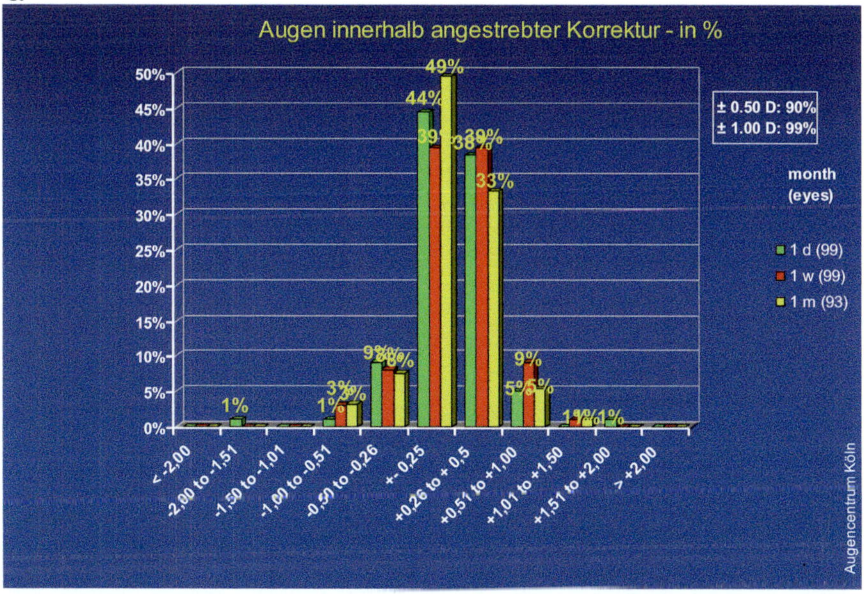

b

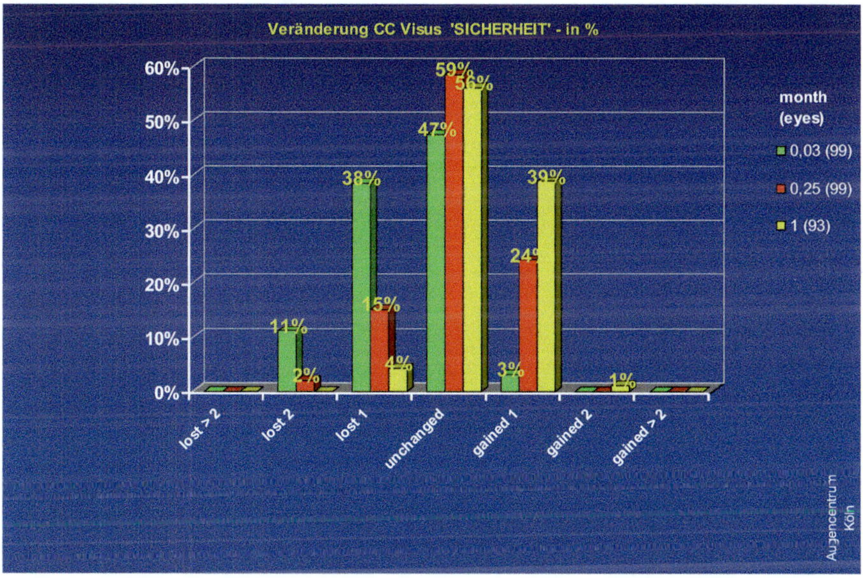

Fig. 10.5 **a** (Left-hand side) The predictability of refractive change. **b** The safety (CDVA; right-hand side) at first day, first week, and first month before adjustment of the laser settings

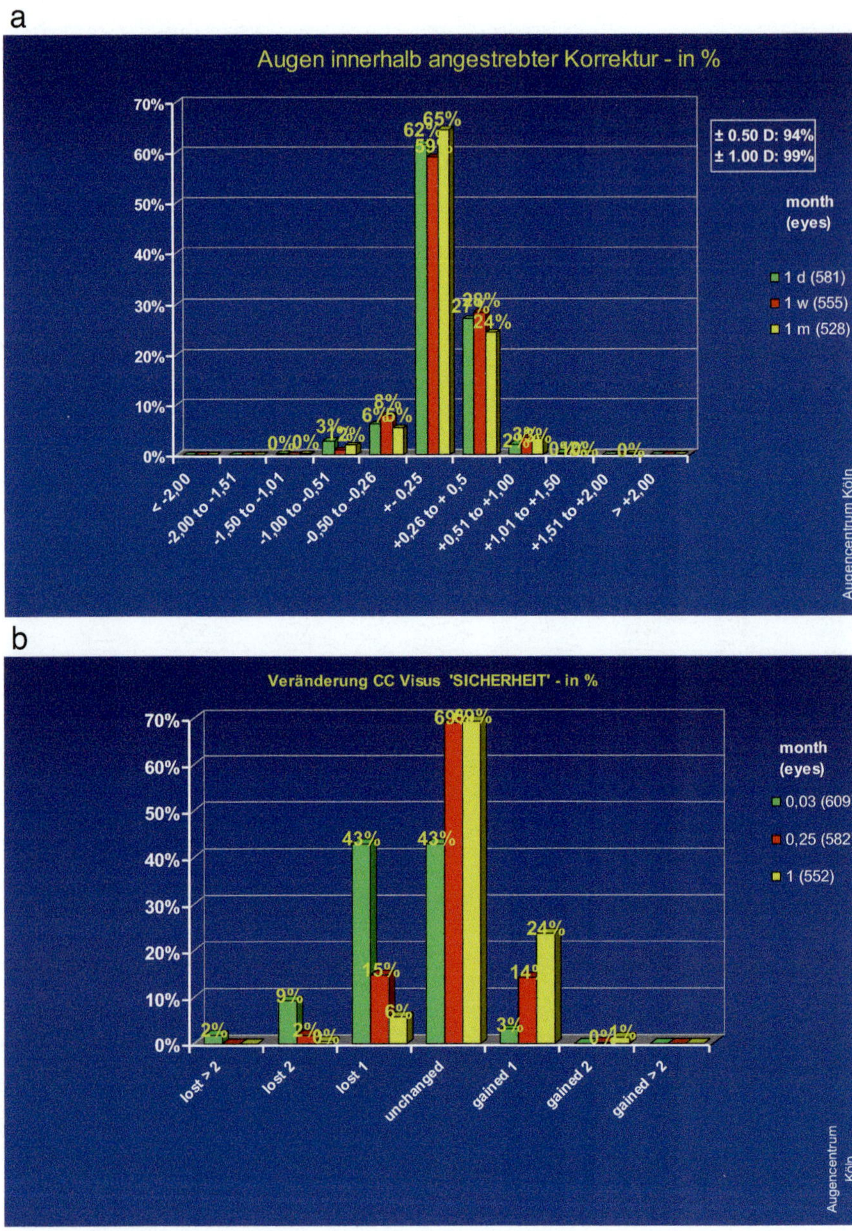

Fig. 10.6 **a** (Left-hand side) The predictability of refractive change. **b** The safety (CDVA; right-hand side) at first day, first week, and first month after adjustment of the laser settings. Higher accuracy and slightly better safety at all early follow-up checks

threshold (meaning almost no bubble pattern seen) will provide the best possible result, it creates the danger of poor separability leading to manual tissue distortion. A nice study that looked at correlation of the surface quality by scanning electron microscopy and visual acuity was conducted by Ji et al. in 2017 [2] and later confirmed by Lin et al. in 2020 when analyzed the uncut ("black") areas on the video footage [3]. Both studies showed that with a track/spot distance of 4.5 μm, the lowest energy level possible is 110 nJ (VisuMax index = 21) (Fig. 10.7).

In fact, the vast majority of surgeons would use energy levels between 24 and 27 when the spot/track distance is fixed at 4.5 μm and the cap thickness is between 110 and 130 μm when using VisuMax 500.

Another important finding associated with the energy levels is the occurrence of opaque bubble layer (OBL). OBL significantly decreases the easiness of tissue dissection. Sri Ganesh explains in Chap. 6 how to reduce the incidence of OBL.

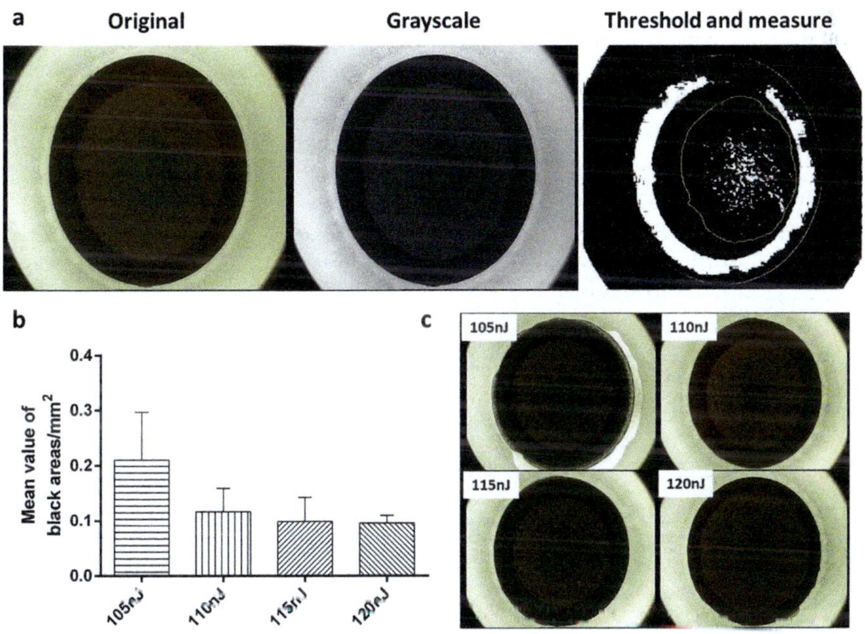

Fig. 10.7 Analysis of black areas of different energy levels. **a** Process of black area measurement quantitatively. **b** Mean proportion of black areas in different energy groups. Data showed that 105 nJ caused the largest black area. Data were represented as mean ± standard error of the mean. **c** Maximum proportion of black areas of each group. [3] Reproduced with permission from Lin et al., Wolters Kluwer, 2020

10.4 Subsequent Study with High-Speed Laser

The introduction of a super-fast laser, currently known as VisuMax 800, is also a result of thorough investigations where the triple speed was compared with the above-mentioned established VisuMax 500 settings. Our assumption was that a tighter spot spacing while reducing energy level should lead to a better separability without the loss of visual recovery. In 2020, Sri Ganesh and Rupal Shah conducted an internal, non-published contralateral, and randomized study to investigate the impact of energy levels on lenticule separability and visual recovery time. The study design involved treating one eye with a "reference regime," using standard energy levels, a conventional surgery technique, and wide track/spot spacings. Simultaneously, the fellow eye of the same patient underwent treatment with an "experimental regime," incorporating varied energies, diverse surgery techniques, and narrow track/spot spacings.

The findings of the study revealed that both regimes resulted in safe and effective outcomes at the three-month postoperative mark. As expected, tissue separation and extraction of the lenticule was significant easier in the experimental group with narrow spot/track spacing and increased energy per unit area (Table 10.3).However, the experimental group with tight laser spots exhibited a slower visual recovery (Fig. 10.8).

Surprisingly, the occurrence of the opaque bubble layer (OBL) was significantly lower in the experimental group due to the high cutting speed of the new laser. Despite the experimental regime's higher energy density compared to the reference regime, the absence of OBL did not provide an explanatory framework for the observed differences in early visual acuity in the experimental group. These insights contribute to the ongoing exploration and refinement of laser settings in refractive surgery procedures.

With the introduction of the new VisuMax 800, we now benefit from its ultra-fast speed, leading to remarkably short treatment times ranging from 8 to 11 s.

Table 10.3 Statistics of separation/extraction stratified by regime and site

Site	Parameter separation/ extraction (score)	Mean	SD	Min	Max	N	Median	IQR	Lower 95% CL for Mean	Upper 95% CL for Mean
BA	REF	5.27	0.72	4.00	7.50	66	5.00	0.50	5.10	5.45
	EXP	7.27	0.99	5.00	9.00	66	7.50	1.00	7.03	7.51
	EXP-REF difference	2.00	1.22	−2.50	3.50	66	2.25	2.00	1.70	2.30
VA	REF	5.89	0.49	4.00	6.50	64	6.00	0.00	5.77	6.01
	EXP	8.67	0.68	6.00	9.50	64	8.75	0.50	8.50	8.84
	EXP-REF difference	2.78	0.72	0.00	5.00	64	3.00	0.50	2.60	2.96

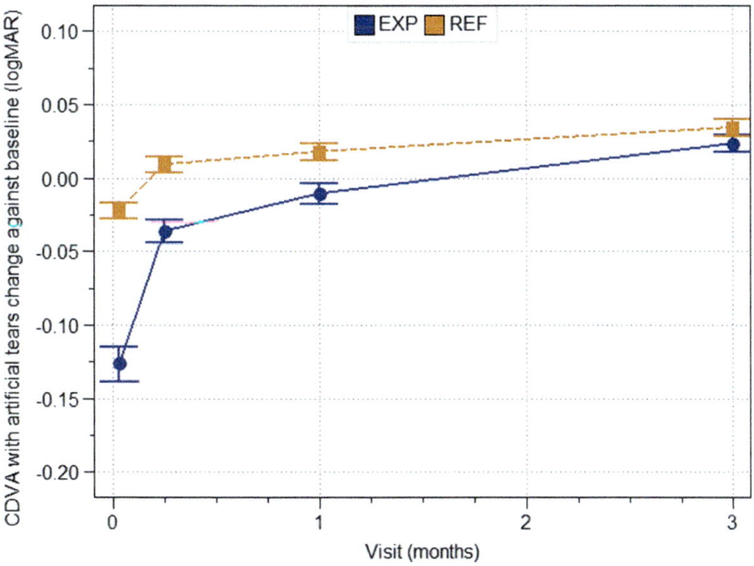

Fig. 10.8 Mean and std. error of CDVA change with artificial tears against baseline for different visits and regimes

This advancement allows us to significantly reduce the spot and tracking distances while concurrently lowering the energy per spot, all without a substantial increase in treatment time (e.g., energy setting: 110 nJ at a spot distance of 3.0 μm). Moreover, with this new laser, it is possible (and advisable) to use different spot/track distances at the lower and the upper plane (e.g., 4.1/4.5 μm). Because of the energy dispersion, the deeper plane is more difficult to dissect as compared to the cap plane. By tightening the laser spots at the deeper tissue level, the separation of both planes becomes easy. The use of a lower energy level at high cutting speed contributes to the formation of smaller and more homogeneous bubble patterns, with minimal impact on the surrounding tissue. Furthermore, the high firing frequency of the VisuMax 800 results in reduced interaction among the bubble patterns and virtually free of OBL.

10.5 Conclusion

It is essential to note that the specific energy settings can vary between devices and even patients. Therefore, the surgeon cannot rely on the standard settings of the new machine after installation. Like a violin player, the surgeon needs to fine-tune the instrument (laser machine) to get best possible results. Or instance, with the VisuMax 500, the Zeiss engineer would usually start with spot/track distance of 4.5 μm in the plane and 2.0 μm for the side cut (lenticule border and the entering incision) at the energy index of 32 (160 nJ). From there on, the surgeon should slowly reduce the energy in 5 nJ increments (1 index unit) as long as the bubble pattern is uniform and the dissection acceptable. The surgeon should also learn to adjust the energy to the thickness of the expected lenticule thickness. As mentioned above, the energy dissipates the deeper is the lower refractive cut. For instance, when using the energy index of 25 for low myopia of −1.5 D, the surgeon is advised to increase the energy index to 26–27 when he/she approaches a −9D correction. Vice versa, because there are also variations between patients, the surgeon can use the first eye to optimize the outcome of the fellow eye. For example, a patient with both eyes of −3.0 D in the main meridian (not the spherical equivalent!) is treated with the energy index of 26 resulting in super-easy separation. The surgeon is encouraged to reduce the energy for the fellow eye by one click. The separation usually will not differ much, but the total energy introduced into the cornea will be significantly decreased.

References

1. Shah R, Shah S. Effect of scanning patterns on the results of femtosecond laser lenticule extraction refractive surgery. J Cataract Refract Surg. 2011;37:1636–47.
2. Ji YW, Kim M, Kang DSY, et al. Effect of lowering laser energy levels lead to better visual recovery after small incision lenticule extraction: prospective, randomized clinical trial. Am J Ophthalmol. 2017;179:159–70.
3. Lin L, Weng S, Liu F, et al. Development of low level energy levels in small incision lenticule extraction: clinical results, black areas, and ultrastructural evaluation. J Cataract Refract Surg. 2020;46(3):410–8.

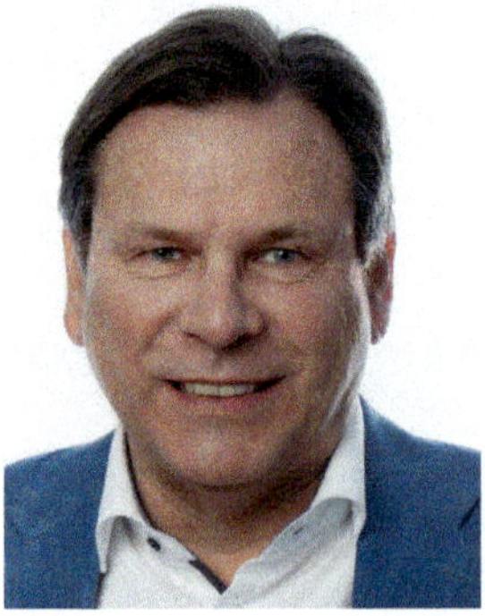

Bertram Meyer is a specialist in laser refractive surgery, with a career spanning over three decades since he began his practice in 1992. Notably, he has been performing SMILE (Small Incision Lenticule Extraction) procedures since 2010. Bertram Meyer offers his expertise in private clinics located in Cologne, Germany, and Dubai, UAE. His professional contributions extend beyond clinical practice. Bertram Meyer regularly shares his knowledge and advancements in the field through lectures and updates at prominent annual meetings, including those organized by the German Ophthalmological Society (DOG), the German Society of Cataract and Refractive Surgery (DOC), the German-speaking Society of Intraocular Lens Implantation (DGII), and the European Society of Cataract and Refractive Surgeons (ESCRS). These presentations primarily focus on Femto-Lasik and Laser-Assisted-Lenticule-Extraction e.g. ReLEx®SMILE, reflecting his deep expertise and commitment to advancing laser refractive surgery.

Advantages and Disadvantages of Different Cap Thicknesses

11

José L. Güell, Nuno Moura-Coelho, Paula Verdaguer, Honorio Pallás, Daniel Elies, Oscar Gris, and Felicidad Manero

Abstract

This chapter explores the impact of different cap thicknesses in small incision lenticule extraction (SMILE) procedures, a minimally invasive corneal lenticule extraction technique using femtosecond laser technology.

Keywords

Small incision lenticule extraction surgery (SMILE) • Cap thickness • Femtosecond laser technology • Refractive outcomes • Visual acuity • Corneal biomechanics

Supplementary Information The online version contains supplementary material available at https://doi.org/10.1007/978-3-031-60424-9_11.

The authors have equally contributed to this chapter.

J. L. Güell
Cornea and Refractive Surgery Unit, Instituto Microcirugia Ocular, Barcelona, Spain

J. L. Güell · N. Moura-Coelho (✉) · N. Moura-Coelho (✉) · P. Verdaguer · H. Pallás · D. Elies · O. Gris · F. Manero
Cornea and Refractive Surgery Unit, Instituto de Microcirugia Ocular (IMO), Barcelona, Spain
e-mail: nunomouracoelho.oft@gmail.com

J. L. Güell
Ophthalmology at the "Universitat Autònoma de Barcelona" (UAB), Barcelona, Spain

P. Verdaguer · D. Elies · O. Gris
Universitat Autònoma de Barcelona (UAB), Barcelona, Spain

W. Sekundo and F. M. Wagner (eds.), *Femtosecond Laser Assisted Lenticule Extraction*,
https://doi.org/10.1007/978-3-031-60424-9_11

11.1 Introduction

Advanced, minimally invasive corneal lenticule extraction using femtosecond laser technology procedure, or "Keratorefractive Lenticule Extraction" (KLEx) as jointly proposed by the editors of Journal of Refractive Surgery and Journal of Cataract and Refractive Surgery, is an all-in-one technology for correcting refractive errors that has become available for intrastromal lenticule cutting and subsequent lenticule extraction. These technologies have exhibited excellent efficacy, safety, and predictability for the correction of myopia and astigmatism [1–3].

We started using the Small Incision Lenticule Extraction (SMILE) technique (SMILE Zeiss VisuMax 500, Carl Zeiss Meditec, Germany) in 2011, with progressively better visual and refractive results. Novel platforms for second generation KLEX procedures include the updated SMILE Pro (Zeiss VisuMax 800, Carl Zeiss Meditec, Germany), the Corneal Lenticule Extraction for Advanced Refractive Correction (CLEAR, Femto LDV Z8 NEO, Ziemer Ophthalmic Systems AG, Germany), SmartSight (Schwind ATOS, Schwind eye-tech solutions, Germany), Smooth Incision Lenticule Keratomileusis (SILK Procedure, ELITA Femtosecond Laser System, Johnson & Johnson) which are described in appropriate chapters in this book.

Considering the theoretically lower impact on corneal biomechanics with deeper cuts and with the concept in mind of a secondary more superficial retreatments (re-SMILE procedures), we decided to study the refractive and visual results of deeper lenticule depths. The procedure was performed using 4 different lenticule depths in a prospective, non-randomized way (130, 140, 150 and 160 μm).

11.2 Surgical Procedure

A standard SMILE surgery sequence as described in Chaps. 6 and 7 was carried out. At the conclusion of the laser scan, an opening incision of 30° length (approx. 2 mm) was created at the 10.30 -o'clock position for lenticule extraction. The shape of the lenticule generated was designed to correct the refractive error. The femtosecond laser parameters were adjusted for: 130, 140, 150 or 160 μmcap thickness, 7.5 mm diameter of anterior lenticule surface (cap), 6.5 mm diameter of posterior lenticule surface and at the VisuMax 500 energy level of 26 and spot/track distance of 3 μm for both the lenticule and cap cuts. We increased the spherical equivalent of the correction by 3% for every 10 μm of higher depth in relation to the 130 μm cap. After completion of the laser sequence, a blunt spatula (G-33954 Güell Femto Double-Ended instrument, Geuder GmbH, Germany) was inserted through the small incision over the roof of the refractive lenticule dissecting this plane, followed by the bottom of the lenticule. The lenticule was subsequently grasped and removed with micro forceps. After removal of the lenticule, the stromal pocket was flushed with BSS using a Güell flap hydrodissection cannula 25G (AE-7288) (Video of 160 μm depth SMILE procedure).

11.3 Postoperative Treatment

Standard postoperative treatment was tobramycin antibiotic and dexamethasone steroid eye drops (Tobradex™, Alcon) three times a day for a week then slowly tapered off over a 4-week period, plus preservative-free artificial tears five times a day for almost a month.

11.4 Statistical Analysis

Microsoft Excel (Microsoft; Redmond, Washington, USA) was used for data collection and for performing descriptive statistics. Continuous variables were described with mean and standard deviation (SD).

The results were analyzed using SPSS software version 17.0 (SPSS Inc., Chicago, Illinois, USA). Comparison between preoperative and postoperative data was performed using Wilcoxon-Signed-Rank tests for non-parametric data. The tests were performed before surgery, at 4 weeks (1 month), 3 months, 6 months and at 1 year after the surgery. A p-value lower than 0.05 was considered to be statistically significant.

11.5 Results

Ninety-four eyes of 47 patients with myopia with and without myopic astigmatism were recruited for this study. The number of eyes in the 4 different lenticule depth groups was: 130 μm ($n = 44$), 140 μm ($n = 14$), 150 μm ($n = 12$) and 160 μm ($n = 24$). Mean preoperative logMAR uncorrected visual acuity (UCVA) was 1.21 (SD 0.35). Mean postoperative logMAR UCVA was: 0.15 (SD 0.20) at 1 month; 0.08 (SD 0.12) at 3 months; 0.07 (SD 0.12) at 6 months and 0.07 (SD 0.12) at 1 year. There were no statistically significant differences in the UCVA variables between the 4 groups ($p < 0.05$).

Mean preoperative spherical equivalent (SE) was −4.89 (SD 1.48). Mean postoperative SE was: −0.26 (SD 0.42) at 1 month; −0.24 (SD 0.39) at 3 months; 0.09 (SD 0.62) at 6 months and 0.07 (SD 0.57) at 1 year. There were no statistically significant differences in the SE variable between the 4 groups ($p < 0.05$).

Mean preoperative cylinder (CYL) was −0.63 (SD 0.54). Mean postoperative CYL was: −0.28 (SD 0.47) at 1 month; −0.21 (SD 0.41) at 3 months; −0.33 (SD 0.42) at 6 months and −0.16 (SD 0.34) at 1 year. There were no significant statistical differences in CYL when the different groups were compared for the same periods of time ($p < 0.05$).

We did not observe statistically significant differences using the SMILE technique at 4 different lenticule depths in a random manner (130, 140, 150 and 160 μm) in visual acuity or refractive outcomes (Figs. 11.1, 11.2 and 11.3) with a minimum follow-up time of 1 year.

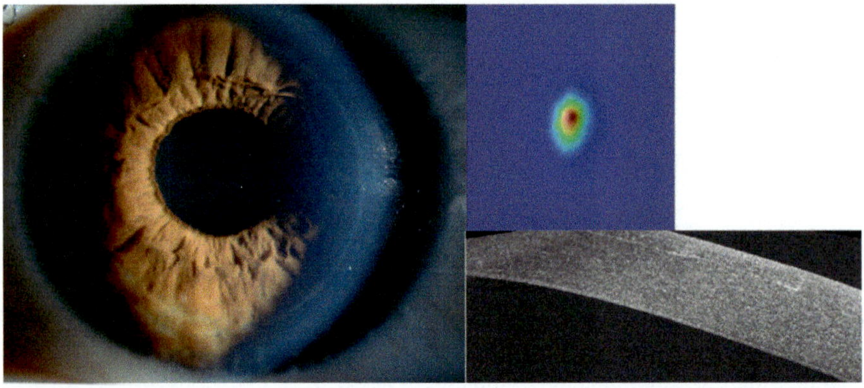

Fig. 11.1 Anterior segment photography of an eye 3 months post 130 μm SMILE procedure. Anterior segment optical coherence tomography and Optical Quality Analysis System (OQAS) (Visometrics SL, Terrassa, Barcelona) of the same eye

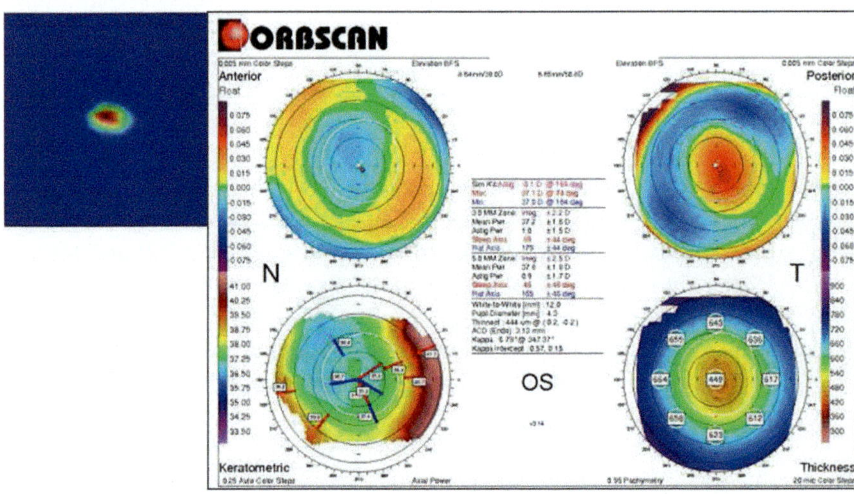

Fig. 11.2 Orbscan (Orbtek Inc./Bausch & Lomb, Tampa, FL, USA) corneal topography and OQASofoneleft eye 3 months post 140 μm SMILE procedure

We certainly had more difficulties in dissecting the stroma as deeper was the cut in some cases but not in all of them. That is why we cannot make a significant difference also in this point.

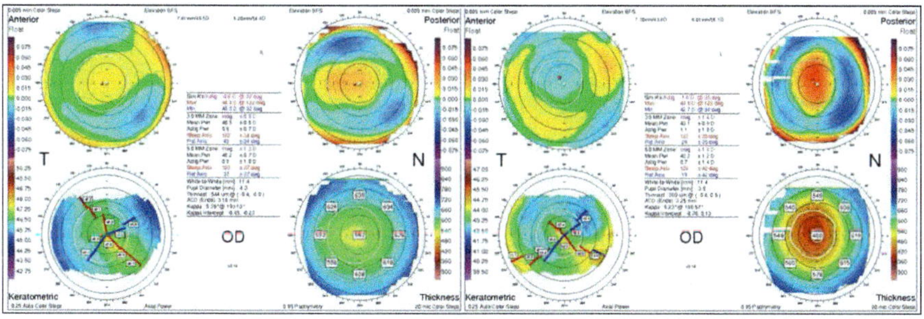

Fig. 11.3 Orbscan (Orbtek Inc./Bausch & Lomb, Tampa, FL, USA) corneal topography of one right eye pre- and 3 months post 160-μm procedure

No complications were observed during the surgery and the immediate postoperative period.

11.6 Discussion

KLEX has good refractive outcomes and other benefits such as reduction in scatter. This procedure induces fewer higher-order aberrations and exerts a minimal negative impact on the quality of the retinal image leading to good vision [4–7]. Moreover, it is less invasive and there is a reduction in postoperative irritation, less loss of corneal sensitivity, less inflammation and less impact on tear production, because the short incision cuts fewer corneal nerves (see Chaps. 2 and 3). In addition, tissue extraction is more precise and repeatable regardless of the treatment prescription. As no flap is created, there is a potential better postoperative biomechanical stability and a lesser risk of secondary corneal ectasia, due to the preservation of the anterior corneal stromal layer, which in turn preserves corneal resistance (see Chap. 14) [8–10].

Dry eye is a common complaint among patients who have undergone refractive surgery, including laser in situ keratomileusis (LASIK), photorefractive keratectomy and femtosecond LASIK whereby and the incidence of dry eye varies among these patients [8–12]. It has been reported that patients who develop dry eye after refractive surgery also have elevated risks of developing subsequent refractive regression and ocular surface damage. In addition, refractive surgery procedures also interrupt the normal organization and regeneration of the corneal nerves, which in turn lead to a prolonged reduction in corneal sensation (see Chap. 3).

A recent study added an important issue that surgery could result in dry eye symptoms, tear film instability, and decreased corneal sensitivity. Furthermore, SMILE has superiority over femto-LASIK in lower risk of postoperative corneal fluorescein staining and less reduction of corneal sensation [13]. The corneal nerve anatomy could also be taken into consideration in lenticule extraction procedures, as more superficial caps could theoretically impose more damage to the corneal nerves.

As no flap is created with SMILE technique, there is theoretically a higher postoperative biomechanical stability and a lower risk of secondary corneal ectasia due to the anatomical preservation of the anterior corneal stromal layer. The treatment is carried out under Bowman's layer, which creates greater corneal resistance. Several authors argue that—from the biomechanical point of view—in a cornea operated on by LASIK surgery, the useful corneal thickness is that of the residual stromal bed, as the flap thickness is not important when it comes to maintaining the corneal structure: corneal weakening is greater when the residual stromal thickness is thinner (the recommended residual stromal thickness is 250–300 μm) [13–15]. With the SMILE technique, this concept changes: because of the preservation of Bowman's layer a greater lenticule depth (=a thicker cap) shell go along with more corneal resistance [14, 15]. A recent, randomized prospective contralateral eye study of 34 patients compared 110-μm versus 145-μm cap thickness [16]. The authors found that thicker SMILE corneal caps showed no advantage regarding visual outcomes and higher-order aberrations, but observed that the Corvis ST biomechanical index changes at 3 months postoperative follow-up favored the deeper cap thickness, confirming that cap thickness influences postoperative biomechanical properties [16]. Another study (prospective, case–control study) reported similar findings suggesting that a 130-μm cap had advantages in terms of corneal biomechanics in comparison with 110- or 120-μm caps, without statistically significant differences in visual outcomes at 3-month follow-up [17]. However, some authors have reported conflicting results regarding corneal biomechanics and different cap thicknesses [18].

Conversely, it is possible that being deeper leads to a lower precision of the femtosecond laser cut diminishing the refractive predictability of the procedure. To overcome this possible energy loss and following discussions with the company, we decided to increase 3% of the spherical equivalent correction for every 10 μm of higher depth in relation to the 130 μm cap. That regularly meant that for all of our 160 μm depth SMILE, we were correcting 10% higher.

Despite different cap thicknesses, there were no additional complications either in regard to the surgical technique or any parameters of visual quality or refraction, safety and predictability between the 4 lenticule depth groups (130, 140, 150 and 160 μm) at the different follow-ups. This has been confirmed in several recent studies [16, 17, 19]. Importantly, more superficial caps may induce stronger wound-healing reactions compared with deeper caps, at least in eyes with thick corneas [20].

Another aim of the study was to find out if we could perform a second more superficial SMILE procedure in case of a possible retreatment. Current retreatment techniques are summarized in Chap. 12. We consider that perhaps the best option at present is to perform a thin-flap LASIK; however, conceptually, after a SMILE procedure at 160 μm depth, one could repeat SMILE at 130 μm. This concept has already been tested by our group in 2 cases of primary SMILE at 160 μm and retreatment with re-SMILE at 130 μm achieving good refractive and visual results. As a matter of fact these 2 cases showed a residual refraction of> − 1D (which in our opinion is the minimum refraction needed to perform a SMILE treatment), because we initially aimed for monovision, but the patients complained of discomfort in binocular vision (submitted for publication as case report).

Our study also confirmed the assumption that in order to obtain the same refractive results at 160 μm as compared to 130 μm it was necessary to apply an additional 10% of correction without changes in laser energy settings.

In summary, the present study shows no differences in visual acuity, refractive outcomes and optical visual quality using the 4 different cap thicknesses. Setting a primary SMILE procedure at 160 μm might lead to a better corneal stability and leave enough anterior stroma for a secondary SMILE retreatment at 130 μm or thinner.

Further, comparative studies are required to support these conclusions in order to decide the ideal depth for primary and secondary SMILE procedures.

References

1. Vestergaard A, Ivarsen A, Asp S, Hjortdal J. Femtosecond (FS) laser vision correction procedure for moderate to high myopia: a prospective study of ReLEx Flex and comparison with a retrospective study of FS-laser in situ keratomileusis. Acta Ophthalmol. 2013;91(4):355–62.
2. Verdaguer P, El-Husseiny MA, Elies D, Gris O, Manero F, Biarnés M, Güell JL. Small incision lenticule extraction (SMILE) procedure for the correction of myopia and myopic astigmatism. J Emmetropia. 2013;4:191–6.
3. Papa-Vettorazzi MR, Güell-Villanueva JL, Cruz-Rodriguez JB, Moura-Coelho N, Artells-de Jorge N, Elies-Amat D. Long-term efficacy and safety profiles following small incision lenticule extraction in eyes with ≥ 5-year follow-up. Eur J Ophthalmol. 2022;32(6):3333–9. https://doi.org/10.1177/11206721221077541 3.
4. Sekundo W, Kunert KS, Blum M. Small incision corneal refractive surgery using the small incision lenticule extraction (SMILE) procedure for the correction of myopia and myopic astigmatism: results of a 6 month prospective study. Br J Ophthalmol. 2011;95(3):335–9.
5. Vestergaard A, Ivarsen A, Asp S, Hjortdal J. ReLEx smile for moderate to high myopia: a prospective study of predictability, safety and patient satisfaction. J Cataract Refract Surg. 2012;38(11):2003–10.
6. Hjortdal J, Vestergaard AH, IvarsenA, Ragunathan S, Sven Asp. Predictors for the outcome of small incision lenticule extraction for myopia. J Refract Surg. 2012;28(12):865–71.
7. Miao H, He L, Shen Y, Li M, Yu Y, Zhou X. Optical quality and intraocular scattering after femtosecond laser small incision lenticule extraction. J Refract Surg. 2014;30(5):296–302.
8. Wu D, Wang Y, Zhang L, Wei S, Tang X. Corneal biomechanical effects: small-incision lenticule extraction versus femtosecond laser-assisted laser in situ keratomileusis. J Cataract Refract Surg. 2014;40(6):954–62.
9. Kamiya K, Shimizu K, Igarashi A, Kobashi H. Visual and refractive outcomes of femtosecond lenticule extraction and small-incision lenticule extraction for myopia. Am J Ophthalmol. 2014;157(1):128–34.
10. Gatinel D, Chaabouni S, Adam PA, Munck J, Puech M, Hoang-Xuan T. Corneal Hysteresis, resistance factor, topography, and pachymetry after corneal lamellar flap. J Refract Surg. 2007;23:76 81.
11. Chang DH, Stulting RD. Change in intraocular pressure measurements after LASIK the effect of the refractive correction and the lamellar flap. Ophthalmology. 2005;112:1009–16.

12. Ivarsen A, Asp S, Hjortdal J. Safety and complications of more than 1500 small-incision lenticule extraction procedures. Ophthalmology. 2014;121(4):822–8.
13. Li M, Zhao J, Shen Y, Li T, He L, Xu H, Yu Y, Zhou X. Comparison of dry eye and corneal sensitivity between small incision lenticule extraction and femtosecond LASIK for myopia. PLoS One. 2013;8(10).
14. Sekundo W, Gertnere J, Bertelmann T, Solomatin I. One-year refractive results, contrast sensitivity, high-order aberrations and complications after myopic small-incision lenticule extraction (ReLEx SMILE). Graefes Arch Clin Exp Ophthalmol. 2014;252(5):837–43.
15. Kamiya K, Shimizu K, Igarashi A, Kobashi H, Sato N, Ishii R. Intraindividual comparison of changes in corneal biomechanical parameters after femtosecond lenticule extraction and small-incision lenticule extraction. J Cataract Refract Surg. 2014;40(6):963–70.
16. Zarei-Ghanavati S, Jafarzadeh SV, Es'haghi A, Kiarudi MY, Hassanzadeh S, Ziaei M. Comparison of 110- And 145-μM small-incision lenticule extraction cap thickness: a randomized contralateral eye study [published online ahead of print, 2023 May 4]. Cornea. 2023;https://doi.org/10.1097/ICO.0000000000003294. https://doi.org/10.1097/ICO.0000000000003294
17. Lv X, Zhang F, Song Y, et al. Corneal biomechanical characteristics following small incision lenticule extraction for myopia and astigmatism with 3 different cap thicknesses. BMC Ophthalmol. 2023;23(1):42. Published 2023 Jan 30. https://doi.org/10.1186/s12886-023-02786-8
18. Jun I, Kang DSY, Roberts CJ, et al. Comparison of clinical and biomechanical outcomes of small incision lenticule extraction with 120- and 140-μM cap thickness. Transl Vis Sci Technol. 2021;10(8):15. https://doi.org/10.1167/tvst.10.8.15.
19. Wu D, Liu C, Li B, Wang D, Fang X. Influence of cap thickness on corneal curvature and corneal biomechanics after smile: a prospective contralateral eye study. J Refract Surg. 2020;36(2):82–8. https://doi.org/10.3928/1081597X-20191216-01.
20. Liu M, Zhou Y, Wu X, Ye T, Liu Q. Comparison of 120- and 140-μm SMILE cap thickness results in eyes with thick corneas. Cornea. 2016;35(10):1308–14. https://doi.org/10.1097/ICO.0000000000000924.

Complications During and After SMILE and Its Management Including Re-treatment Techniques

12

Rupal Shah and Walter Sekundo

Abstract

This chapter provides a comprehensive overview of potential issues encountered in small incision lenticule extraction (SMILE) surgery and the corresponding management strategies. The authors emphasize the importance of surgeon awareness regarding complications and their prevention or appropriate response. The chapter covers preoperative considerations, detailed insights into dissection-related complications, and postoperative complications. The authors provide recommendations for enhancements after SMILE, considering factors like myopic drift, over or under-correction. The chapter serves as a practical guide, aiming to offer valuable insights for surgeons dealing with SMILE procedures.

Keywords

Small incision lenticule extraction surgery (SMILE) • Pre-operative considerations • Post-operative complications

Any surgery has some potential complications. Awareness of these can help to develop strategies to avoid them or—if they happen—to react appropriately. If the surgeon is aware of potential complications and ways to mitigate them or recover

Supplementary Information The online version contains supplementary material available at https://doi.org/10.1007/978-3-031-60424-9_12.

R. Shah
New Vision Laser Centers-Centre for Sight, Mumbai, India

W. Sekundo (✉)
Department of Ophthalmology, Philipps University of Marburg, Marburg, Germany
e-mail: sekundo@med.uni-marburg.de

W. Sekundo and F. M. Wagner (eds.), *Femtosecond Laser Assisted Lenticule Extraction*,
https://doi.org/10.1007/978-3-031-60424-9_12

from them, it is easy to react quickly during and after surgery. Moreover, relative to LASIK or Femto LASIK, the SMILE procedure requires more surgical dexterity and more skill. This can lead to complications from which it is not easy to recover. In the present chapter, we give a short overview of the hitherto known complications and our subjective opinion on their management. It is obvious, that despite our best efforts, this chapter cannot raise a claim to cover all the complications or to give the best possible solutions. Rather, it should be treated as a useful practical guide and starting point. For those who are interested in exact incidence numbers, we recommend a meta-analysis by Asif et al. [1].

12.1 Preoperative Considerations for Prevention of Complication

A beginning SMILE surgeon should always start with easy cases. Those are moderate myopias between −3 and −6 D in the main meridian, relatively large corneas with white-to white of ≥ 11.9 mm and a rather small angle κ. Choose a large zone of up to 7 mm to counteract for possible minor decentrations. Allow for a large clearance zone between the lenticule and the cap of roughly 1 mm (e.g. 6.8 mm zone and 7.8 mm cap) to help with the lenticule border identification. Also avoid steep corneas with K-readings over 47 D. Choose eyes with relatively wide lid aperture. In the first cases, a large entering incision of ≥ 4 mm is acceptable. One will reduce the incision length with the increasing experience. Depending on the surgeon's hand dominance, choose the location of the incision in order to have comfortable intracorneal manipulations. For instance, for a right-handed surgeon a location at around 140° is often advantageous (40° for a left-handed surgeon).

To hold the globe, use a fine-toothed forceps with your non-dominant hand, as explained in the "Instrumentation" chapter. Use either a closed blade speculum (however, it reduces the space to approach the eye) or meticulously cover the eyelid margins including eyelashes with a sterile drape to avoid any Meibum secret spillage onto the surface. In fact, one of the authors uses an aspirating speculum in addition to draping to reduce the "lake" (particularly in deep set eyes) around the cornea, while maintaining the wet surface of the cornea during the docking process using a saturated wet sponge. For further details the reader is referred to the Chap. 5 of this book.

12.2 Intraoperative Complications

There are a number of intraoperative complications that can occur during the SMILE procedure. Some of these include:

12.2.1. A suction loss wherein the contact glass and cornea become detached during the procedure, and the procedure is then aborted by the laser

12.2.2. A poor laser cut with uncut areas, particularly in the optical zone, the so-called black spots.
12.2.3. Opaque bubble layer (OBL)
12.2.4. Obvious intraoperative decentration (≥0.6 mm)
12.2.5. Entering incision-related complications
   a. Para incisional epithelial defect
   b. Tear of the incision
   c. Cap perforation
   d. Incisional bleeding
12.2.6. Dissection-related complications
   a. Inadvertent initial dissection of the deeper plane.
   b. Incomplete removal of the lenticule or *partial lenticule tearing*
   c. Creation of a wrong deeper dissection plane (so-called via falsa) by forceful manual dissection
   d. Epithelial implantation.

In our opinion, with the exception of via *falsa* none of these are vision threatening and if managed well allow the procedure to be completed or converted to another laser vision correction (LVC) surgery with a satisfactory result.

12.2.1 Suction Loss Wherein the Contact Glass and the Cornea Become Detached During the Laser Firing Procedure

This can happen due to several reasons.:

a. Most commonly, the patient squeezes the eye or moves suddenly.
b. There could be fluid ingress between the suction ports of the contact glass and the cornea.
c. Gas bubble migration and subsequent compressive forces against the contact glass.

In this situation, the VisuMax® automatically goes into a specific mode, based on the stage of the procedure at which the suction loss occurred. The below described management is based on SMILE lenticule geometry with a refractive bottom cut and surface parallel upper cut (see Chap. 1 for details).

In case the suction loss occurs during the *first pass* of the laser (i.e. the pass which defines the posterior surface of the lenticule), the user is not given the option to complete the procedure and is asked to convert the procedure into a Femto LASIK or PRK procedure, unless the initial cut is less than 10% (then the wizard will suggest to immediately restart) The user can convert the procedure in the same surgical session, if the patient is not too nervous (Video 1). In our experience, it is safer to postpone the procedure for a few minutes or days and then complete the procedure from scratch (Video 2). However, if one decides to redo SMILE, a different depth of the lenticule's bottom may be considered in order to avoid entering of the old incision. This measure is important, since one does not want the existing cleavage plane to interact with the new cleavage plane being created for the posterior surface of the lenticule in an unpredictable fashion. The decision to go deeper or shallower as the initial plane depends on following parameters: (1) Cap thickness, (2) Total corneal thickness, and (3) the magnitude of correction = the depth of the refractive cut. It is considered safe to redo the cut placing the new cut either 30 μm above or below the aborted cleavage plane. For instance in a thick cap SMILE (cap ≥ 140 μm) the surgeon can re-program the same refraction with a 105–110 μm cap. In primary thin caps of 110–120 μm, one can re-program the laser with a new cap of 150 μm only if the residual stromal thickness (RST) is at least 280 μm (some surgeons would except 250 μm RST despite a slightly higher risk of keratectasia).

If the suction loss occurs at any other stage during the laser firing procedure, the laser allows the option of completing the procedure in the same surgical session after re-docking of the contact glass (Videos 3 and 4). The general challenge in this situation is re-docking of the contact glass interface to the eye, while still retaining the original centration. This is because the pupil is obscured by the gas bubbles from the earlier pass(es). It is preferable to use the same contact glass, so that the foot prints of the contact glass match. Proper centration during re-docking is extremely important. Once re-docking is completed, depending on the stage at which suction loss occurs, the laser repeats both femtosecond passes, only the "cap" pass or only the side cut incision. The laser wizard assists you in the choice of the cap diameter. In fact, it is prudent to choose a larger then initial cap: in case of cap decentration related to the lenticule one would still have enough clearance for dissection. The lenticule separation and removal is then carried out as usual.

If the main reason for suction loss is an extremely poor patient's compliance with no hope for compliance's improvement, an ICL implantation under general anaesthesia might be a safer solution.

12.2.2 Black Spots

Black spots are seen best in the infrared cutting mode. In reality "black spots" are areas of poor or non-existing laser cut (Fig. 12.1a, b). In the vast majority of cases, black spots occur when the laser optical path is hindered by non-transparent obstacles. These are: Meibum secretion from the eyelids, cotton fibre from the surgical cover or dry areas of the applanated cornea. In rare instances of very low energy black spots appear as small snake-like spots. If the uncut areas are small and not located in the central optical zone, a thorough dissection usually leads to a satisfactory result. However, in large and/or central "black spots" forceful dissection might lead to stromal scarring and/or uneven cleavage plane resulting in poor outcomes. In these circumstances, the case should be aborted and converted to PRK/Femto-Lasik/ SMILE at a different level.

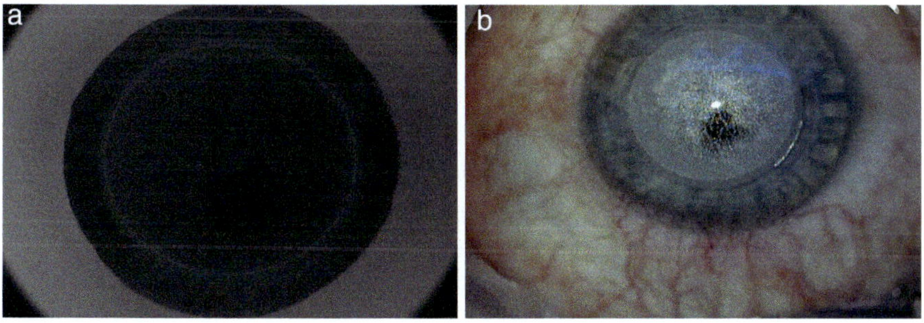

Fig. 12.1 **a** "Black spot" is seen in this infrared image. **b** After the release of suction the "black spot" is seen as an uncut area of cornea with no gas bubbles at all. The surgery was aborted and converted to Femto LASIK at a later stage

12.2.3 Opaque Bubble Layer (OBL)

The opaque bubble layer (OBL) is usually a consequence of too high energy leading to expandable gas bubbles. Chapter 6 provides an in-depth explanation and tips of laser energy adjustment as does Chap. 10 of this book. A successful dissection can be achieved even in presence of OBL, but it tends to be more forceful. While midperipheral or peripheral OBLs can be dissected without great fear of stromal damage, it might be prudent to abort the procedure if prominent OBLs are present over the central pupil. The choice of instruments is also important. Usually blunt dissectors such as Chansue, Reinstein, or Sekundo dissectors are good instruments even in moderate OBL. However, when the stromal adherence is quite strong, the original semi-sharp dissectors, such as "Blum Spoon", are very helpful rescue instruments (see Chap. 5 for details and photographs).

12.2.4 Intraoperative Decentration

Sometimes the anatomy of the eye or the cornea or very poor compliance (Bell's phenomenon) creates obstacles to apply suction at the desired centration. The VisuMax 800 with its centration tool displays different colours, which are wonderfully appreciated in infrared mode: as long as the centration spot turns blue the centration is adequate. With the VisuMax 500, the surgeon has to judge the centration prior to pushing the pedal (see also Chap. 15). If there is a decentration over 0.6 mm, one should either re-centre or abort the procedure. In those cases, a Femto LASIK with an active eye tracker might be a safer option.

12.2.5 Entering Incision-Related Complications

(a) *Para-incisional epithelial defect* happens usually during the dissection of the lenticule by pushing the shaft of the dissector against the epithelium. The best way to reduce the incidence is to adequately wet the surface of the cornea before entering the intrastromal space. Basement membrane dystrophy and older patient's age predispose to epithelial defects. If the epithelium is fairly loos and a defect happens, one should try not to go in and out, but rather stay with the dissector intrastromally because of the increased probability of epithelial implantation. Once the dissection has been completed, one would readjust the epithelium and place a bandage contact lens. Alternatively, if the epithelium is very loose, it may be a good idea to carefully remove the juxta-incisional epithelium to prevent ingrowth and place a bandage contact lens (BCL) (Fig. 12.2). Particularly in larger defects there is a high chance of developing localized DLK. To reduce the risk of DLK, we advise the patients to double the frequency of topical steroid drops on the day of surgery.

(b) *Tear of the incision* happens more frequently with very small incisions. It is important to consider the entering incision size in accordance with the cap diameter, as large diameter lenticules and caps require more lateral movements. As a rule of thumb a 2 mm, incision is well situated for the lenticle/cap combination 6.0/7.0 mm. In contrast, in a 7.0/7.9 mm combination, an entering incision of 3 mm is in our opinion a better choice. Other factors are the thickness of the cap: in thinner caps of 100–110 μm a tear along the incision is in our hands more frequent compared to 130 or 140 μm cap. In the vast majority of cases, a tear along the border of the cap does not create any problems. It is re-adapted in the same way as the laser pre-cut incision, even without the need for a bandage contact lens. A radial tear can develop when the eye jerks while the dissector is in the pocket. The surgeon would carefully readapt the torn cap and place a BCL. The visual result will remain favourable as long as the optical axis is not affected. However, this complication can be

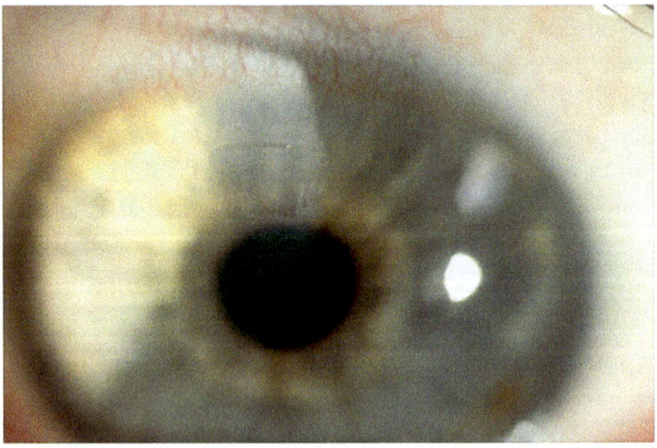

Fig. 12.2 Epithelial abrasion around the entering incision as shown in this example is usually fully epithelialized within 24 h. However, the surgeon should carefully observe the interface for the development of localized DLK and increase topical steroids, if necessary

effectively prevented, when the surgeon uses bimanual technique firmly taking control of the globe by holding it with the non-dominant hand using a fine-toothed forceps (see chapter "Instrumentation").

(c) *Cap perforation* can happen due to a forceful dissection in the area of poor laser cut ("black spot"). Again, adjusting the bits back to their anatomical location using fine spear sponges and placing a BCL is all one can do. Topical steroids are increased and tapered off over a period of 1–3 months. If no scarring occur, the visual outcome remains quite good. If the vision remains poor even after 1 year a topography and OCT-guided surgical intervention is warranted (see Chap. 13). As an *ultima ratio,* a superficial lamellar keratoplasty might elevate the symptoms.

(d) *Incisional bleeding* is less common then with Lasik flaps, since SMILE caps are usually smaller. Still, in small corneas or in extensively large caps (such as in hyperopic SMILE, see Chap. 9) a bleeding can occur. Thoroughly rinse the interface with BSS and press a sponge onto the bleeding site. A sponge soaked in a local anaesthetic provides some additional help due to pharmacological constriction of the vessels. Particularly, if there is an influx of blood into the pocket (which needs to be prevented) push the sponge as long as necessary on the incision (sometimes up to 2–5 min). Afterward, apply a BCL and increase the frequency of preservative-free steroid drops to prevent DLK.

12.2.6 Dissection-Related Complications

(a) *Inadvertent initial dissection of the deeper plane* represents a notable challenge. This complication arises when, in the first step of the lenticule separation procedure, the surgeon unintentionally selects the wrong plane while attempting to separate the anterior lenticule surface from the overlying cornea. Consequently, this leads to the separation of the posterior part of the lenticule instead. In this scenario, the lenticule adheres to the underside of the cap rather than lying on the stromal bed, presenting a significant surgical challenge. The absence of the posterior cornea's anchoring complicates the entry into the anterior cleavage plane for lenticule separation. However, once this issue is identified, lenticule separation and removal are still feasible. Our preferred method involves using the hook end of the double-sided dissector to gently scrape a small edge of the lenticule from the anterior cap, employing an upward twisting motion along the clearance corridor. Once a small edge is accessible, it is grasped with ultrafine forceps, such as Shah SMILE forceps (refer to the chapter "Instrumentation"), to hold and peel off more of the lenticule. When enough space is created, a separation spatula is used to dissect and remove the lenticule in the standard manner. If the initial incision is too narrow, it may be widened slightly along the cap border using a preset diamond knife or an MVR-blade. Notably, the Mehta group in Singapore developed specific rescue instruments to address this complication (also see Chap. 5). These tools, including a rake, wedge, or hook, enable the surgeon

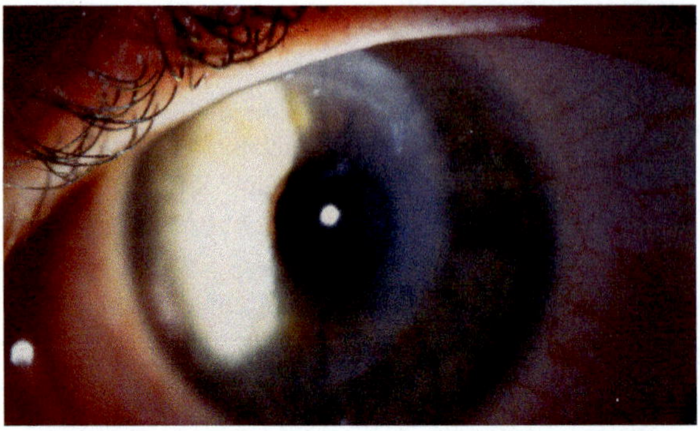

Fig. 12.3 Typical tear along the border of the cap. No problems are anticipated in such a case

to approach the lenticule's edge at the inferior part of the cornea, facilitating separation from that end and progressively removing the lenticule along its entire circumferential edge. (Videos 5, 6, 7)

(b) *Incomplete removal of the lenticule or partial lenticule tearing* can arise, particularly with thin lenticules or suboptimal laser separation. Surgeons might inadvertently leave behind remnants of the lenticule, especially at the edges. Utilizing specialized dissectors designed for backward cutting (see Fig. 12.3, Chap. 5) significantly reduces this risk. Remaining lenticule portions can lead to irregular astigmatism and unsatisfactory results. Therefore, ensuring complete separation in the initial attempt is crucial. The spatula/dissector should be used to fully detach the lenticule from both surfaces along the entire circumference. Attempting only partial separation before using forceps to grasp and pull at unseparated sections heightens the risk of lenticule tearing and residual tags. If there is any doubt about lenticule integrity or remaining tags, it is advisable to unroll the lenticule on the corneal epithelial surface post-removal and verify if its size corresponds with the original laser separation diameter. Should suspicions of leftover lenticule tags persist, subsequent dissection to remove them is possible. Depending on the size of the remaining lenticule, discernible through OCT scans of the cornea, three approaches are available:

1. Re-enter through the same incision site to remove the tags.
2. Create an additional entry incision adjacent to the tag using CIRCLE software.
3. Convert the cap into a flap with CIRCLE software and remove the remnants in an "open sky" manner.

(c) *Creation of a wrong deeper dissection plane (so-called* via *falsa) by forceful manual dissection* of the wrong plane deeper than the cleavage plane created by the laser. This extremely rare complication was referred to us twice for a second opinion. In both cases the surgeon was novel to the procedure. This complication, in our view, is a result of a totally improper handling of the tissue. Little resistance to the dissection spatula is normal. However, if the surgeon encounters sever resistance reminiscent of lamellar keratoplasty, the procedure should be abandoned, and no tissue removed from within the cornea.

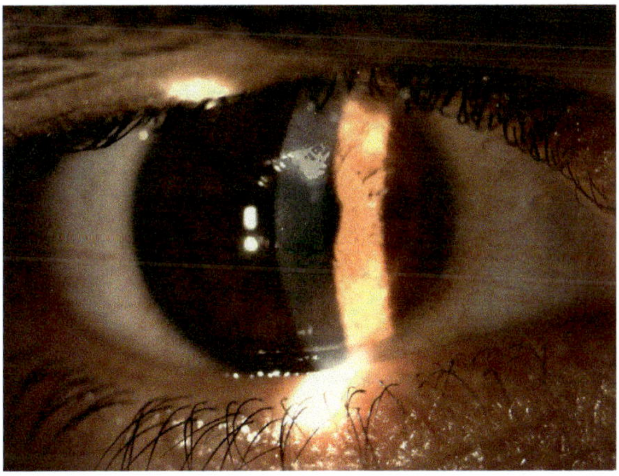

Fig. 12.4 Prominent area of progressive epithelial ingrowth encroaching the visual axis and also clearly seen as anterior elevation on topography. Such an epithelial nest must be removed swiftly, the interface flushed and the entering incision temporally closed by a 10.0 Nylon suture

Otherwise a permanent damage will occur, relievable only by an anterior or deep anterior lamellar keratoplasty.

(d) *Epithelial implantation* is a result of loose and/or dry epithelium brought inside the pocket by the dissecting instrument. If encountered during slit-lamp examination immediately after surgery the epithelium needs to be flushed out right away. If the original incision appears to have a gap, an additional placement of a 10.0 cross-stich suture might be required.

12.3 Post-operative Complications After SMILE

12.3.1 Epithelial Ingrowth

Sometimes epithelial ingrowth can be observed, after SMILE. Unlike with LASIK, where ablation of the hinge can sometimes result in a path for the epithelium to encroach under the flap, in SMILE, it is usually an isolated nest of cells (Fig. 12.4). They can either be left alone, if the nest is silent, or it can be scraped off by entering with an epithelial scraper from the original incision. While some surgeons advocate Nd:YAG laser treatment of the nest, the authors prefer surgical removal either by scraping or by scraping followed by flashing. If two small incisions are in place and the nest is quite central, a bimanual irrigation-aspiration set (as used for cortex removal in cataract surgery) can prove useful. The often forgotten trick, however, is to close the entering incision gap either by a 10.0 Nylon stich for 1–2 weeks or by using corneal glue to prevent the ingrowth recurrence.

12.3.2 Irregular Astigmatism Consequent to Decentration

Sometimes, if the docking procedure is not correct, it can result in decentration of the treatment and consequent irregular astigmatism and/or induction of aberrations, such as coma. In our opinion, it is best to prevent this complication. Following the proper docking procedure is essential. We also find it useful to switch to infrared illumination for a brief period after docking (and before initiating the laser pass), to verify that the pupil dilates around the centre of the contact glass. In case decentration occurs, and it is visually significant, then it is best to perform a topography guided excimer laser correction using PRK with mitomycin C, keeping in mind the cap thickness and epithelial map. An in-detail guide to the treatment of irregular corneas is given in the following chapter by Reinstein et al.

12.3.3 Other Post-operative Complications

a. In some cases, a fine *scarring* is observed at the cap edge or the lenticule edge. However, this is outside the pupillary zone and is visually non-significant.
b. Some patients, especially chronic contact lens users before the procedure, experience dry eyes after the procedure. Fortunately the *dry eye problem* is less severe in SMILE compared to LASIK or PRK. However, even with SMILE in larger corrections neurotrophic keratopathy can persist for a long time. The treatment is directed at the main cause of the problem. Lubricants, eye lid scrubs (manual and mechanical), Cyclosporin A eye drops, intense pulse light therapy (IPL), punctum plugs (temporary and permanent), and even autologous serum eye drops are used depending on the type of dry eye (evaporative; blepharitis; purely neutrotrophic)
c. We have noted a few instances of fine interface haze occurring several months post-procedure, which in the majority of cases does not significantly impact vision. The haze is sometimes associated with the difficulty of dissection. As a result, some surgeons opt to extend and intensify their steroid treatment following challenging dissections. In cases where a prolonged course of topical steroids is necessary, it is advisable to select agents with lower IOP-inducing potential, such as fluorometholone or loteprednol etabonate drops. Regular monitoring of intraocular pressure (IOP) is essential in these situations. If a prolonged steroid regimen is not preferred, for instance in patients who are steroid responders, administering 1% Cyclosporin A (CSA) eye drops twice daily for several months can be effective in mitigating the haze.
d. Due to a geometrical mismatch between the undersurface of the cap and the stromal bed after lenticule removal, some microstriae, named "*Bowman's layer microdistortions*" (BLMD), have been described particularly after highly myopic SMILE [2] (Fig. 12.5). In the majority of cases, these microfolds are smoothed out by the epithelium as time goes by. If desired, an early intervention with pressurized flushing of the pocket can be attempted (B.Meyer, personal communication). Prior to such radical measures, an anterior high-resolution OCT scan is of value. To prevent visually significant folds in the optical zone, one is advised to gently massage the cap centrifugally as suggested by Reinstein et al. [3].

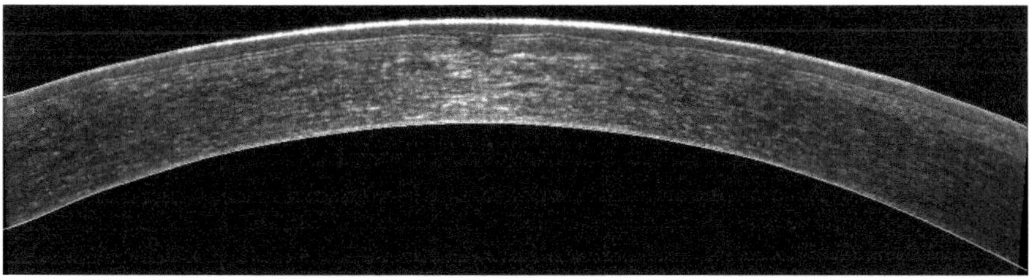

Fig. 12.5 High resolution corneal OCT (Optovue Inc., USA) depicts fine undulations of Bowman's layer centrally following a high myopic correction. These so called Bowman's Layer Microdistorsions (BMLD) are smoothened by the overlaying hyperplastic epithelium

e. Unlike in FS-Lasik surgery sterile keratitis, also called *diffuse lamellar keratitis* (DLK) is rare after SMILE. But sterale inflammation has been observed after the procedure, especially if
   - the energy settings of the laser are too high, or
   - one has a large periincisional epithelial abrasion (Fig. 12.2) or even an intraoperative epithelial slough off (usually in eyes with epithelial basement membrane dystrophy) or
   - some debris were left behind in the pocket.

Usually this resolves on frequent topical steroids such as prednisolone acetate that can be augmented by oral steroids with no visual significance. Only if the DLK progresses from stage 2 to stage 3, the interface flushing with preservative-free steroids becomes necessary. An exception is a secondary interlamellar keratitis due to steroid-induced IOP rise. Here, flushing of the pocket, discontinuation of steroids, and temporary antiglaucomatous drugs will resolve the problem.

(a) *Infection*, like with any other procedure, can also occur and spread rapidly because of the pocket. Any intra-pocket infection is best managed by pocket flushing and drug injection into the interface along with microbiological cultures.
(b) Lastly, like any corneal subtraction procedure, there is also risk of *Corneal Ectasia*. The reader is referred to the Chap. 20 on corneal ectasia by Wagner & Sekundo in this book.

12.4 Enhancements After SMILE

Similar to other refractive surgery procedures, there is sometimes a need for enhancements following the initial operation. This can be because of a myopic drift several years after the procedure, or because of a primary over or under correction. This presents a peculiar problem after the SMILE procedure, because it does not offer the chance of lifting the flap and performing excimer laser reshaping, which is relatively easy after LASIK. Enhancements after SMILE can be accomplished by.

- using excimer laser PRK, however, additional use of Mitomycin C is recommended, even in very small corrections to prevent haze formation [4].
- The "CIRCLE" software was developed to convert the original SMILE cap into a complete flap, with a hinge and a 270–330 degree side cut incision. In the CIRCLE procedure, the femtosecond laser is used to create a) an incision plane encircling the original "cap" cut as a lamellar ring and b) a side cut with hinge around the new incision plane and c) a "junction cut" which allows the original "cap" and the new incision plane to be part of one larger surface. (Fig. 12.6). In our own clinical experience, the CIRCLE software is easy to use and reliably creates flaps which can be lifted easily to perform excimer laser reshaping. The mid-term clinical outcomes are similar for both the PRK with MMC and conversion to Femto LASIK by CIRCLE procedure [4]. However, creating a flap substantially reduces the biomechanical strength of the cornea (**Video 8**) [5].

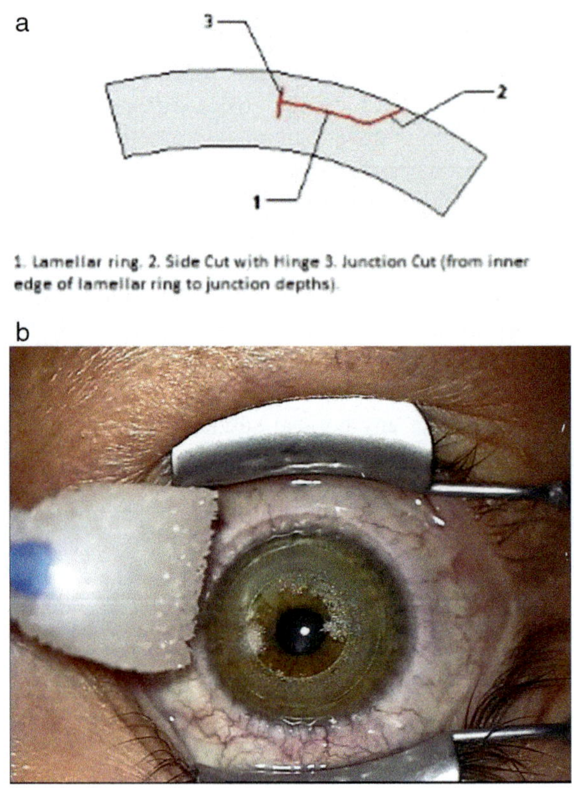

Fig. 12.6 **a** Diagram of the CIRCLE cut. The laser creates a lamellar ring (1) with a typical flap side cut (2) and a hinge located away from the original SMILE incision. The junction cut goes 10 μm above and below the original interface to get a smooth entry into the old SMILE pocket.
b Intraoperative view of the CIRCLE procedure with a ring of bubbles reaching the old interface. The hinge of this new 8.7 mm flap is at 12 o'clock, while the old SMILE incision of the 7.5 mm cap was at 9 o'clock

- For mixed residual astigmatism, a paired limbal relaxing incisions (LRI) or even astigmatic keratotomy (AK) at the 9 mm zone provide an inexpensive and fast way to resolve the problem. Although there is a negative impact on corneal biomechanics (depending on the zone used and the extent of the vertical relaxing incisions), the visual recovery is extremely fast, and the post-operative comfort is excellent. One of the authors (WS) favours LRI for residual manifest refractive (not topographical) astigmatism up to 1.5 D cyl. The aim is to get the refractive cylinder $\leq$ 0.5 D cyl. A guarded diamond knife or a single use pre-set knife can be used. If available, femtosecond laser AKs are a more sophisticated and expensive option. The surgeon can use the nomogram he is most familiar with. The nomograms exist both, as printed tables and as online applications (e.g. www.lricalculator.com, www.eyelri.com, www.lricalc.com)
- The authors do not have experience with thin flap Femto LASIK in the cap or a second SMILE in a thick cap or below the original incision for performing enhancements, though some surgeons have done this successfully. The prerequisites is a fairly thick cap, preferably of not less than 135 μm. In that case, a 100 μm flap can be cut above the cap [6]. The rational of this procedure is to have the comfort of flap-based surgery while less affecting the biomechanics of the cornea than in the CIRCLE procedure.
- A "capless" SMILE (also called "SMILE after SMILE" or "Sub-Cap-SMILE") was proposed by Donate and Thaëron as early as 2015 [7]. This method only creates a lenticule base and the edge cut. The operator then stops the laser process. The old interface forms the "roof" of the lenticule. The new lenticule is removed through the original small incision. The procedure is an elegant off-label method for higher corrections of at least 1 D. However, with the high precision of nowadays SMILE regressions or undercorrections of 1 D or even higher are extremely rare. The usual enhancements range between 0.5 and 1.0 D. Such small corrections can be done when the lenticule is extra "thickened" in order to have enough tissue for the extraction. As a result, the tissue consumption is usually at least 20 μm higher than necessary. In addition, the procedure is surgically challenging and only applies to myopic corrections. Particularly with the VisuMax 500 to achieve the same centration as with the initial procedure is an issue. Therefore, the diameter of the second lenticule is usually smaller compared to the first SMILE. With the introduction of the VisuMax 800 this problem can be addressed by its CetraLign tool, though. The advantage is the retention of a flapless procedure with a high level of comfort and almost unchanged biomechanics [5]. In addition, Riau et al demonstrated the lowest level of inflammation with the sub-cap SMILE in comparison with excimer-based enhancement procedures [8].

Financial Disclosure The authors are consultants for Carl Zeiss Meditec AG.

References

1. Asif MI, Bafna RK, Mehta JS, Reddy J, Titiyal JS, Maharana PK, Sharma N. Complications of small incisions lenticule extraction. Indian J Ophthalmol. 2020;68(12):2711–22.
2. Yao P, Zhou J, Meiyan L, Shen Y, Dong Z, Zhou X. Microdistortions in bowman's layer following femtosecond laser small incision lenticule extraction observed by fourier-domain OCT. J Refract Surg. 2013;29(10):668–74.
3. Reinstein DZ, Archer TJ, Gobbe M. Small incision lenticule extraction (SMILE). History, fundamentals of a new refractive surgery technique and clinical outcomes. Eye and Vision.2014;1:3.
4. Siedlecki J, Siedlecki J, Luft N, Kook D, Meyer B, Bechmann M, Wiltfang R, Sekundo W, Pringlinger SG, Dirisamer M. Surface ablation versus CIRCLE for myopic enhancement after SMILE: a matched comparative study. J Refract Surg. 2019;35:294–300.
5. Kling S, Spiru B, Hafezi F, Sekundo W. Biomechanical weakening of different re-treatment options after small incision lenticule extraction (SMILE). J Refract Surg. 2017;33(3):193–8.
6. Reinstein DZ, Carp GI, Archer TJ, Vida RS. Outcomes of re-treatment by LASIK after SMILE. J Refract Surg. 2018;24:578–88.
7. Donate D, Thaëron R. Preliminary Evidence of successful enhancement after a primary SMILE procedure with the Sub-Cap-Lenticule Extraction technique. J Refract Surg. 2015;31:708–10.
8. Riau AK, Liu YC, Lim CHL, Lwin NC, Teo EP, Yam HG, Tan DT, Mehta JS. Retreatment strategies following SMILE: In vivo tissue response. PLoS One 2017;14:12(7).

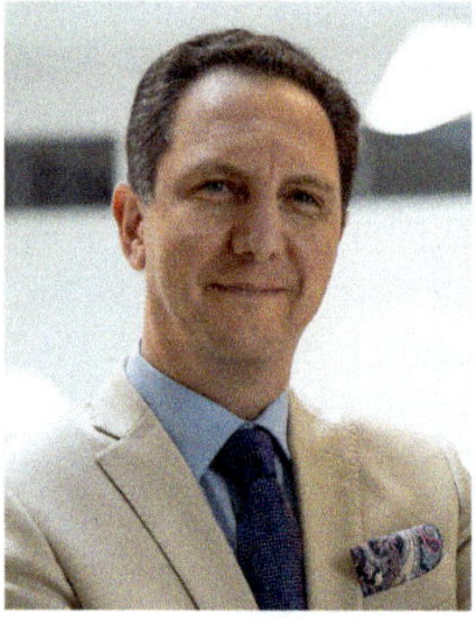

Walter Sekundo MD, PhD is Professor and Chairman, Department of Ophthalmology, Philipps University of Marburg, Germany. He studied Medicine in Frankfurt (Germany), New Orleans and Durham (US). He was a resident at the University of Bonn in Germany and a Fellow in Corneal and Refractive surgery at Moorfields Eyes Hospital and Ocular Pathology at the University of Glasgow in UK. He received his vitreoretinal training in Marburg and glaucoma training in Mainz (Germany). He also holds a degree of "Health Care Manager" from the Faculty of Economics in Marburg. Prof. Sekundo has published 200+ original papers, over 50 book chapters and edited the first international book on SMILE surgery. He gave countless presentations at national and international meetings. He is a reviewer for 21 Ophthalmic Journals and a Board Member of "Die Ophthalmologie". Prof. Sekundo is a busy surgeon with over 30,000 procedures in the anterior and posterior segment and has been repeatedly named as one of the 30 top refractive and cataract surgeons in Germany. Together with Marcus Blum he largely contributed to the development of KLEx. In fact, he was the first surgeon in the world who performed FLEx and SMILE. He received several prestigious prizes for the contribution to the field of ophthalmic surgery. In the last 25 years his research has been focused on corneal, cataract and refractive surgery.

Therapeutic Excimer Laser-Based Surgery for SMILE Complications

13

Dan Z. Reinstein and Timothy J. Archer

Abstract

In this chapter, we describe the diagnostic approach in cases of irregular astigmatism using front surface corneal topography and epithelial thickness mapping. Topography-guided custom ablation is an appropriate, safe and effective method for the treatment of global irregularities such as a zone enlargement or decentration. In cases of irregularly irregular astigmatism with localised irregularities, the natural compensatory mechanism of epithelial remodelling acts to mask a proportion of the stromal surface irregularity from front surface corneal topography. In these cases, the more appropriate and effective treatment is a trans-epithelial phototherapeutic keratectomy (PTK), which uses the epithelium as a natural masking agent to target the ablation onto the raised areas of stroma where the epithelium is thinnest.

Keywords

Irregular astigmatism • Therapeutic excimer laser-based surgery • Small incision lenticule extraction surgery (SMILE) • Topography-guided • Trans-epithelial phototherapeutic keratectomy (PTK) • Front surface corneal topography • Epithelial thickness mapping • Custom ablation

D. Z. Reinstein (✉) · T. J. Archer
London Vision Clinic, 138 Harley Street, London W1G 7LA, UK
e-mail: dzr@londonvisionclinic.com

D. Z. Reinstein
Department of Ophthalmology, Columbia University Medical Center, New York, NY, USA

Sorbonne Université, Paris, France

Biomedical Science Research Institute, University of Ulster, Coleraine, UK

W. Sekundo and F. M. Wagner (eds.), *Femtosecond Laser Assisted Lenticule Extraction*,
https://doi.org/10.1007/978-3-031-60424-9_13

13.1 Introduction

In this chapter, we describe the diagnostic approach in cases of irregular astigmatism using front surface corneal topography and epithelial thickness mapping. Topography-guided custom ablation is an appropriate, safe, and effective method for the treatment of global irregularities such as a zone enlargement or decentration. In cases of irregularly irregular astigmatism with localized irregularities, the natural compensatory mechanism of epithelial remodeling acts to mask a proportion of the stromal surface irregularity from front surface corneal topography. In these cases, the more appropriate and effective treatment is a trans-epithelial phototherapeutic keratectomy (PTK), which uses the epithelium as a natural masking agent to target the ablation onto the raised areas of stroma where the epithelium is thinnest.

13.2 Diagnosis of Irregularly Irregular Astigmatism

Visual symptoms such as reduced CDVA and contrast sensitivity, halos and starbursts, ghosting, and diplopia after corneal refractive surgery are usually found to be caused by irregular astigmatism. Irregular astigmatism can be classified in two categories: *regularly* irregular astigmatism and *irregularly* irregular astigmatism. The main examples of regularly irregular astigmatism are high spherical aberration (i.e., a small achieved optical zone) and decentration. In these situations, there is effectively one large 'global' irregularity, but the topographic optical zone is otherwise symmetrical and round. On the other hand, in cases of irregularly irregular astigmatism, irregularities are localized to small regions resulting in an asymmetric or distorted topography and often within the boundary of the optical zone.

The most important aspect of treating complications is to first make a confident diagnosis of the problem since some treatment options could actually be detrimental in certain circumstances. The introduction of custom ablation based on either topography or wavefront promised to be the answer to postop complications. However, neither topography nor wavefront can measure the true source of the irregularity, the stromal surface. The natural compensatory mechanism of epithelial remodeling acts to mask a proportion of the stromal surface irregularity from front surface corneal topography (or from the wavefront) [1–5]. If there is irregular astigmatism on the topography, then by definition there will be irregular epithelium; the epithelium overlying bumps in the stromal surface becomes progressively thinner, and the epithelium overlying troughs in the stromal surface become progressively thicker. Further, the amount of epithelial remodeling has been shown to be correlated to the local curvature gradient of the stromal surface, with greater epithelial compensation for more localized irregularities [1, 6–8]. In 1994, we summarized this phenomenon in the Law of Epithelial Compensation for irregular astigmatism: 'Irregular astigmatism results in irregular epithelium [9].'

Therefore, in cases of local irregularities (irregularly irregular astigmatism) the majority of the stromal irregularity will be masked from topography by epithelial remodeling. In contrast, the stromal curvature gradient is more gradual for global irregularities, which reduces the amount of compensatory epithelial remodeling such that the majority of the stromal irregularity will be detectable on front surface corneal topography. Therefore, a topography-guided treatment can only be expected to be effective when used to treat global irregularities and minimally effective in irregularly irregular astigmatism—which is exactly what has been reported for topography-guided custom ablation[10]. In some cases of irregularly irregular astigmatism, a topography-guided treatment can even make the irregularity worse [1, 2, 4].

For this reason, an epithelial thickness profile is vital for an accurate diagnosis in cases of irregular astigmatism. In cases with localized irregularities where the epithelium has compensated for the majority of the irregularity, a different treatment option is required. Trans-epithelial PTK offers a solution by using the epithelium as a natural masking agent to focus the ablation onto the relative peaks in the stromal surface.

Thus, the decision process (Fig. 13.1) for irregular astigmatism can be summarized as:

- 'Global' regularly irregular astigmatism—dominant irregularity on topography – topography-guided custom ablation
- 'Local' irregularly irregular astigmatism—dominant irregularity masked by epithelium – trans-epithelial PTK

13.3 Topography-Guided Custom Ablation

Since the introduction of topography-guided custom ablation in the late 1990s, [11, 12] most modern excimer laser platforms include a topography-guided option [10, 13–15]. As described above, topography-guided custom ablation has proved to be very effective for treating global irregularities such as small optical zone and decentration.

13.3.1 Topography-Guided Treatment Planning

Topography-guided algorithms import the front surface corneal topography and calculate the ablation profile that would result in a smooth aspheric surface with a large optical zone. Our experience is with the Carl Zeiss Meditec topography-guided option, which is part of the CRS-Master software and can be used with the MEL 80 or MEL 90 excimer lasers. The CRS-Master is linked to the Atlas Placido topographer, which remains one of the most reliable Placido topography systems [16, 17].

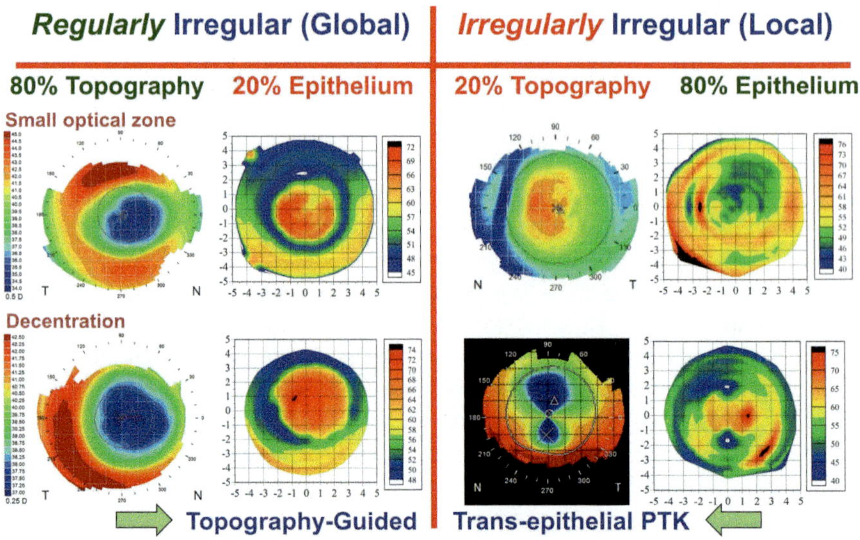

Fig. 13.1 Diagram outlining the decision process for choosing the appropriate therapeutic treatment type for an eye that presents with irregular astigmatism after corneal laser refractive surgery. Topography-guided treatment is more effective for 'global' irregularities such as small optical zones and decentration where the majority of the irregularity is on the topography. On the other hand, if there is irregularly irregular astigmatism, characterized by local irregularities, a significant proportion will have been compensated for by epithelial remodeling. Therefore, trans-epithelial PTK is a more effective treatment in these cases than topography-guided custom ablation. Reproduced with permission from Reinstein DZ, Archer TJ, Carp GI. The Surgeon's Guide to SMILE. SLACK Inc, 2018

When performing a topography-guided treatment, the most important part is the planning—of which, the most important part is the topography acquisition. The efficacy of the treatment depends entirely in the quality and reliability of the topography exam that the treatment was based on. The following factors should be considered when obtaining the topography scan:

- Ensure that the scans are well focused—in most topographers, focusing is determined by the focusing ring being equidistant from the adjacent rings (Fig. 13.2).
- Ensure that the scans are well centered—refer to the eye image to check that the patient was fixating on the target, although it can still be very difficult to detect a patient with poor fixation (Fig. 13.2).
- Carefully review the quality of the mires rings to check for any distortion due to tear film discontinuities—use artificial tear drops if the mires rings are consistently poor quality (Fig. 13.3 shows some examples of topography scans on the same eye being distorted by the tear film).
- Select the scan with the largest area of continuous data—superior data is often obstructed by the eyelashes, which can be resolved by holding the upper the

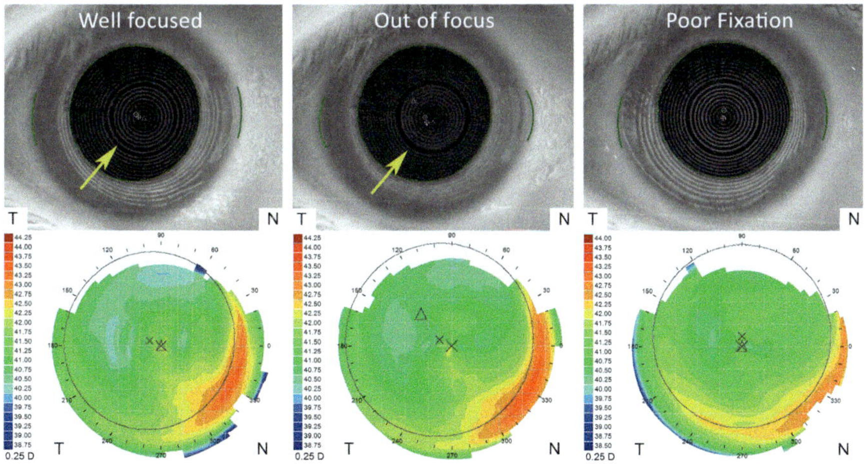

Fig. 13.2 When obtaining a topography scan, it is important to ensure that the system was well focused (left), indicated by the focusing ring being equidistant from the adjacent rings (yellow arrows). If the scan is out of focus (middle), this can lead to an inaccurate and unreliable measurement. The second factor that can affect the quality of a topography scan is the patient's fixation, as this can cause a significant error if the patient is not fixating properly on the target, particularly in an eye with irregular astigmatism. However, this can be very difficult to detect as demonstrated by this example (right)—there is no obvious sign that the patient was fixating on the target in the left image, whereas the patient was looking off to the side in the right image. Reproduced with permission from Reinstein DZ, Archer TJ, Carp GI. The Surgeon's Guide to SMILE. SLACK Inc, 2018

eyelid or tilting the patients head slightly upwards—we find that asking patients to rest their chin on *top* of the chinrest is very effective in exposing the superior cornea. Figure 13.4 shows an example of before and after changing the patient's chin position.

- Obtain numerous scans to verify that the irregularity is repeatable (Fig. 13.5).
- Ensure that the data are continuous—discard scans with patches of missing data as these can be misinterpreted by the algorithm, often presenting as 'spikes' in the ablation profile (Fig. 13.6).
- The final exam selection for treatment must be done personally by the surgeon.
- The surgeon should also carefully review the final ablation profile to confirm that it makes sense in the context of the topography and other diagnostic data available.

The CRS-Master allows for simultaneous correction of topographical irregularities (higher order aberrations) and control of sphere and cylinder (lower order aberrations). The algorithm uses corneal elevation and wavefront data to calculate the refractive effect due to the intended change in topography, which is combined with the manifest refraction to derive the final refractive correction. The user also has the 'topography-smooth' option to address only the corneal irregularity, leaving

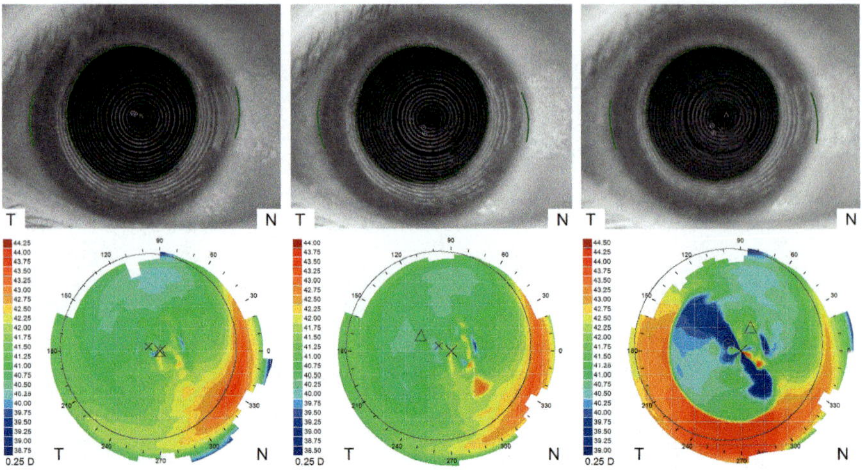

Fig. 13.3 Eye image and axial curvature map for three scans of the same eye with varying degrees of tear film distortion from severe (left) to mild (right). A severe distortion will present as an obvious topographic irregularity (right); however, more subtle distortions can appear as plausible topographic irregularities (middle and left). This highlights the importance of reviewing the quality of the Mires rings before using a scan to plan a topography-guided treatment. Tear film irregularities can usually be managed by asking the patient to blink; otherwise, artificial tears can be used. Reproduced with permission from Reinstein DZ, Archer TJ, Carp GI. The Surgeon's Guide to SMILE. SLACK Inc, 2018

corneal sphere and cylinder unchanged. The CRS-Master algorithm will therefore aim to leave a toric corneal surface if there is a significant discrepancy between the manifest refractive cylinder and the calculated astigmatic change according to the topography. This assumes that the difference is due to ocular residual astigmatism (ORA), i.e., from the posterior corneal surface or the lens. However, manifest refraction can be challenging in patients with irregular astigmatism as the patient may ask for refractive cylinder to partially compensate for coma or secondary astigmatism. Alternatively, the manifest refraction that achieves the best CDVA may not be the same as the refraction that minimizes the point spread function. Therefore, it is very important to review the target curvature map. If this target surface has significant corneal astigmatism, then the manifest refraction should be reconsidered as it is rare for an eye to truly have significant ORA.

The main aim of a topography-guided treatment is to enlarge and/or re-center the optical zone, so the topography-guided optical zone should be set as large as possible according to residual stromal thickness safety limits. As topography-guided ablations are not symmetrical, the location of maximum ablation is rarely central, so safety planning should consider this location in addition to the center and the location of the thinnest pachymetry. In this way, a topography-guided ablation can often be safe to perform even in cases with low central tissue reserves. An example of residual stromal thickness planning for a topography-guided treatment is shown in Fig. 13.7.

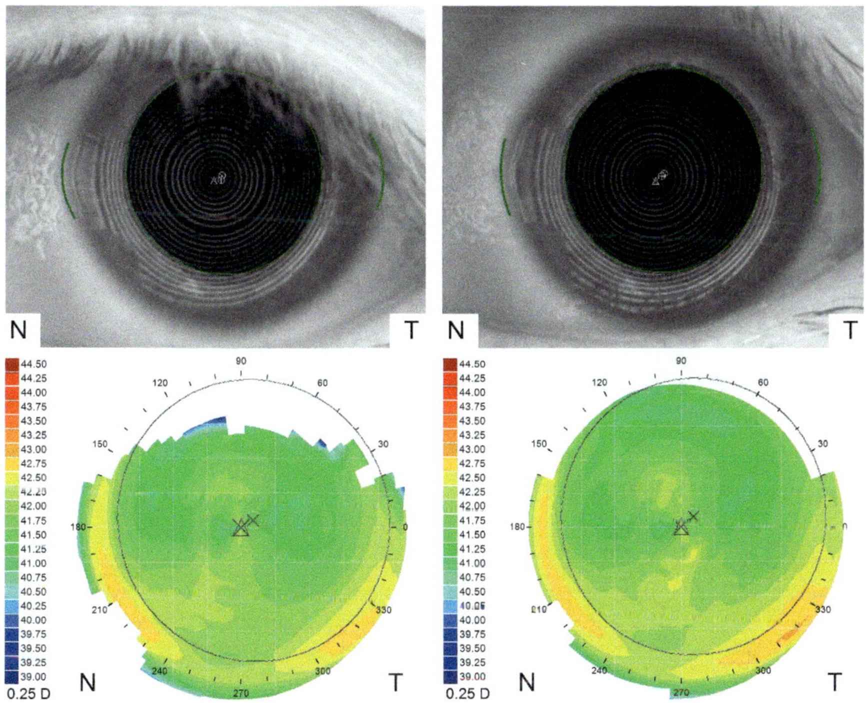

Fig. 13.4 Pair of topography scans for the same eye demonstrating the successful management of a patient where the eyelid was obscuring the superior cornea (left). The patient was asked to rest their chin on *top* of the chinrest, which tilted the head and exposed the superior cornea, enabling the full corneal diameter to be captured. Reproduced with permission from Reinstein DZ, Archer TJ, Carp GI. The Surgeon's Guide to SMILE. SLACK Inc, 2018

The CRS-Master initially selects the center of the pupil as found by the Atlas to use as the center for the ablation generation algorithms. It is preferable that the surgeon then shift this location to the corneal vertex, identified as the center of the topography mires and center of the overlaid cross-hairs (Fig. 13.8). During surgery, the corneal vertex can be determined as the first Purkinje reflex, with the patient fixating coaxially to the aiming beam so that the topography, the ablation profile, and the eye tracker are all coaxially registered to the best approximation of the visual axis.

13.3.2 Small Optical Zone

A small achieved optical zone will be associated with elevated spherical aberration and may cause night vision disturbances, notably halos. In these cases, either a topography-guided or wavefront-guided custom ablation might be used, depending on what excimer laser platform is available for the treatment. A wavefront-guided

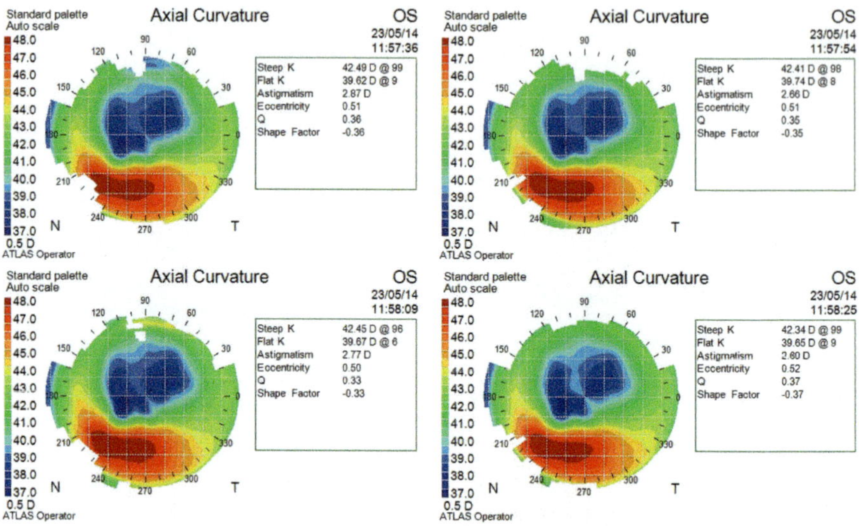

Fig. 13.5 Series of four topography scans demonstrating that the irregular topography was repeatable, hence confirming that the measurement was reliable and could be used for treatment planning. Reproduced with permission from Reinstein DZ, Archer TJ, Carp GI. The Surgeon's Guide to SMILE. SLACK Inc, 2018

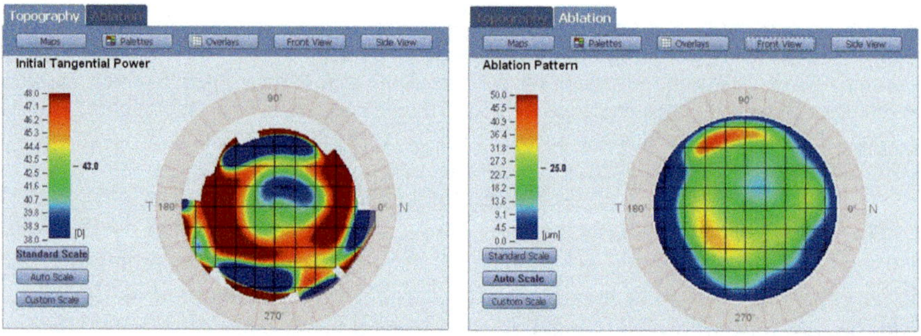

Fig. 13.6 Example of a 'spike' in a topography-guided profile (right) caused by using a scan with an area of missing data (left) for treatment planning. Reproduced with permission from Reinstein DZ, Archer TJ, Carp GI. The Surgeon's Guide to SMILE. SLACK Inc, 2018

ablation will aim to treat the spherical aberration directly, whereas a topography-guided treatment will aim to expand the topographic optical zone, which will reduce the spherical aberration as a consequence.

In our experience with both approaches in eyes with high spherical aberration, topography-guided ablations are significantly more effective in reducing spherical aberration. In our first study using the MEL 80 topography-guided system for

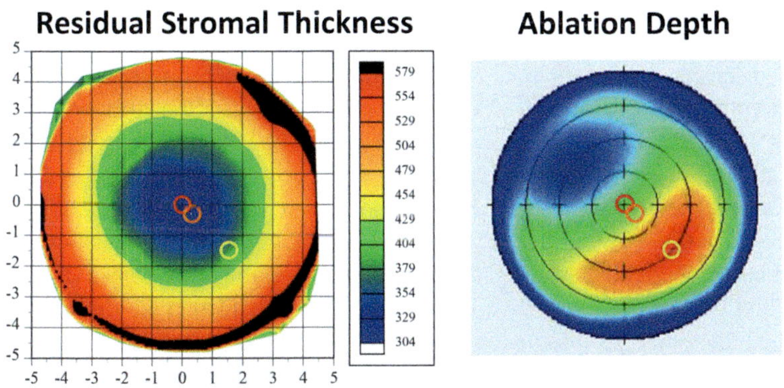

Location	RST	Ablation	Pred. RST
Central	316	22	294
Thinnest Point	304	31	273
Max Ablation	375	75	300

Fig. 13.7 Example of safety assessment for a topography-guided treatment (right) using an Artemis Insight 100 VHF digital ultrasound residual stromal thickness map (left). As the maximum ablation is not central in a custom ablation, the residual stromal thickness calculation should be performed in three locations: at the location of the maximum ablation, centrally, and at the location of the thinnest residual stromal thickness. Reproduced with permission from Reinstein DZ, Archer TJ, Carp GI. The Surgeon's Guide to SMILE. SLACK Inc, 2018

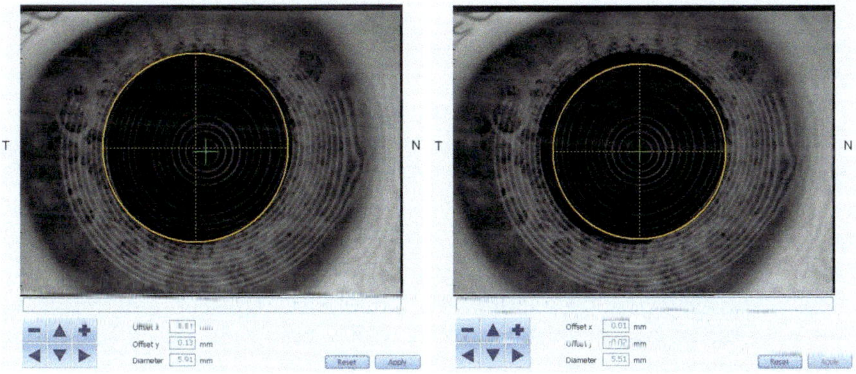

Fig. 13.8 In the CRS-Master, the center for the topography-guided ablation algorithm is selected by the user placing the cross-hairs in the desired location on the topography eye image. Our protocol is to use the corneal vertex (the center of the Mires rings) as the treatment center. Reproduced with permission from Reinstein DZ, Archer TJ, Carp GI. The Surgeon's Guide to SMILE. SLACK Inc, 2018

highly aberrated eyes following complications of refractive surgery, the spherical aberration was reduced by 41% on average [10]. In a second study, [18] we analyzed the results for 73 eyes where a topography-guided retreatment was performed to expand the optical zone or correct a decentration, following primary myopic LASIK with the MEL 80. In this group, we achieved an 11% increase in the topographic optical zone diameter, which contributed a 46% reduction in spherical aberration (Table 13.1).

In comparison, we found that wavefront-guided treatment only achieved a 27% reduction in spherical aberration, although this was enough to subjectively improve vision and restore contrast sensitivity to normal levels [19]. This finding was corroborated by other studies using wavefront-guided custom ablation, where the average reduction of spherical aberration across studies was only 32%, [19–31] although a subjective improvement was reported in all studies despite this modest reduction in spherical aberration.

This is an interesting result and one that suggests we do not need to 'flatten the wavefront' to improve the visual quality. This suggests that there is a tolerable level below which the brain can filter out the aberrations. In our study, we estimated the tolerable level of spherical aberration to be about 0.56 μm (OSA notation), by comparison to a post-LASIK control group with no visual quality symptoms [19].

13.3.3 Decentration

Decentration is the other most common complication in corneal laser refractive surgery. In SMILE, there will be a higher incidence of decentration if the surgeon attempts to center the lenticule using the pupil center. In eyes with a large angle kappa, centering the lenticule on the entrance pupil center will result in the creation of a new vertex, whereas the natural vertex is maintained if centration is on the corneal vertex [32–34].

Wavefront-guided ablations have been used to successfully correct decentrations, [22, 35] however, the angle kappa must always be considered before using a wavefront-guided treatment in a decentration case. Whole eye wavefront is calculated centered on the entrance pupil center, since wavefront data can only be obtained within the pupil. Therefore, in an eye with a large angle kappa, the wavefront will not represent the patient's natural vision since the patient is not 'looking' through the center of the pupil (where the wavefront is centered). This means that using a wavefront custom ablation in eyes with a large angle kappa could result in a worsening of the visual symptoms; such a treatment results in shifting the corneal vertex away from the nascent position.

For these reasons, a topography-guided ablation is a much more reliable and effective treatment option for decentration [36]. As described previously, the main aims for topography-guided custom ablation are to regularize the topography, hence providing an improvement in quality of vision. Specifically, the aims are to increase the optical zone diameter, shift the optical zone center closer to the corneal vertex, and reduce higher order aberrations as a consequence. Figure 13.9

Table 13.1 Change in optical zone diameter and higher order aberrations after topography-guided custom ablation for optical zone enlargement and recentration treatments following primary LASIK

	Optical zone diameter	Spherical aberration	Coma	HO RMS
Pre	5.65 ± 0.52 mm (4.80 to 7.00 mm)	0.69 ± 0.21 μm (0.33 to 1.33 μm)	0.60 ± 0.35 μm (0.01 to 1.73 μm)	0.97 ± 0.34 μm (0.50 to 1.95 μm)
Post	6.32 ± 0.52 mm (5.00 to 7.60 mm)	0.38 ± 0.24 μm (−0.01 to 1.12 μm)	0.28 ± 0.17 μm (0.02 to 0.79 μm)	0.59 ± 0.23 μm (0.24 to 1.39 μm)
Change	0.67 ± 0.52 mm (−0.40 to 2.00 mm) 11% increase	−0.30 ± 0.23 μm (−0.88 to 0.39 μm) 44% reduction	−0.32 ± 0.35 μm (−1.29 to 0.29 μm) 53% reduction	−0.39 ± 0.32 μm (−1.16 to 0.15 μm) 39% reduction

shows some example cases where a topography-guided treatment has been used to correct a decentration after myopic LASIK.

In our study of 73 eyes treated by topography-guided custom ablation following primary myopic LASIK, size and centration of the topographic optical zone was assessed by overlaying paracentral rings and a central grid onto Atlas tangential curvature difference maps [18]. The two plots in Fig. 13.10 show the

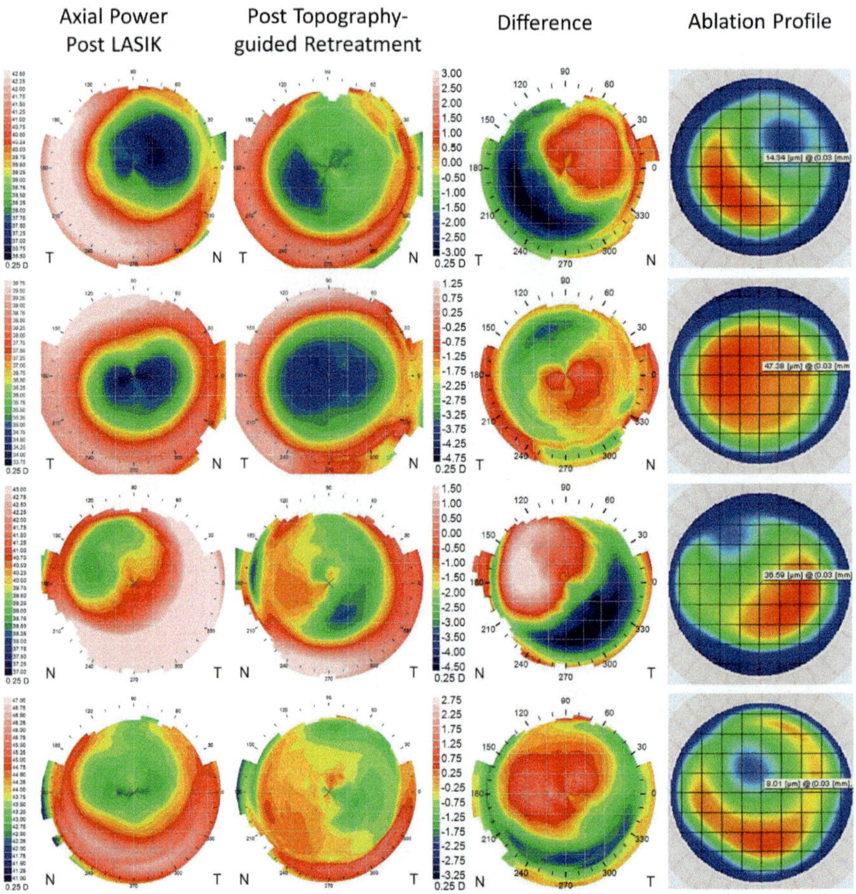

Fig. 13.9 Four examples of topography-guided retreatment for decentration and small optical zone following primary myopic LASIK. The post-LASIK topography that was used to calculate the topography-guided treatment is shown in the first column. The second column shows the postoperative topography, demonstrating a significant improvement in centration and optical zone diameter. The third column shows the difference map, which correlated to the intended ablation profile (fourth column). The difference map showed an area of flattening in the region of maximum ablation. Reproduced with permission from Reinstein DZ, Archer TJ, Carp GI, Stuart AJ, Rowe EL, Nesbit A, Moore T. Incidence and outcomes of optical zone enlargement and recentration after previous myopic LASIK by topography-guided custom ablation. J Refract Surg. 2018;34:121–130

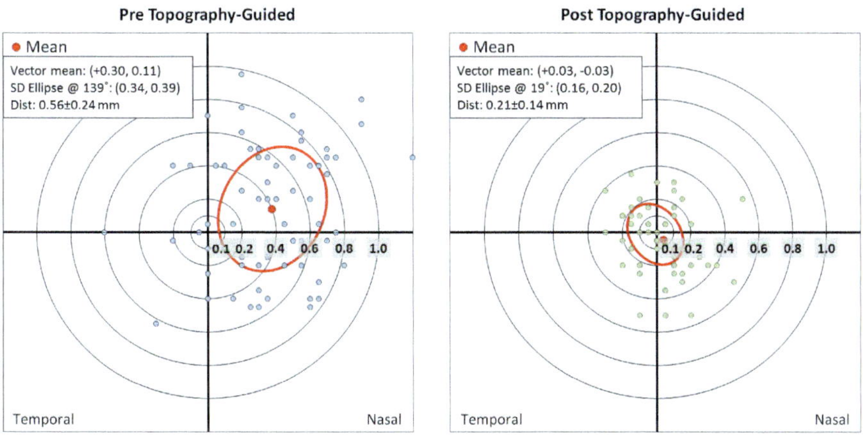

Fig. 13.10 Plots of the optical zone center before (left) and after (right) a topography-guided retreatment. The red dot represents the vector mean, and the red line represents the standard deviation ellipse. The topography-guided treatment achieved a significant improvement in centration, reducing the optical zone offset by 63% from 0.56 mm to 0.21 mm on average. Reproduced with permission from Reinstein DZ, Archer TJ, Carp GI, Stuart AJ, Rowe EL, Nesbit A, Moore T. Incidence and outcomes of optical zone enlargement and recentration after previous myopic LASIK by topography-guided custom ablation. J Refract Surg. 2018;34:121–130

topographic optical zone center relative to the corneal vertex (0, 0) before and after the topography-guided treatment. This analysis found that decentration from the corneal vertex was reduced by 64% from 0.58 ± 0.26 mm (0.05 to 1.28 mm) to 0.21 ± 0.14 mm (0.00 to 0.54 mm).

These results demonstrate the effectiveness of topography-guided treatments for regularly irregular astigmatism such as decentration and optical zone enlargement. However, before a decentration is treated by topography-guided ablation, it is important to have first made a confident diagnosis and in particular to have considered the effect of epithelial thickness changes. The next section describes how common diagnostic technologies like topography and wavefront can be misleading and may result in the wrong treatment being performed.

It is also important to realize that topography-guided ablation (and wavefront-guided) can never be a complete solution because it does not account for epithelial thickness changes. However, in many cases a reduction in aberrations is sufficient to alleviate patient symptoms, as the remainder can be masked by epithelial remodeling, or filtered by neural processing.

13.4 Trans-epithelial Phototherapeutic Keratectomy

13.4.1 Understanding Epithelial Remodeling

As introduced earlier, epithelial remodeling is a well-known phenomenon and has been shown to occur in a wide range of situations. Somewhat surprisingly, we found that the epithelium was not uniform in thickness for a normal virgin eyes as had previously been thought, but followed a very distinct pattern; on average the epithelium was 5.7 μm thicker inferiorly than superiorly, and 1.2 μm thicker nasally than temporally, with a mean central thickness of 53.4 μm (Fig. 13.11) [37]. This non-uniformity seemed to provide evidence that epithelial thickness is regulated by eyelid mechanics and blinking, as we suggested in 1994 [38].

Further evidence for this theory is provided by the epithelial thickness changes observed in orthokeratology [39]. In orthokeratology, a reversed geometry contact lens is placed on the cornea overnight that sits tightly on the cornea centrally, but leaves a gap in the mid-periphery. Therefore, the natural template provided by the posterior surface of the semi-rigid tarsus of the eyelid is replaced by an artificial contact lens template designed to fit tightly to the center of the cornea and loosely paracentrally. We found significant epithelial thickness changes with central thinning and mid-peripheral thickening (Fig. 13.11) showing that the epithelium has remodeled according to the template provided by the contact lens, i.e., the epithelium is chafed and squashed by the lens centrally while the epithelium is free to thicken paracentrally where the lens is not so tightly fitted.

Epithelial thickness changes have been described after myopic excimer laser ablation [40–43], hyperopic excimer laser ablation, [44] radial keratotomy, [45] intra-corneal ring segments,[46] irregularly irregular astigmatism after corneal refractive surgery, [1–4, 47, 48] and in keratoconus [49–53] and ectasia [54]. Figure 13.11 shows the epithelial thickness profile in a number of different situations.

In all of these cases, the epithelial thickness changes are clearly a compensatory response to the change to the stromal surface and can all be explained by the theory of eyelid template regulation of epithelial thickness. A further example is the epithelial thickness changes reported following the rotation of a LASIK free cap, in which dramatic changes were observed overnight once the asymmetric free cap was replaced in the correct anatomical position, demonstrating that the original stromal surface curvature had been restored [55]. Compensatory epithelial thickness changes can be summarized by the following rules:

1. The epithelium thickens in areas where tissue has been removed or the curvature has been flattened (e.g. central thickening after myopic ablation [40–42] or radial keratotomy [45] and peripheral thickening after hyperopic ablation [44]).
2. The epithelium thins over regions that are relatively elevated or the curvature has been steepened (e.g. central thinning in keratoconus, [49–53] ectasia [54] and after hyperopic ablation [44]).

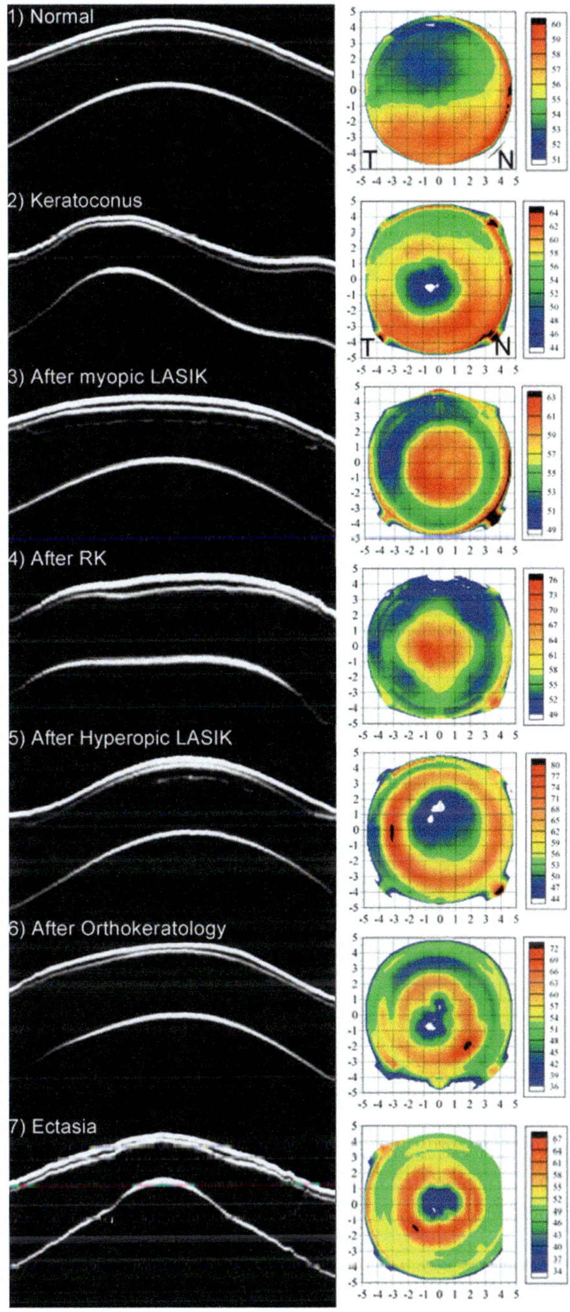

Fig. 13.11 Artemis Insight 100 VHF digital ultrasound non-geometrically corrected B-scan (left) and epithelial thickness profile (right) for: (1) a population of 110 normal untreated eyes, (2) a population of 54 keratoconic eyes, (3) a population of 24 eyes after myopic LASIK, (4) a population of 14 eyes after radial keratotomy, (5) a population of 65 eyes after hyperopic LASIK, (6) a case example of an eye after 2 weeks wear of an orthokeratology lens, and (7) a case of post-LASIK ectasia. Reproduced with permission from Reinstein DZ, Archer TJ, Carp GI. The Surgeon's Guide to SMILE. SLACK Inc, 2018

3. The magnitude of epithelial changes correlates to the magnitude of the change in curvature (e.g. more epithelial thickening for higher myopia, [40, 41, 43] higher hyperopia, and [44] more advanced keratoconus [49–53]).
4. The amount of epithelial remodeling is defined by the curvature gradient of an irregularity; there will be more epithelial remodeling for a more localized irregularity [1–4, 6–8]. The epithelium effectively acts as a low pass filter, smoothing small changes almost completely, but only partially smoothing large changes.

13.4.2 Trans-epithelial PTK Treatment

As described earlier, despite all the advances in corneal topography and ocular wavefront measurement, it is not always possible to diagnose the cause of subjective visual complaints by these means alone because of the compensatory epithelial thickness changes that partially mask the true stromal surface irregularity. In applying the *Law of Epithelial Compensation*, if a patient presents with stable irregular astigmatism, by definition the epithelium has reached its maximum compensatory function. The epithelium can compensate almost completely for very localized irregularities. Therefore, topography or wavefront-guided treatments may lead to a sub-optimal treatment plan and potentially make things worse [2–4]. Instead, we need a method to target the irregularities masked by the epithelium, something that is achieved, by definition, by trans-epithelial PTK [1–4].

We have described our treatment protocol for trans-epithelial PTK in detail in previous publications (Fig. 13.12) [1–4]. When planning these cases, we always obtain an epithelial thickness map in order to simulate the stromal ablation profile. We refer to this technique as Digital Subtraction Pachymetry (DSP) as demonstrated in Fig. 13.13, in which the breakthrough pattern and remaining epithelium at regular lamellar depths of trans-epithelial PTK ablation are simulated. This pattern can also be used to estimate the refractive effect; for example, a hyperopic shift would be expected if central stroma was being removed primarily. In our study, we found that trans-epithelial PTK resulted in a refractive shift of more than 0.50 D in 59% of eyes, equally split between myopic and hyperopic shifts [1].

The PTK ablation is a uniform depth applied over a large diameter zone—the maximum zone is 8.0 mm for the MEL 80/90. Stromal tissue removal is defined by the epithelial thickness profile, so the optical zone diameter does not increase the ablation depth as for a refractive ablation. The ablation is centered in the same way as a refractive ablation, by centering the eye tracker on the coaxially sighted corneal light reflex. However, there is effectively no concern about centration as the PTK ablation is uniform depth across a wide 8 mm diameter. In contrast, if a topography-guided ablation is slightly misaligned, then this may increase the irregularity, particularly in cases of very localized irregularities. This makes trans-epithelial PTK extremely easy to perform.

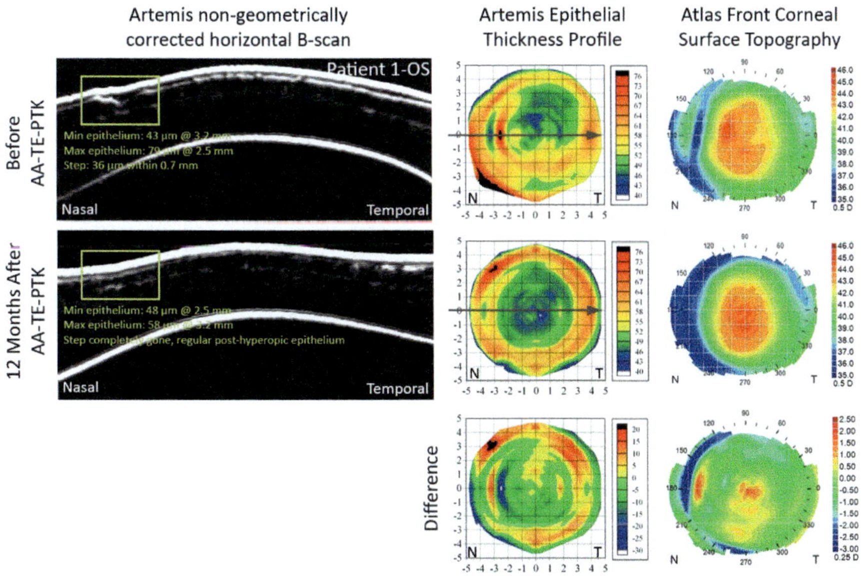

Fig. 13.12 (Left column) Artemis Insight 100 non-geometrically corrected horizontal B scans before and after an Artemis-assisted trans-epithelial PTK (AA-TE-PTK) procedure. The yellow box highlights the nasal region where the flap interface can be seen to stop abruptly. In this area, there is a crevice on the stromal surface over which the epithelium has thickened with thin epithelium overlying the adjacent ridge. (Middle column) Artemis Insight 100 epithelial thickness maps before and after the AA-TE-PTK procedure plotted on the same scale. These show that the nasal step in epithelial thickness has been completely smoothed after the procedure. The difference map is plotted underneath, which shows the significant epithelial remodeling in the nasal region after the procedure. (Right column) Atlas corneal front surface topography before and after the AA-TE-PTK procedure plotted on the same scale. The difference map is plotted underneath, which demonstrates the significant improvement in the topographic irregularity after the procedure. Reproduced with permission from Reinstein DZ, Archer TJ, Gobbe M. Improved effectiveness of trans-epithelial phototherapeutic keratectomy versus topography-guided ablation degraded by epithelial compensation on irregular stromal surfaces [plus video]. J Refract Surg. 2013;29:526–533

In our protocol, the first trans-epithelial PTK ablation is planned to expose a small area of stroma in the region of the thinnest epithelium. The initial trans-epithelial ablation depth data entry is calculated using a conversion factor of 1.14 times the intended depth based on our previous experience with the MEL 80 and MEL 90 excimer lasers. After the initial ablation the epithelial DSP maps are compared to the observed epithelial breakthrough pattern to estimate the actual achieved ablation depth. This allows the conversion factor used for subsequent ablations to be calibrated individually for each case. Based on the remaining thickness of epithelium, trans-epithelial PTK ablations are applied in steps of 10–20 μm with the final goal of removing almost all of the epithelium up to the maximum thickness. In cases with very localized irregularities, we often choose not to remove the full thickness of epithelium in order to conserve stromal tissue.

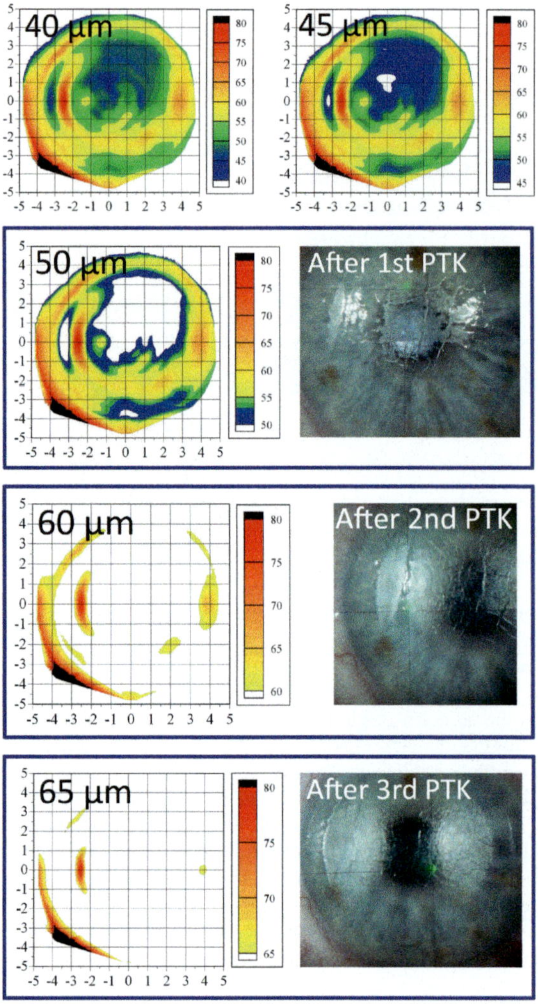

Fig. 13.13 Digital subtraction pachymetry simulation of the pattern of remaining epithelium that would be expected after increasing trans-epithelial PTK ablations from 40 to 65 μm in 5 μm steps. The white represents regions where all the epithelium would have been ablated after the labeled trans-epithelial PTK ablation and hence the regions where ablation of stromal tissue would occur. Due to the epithelial masking, the stromal ablation was concentrated onto a nasal ridge immediately adjacent to a crevice on the stromal surface. During the procedure, the trans-epithelial PTK ablation was performed in three steps, with a planned 50 μm ablation as the first step. After the first ablation, the cornea was examined (as shown in the intraoperative photograph), and the areas of exposed stroma were compared to the Artemis simulated maps, which confirmed that the first ablation was close to 50 μm. The second and third trans-epithelial PTK ablations could then be planned to reach the intended end point of 65 μm accurately. The intraoperative photographs show that the pattern of remaining epithelium was similar to the predicted pattern with only a small line of epithelium remaining overlying the stromal crevice. Reproduced with permission from Reinstein DZ, Archer TJ, Gobbe M. Improved effectiveness of trans-epithelial phototherapeutic keratectomy versus topography-guided ablation degraded by epithelial compensation on irregular stromal surfaces [plus video]. J Refract Surg. 2013;29:526–533

On completion of the trans-epithelial PTK ablations, the stromal surface quality and smoothness is assessed. If there are fine irregularities visible, such as microfolds, a series of 'wet' PTK ablations can be performed to smooth and polish the stromal surface [2]. The 'wet' PTK ablations are done by first flooding the cornea with balanced salt solution (BSS) immediately followed by a PTK ablation of eight seconds duration in an 8-mm zone (equivalent to a readout of 20 μm on the MEL 80 PTK mode). The tendency for BSS surface tension to break up means that such PTK bursts must be kept short to avoid inadvertently ablating other areas of the stroma, which is why we limit each ablation to approximately 8 s. The BSS acts as a masking agent, in a similar way to the epithelium previously, and naturally spreads across the surface leaving the ridges of any microfolds closer to the surface. The shockwaves of the excimer laser expose the peaks of the microfolds allowing them to be ablated in isolation of the rest of the stromal surface. This process is usually repeated 2–4 times until the surface is visibly smoothed of microfolds on drying. In our population of eyes treated by trans-epithelial PTK, a 'wet' PTK was performed in approximately half of the cases [1].

In addition, a standard refractive, topography-guided or wavefront guided ablation might be performed immediately following trans-epithelial PTK in selected cases. As described above, the DSP simulation can be used to estimate the refractive effect of the trans-epithelial PTK ablation, so a refractive ablation can be used in cases where the refractive shift is considered to be predictable. If the patient has a significant refractive error, then this might be treated simultaneously. Alternatively, if there is an obvious large-scale global irregularity in addition to the localized irregularities, then these might be treated by a topography-guided ablation. In theory, performing both a trans-epithelial PTK and a topography-guided treatment will correct the total stromal surface irregularity. However, if in doubt, it is preferable to do less and conserve tissue for future treatments.

13.4.3 Trans-epithelial PTK Without an Epithelial Thickness Measurement

While an epithelial thickness map and DSP can provide a confirmed diagnosis and expected treatment outcome, these are not compulsory for performing a trans-epithelial PTK treatment. As long as there is irregularly irregular topography, the epithelium must also be irregular, meaning that a trans-epithelial PTK treatment will afford some smoothing of the stromal surface. The mean central epithelial thickness in a normal eye is 53 μm, [37] so by definition the thinnest epithelium in an irregularly irregular cornea will most likely be less than this (as there must be compensatory thinning for an irregularity). This is confirmed by the distribution of minimum and maximum epithelial thicknesses in our trans-epithelial PTK population as shown in Fig. 13.14 [1]. The mean thinnest epithelial thickness was 43 μm (significantly thinner than normal), and the mean thickest epithelial thickness was 79 μm (significantly thicker than normal).

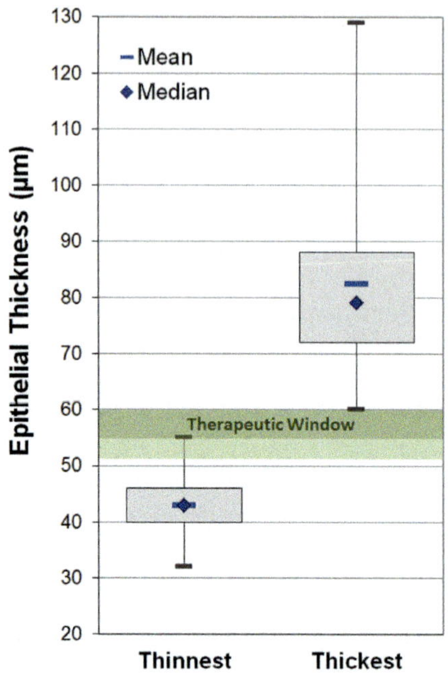

Fig. 13.14 Boxplot displaying preoperative Artemis Insight 100 VHF digital ultrasound epithelial thickness range for a population of 41 eyes with irregularly irregular astigmatism. The 'therapeutic window' is defined as the region between the population's maximum thinnest epithelium and minimum thickest epithelium. Dark green indicates the narrow 'therapeutic window' including an anomalously high thinnest epithelium, and light green indicates a wider 'therapeutic window' without this outlier. Reproduced with permission from Reinstein DZ, Archer TJ, Dickeson ZI, Gobbe M. Trans-epithelial phototherapeutic keratectomy protocol for treating irregular astigmatism based on population epithelial thickness measurements by Artemis very high-frequency digital ultrasound. J Refract Surg. 2014;30:380–387

The goal of the initial trans-epithelial PTK ablation is to break through the epithelium in the region where it is thinnest to expose the peaks in the stromal surface to be ablated. The secondary goal of the initial trans-epithelial PTK ablation is to avoid removing the full thickness of epithelium as any ablation after complete removal of the epithelium will have no effect on stromal surface irregularities. This method therefore avoids wasting stromal tissue.

If no epithelial thickness measurement is available, the following standardized treatment method can be used based on the population minimum and maximum epithelial thicknesses. The highest minimum epithelial thickness was 54 µm, but as this was a single outlier, the next lowest value of 51 µm is considered for this protocol. The lowest maximum epithelial thickness was 60 µm. Therefore, to achieve breakthrough but not complete removal of the epithelium, the first ablation should be targeted within the 'therapeutic window' of 51–60 µm. We suggest an initial ablation depth of 55 µm, although this should be adjusted to take into account the epithelial ablation rate for the excimer laser being used (if this can be measured). Subsequent ablations can be performed in 10–20 μm steps, chosen intraoperatively after reviewing the coverage and pattern of epithelium remaining after each ablation. During this process, the pattern of remaining epithelium can be observed to identify the areas where the stroma is being ablated. The pattern of stromal ablation can then be correlated to corneal topography and wavefront to gain an understanding of the stromal surface irregularity being treated and evaluate potential postoperative changes. These stepwise ablations can be continued until the epithelium is completely removed or is restricted to an isolated area.

13.4.4 Irregular Astigmatism Due to Lenticule Remnants or False Planes

In SMILE, irregularly irregular astigmatism after SMILE can be caused by lenticule remnants or by cases of difficult interface separation where false planes are created. In this example, the patient underwent a FLEx procedure for the correction of approximately −2.00 D. The flap was lifted without significant difficulty; however, there was very high resistance in the lenticule interface. The surgeon tried using a variety of different instruments including a straight spatula, a forceps, a Blum femto-spoon, and a LASIK flap lifter (Fig. 13.15). This example highlights the importance of immobilizing the eye during SMILE; otherwise, the eye simply rolls to one side when pressure is applied by the separating instrument. This makes it virtually impossible to make precise and controlled movements.

The surgeon settled on a technique of lifting the edge of the lenticule with the forceps and using the Blum femto-spoon to cut through the exposed unseparated interface. This was successful for about 75% of the interface, but the infero-nasal region proved to be inaccessible. It is not entirely clear from the video what happened, although it is likely that a false plane was created meaning that it was not

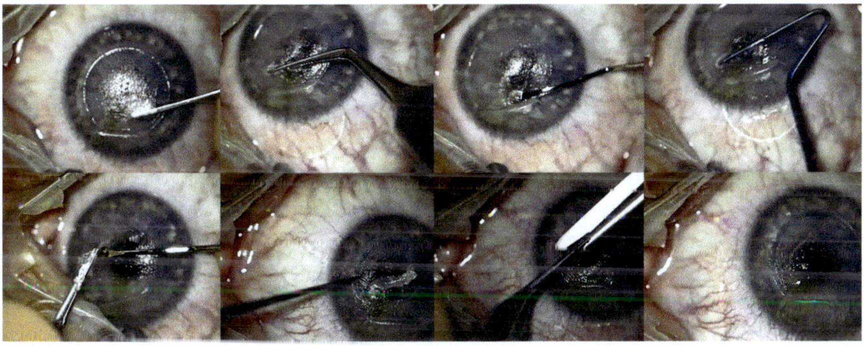

Fig. 13.15 Series of images showing the various surgical instruments and techniques used while trying to separate a highly resistant interface during a FLEx procedure. Ultimately, it was not possible to extract a large portion of the lenticule infero-nasally. Reproduced with permission from Reinstein DZ, Archer TJ, Carp GI. The Surgeon's Guide to SMILE. SLACK Inc, 2018

possible to complete the separation. The surgeon then tried accessing the edge of the lenticule interface from the nasal side using a Sinskey hook, but was unsuccessful. In the end, the separated portion of the lenticule was cut free, leaving a large lenticule remnant in the eye.

As expected, the patient ended up with irregularly irregular astigmatism (Fig. 13.16), reduction in CDVA, severe night vision disturbances and ghost images, and almost total loss of contrast sensitivity. Six months after surgery, the UDVA was $20/63^{-1}$ with a manifest refraction of + 1.25 −2.25 × 76 ($20/25^{-1}$). The corneal topography showed a temporal-nasal asymmetry of 10 D, and VHF digital ultrasound B-scans showed large undulations on the stromal surface, with a significant step infero-nasally (Fig. 13.17). The SMILE interface can be seen to stop abruptly in the location of the step, indicating the border of the lenticule remnant that was responsible for the discontinuity in stromal surface curvature. However, the front corneal surface was relatively smooth due to compensatory epithelial remodeling. The magnitude of the epithelial remodeling can be appreciated by the 80 μm thickness difference in the region of the step; the epithelial thickness was 116 μm overlying the trough compared to 36 μm overlying the adjacent ridge, with these points separated by less than 1 mm.

Obviously, the aim of a therapeutic treatment would be to remove stromal tissue from the region of the lenticule remnant to complete the original intended treatment. This is very similar to the LASIK complication of performing an ablation with an incomplete flap, meaning that the ablation is truncated [2]. Given the extreme degree of epithelial remodeling, the majority of the stromal surface irregularity was being masked by the epithelium. Therefore, a trans-epithelial PTK would be a more appropriate treatment than a topography-guided ablation. To demonstrate this, we simulated the predicted stromal ablation due to a trans-epithelial PTK and compared this to the topography-guided ablation profile (Fig. 13.18). This comparison showed that a topography-guided ablation would remove only a small amount of tissue from the region of the step, whereas this area was the primary focus of the trans-epithelial PTK.

A trans-epithelial PTK treatment was performed using the protocol as described above. Nine months later, the topographic irregularity had been reduced with a change in curvature of 2.50 D in the infero-nasal region (Fig. 13.16). VHF digital ultrasound B-scans (Fig. 13.17) showed that the undulations in the stromal surface had been completely smoothed and the step had been halved as quantified by the epithelial thickness difference reducing from 80 to 43 μm. As expected, there was no refractive improvement—UDVA was 20/50 with a manifest refraction of + 4.00 −3.25 × 88 ($20/25^{-1}$). Contrast sensitivity was also still virtually nonexistent.

A second trans-epithelial PTK procedure was planned to target the remaining localized step irregularity on the stromal surface. This treatment was performed following the same protocol including DSP simulations to calibrate the progress of the ablation through the epithelium (Fig. 13.19).

At the 1 year visit, another significant step forward in regularizing the topography had been achieved, again showing a 2.00 D change on the difference map

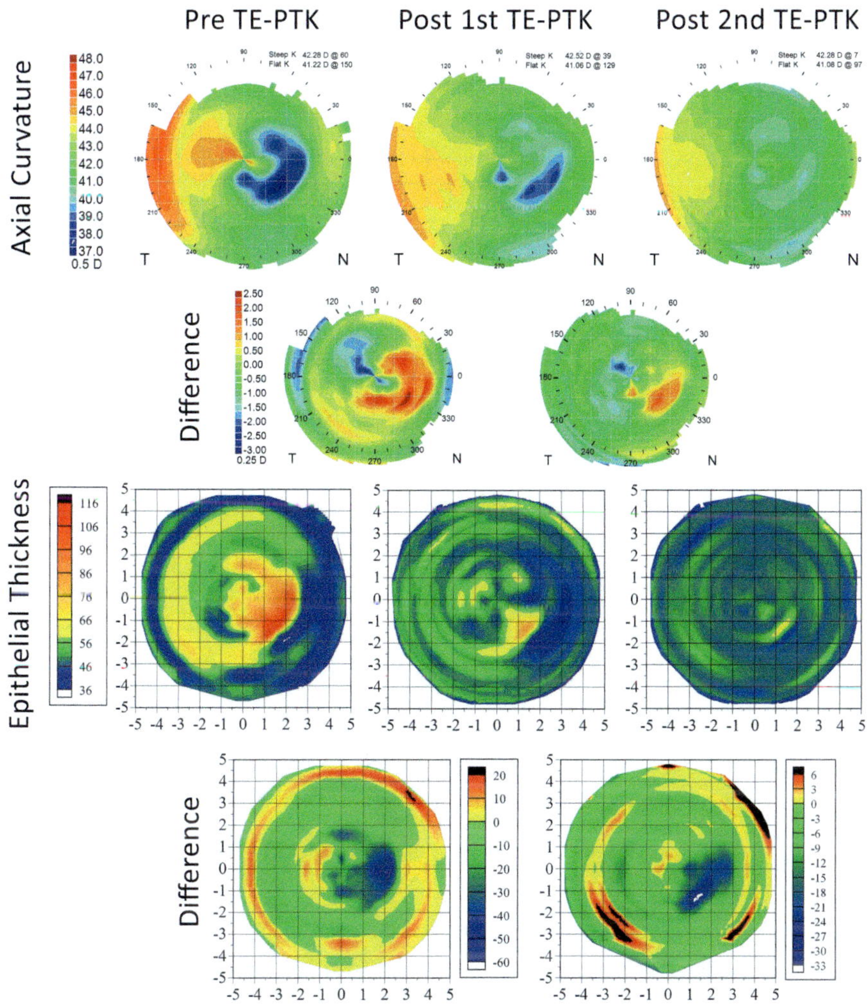

Fig. 13.16 Corneal topography (top) and epithelial thickness (bottom) before and after a series of two trans-epithelial PTK treatments. The difference maps are also shown between each time point. Reproduced with permission from Reinstein DZ, Archer TJ, Carp GI. The Surgeon's Guide to SMILE. SLACK Inc, 2018

infero-nasally (Fig. 13.16). This was correlated with further smoothing of the stromal surface, with the epithelial thickness difference over the step now only 18 μm (Fig. 13.17). Again, no improvement in refraction was expected—UDVA was 20/ 63^{-1} with a manifest refraction of + 3.00 –2.50 × 68—but CDVA improved to 20/ 16^{-1} and contrast sensitivity to mid-normal range.

Now that the localized irregularities had been adequately smoothed by trans-epithelial PTK, a topography-guided ablation was the next logical step as this

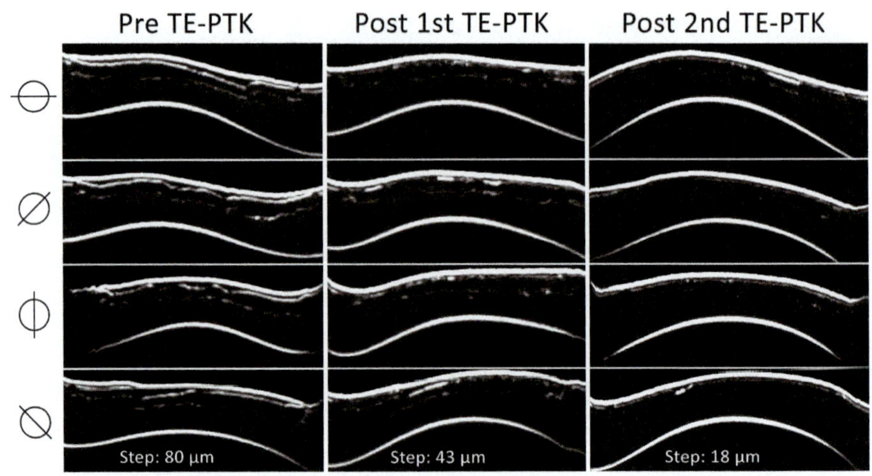

Fig. 13.17 Artemis Insight 100 VHF digital ultrasound B-scans before and after a series of two trans-epithelial PTK treatments to remove a large lenticule remnant following a FLEx procedure. The trans-epithelial PTK succeeded in significantly regularizing the stromal surface reducing the largest step irregularity from 80 μm to 18 μm. An interesting incidental observation are the bright patches on Bowman's layer after the first treatment, indicating the regions of thickest epithelium where the PTK had been stopped before full epithelial removal. Reproduced with permission from Reinstein DZ, Archer TJ, Carp GI. The Surgeon's Guide to SMILE. SLACK Inc, 2018

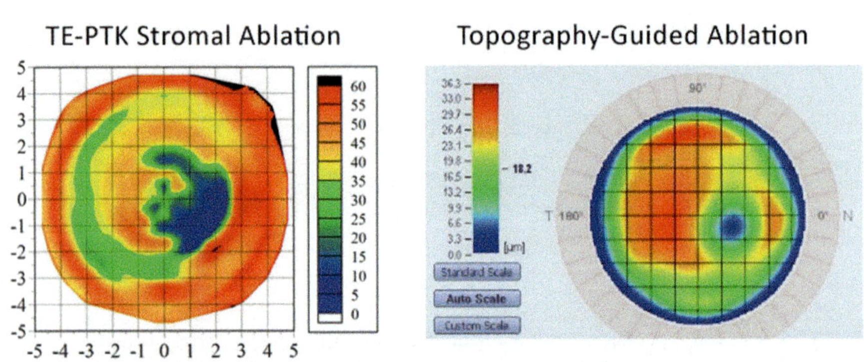

Fig. 13.18 Predicted stromal ablation calculated for a trans-epithelial PTK treatment (left) compared to the topography-guided ablation profile (right). Due to epithelial masking of the stromal irregularity, the topography-guided ablation did not focus the ablation onto the location of the lenticule remnant infero-nasally. Reproduced with permission from Reinstein DZ, Archer TJ, Carp GI. The Surgeon's Guide to SMILE. SLACK Inc, 2018

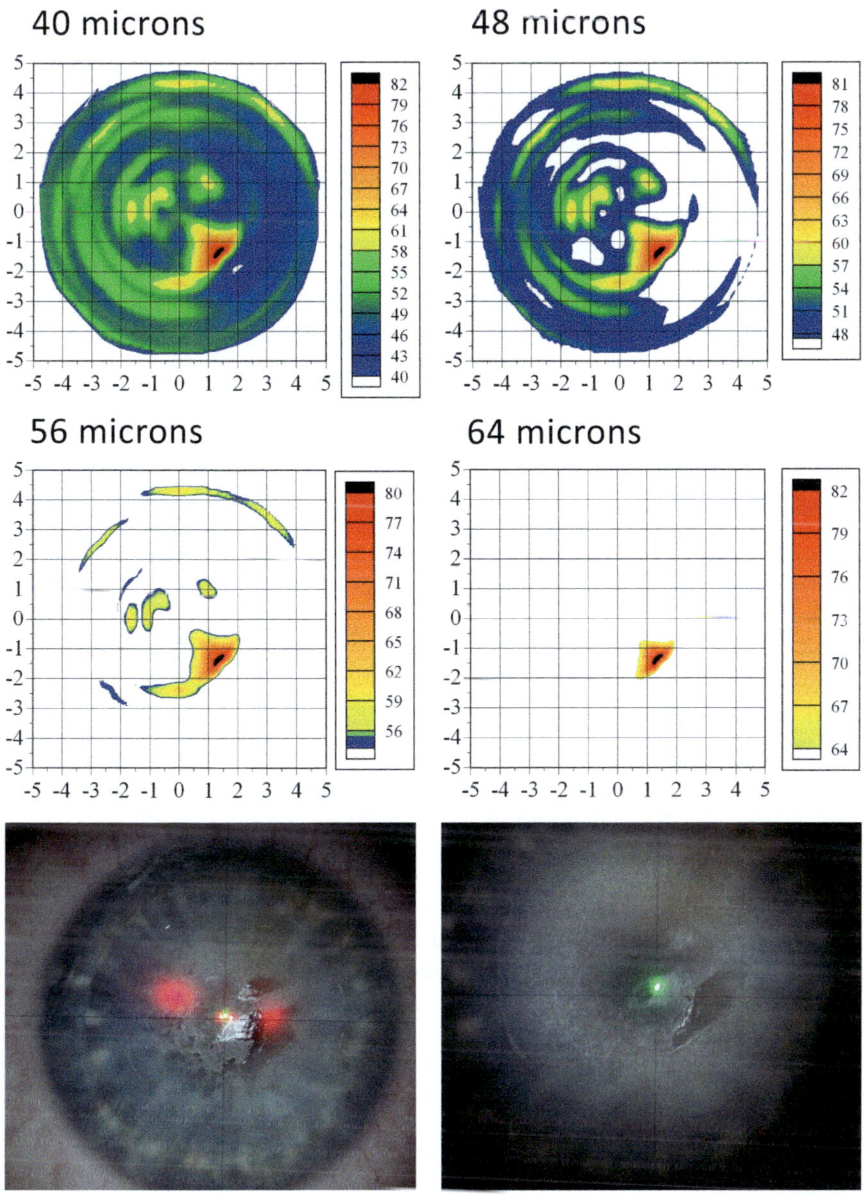

Fig. 13.19 Digital subtraction pachymetry maps that were used to assess the progress of the trans-epithelial PTK intraoperatively. A series of maps are generated representing the predicted pattern of remaining epithelial thickness after different ablation depths (top row). The intraoperative appearance (bottom row) was compared to the maps to determine the true effective ablation so that subsequent PTK ablations could be calibrated to the epithelial ablation rate for that individual eye. Reproduced with permission from Reinstein DZ, Archer TJ, Carp GI. The Surgeon's Guide to SMILE. SLACK Inc, 2018

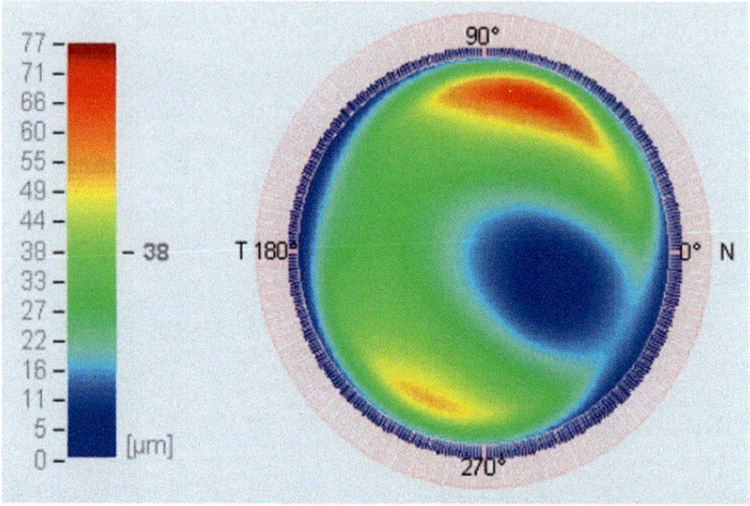

Fig. 13.20 Topography-guided ablation profile used for the third therapeutic treatment to correct the global irregularity remaining following two trans-epithelial PTK procedures to smooth the local irregularities. Reproduced with permission from Reinstein DZ, Archer TJ, Carp GI. The Surgeon's Guide to SMILE. SLACK Inc, 2018

would address a larger proportion of the remaining irregularities than a third trans-epithelial PTK. Indeed, the topography-guided ablation (Fig. 13.20) showed an asymmetric hyperopic astigmatism profile indicating that it was aiming to address global, rather than localized, irregularities. This treatment was performed by creating a new 110-μm LASIK flap.

One year postoperatively, UDVA was 20/50 with a manifest refraction of + 3.00 -- 3.00 × 102 ($20/16^{-2}$). The refractive cylinder magnitude had not changed; however, the topography now had the appearance of regular orthogonal astigmatism, and the nasal/temporal asymmetry had been resolved (Fig. 13.21).

A final treatment was then planned as a standard refractive ablation to correct the hyperopic astigmatism. Seven months later, UDVA was $20/20^{-1}$ with a manifest refraction of + 0.25 DS ($20/20^{-1}$). There was still more than 2.00 D of corneal astigmatism, but this was compensated for by posterior corneal astigmatism. The patient still reported some distortion and ghosting, albeit greatly improved from before the therapeutic treatments.

13.4.5 Irregular Astigmatism Due to Distorted Femtosecond Interface Creation

The other cause of irregularly irregular astigmatism after SMILE is in cases where the one or both of the lenticule interfaces were distorted during the femtosecond cutting, possibly due to eye movements, but more likely associated with black

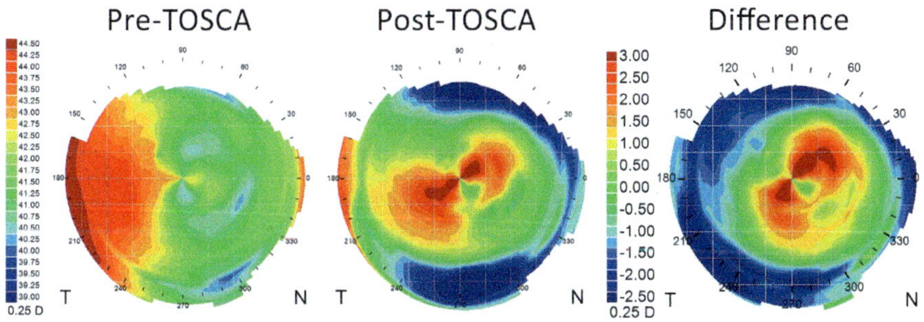

Fig. 13.21 Corneal topography and difference map before and one year after the topography-guided treatment. This ablation corrected the irregular astigmatism, leaving only orthogonal astigmatism. Reproduced with permission from Reinstein DZ, Archer TJ, Carp GI. The Surgeon's Guide to SMILE. SLACK Inc, 2018

spots. In total, we have had 5 eyes (3 patients) where a trans-epithelial PTK has been required to treat localized stromal irregularities (i.e., incidence 0.13% for a 4,000 eye population).

The first example was described earlier in Chap. 7.4, where the appearance of linear translucent areas in the lenticule interface centrally (Fig. 13.22) resulted in abrupt distortions in Bowman's layer and irregular astigmatism on topography (Fig. 13.23). Having been –3.25 –0.50 × 30 ($20/12.5^{-2}$) before surgery, the irregular topography had induced a loss of three lines CDVA and reduction in contrast sensitivity. At eight months, UDVA was 20/25 with a manifest refraction of + 1.50 -0.50 × 127 ($20/25^{+1}$).

A trans-epithelial PTK treatment was performed using the standard protocol with the aim of smoothing the stromal surface, based on the DSP epithelial thickness maps. Four months after the procedure, the topography was significantly more

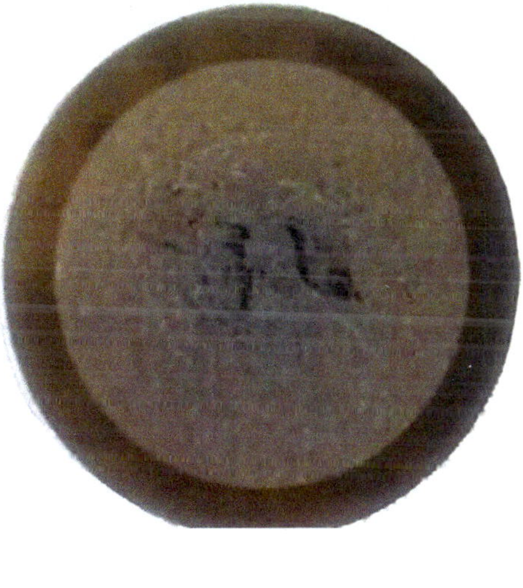

Fig. 13.22 Femtosecond bubble pattern showing linear translucent regions centrally in the lenticule interface, which caused irregularly irregular astigmatism after surgery. Reproduced with permission from Reinstein DZ, Archer TJ, Carp GI. The Surgeon's Guide to SMILE. SLACK Inc, 2018

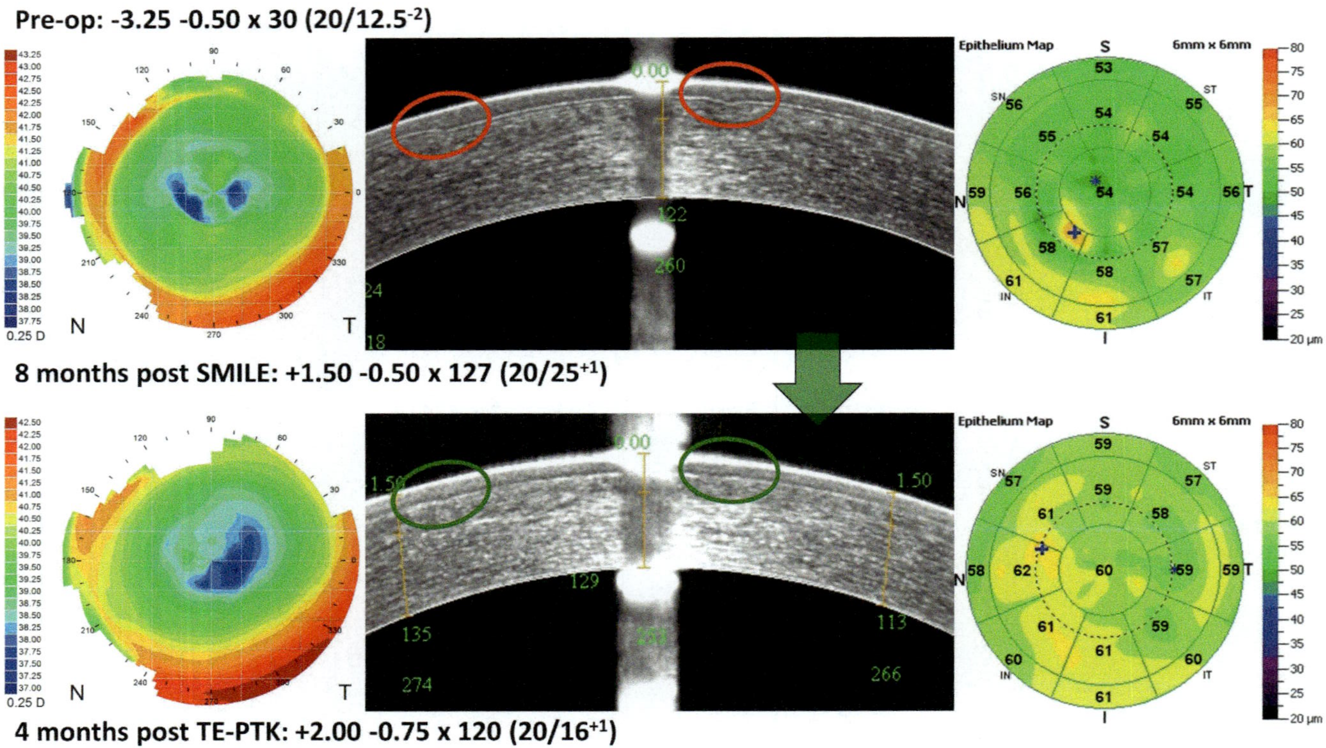

Fig. 13.23 Corneal topography (left), OCT B-scan (middle), and OCT epithelial thickness (right) for an eye with irregularly irregular astigmatism 8 months after SMILE (top). The irregularities on Bowman's layer are highlighted in red, which were correlated to the translucent lines in the femtosecond bubble patter of the lenticule interface. A trans-epithelial PTK treatment achieved a significant improvement in the stromal surface regularity, which was mirrored by an improvement in the topography and restoration of CDVA. Regularization of the epithelial thickness profile was further evidence that the stromal surface was more regular. Reproduced with permission from Reinstein DZ, Archer TJ, Carp GI. The Surgeon's Guide to SMILE. SLACK Inc, 2018

regular, as was the stromal surface on the OCT B-scan, as well as the epithelial thickness profile (Fig. 13.23). The UDVA was 20/32 with a manifest refraction of + 2.00 −0.75 × 120 (20/16^{+1}), so the CDVA had recovered to within two letters of the preoperative vision, and contrast sensitivity had also recovered to the preoperative level.

13.4.6 Alternatives and Weaknesses of Trans-epithelial PTK

The effectiveness of trans-epithelial PTK is defined by the proportion of the irregularity that has been masked by the epithelial remodeling. A trans-epithelial PTK will therefore not treat the irregularity that is visible on front surface corneal topography, which in theory would become the postoperative stromal surface. After a trans-epithelial PTK treatment, the epithelium then remodels according to this new stromal surface, hence partially masking the remaining irregularity. In some cases, the remaining irregularity is small enough to be masked almost completely by the epithelium, resulting in an apparently normal front corneal surface topography, and no further therapeutic treatment is required. In other cases, the remaining irregularity is large enough that it cannot be completely compensated by the epithelium, in which case further treatment would be needed if the patient reports subjective symptoms. Depending on whether the remaining irregularity is global or local, further treatment can be performed as a topography-guided ablation or trans-epithelial PTK.

Another approach, described by Chen et al. [56, 57] is to combine a trans-epithelial PTK with a topography-guided ablation into a single treatment. The concept is that trans-epithelial PTK will treat the irregularity masked by the epithelium and the topography-guided treatment will treat the irregularity detectable on the front surface corneal topography, thereby treating the whole of the stromal surface irregularity. This treatment protocol has been used successfully in cases of flap and interface complications [56, 57]. However, performing a trans-epithelial PTK alone can be a more conservative approach because the cornea can be regularized with less tissue removal by taking advantage of the epithelium masking the remaining irregularity that was not treated by the PTK. Also if the procedure is performed in one step, the predictability of the refractive outcome is likely to be less accurate given the power shifts that can be induced by epithelial compensation [1–4].

Another method of treating irregular astigmatism has been described by Vinciguerra et al. [5] In their custom phototherapeutic keratectomy protocol, a topography-guided ablation is generated from a topography scan obtained after removing the epithelium, i.e., a topography of the stromal surface. After applying this ablation, another topography scan is obtained, and a second topography-guided ablation is generated and applied. This process can be repeated numerous times, each time improving the regularity of the stromal surface.

The advantages of trans-epithelial PTK are that it is straight forward to perform, very low risk, and conservative. All excimer lasers include a PTK mode, so no extra repair software is required, and consequently no complicated ablation profile programming. By definition, the epithelium will be masking a proportion of the stromal surface irregularity, so it can be assumed that a trans-epithelial PTK will afford some smoothing of the stromal surface, but probably not as much as with other more complex techniques. Another advantage is that there is no concern about centration as the PTK ablation has a uniform depth across the whole diameter. In contrast, if a topography-guided ablation is slightly misaligned, then this may increase the irregularity, particularly in cases of very localized irregularities.

The weakness of trans-epithelial PTK is that the refractive shift is currently unpredictable, as demonstrated by our study reporting outcomes for a population of 41 eyes treated by trans-epithelial PTK [1]. A myopic shift was as likely as a hyperopic shift, and the change in spherical equivalent refraction was within ± 0.50 D in only 41% of cases after a trans-epithelial PTK alone. In one case, a trans-epithelial PTK treatment induced a refractive change of $+\ 2.24\ -3.97 \times 120$[4].

13.5 Therapeutic Refractive Surgery: State of the Technology and Geography

In summary, there are now a number of different treatment options for therapeutic refractive surgery, meaning that virtually all refractive surgery complications can be resolved, or at least the visual quality can be improved. Topography-guided custom ablation provides a very effective solution for regularly irregular astigmatism, such as decentration and small optical zone, and trans-epithelial PTK provides a treatment option in even the most irregular corneas. Both procedures have now matured to the point where they can become part of mainstream refractive surgery; all surgeons should at least be aware of these and feel comfortable in referring patients to specialist therapeutic centers if they do not have the tools available. Epithelial thickness mapping plays a critical role for diagnostics in therapeutic cases due to the significant epithelial remodeling that occurs to compensate for stromal surface irregularities. Fortunately, this remodeling can be turned to our advantage as a natural masking agent to use trans-epithelial PTK to target the stromal irregularities.

Financial Disclosure Dr Reinstein is a consultant for Carl Zeiss Meditec (Jena Germany) and CSO Italia (Florence Italy) and has a proprietary interest in the Artemis technology (ArcScan Inc Morrison Colorado) and is an author of patents related to VHF digital ultrasound administered by the Cornell Center for Technology Enterprise and Commercialization (CCTEC) Ithaca New York. the remaining authors have no proprietary or financial interest in the materials presented herein.

References

1. Reinstein DZ, Archer TJ, Dickeson ZI, Gobbe M. Trans-epithelial phototherapeutic keratectomy protocol for treating irregular astigmatism based on population epithelial thickness measurements by Artemis very high-frequency digital ultrasound. J Refract Surg. 2014;30(6):380–7.
2. Reinstein DZ, Archer TJ, Gobbe M. Improved effectiveness of trans-epithelial phototherapeutic keratectomy versus topography-guided ablation degraded by epithelial compensation on irregular stromal surfaces [plus video]. J Refract Surg. 2013;29(8):526–33.
3. Reinstein DZ, Archer T. Combined Artemis very high-frequency digital ultrasound-assisted transepithelial phototherapeutic keratectomy and wavefront-guided treatment following multiple corneal refractive procedures. J Cataract Refract Surg. 2006;32(11):1870–6.
4. Reinstein DZ, Archer TJ, Gobbe M. Refractive and topographic errors in topography-guided ablation produced by epithelial compensation predicted by three-dimensional Artemis very high-frequency digital ultrasound stromal and epithelial thickness mapping. J Refract Surg. 2012;28(9):657–63.
5. Vinciguerra P, Camesasca FI. Custom phototherapeutic keratectomy with intraoperative topography. J Refract Surg. 2004;20(5):S555-563.
6. Reinstein DZ, Archer TJ, Gobbe M. Rate of change of curvature of the corneal stromal surface drives epithelial compensatory changes and remodeling. J Refract Surg. 2014;30(12):800–2. https://doi.org/10.3928/1081597x-20141113-02.
7. Vinciguerra P, Azzolini C, Vinciguerra R. Corneal curvature gradient determines corneal healing process and epithelial behavior. J Refract Surg. 2015;31(4):281–2. https://doi.org/10.3928/1081597x-20150319-08.
8. Vinciguerra P, Roberts CJ, Albe E, Romano MR, Mahmoud A, Trazza S, et al. Corneal curvature gradient map: a new corneal topography map to predict the corneal healing process. J Refract Surg. 2014;30(3):202–7. https://doi.org/10.3928/1081597x-20140218-02.
9. Reinstein DZ, Aslanides IM, Silverman RH, Najafi DJ, Brownlow RL, Belmont S, et al. Epithelial and Corneal 3D ultrasound pachymetric topography post excimer laser surgery. Invest Ophthalmol Vis Sci. 1994;35(4):1739.
10. Reinstein DZ, Archer TJ, Gobbe M. Combined corneal topography and corneal wavefront data in the treatment of corneal irregularity and refractive error in LASIK or PRK using the Carl Zeiss Meditec MEL80 and CRS Master. J Refract Surg. 2009;25(6):503–15.
11. Kymionis GD, Panagopoulou SI, Aslanides IM, Plainis S, Astyrakakis N, Pallikaris IG. Topographically supported customized ablation for the management of decentered laser in situ keratomileusis. Am J Ophthalmol. 2004;137(5):806–11.
12. Wiesinger-Jendritza B, Knorz MC, Hugger P, Liermann A. Laser in situ keratomileusis assisted by corneal topography. J Cataract Refract Surg. 1998;24(2):166–74.
13. Lin DT, Holland SR, Rocha KM, Krueger RR. Method for optimizing topography-guided ablation of highly aberrated eyes with the ALLEGRETTO WAVE Excimer Laser. J Refract Surg. 2008;24(4):S439-445.
14. Alio J, Galal A, Montalban R, Pinero D. Corneal wavefront-guided LASIK retreatments for correction of highly aberrated corneas following refractive surgery. J Refract Surg. 2007;23(8):760–73.
15. Toda I, Yamamoto T, Ito M, Hori-Komai Y, Tsubota K. Topography-guided ablation for treatment of patients with irregular astigmatism. J Refract Surg. 2007;23(2):118–25.
16. Jeandervin M, Barr J. Comparison of repeat videokeratography: repeatability and accuracy. Optom Vis Sci. 1998;75(9):663–9.
17. Belin MW, Ratliff CD. Evaluating data acquisition and smoothing functions of currently available videokeratoscopes. J Cataract Refract Surg. 1996;22(4):421–6.
18. Reinstein DZ, Archer TJ, Carp GI, Stuart AJ, Rowe EL, Nesbit A, et al. Incidence and outcomes of optical zone enlargement and recentration after previous myopic LASIK by topography-guided custom ablation. J Refract Surg. 2018;34(2):121–30. https://doi.org/10.3928/1081597x-20171215-01.

19. Reinstein DZ, Archer TJ, Couch D, Schroeder E, Wottke M. A new night vision disturbances parameter and contrast sensitivity as indicators of success in wavefront-guided enhancement. J Refract Surg. 2005;21(5):S535-540.
20. Steinert RF, Fynn-Thompson N. Relationship between preoperative aberrations and post-operative refractive error in enhancement of previous laser in situ keratomileusis with the LADARVision system. J Cataract Refract Surg. 2008;34(8):1267–72.
21. Bababeygy SR, Zoumalan CI, Chien FY, Manche EE. Wavefront-guided laser in situ keratomileusis retreatment for consecutive hyperopia and compound hyperopic astigmatism. J Cataract Refract Surg. 2008;34(8):1260–6.
22. Hiatt JA, Grant CN, Wachler BS. Complex wavefront-guided retreatments with the Alcon CustomCornea platform after prior LASIK. J Refract Surg. 2006;22(1):48–53.
23. Carones F, Vigo L, Scandola E. Wavefront-guided treatment of abnormal eyes using the LADARVision platform. J Refract Surg. 2003;19(6):S703-708.
24. Carones F, Vigo L, Scandola E. Wavefront-guided treatment of symptomatic eyes using the LADAR6000 excimer laser. J Refract Surg. 2006;22(9):S983-989.
25. Montague AA, Manche EE. CustomVue laser in situ keratomileusis treatment after previous keratorefractive surgery. J Cataract Refract Surg. 2006;32(5):795–8.
26. Chalita MR, Xu M, Krueger RR. Alcon CustomCornea wavefront-guided retreatments after laser in situ keratomileusis. J Refract Surg. 2004;20(5):S624-630.
27. Kashani S, Rajan M, Gartry D. Wavefront-guided retreatment after primary wavefront-guided laser in situ keratomileusis in myopes and hyperopes: long-term follow-up. Am J Ophthalmol. 2009;147(3):417–423 e412.
28. Alio JL, Montes-Mico R. Wavefront-guided versus standard LASIK enhancement for residual refractive errors. Ophthalmology. 2006;113(2):191–7.
29. Jin GJ, Merkley KH. Conventional and wavefront-guided myopic LASIK retreatment. Am J Ophthalmol. 2006;141(4):660–8.
30. Kanellopoulos AJ, Pe LH. Wavefront-guided enhancements using the wavelight excimer laser in symptomatic eyes previously treated with LASIK. J Refract Surg. 2006;22(4):345–9.
31. Gimbel HV, Sofinski SJ, Mahler OS, van Westenbrugge JA, Ferensowicz MI, Triebwasser RW. Wavefront-guided multipoint (segmental) custom ablation enhancement using the Nidek NAVEX platform. J Refract Surg. 2003;19(2 Suppl):S209-216.
32. Reinstein DZ, Gobbe M, Archer TJ. Coaxially sighted corneal light reflex versus entrance pupil center centration of moderate to high hyperopic corneal ablations in eyes with small and large angle kappa. J Refract Surg. 2013;29(8):518–25. https://doi.org/10.3928/1081597x-20130719-08.
33. de Ortueta D, Schreyger FD. Centration on the cornea vertex normal during hyperopic refractive photoablation using videokeratoscopy. J Refract Surg. 2007;23(2):198–200.
34. Wu L, Zhou X, Chu R, Wang Q. Photoablation centration on the corneal optical center in myopic LASIK using AOV excimer laser. Eur J Ophthalmol. 2009;19(6):923–9.
35. Durrie DS, Stahl JE, Schwendeman F. Alcon LADARWave customcornea retreatments. J Refract Surg. 2005;21(6):S804-807.
36. Reinstein DZ, Archer TJ, Gobbe M. Is topography-guided ablation profile centered on the corneal vertex better than wavefront-guided ablation profile centered on the entrance pupil? J Refract Surg. 2012;28(2):139–43.
37. Reinstein DZ, Archer TJ, Gobbe M, Silverman RH, Coleman DJ. Epithelial thickness in the normal cornea: three-dimensional display with Artemis very high-frequency digital ultrasound. J Refract Surg. 2008;24(6):571–81.
38. Reinstein DZ, Silverman RH, Coleman DJ. High-frequency ultrasound measurement of the thickness of the corneal epithelium. Refract Corneal Surg. 1993;9(5):385–7.
39. Reinstein DZ, Gobbe M, Archer TJ, Couch D, Bloom B. Epithelial, stromal, and corneal pachymetry changes during orthokeratology. Optom Vis Sci. 2009;86(8):E1006-1014.
40. Gauthier CA, Holden BA, Epstein D, Tengroth B, Fagerholm P, Hamberg-Nystrom H. Role of epithelial hyperplasia in regression following photorefractive keratectomy. Br J Ophthalmol. 1996;80(6):545–8.

41. Reinstein DZ, Srivannaboon S, Gobbe M, Archer TJ, Silverman RH, Sutton H, et al. Epithelial thickness profile changes induced by myopic LASIK as measured by Artemis very high-frequency digital ultrasound. J Refract Surg. 2009;25(5):444–50.
42. Reinstein DZ, Archer TJ, Gobbe M. Change in epithelial thickness profile 24 hours and longitudinally for 1 year after myopic lasik: three-dimensional display with artemis very high-frequency digital ultrasound. J Refract Surg. 2012;28(3):195–201.
43. Kanellopoulos AJ, Asimellis G. Longitudinal postoperative lasik epithelial thickness profile changes in correlation with degree of myopia correction. J Refract Surg. 2014;30(3):166–71. https://doi.org/10.3928/1081597x-20140219-01.
44. Reinstein DZ, Archer TJ, Gobbe M, Silverman RH, Coleman DJ. Epithelial thickness after hyperopic LASIK: three-dimensional display with artemis very high-frequency digital ultrasound. J Refract Surg. 2010;26(8):555–64.
45. Reinstein DZ, Archer TJ, Gobbe M. Epithelial thickness up to 26 years after radial keratotomy: three-dimensional display with artemis very high-frequency digital ultrasound. J Refract Surg. 2011;27(8):618–24.
46. Reinstein DZ, Srivannaboon S, Holland SP. Epithelial and stromal changes induced by intacs examined by three-dimensional very high-frequency digital ultrasound. J Refract Surg. 2001;17(3):310–8.
47. Reinstein DZ, Silverman RH, Sutton HF, Coleman DJ. Very high-frequency ultrasound corneal analysis identifies anatomic correlates of optical complications of lamellar refractive surgery: anatomic diagnosis in lamellar surgery. Ophthalmology. 1999;106(3):474–82.
48. Reinstein DZ, Gobbe M, Archer TJ, Youssefi G, Sutton HF. Stromal surface topography-guided custom ablation as a repair tool for corneal irregular astigmatism. J Refract Surg. 2015;31(1):54–9.
49. Reinstein DZ, Archer TJ, Gobbe M, Silverman RH, Coleman DJ. Epithelial, stromal and corneal thickness in the keratoconic cornea: three-dimensional display with Artemis very high-frequency digital ultrasound. J Refract Surg. 2010;26(4):259–71.
50. Li Y, Tan O, Brass R, Weiss JL, Huang D. Corneal epithelial thickness mapping by fourier-domain optical coherence tomography in normal and keratoconic eyes. Ophthalmology. 2012;119(12):2425–33. https://doi.org/10.1016/j.ophtha.2012.06.023.
51. Rocha KM, Perez-Straziota CE, Stulting RD, Randleman JB. SD-OCT analysis of regional epithelial thickness profiles in keratoconus, postoperative corneal ectasia, and normal eyes. J Refract Surg. 2013;29(3):173–9. https://doi.org/10.3928/1081597x-20130129-08.
52. Kanellopoulos AJ, Aslanides IM, Asimellis G. Correlation between epithelial thickness in normal corneas, untreated ectatic corneas, and ectatic corneas previously treated with CXL; is overall epithelial thickness a very early ectasia prognostic factor? Clin Ophthalmol. 2012;6:789–800. https://doi.org/10.2147/opth.s31524.
53. Sandali O, El Sanharawi M, Temstet C, Hamiche T, Galan A, Ghouali W, et al. Fourier-domain optical coherence tomography imaging in keratoconus: a corneal structural classification. Ophthalmology. 2013;120(12):2403–12. https://doi.org/10.1016/j.ophtha.2013.05.027.
54. Reinstein DZ, Gobbe M, Archer TJ, Couch D. Epithelial thickness profile as a method to evaluate the effectiveness of collagen cross-linking treatment after corneal ectasia. J Refract Surg. 2011;27(5):356–63.
55. Reinstein DZ, Archer TJ, Gobbe M, Rothman RC. Epithelial thickness changes following the realignment of a malpositioned free cap. J Cataract Refract Surg. 2014;40(7):1237–9.
56. Chen X, Stojanovic A, Zhou W, Utheim TP, Stojanovic F, Wang Q. Transepithelial, topography-guided ablation in the treatment of visual disturbances in LASIK flap or interface complications. J Refract Surg. 2012;28(2):120–6.
57. Chen X, Stojanovic A, Nitter TA. Topography guided transepithelial surface ablation in treatment of recurrent epithelial ingrowths. J Refract Surg. 2010;26(7):529–32.

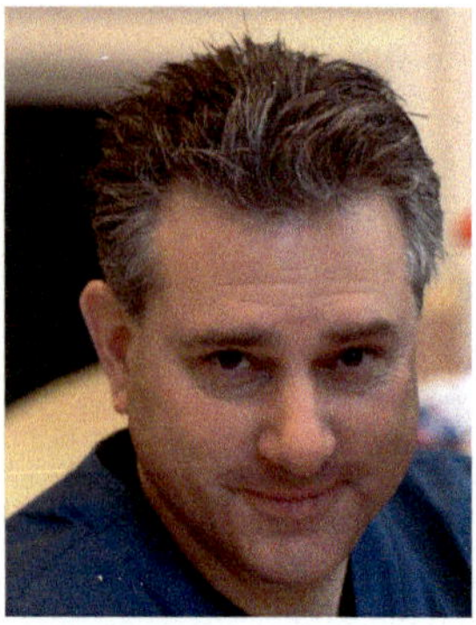

Dan Z. Reinstein Professor Dan Z. Reinstein, Founder and Medical Director of the London Vision Clinic and part of the EuroEyes Group, is a board-certified ophthalmologist in the US and Canada, with professorships in the UK, New York, and Paris. Dedicated solely to Refractive Surgery since the 1990s, he has pioneered epithelium mapping and corneal 3D pachymetric imaging with VHF digital ultrasound and OCT. His extensive contributions include over 215 scientific papers, 1,000+ lectures globally, and significant roles in Therapeutic Refractive Surgery and as the Section Editor for the Journal of Refractive Surgery. He authored a definitive textbook on SMILE, contributed to 44 book chapters, and holds patents for VHF digital ultrasound technology, commercialized as the Insight 100 by ArcScan Inc., which is pivotal for the most accurate ICL sizing. Reinstein developed PRESBYOND Laser Blended Vision, now a part of the Carl Zeiss Meditec platform, and has been their Lead Refractive Surgery consultant since 2001. His achievements have earned him numerous awards, including the Waring Medal (2006), the Kritzinger Award (2013), the ISRS President's and AAO Senior Achievement Awards (2020), the Lifetime Achievement Award from UKISCRS (2023), and the Barraquer Award from AAO (2024). An accomplished saxophonist, he has maintained a monthly residency at the 606 Club in Chelsea for over 20 years.

Part III

Small Incision Lenticule Extraction (SMILE® and SMILE pro®): Clinical Science Related to SMILE

The Key Characteristics of Corneal Refractive Surgery: Biomechanics and Corneal Sensitivity After SMILE

14

Dan Z. Reinstein, Timothy J. Archer, and Felix Mathias Wagner

Abstract

This chapter focuses on the biomechanical and sensory aspects of Small Incision Lenticule Extraction (SMILE) in corneal refractive surgery. It explores the procedure's impact on corneal strength, comparing it to other techniques such as LASIK, and highlights how SMILE preserves the anterior stroma, contributing to better biomechanical stability. The chapter also delves into the effects of SMILE on corneal nerve integrity and sensitivity, addressing postoperative recovery and complications like dry eye. Through a review of key studies, the chapter provides insights into the biomechanical advantages and clinical outcomes associated with SMILE.

Keywords

Small incision lenticule extraction surgery (SMILE) • Corneal biomechanics • Corneal sensitivity • Corneal tensile strength

D. Z. Reinstein · T. J. Archer
London Vision Clinic, London, UK

D. Z. Reinstein
Department of Ophthalmology, Columbia University Medical Center, New York, NY, USA

Centre Hospitalier National d'Ophtalmologie, Paris, France

F. M. Wagner (✉)
Department of Ophthalmology, University Medical Center of the Johannes Gutenberg University, Langenbeckstr. 1, 55131 Mainz, Germany
e-mail: felix.mathias.wagner@gmail.com

W. Sekundo and F. M. Wagner (eds.), *Femtosecond Laser Assisted Lenticule Extraction*,
https://doi.org/10.1007/978-3-031-60424-9_14

14.1 Biomechanical Advantages of SMILE

Approximately 200 collagen lamellae compose the cornea, which contain crucial collagen fibers for maintaining its shape [1, 2]. The biomechanical strength of the cornea is ensured by the intertwining of these lamellae and the cornea's natural cross-linking, with the strongest part being the anterior third [3]. After an incision, the tensile strength in the corneal lamellae decreases and does not contribute to the cornea's overall resistance to intraocular pressure. A vertical incision, due to the lamellae's orientation, causes a greater reduction in biomechanical stability compared to an incision that is parallel to the corneal surface [4].

14.1.1 Vertical Cuts Have More Biomechanical Impact Than Horizontal Cuts

The cornea is composed of layers of collagen lamellae, which run from limbus to limbus and are oriented at precise angles relative to adjacent lamellae, contributing to corneal transparency and strength. The stromal collagen lamellae, primarily type I collagen, are uniformly sized and regularly spaced in over 200 thin layers, a feature unique to the cornea and pivotal for light transmission. These lamellae are enveloped by several proteoglycans, including keratocan, lumican, and decorin. These macromolecules, with their glycosaminoglycan chains such as keratan sulfate and chondroitin sulfate, ensure proper spacing of the collagen fibers and maintain stromal hydration. In LASIK, the sidecut disrupts the anterior corneal lamellae. Consequently, the peripheral anterior lamellae, no longer under tension, relax and spread out, leading to peripheral stromal thickening (as shown in Fig. 14.1). This expansion exerts a pulling force on the posterior lamellae, causing central flattening of the cornea. However, these posterior lamellae must also contend with an unchanged intraocular pressure (IOP), which may result in some forward bowing of the cornea. SMILE preserves the structural integrity of the anterior cornea better, leading to less biomechanical compromise due to the smaller vertical incision that impacts the corneal biomechanics to a lesser extent.

In a study on cadaver eyes in organ culture, Knox Cartwright et al. [4] demonstrated the greater influence of vertical incisions on biomechanical stability. The study compared the corneal strain produced by a LASIK flap, a sidecut only, and a delamination cut only, with each incision type performed at both 90 μm and 160 μm. Table 14.1 summarizes the results, which found that the increase in strain was equivalent between a LASIK flap and a sidecut alone at both depths with a significantly greater increase for the 160 μm depth. In contrast, the increase in strain after a delamination/bed cut only (i.e., no vertical sidecut—only horizontal intrastromal cut) was significantly lower than after a LASIK flap or sidecut only. Also, the strain did not increase when a delamination/bed cut only was performed at the greater 160 μm depth. A similar result has also been found in a study by Medeiros et al. [9] who showed in pig eyes that there was significant greater

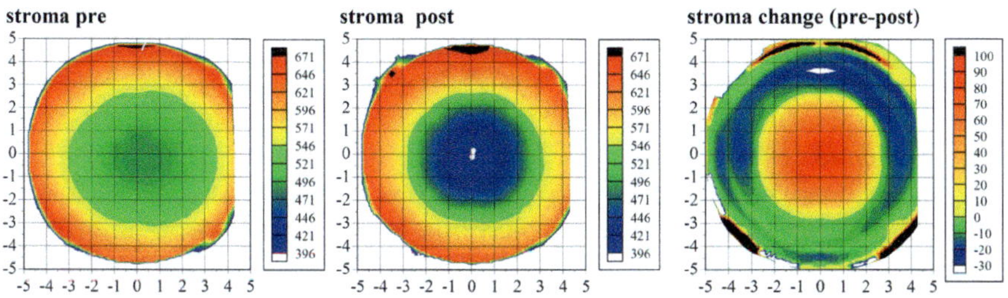

Fig. 14.1 Artemis® very high-frequency digital ultrasound (ArcScan Inc.) stromal thickness maps before (left) and 3 months after (middle) LASIK for −9.00 D myopia with a 6 mm optical zone. The color scales are thickness in μm, and a Cartesian grid is superimposed at 1 mm intervals for the 10 mm diameter. Scans were centered on the corneal vertex. The difference map (right) shows the change in stromal thickness (red/orange represents stromal thinning, and blue/green represents stromal thickening) demonstrating the tissue removed by the ablation centrally with less tissue removal radially as expected for a myopic ablation. However, outside the 6 mm optical zone, the stroma was actually thicker after LASIK

Table 14.1 Percentage increase in central corneal strain (to an intraocular pressure change from 15 mmHg to 15.5 mmHg) after the creation of a LASIK flap, a sidecut or delamination at both 90 μm and 160 μm

	90 μm (%)	160 μm (%)
LASIK flap	9	32
Sidecut only	9	33
Delamination only	5	5

Data obtained from Knox Cartwright NE, Tyrer JR, Jaycock PD, Marshall J. Effects of Variation in Depth and Side Cut Angulations in LASIK and Thin-flap LASIK Using a Femtosecond Laser: A Biomechanical Study. J Refract Surg. 2012;28:419–425

biomechanical changes following the creation of a thick flap of 300 μm compared to a thin flap of 100 μm.

Applying this finding to SMILE, since no anterior corneal sidecut is created, there will be slightly less increase in corneal strain in SMILE compared to thin flap LASIK and a significant difference in corneal strain compared to LASIK with a thicker flap.

14.1.2 Anterior Stromal Lamellae are Stronger Than Posterior Stromal Lamellae

Randleman et al. [3] demonstrated that the cohesive tensile strength (i.e., how strongly the stromal lamellae are held together) of the stroma decreases from anterior to posterior within the central corneal region (Fig. 14.2). In an experiment in which the cohesive tensile strength was measured for strips of stromal lamellae cut from different depths within donor corneoscleral buttons, a strong negative correlation was found between stromal depth and cohesive tensile strength. The anterior 40% of the central corneal stroma was found to be the strongest region of the cornea, whereas the posterior 60% of the stroma was at least 50% weaker. A number of other authors have reached this conclusion by other indirect means.

In addition to cohesive tensile strength, tangential tensile strength (i.e., stiffness along the stromal lamellae) and shear strength (i.e., resistance to torsional forces) have both been found to vary with depth in the stroma. Kohlhaas et al. [16] and Scarcelli et al. [17] found that the tangential tensile strength was greater for anterior stroma than posterior stroma, each using different methodology. Petsche et al. [18] found a similar result for transverse shear strength to decrease with stromal depth. The same group have used nonlinear optical high-resolution macroscopy to image the three-dimensional distribution of transverse collagen fibers and have shown that the nonlinearity of tensile strength through the stroma is caused by the greater interconnectivity of the collagen fibers in the anterior stroma compared to the posterior stroma where the collagen fibers lie in parallel to each other [19].

An interesting finding of these studies is the nonlinear nature of the change in tensile strength through the stroma. The cohesive tensile strength appears to decrease rapidly for the anterior-most 30% [3]. There is then a region between 70 and 20% depth where the cohesive tensile strength decreases slowly, but then drops off sharply again for the posterior-most 20% (as seen in Fig. 14.2). This nonlinearity may be associated with the known different collagen organizational layers within the stroma [12, 20, 21]. Of note is the remarkable similarity of this curve to that reported for tangential tensile strength by Scarcelli et al. [17] (Fig. 14.3), which demonstrates the strong correlation between corneal biomechanical properties with stromal depth. This finding also agrees with studies that have found other depth-dependent properties of the corneal stroma such as decreasing refractive index [22], greater UV-B absorption in the anterior stroma [23], and varying excimer laser ablation rates [24, 25].

14.1.3 Residual Stromal Thickness Calculation in SMILE

The approach to calculating residual stromal thickness (RST) has evolved with advancements in techniques, particularly with the introduction of SMILE. In our opinion, this rational can also be applied to other keratorefractive lenticule extraction (KLEX) procedures. Unlike in LASIK, where RST is gauged as the stromal tissue remaining beneath the flap, SMILE requires a different assessment due to its unique procedure. In SMILE, due to preservation of the anterior stromal lamellae, the true RST in SMILE is determined by the full thickness of uncut stromal tissue, combining the stroma beneath the posterior lenticule interface and the untouched stroma above the anterior lenticule interface up to Bowman's layer.

$$\text{RST} = \text{Preoperative Corneal Thickness} - \text{Lenticule Thickness}$$

Considering that SMILE leaves the anterior corneal stroma intact, while keratomileusis is performed in the deeper and weaker portion of the cornea, it is

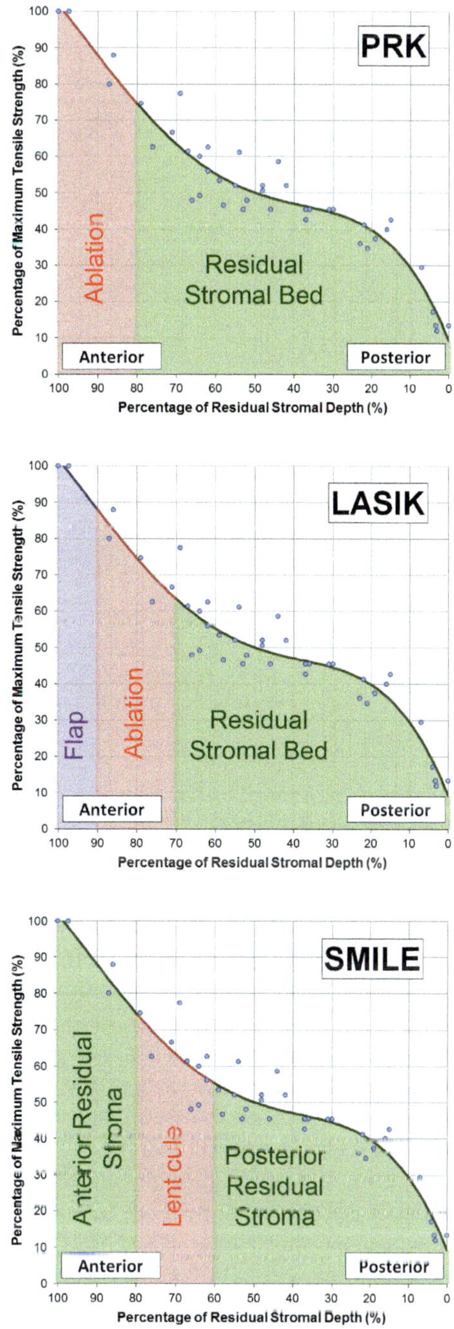

Fig. 14.2 Scatter plots of the percentage of maximum cohesive tensile strength against the percentage of residual stromal depth using data from the study by Randleman et al. [3] Regression analysis found that a fourth-order polynomial provided the closest fit to the data and the R^2 of 0.93 demonstrated the high correlation achieved. The fourth-order polynomial regression equation was integrated to calculate the area under the curve for the relevant stromal depths after photorefractive keratectomy (PRK), LASIK, and small incision lenticule extraction (SMILE) as demonstrated by the green shaded regions. The red areas represent the tissue removed (excimer laser ablation/lenticule extraction) and the purple area in LASIK represents the LASIK flap. Reprinted with permission from Reinstein DZ, Archer TJ, Randleman JB. Mathematical model to compare the relative tensile strength of the cornea after PRK, LASIK, and small incision lenticule extraction. J Refract Surg. 2013 Jul;29(7):454–60

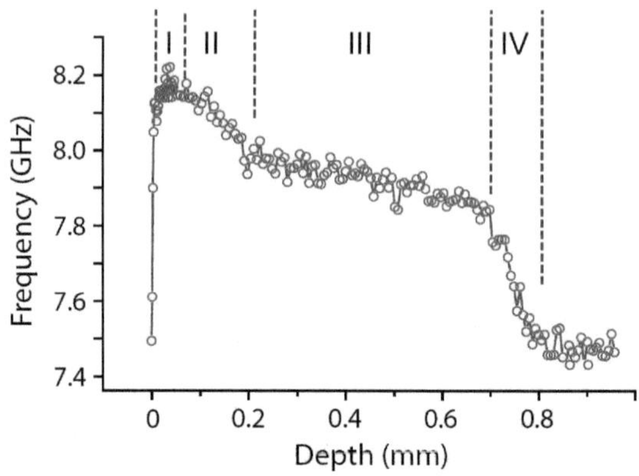

Fig. 14.3 Tangential tensile strength (longitudinal modulus of elasticity) measured by Brillouin microscopy at different depths in a (bovine) cornea including the epithelium (I), anterior stroma (II), posterior stroma (III), and the innermost region near the endothelium (IV). Reprinted with permission from Scarcelli G, Pineda R, Yun SH. Brillouin optical microscopy for corneal biomechanics. Invest Ophthalmol Vis Sci. 2012;53:185–190

reasonable to assume that SMILE will leave the cornea with greater tensile strength than LASIK or PRK for any given refractive correction. Therefore, it may be helpful to consider tensile strength rather than residual stromal thickness.

14.1.4 Biomechanics Model—Comparing SMILE to PRK and LASIK

Reinstein et al. developed a mathematical model based on Randleman's [3] depth-dependent tensile strength data for postoperative tensile strength comparison in PRK, LASIK, and SMILE [26]. This model assumes cohesive tensile strength as a representative metric for overall corneal biomechanics. Using a nonlinear regression analysis of Randleman's data, the model calculates the total tensile strength of the untreated cornea and compares it postoperatively for each refractive surgery type. In SMILE, the model accounts for both the untouched anterior stroma and the tissue below the lenticule, suggesting that SMILE maintains greater tensile strength than LASIK or PRK for equivalent refractive corrections.

The model's application to various scenarios revealed that SMILE consistently maintains higher postoperative tensile strength. It also demonstrated that thicker caps, leaving more anterior stroma intact, result in greater tensile strength. Conversely, in LASIK, thicker flaps correlate with lower postoperative strength. The model also indicates that corneal tensile strength decreases with thinner corneas, with a more pronounced difference between procedures. The results are quantified in an example scenario shown in Fig. 14.4.

This model, while focused on the central corneal point, suggests a different approach in assessing the safety of subtractive corneal refractive surgeries.

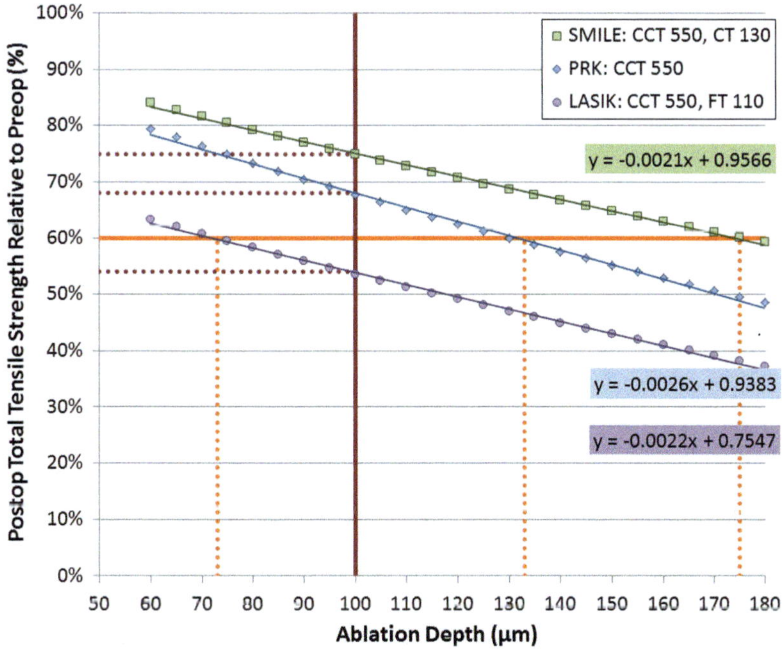

Fig. 14.4 This graph shows the relative total tensile strength after LASIK (purple), photorefractive keratectomy (PRK) (blue), and small incision lenticule extraction (SMILE) (green) plotted against a range of ablation depths for a fixed central corneal thickness of 550 μm, a LASIK flap thickness of 110 μm, and a SMILE cap thickness of 130 μm. The orange lines indicate that the postoperative relative total tensile strength reached 60% for an ablation depth of 73 μm in LASIK (approximately −5.75 diopters [D]), 132 μm in PRK (approximately −10.00 D), and 175 μm in SMILE (approximately −13.50 D), translating to a 7.75 D difference between LASIK and SMILE for a cornea of the same postoperative relative total tensile strength. The red lines indicate that the postoperative relative total tensile strength after a 100 μm tissue removal would be 54% in LASIK, 68% in PRK, and 75% in SMILE. Reprinted with permission from Reinstein DZ, Archer TJ, Randleman JB. Mathematical model to compare the relative tensile strength of the cornea after PRK, LASIK, and small incision lenticule extraction. J Refract Surg. 2013 Jul;29(7):454–60

It proposes that total tensile strength, acknowledging the nonlinearity of stromal strength, is a more appropriate measure than just residual stromal thickness.

14.2 Evidence for Biomechanical Advantages of SMILE

Measuring the biomechanical differences between SMILE and LASIK in vivo is a challenging task, despite the increasing number of devices that indirectly quantify the biomechanical properties. There are multiple studies where the Ocular Response Analyzer (Reichert Inc, Depew, NY, USA) or the high-speed Scheimpflug camera (Corvis ST, Oculus, Wetzlar, Germany) have been used to measure viscoelastic parameters, such as corneal hysteresis (CH) and corneal resistance factor (CRF) or elastic properties of the cornea. These studies show no or only slight differences between the SMILE and LASIK groups [36–43]. These results do not agree with the expected increased biomechanical strength after SMILE in comparison with flap-based procedures. However, it is likely corneal hysteresis and corneal resistance are not ideal parameters for measuring corneal biomechanics [44] given that many studies show no change in CH and CRF after cross-linking [45]. It is also well-known that CH and CRF are correlated with corneal pachymetry [46], so it would be expected for CH and CRF to be reduced after SMILE due to tissue removal.

The biomechanical benefits of SMILE, as calculated in the above model, have been confirmed by the experimental work of the team led by Sekundo and Hafezi [47]. In their intra-individual experiments on cadaver eyes, biomechanical properties of human corneas post-Femtosecond Laser-Assisted LASIK (Fs-LASIK) and Small Incision Lenticule Extraction (SMILE) were compared using 11 pairs of human corneas. Corneas from right eyes were treated with Fs-LASIK and left eyes with SMILE. All corneas underwent refractive correction with either a 110 μm flap (Fs-LASIK) or a 130 μm cap (SMILE). Two-dimensional biomechanical measurements were used to characterize the corneas post-Fs-LASIK and SMILE. A three-dimensional test force was applied from the posterior surface using a spherical indenter to mimic intraocular pressure. Each specimen underwent two stress–strain testing cycles, followed by a stress-relaxation test. The study revealed that the effective elastic modulus in stress–strain measurements was 1.47 times higher in corneas treated with SMILE than in those treated with Fs-LASIK (Fig. 14.5), demonstrating greater biomechanical stability with SMILE procedures. This shows that SMILE, which does not sever the anterior stromal lamellae or Bowman's layer, preserves corneal strength more effectively than Fs-LASIK.

14.3 Ocular Surface and Corneal Sensitivity

The cornea is one of the most densely innervated peripheral tissues in humans. Nerve bundles within the anterior stroma grow radially inward from the periphery toward the central cornea [53, 54]. The nerves then penetrate Bowman's layer and create a dense network of nerve fibers, known as the subbasal nerve plexus, by branching both vertically and horizontally between Bowman's layer and basal epithelial cells. In LASIK, subbasal nerve bundles and superficial stromal nerve bundles in the flap interface are cut by the microkeratome or femtosecond laser, with only nerves entering the flap through the hinge region being spared. Subsequent excimer laser ablation severs further stromal nerve fiber bundles. Therefore, corneal sensitivity is decreased while the nerves regenerate. The lower corneal sensitivity can lead to a reduction in the blink rate, resulting in epitheliopathy (known as LASIK-induced neurotrophic epitheliopathy) due to the increased ocular surface

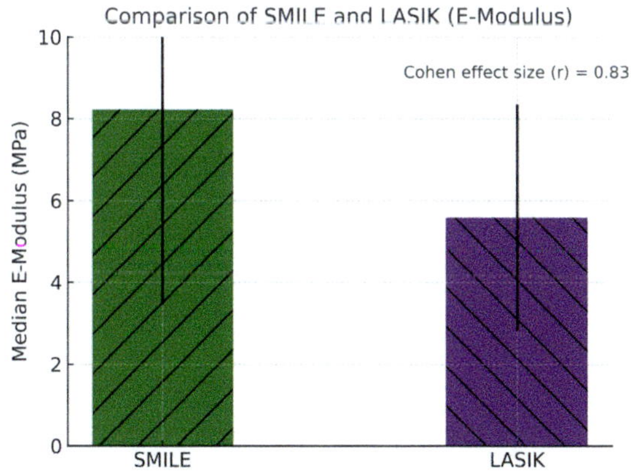

Fig. 14.5 Bar chart of the median e-moduli at 0.5–0.2 strain. Significantly higher e-Module in the SMILE group with 8.22 MPa compared to the LASIKK group with 5.59 MPa ($p = 0.003$). Illustration of data from Spiru B, Kling S, Hafezi F, Sekundo W. Biomechanical Properties of Human Cornea Tested by Two-Dimensional Extensiometry Ex Vivo in Fellow Eyes: Femtosecond Laser-Assisted LASIK Versus SMILE. J Refract Surg. 2018 Jun 1;34(6):419–423

exposure and patients feel 'dry eye' [55, 56]. While there are also other contributing factors, it is generally accepted that corneal denervation is the largest factor [57–59].

While the trunk nerves that ascend into the epithelial layer within the diameter of the cap will still be severed in SMILE, those that ascend outside the cap diameter or that are anterior to the cap interface will be spared. A number of studies have investigated this by measuring corneal sensitivity using aesthesiometry and corneal innervation using confocal microscopy.

A study by Reinstein et al. showed reduced corneal sensitivity in the early postoperative period after SMILE ($n = 156$), but recovery to baseline in 76% of eyes by 3 months and in 89% of eyes by 6 months [60]. Similar results have been reported in other SMILE studies. Wei et al. [61] found significantly higher central corneal sensitivity in the SMILE group ($n = 61$) compared with the LASIK group ($n = 54$) at 1 week, 1 month, and 3 months. Central corneal sensitivity decreased only slightly at 1 week and recovered to baseline 3 months after SMILE, whereas it had not reached baseline in the LASIK group. Similar results were found in a larger study by the same group [62].

Vestergaard et al. [63] performed a contra-lateral eye study comparing central corneal sensitivity after FLEx and SMILE in 35 myopic patients. At the 6-month time point, mean central corneal sensitivity was found to have returned to the baseline level in the SMILE group (1.0 mm less than baseline, $p > 0.05$). In contrast, mean central corneal sensitivity was 3.8 mm less than baseline in the FLEx group ($p < 0.05$) and was statistically significantly lower than the SMILE group.

Demirok et al. [64] performed a contra-lateral eye study comparing central corneal sensitivity after LASIK and SMILE in 28 myopic patients over a 6-month follow-up period. Mean central corneal sensitivity was reduced after both SMILE and LASIK at 1 week, 1 month, and 3 months; however, it was statistically significantly higher in the SMILE group at each of these time points. Central corneal sensitivity had returned to baseline levels at the 6-month time point in both groups. Although there was a difference in corneal sensitivity, other dry eye parameters were not affected including tear break-up time, Schirmer test, and tear film osmolarity.

Li et al. [65, 66] compared the change in central corneal sensitivity between SMILE (n = 38) and LASIK (n = 31) over a 6-month follow-up period. Mean central corneal sensitivity was reduced after both SMILE and LASIK at 1 week, 1 month, 3 months, and 6 months; however, it was statistically significantly higher in the SMILE group at each of these time points. As with the previous study, although there was a difference in corneal sensitivity, there were no real differences between groups for other dry eye parameters, such as tear break-up time, Schirmer test, and the Ocular Surface Disease Index (OSDI) questionnaire. Similar results were found by the same group in a second study [67].

Gao et al. [68] compared the change in central corneal sensitivity between SMILE (n = 30) and LASIK (n = 64) over a 3 month follow-up period. Mean central corneal sensitivity was reduced after SMILE at 1 week and 1 month, but had recovered to baseline by 3 months. The reduction in central corneal sensitivity after LASIK was significantly greater than after SMILE at all time points and was still 39% lower than baseline at 3 months. This study also showed that SMILE resulted in milder ocular surface changes than LASIK in terms of fluorescein staining, tear break-up time, OSDI scores, IL-6 and NGF levels, and TNF-α and ICAM-1 concentrations.

Figure 14.6 shows the average corneal sensitivity (across all eight studies after SMILE) plotted over time [60–68]. For comparison, the graph also shows the average corneal sensitivity (across twenty one studies [60] after LASIK where the Cochet–Bonnet aesthesiometer had been used) plotted over time.

A few studies have also investigated the change in corneal innervation using confocal microscopy. Vestergaard et al. [63] demonstrated that the decrease in

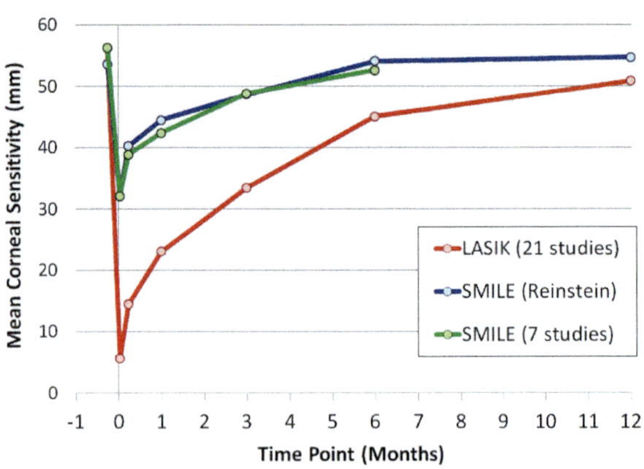

Fig. 14.6 Line graph showing the mean central corneal sensitivity over the 12-month follow-up period averaged across 7 SMILE studies and 16 LASIK studies following a review of the peer-reviewed literature

corneal nerves was greater after LASIK compared with SMILE at 6 months. Li et al. [67] found that the decrease in subbasal nerve fiber density was less severe in the first 3 months after SMILE than after LASIK. Similarly, Mohamed-Noriega et al. found less nerve damage and faster nerve recovery in rabbit eyes 4 weeks after SMILE compared to LASIK [69]. A detailed review on this topic has been presented in Chap. 3 of this book.

Finally, a recent study by Xu et al. [70] compared dry eye parameters between SMILE and LASIK. They found that all parameters became worse in the early postoperative period in both groups; however, Schirmer's test, tear break-up time, and the McMonnies score were all better in the SMILE group.

14.4 Summary

The evolution of SMILE and KLEX in general created a new method for corneal refractive surgery that minimizes the change in corneal biomechanics compared to PRK and flap-based procedures by leaving the stronger anterior stroma intact. When assessing corneal stability before SMILE tensile strength should be taken into account and RST should include full thickness of uncut stromal tissue. The biomechanical superiority of SMILE surgery over flap-based procedures has now been demonstrated in the laboratory on human corneas following the modeled prediction. The other advantage of the flapless mechanism of SMILE is that there is greater preservation of the anterior corneal nerve plexus resulting in faster recovery of corneal innervation and corneal sensitivity.

Financial Disclosure Dr Reinstein is a consultant for Carl Zeiss Meditec (Jena, Germany) and has a proprietary interest in the Artemis technology (ArcScan Inc, Morrison, Colorado) and is an author of patents related to VHF digital ultrasound administered by the Cornell Center for Technology Enterprise and Commercialization (CCTEC), Ithaca, New York. The remaining authors have no proprietary or financial interest in the materials presented herein.

References

1. Aghamohammadzadeh H, Newton RH, Meek KM. X-ray scattering used to map the preferred collagen orientation in the human cornea and limbus. Structure. 2004;12(2):249–56.
2. Bergmanson JP, et al. Assessment of the number of lamellae in the central region of the normal human corneal stroma at the resolution of the transmission electron microscope. Eye Contact Lens. 2005;31(6):281–7.
3. Randleman JB, et al. Depth-dependent cohesive tensile strength in human donor corneas: implications for refractive surgery. J Refract Surg. 2008;24(1):S85–9.
4. Knox Cartwright NE, et al. Effects of variation in depth and side cut angulations in LASIK and thin-flap LASIK using a femtosecond laser: a biomechanical study. J Refract Surg. 2012;28(6).419–25.
5. Reinstein DZ, et al. Arc-scanning very high-frequency digital ultrasound for 3D pachymetric mapping of the corneal epithelium and stroma in laser in situ keratomileusis. J Refract Surg. 2000;16(4):414–30.

6. Dupps WJ, Roberts C. Effect of acute biomechanical changes on corneal curvature after photokeratectomy. J Refract Surg. 2001;17(6):658–69.
7. Dupps WJ, Roberts C, Schoessler JP. Peripheral lamellar relaxation. In ARVO 1995. Fort Lauderdale, FL, USA:1995.
8. Roberts C. The cornea is not a piece of plastic. J Refract Surg. 2000;16(4):407–13.
9. Medeiros FW, et al. Biomechanical corneal changes induced by different flap thickness created by femtosecond laser. Clinics (Sao Paulo). 2011;66(6):1067–71.
10. MacRae S, et al. Diurnal variation in vision after radial keratotomy. Am J Ophthalmol. 1989;107(3):262–7.
11. Maloney RK. Effect of corneal hydration and intraocular pressure on keratometric power after experimental radial keratotomy. Ophthalmology. 1990;97(7):927–33.
12. Muller LJ, Pels E, Vrensen GF. The specific architecture of the anterior stroma accounts for maintenance of corneal curvature. Br J Ophthalmol. 2001;85(4):437–43.
13. Ousley PJ, Terry MA. Hydration effects on corneal topography. Arch Ophthalmol. 1996;114(2):181–5.
14. Simon G, Ren Q. Biomechanical behavior of the cornea and its response to radial keratotomy. J Refract Corneal Surg. 1994;10(3):343–51; discussion 351–6.
15. Simon G, et al. Effect of corneal hydration on Goldmann applanation tonometry and corneal topography. Refract Corneal Surg. 1993;9(2):110–7.
16. Kohlhaas M, et al. Biomechanical evidence of the distribution of cross-links in corneas treated with riboflavin and ultraviolet A light. J Cataract Refract Surg. 2006;32(2):279–83.
17. Scarcelli G, Pineda R, Yun SH. Brillouin optical microscopy for corneal biomechanics. Invest Ophthalmol Vis Sci. 2012;53(1):185–90.
18. Petsche SJ, et al. Depth-dependent transverse shear properties of the human corneal stroma. Invest Ophthalmol Vis Sci. 2012;53(2):873–80.
19. Winkler M, et al. Three-dimensional distribution of transverse collagen fibers in the anterior human corneal stroma. Invest Ophthalmol Vis Sci. 2013;54(12):7293–301.
20. Dawson DG, et al. Biomechanical and wound healing characteristics of corneas after excimer laser keratorefractive surgery: is there a difference between advanced surface ablation and sub-Bowman's keratomileusis? J Refract Surg. 2008;24(1):S90–6.
21. Roy AS, Dupps WJ Jr. Patient-specific computational modeling of keratoconus progression and differential responses to collagen cross-linking. Invest Ophthalmol Vis Sci. 2011;52(12):9174–87.
22. Patel S. Refractive index of the mammalian cornea and its influence during pachometry. Ophthalmic Physiol Opt. 1987;7(4):503–6.
23. Kolozsvari L, et al. UV absorbance of the human cornea in the 240 to 400-nm range. Invest Ophthalmol Vis Sci. 2002;43(7):2165–8.
24. Seiler T, et al. Ablation rate of human corneal epithelium and Bowman's layer with the excimer laser (193 nm). Refract Corneal Surg. 1990;6(2):99–102.
25. Huebscher HJ, Genth U, Seiler T. Determination of excimer laser ablation rate of the human cornea using in vivo Scheimpflug videography. Invest Ophthalmol Vis Sci. 1996;37(1):42–6.
26. Reinstein DZ, Archer TJ, Randleman JB. Mathematical model to compare the relative tensile strength of the cornea after PRK, LASIK, and small incision lenticule extraction. J Refract Surg. 2013;29(7):454–60.
27. Schmack I, et al. Cohesive tensile strength of human LASIK wounds with histologic, ultrastructural, and clinical correlations. J Refract Surg. 2005;21(5):433–45.
28. Seiler T, et al. Does Bowman's layer determine the biomechanical properties of the cornea? Refract Corneal Surg. 1992;8(2):139–42.
29. Sinha Roy A et al. Linking peripheral stromal thickening after refractive surgery to central cornea flattening and induced spherical aberration. J Cataract Refract Surg 2014 [In Press].
30. Reinstein DZ, Archer TJ, Gobbe M. Spherical Aberration change as a function of pupil size: a comparison between small incision lenticule extraction [SMILE] and non-linear aspheric LASIK in moderate to high myopia. In: ARVO. Fort Lauderdale, USA: 2012.

31. Reinstein DZ, Archer TJ, Gobbe M. LASIK for myopic astigmatism and presbyopia using non-linear aspheric micro-monovision with the carl zeiss meditec MEL 80 platform. J Refract Surg. 2011;27(1):23–37.
32. Ganesh S, Gupta R. Comparison of visual and refractive outcomes following femtosecond laser—assisted lasik with smile in patients with myopia or myopic astigmatism. J Refract Surg. 2014;30(9):590–6.
33. Lin F, Xu Y, Yang Y. Comparison of the visual results after SMILE and femtosecond laser-assisted LASIK for myopia. J Refract Surg. 2014;30(4):248–54.
34. Agca A et al. Comparison of visual acuity and higher-order aberrations after femtosecond lenticule extraction and small-incision lenticule extraction. Cont Lens Anterior Eye, 2014.
35. Reinstein DZ, Archer TJ, Gobbe M. ReLEx SMILE induces significantly less spherical aberration than Wavefront Optimised sub-bowman's LASIK for any given residual postoperative relative tensile strength. In ARVO 2014. Orlando, FL, USA: 2014.
36. Vestergaard AH, et al. Central corneal sublayer pachymetry and biomechanical properties after refractive femtosecond lenticule extraction. J Refract Surg. 2014;30(2):102–8.
37. Agca A, et al. Comparison of corneal hysteresis and corneal resistance factor after small incision lenticule extraction and femtosecond laser-assisted LASIK: a prospective fellow eye study. Cont Lens Anterior Eye. 2014;37(2):77–80.
38. Kamiya K, et al. Intraindividual comparison of changes in corneal biomechanical parameters after femtosecond lenticule extraction and small-incision lenticule extraction. J Cataract Refract Surg. 2014;40(6):963–70.
39. Wu D, et al. Corneal biomechanical effects: small-incision lenticule extraction versus femtosecond laser-assisted laser in situ keratomileusis. J Cataract Refract Surg. 2014;40(6):954–62.
40. Wang D, et al. Differences in the corneal biomechanical changes after SMILE and LASIK. J Refract Surg. 2014;30(10):702–7.
41. Sefat SM, et al. Evaluation of changes in human corneas after femtosecond laser-assisted LASIK and small-incision lenticule extraction (SMILE) using non-contact tonometry and ultra-high-speed camera (Corvis ST). Curr Eye Res. 2016;41(7):917–22.
42. Raevdal P, Grauslund J, Vestergaard AH. Comparison of corneal biomechanical changes after refractive surgery by noncontact tonometry: small-incision lenticule extraction versus flap-based refractive surgery—a systematic review. Acta Ophthalmol. 2019;97(2):127–36.
43. Shen Y, et al. Comparison of corneal deformation parameters after SMILE, LASEK, and femtosecond laser-assisted LASIK. J Refract Surg. 2014;30(5):310–8.
44. Reinstein DZ, Gobbe M, Archer TJ. Ocular biomechanics: measurement parameters and terminology. J Refract Surg. 2011;27(6):396–7.
45. Goldich Y, et al. Can we measure corneal biomechanical changes after collagen cross-linking in eyes with keratoconus?–a pilot study. Cornea. 2009;28(5):498–502.
46. Touboul D, et al. Correlations between corneal hysteresis, intraocular pressure, and corneal central pachymetry. J Cataract Refract Surg. 2008;34(4):616–22.
47. Spiru B, et al. Biomechanical properties of human cornea tested by two-dimensional extensiometry ex vivo in fellow eyes: femtosecond laser-assisted LASIK versus SMILE. J Refract Surg. 2018;34(6):419–23.
48. Reinstein DZ, Archer TJ, Gobbe M. Accuracy and reproducibility of cap thickness in small incision lenticule extraction. J Refract Surg. 2013;29(12):810–5.
49. Reinstein DZ, Archer TJ, Gobbe M. Lenticule thickness readout for small incision lenticule extraction compared to Artemis three-dimensional very high-frequency digital ultrasound stromal measurements. J Refract Surg. 2014;30(5):304–9.
50. Reinstein DZ, Archer TJ, Gobbe M. Corneal ablation depth readout of the MEL80 excimer laser compared to Artemis three-dimensional very high-frequency digital ultrasound stromal measurements. J Refract Surg. 2010;26(12):949–59.
51. Reinstein DZ, et al. Repeatability of layered corneal Pachymetry with the Artemis very high-frequency digital ultrasound arc-scanner. J Refract Surg. 2010;26(9):646–59.

52. Reinstein DZ, et al. Stromal thickness in the normal cornea: three-dimensional display with Artemis very high-frequency digital ultrasound. J Refract Surg. 2009;25(9):776–86.
53. He J, Bazan NG, Bazan HE. Mapping the entire human corneal nerve architecture. Exp Eye Res. 2010;91(4):513–23.
54. Tuisku IS, et al. Dry eye and corneal sensitivity after high myopic LASIK. J Refract Surg. 2007;23(4):338–42.
55. Wilson SE. Laser in situ keratomileusis-induced (presumed) neurotrophic epitheliopathy. Ophthalmology. 2001;108(6):1082–7.
56. Savini G, et al. Ocular surface changes in laser in situ keratomileusis-induced neurotrophic epitheliopathy. J Refract Surg. 2004;20(6):803–9.
57. Solomon R, Donnenfeld ED, Perry HD. The effects of LASIK on the ocular surface. Ocul Surf. 2004;2(1):34–44.
58. Shtein RM. Post-LASIK dry eye. Expert Rev Ophthalmol. 2011;6(5):575–82.
59. Chao C, Golebiowski B, Stapleton F. The role of corneal innervation in LASIK-induced neuropathic dry eye. Ocul Surf. 2014;12(1):32–45.
60. Reinstein DZ et al. Corneal sensitivity after small incision lenticule extraction (SMILE). J Cataract Refract Surg. 2014 [In Press].
61. Wei S, Wang Y. Comparison of corneal sensitivity between FS-LASIK and femtosecond lenticule extraction (ReLEx flex) or small-incision lenticule extraction (ReLEx smile) for myopic eyes. Graefes Arch Clin Exp Ophthalmol. 2013;251(6):1645–54.
62. Wei SS, et al. Early outcomes of corneal sensitivity changes after small incision lenticule extraction and femtosecond lenticule extraction. Zhonghua Yan Ke Za Zhi. 2013;49(4):299–304.
63. Vestergaard AH, et al. Subbasal nerve morphology, corneal sensation, and tear film evaluation after refractive femtosecond laser lenticule extraction. Graefes Arch Clin Exp Ophthalmol. 2013;251(11):2591–600.
64. Demirok A, et al. Corneal sensation after corneal refractive surgery with small incision lenticule extraction. Optom Vis Sci. 2013;90(10):1040–7.
65. Li M, et al. Comparison of dry eye and corneal sensitivity between small incision lenticule extraction and femtosecond LASIK for myopia. PLoS ONE. 2013;8(10): e77797.
66. Li M, et al. Comparison of corneal sensation between small incision lenticule extraction (SMILE) and femtosecond laser-assisted LASIK for myopia. J Refract Surg. 2014;30(2):94–100.
67. Li M, et al. Confocal comparison of corneal reinnervation after small incision lenticule extraction (SMILE) and femtosecond laser in situ keratomileusis (FS-LASIK). PLoS ONE. 2013;8(12): e81435.
68. Gao S, et al. Early changes in ocular surface and tear inflammatory mediators after small-incision lenticule extraction and femtosecond laser-assisted laser in situ keratomileusis. PLoS ONE. 2014;9(9): e107370.
69. Mohamed-Noriega K, et al. Early corneal nerve damage and recovery following small incision lenticule extraction (SMILE) and laser in situ keratomileusis (LASIK). Invest Ophthalmol Vis Sci. 2014;55(3):1823–34.
70. Xu Y, Yang Y. Dry eye after small incision lenticule extraction and LASIK for myopia. J Refract Surg. 2014;30(3):186–90.

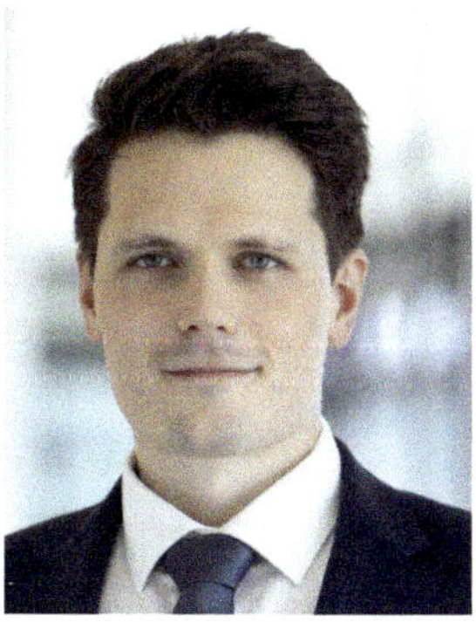

Felix Mathias Wagner is the head of Refractive Laser Surgery and a consultant at the Department of Ophthalmology, University Medical Center of the Johannes Gutenberg University Mainz, Germany. He studied medicine at the Ruperto Carola University Heidelberg and received his doctorate there in 2019. Dr. Wagner completed his residency in ophthalmology at the University Medical Center Mainz, where he became a board-certified ophthalmologist and a Fellow of the European Board of Ophthalmology (FEBO) in 2022. He pursued his clinical fellowship in refractive surgery under Professor Sekundo at the Philipps University of Marburg from 2021 to 2022. Dr. Wagner has published over 30 original research papers.

Centration in SMILE and SMILE Pro 15

Walter Sekundo, Apostolos Lazaridis, and Felix Mathias Wagner

15.1 Introduction

An excellent centration of the treatment zone is of paramount importance in laser vision correction (LVC). Despite the benefits of a pupillary centration [1, 2], it is widely accepted that a centration in regard to the visual axis [3, 4] is the key to optimized visual outcomes while maintaining the functional corneal morphology after the treatment. The advent of eye trackers for excimer lasers led to a significant reduction of extended decentrations and therefore to fewer functional deficits, such as reduced corrected distance visual acuity, irregular astigmatism, halos, glare [5], reduced contrast sensitivity [6], and monocular diplopia [7]. However, despite the efficacy of laser treatments based on eye-tracking systems, the problem of subclinical decentrations (< 1.0 mm) and the induction of higher-order aberrations still remains [8].

15.2 Angle Kappa and the Pattern of the Achieved Centration

A very important issue regarding the achieved centration is its pattern in regard to the visual axis. The visual axis is the line which connects the fovea with the fixation point via the nodal point of the eye. The line of sight is defined as the line connecting the fixation point with the center of the entrance pupil (PC). The

W. Sekundo (✉) · A. Lazaridis
Department of Ophthalmology, Philipps University of Marburg, Marburg, Germany
e-mail: sekundo@med.uni-marburg.de

F. M. Wagner
Department of Ophthalmology, University Medical Center of the Johannes Gutenberg University, Mainz, Germany

W. Sekundo and F. M. Wagner (eds.), *Femtosecond Laser Assisted Lenticule Extraction*,
https://doi.org/10.1007/978-3-031-60424-9_15

pupillary axis is the line passing through the PC perpendicular to the cornea. The definition of angle kappa is the angular distance between visual and pupillary axis [9, 10, 11], which is in myopic eyes approximately 2.0° and is mostly positive [9, 12]. As a result of positive angle kappa, the first image of Purkinje is located nasal to the pupillary center or temporal in cases of a negative angle kappa. Studies conducted in order to assess the distribution of angle K in myopic eyes showed a prevalence of positive angle K in the majority of the tested subjects, while a negative angle K or no angle K were identified in substantially less cases [9, 13]. Figure 15.1 shows the distribution of angle K in our study with typical nasalization pattern since in most eyes angle K was positive. In fact, 76.5% of right eyes and 74.3% of left eyes follow the nasal pattern of angle K. The mean distance of the preoperative CSCLR from the PC was 0.227 ± 0.121 mm, ranging from 0.014 to 0.602 mm [14].

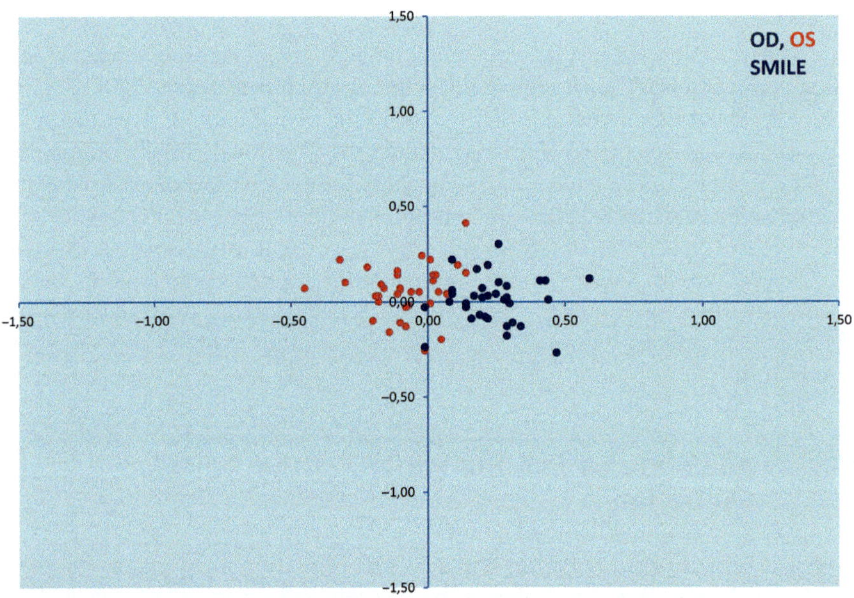

Fig. 15.1 Depiction of the points of the preoperative coaxially sighted corneal light reflex (CSCLR = first image of Purkinje) centration in relation to the pupil center (PC) in SMILE. There is a typical nasalization of the visual axis corresponding to the angle K. Blue dots represent the right eye and red dots the left eye

15.3 Assisting Methods to Intraoperatively Verify Correct Centration/Cyclotorsion

15.3.1 Intraoperative Alignment in SMILE with VisuMax 500 Femtosecond Laser

Unlike excimer laser procedures, where the alignment of the photoablation can be adjusted by the surgeon (objective alignment) and is controlled by eye trackers, in the traditional Small Incision Lenticule Extraction (SMILE) using the VisuMax 500 laser the alignment of the photodisruption is subjective and largely relies on the patient. The patient must fixate on a blinking light during the suction process and the initial stage of the laser scan (after the laser cut of the lenticule's posterior plane the blinking target is obscured by intracorneal gas bubbles). The surgeon controls and encourages the patient to maintain fixation in particular, when the patient's view is obscured by intrastromal gas bubbles during the second half of the laser procedure in order to avoid suction loss. In SMILE correction the centration is targeted at the corneal vertex (CV), which is identified by the coaxially sighted corneal light reflex (CSCLR) or the first image of Purkinje. The initial fears of SMILE without eye tracker to produce higher decentration rates as compared to eye tracker assisted Femtolasik was debunked by our group as early as 2014 (Fig. 15.2) [14]. It was supported by several other studies regardless of the method of decentration measurements as summarized in a recent review by Liang and Yan [15]. Figure 15.3 shows 3 different methods of centration assessment such as videokeratoscopy, axial, or (better) tangential map of Placido-based topographers or pachymetry map using Scheimpflug technology. In addition, Liu et al. unequivocally showed the superiority of CV centered myopic SMILE procedures compared to pupil center (PC)-based procedures in terms of both, refractive outcomes and induction of high-order aberrations (HOA) [16].

The issue of centration in SMILE and other corneal refractive procedures for myopia correction is considered to be less critical compared to hyperopic treatments. Still, with proper centration techniques, excellent centration can easily be achieved in hyperopic SMILE [17] (see Chap. 9).

Theoretically if the patient keeps the gaze at the green blinking light, one will get a perfect centration. In reality, several factors might counteract this concept: (1) not every patient is capable of maintaining gaze during the docking procedure. Unfortunately, Bell's phenomenon is frequently encountered during procedure. (2) In steep corneas and other anatomical deviations from an ideal eye, the docking itself might lead to a "twist" of the cornea when touching the inner surface of the treatment cone ("contact glas"). This all requires a certain degree of surgeon control to assure proper centration.

The simplest way is to ask the patient to look at the coaxial light of the surgical microscope while in the primary position. The surgeon observes the position of the 1st Purkinje reflex and matches its location with the location of the green

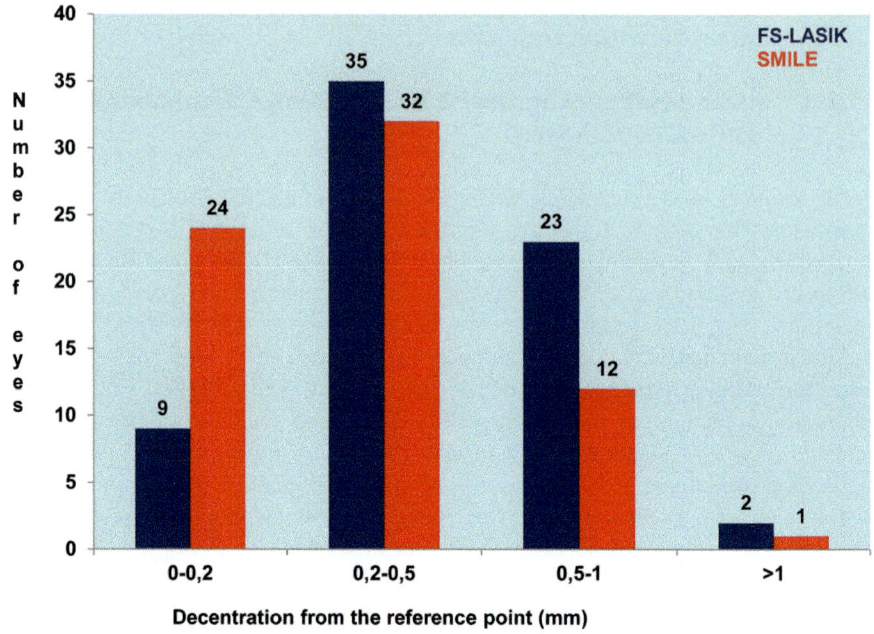

Fig. 15.2 Difference in centration between SMILE using VisuMax 500 and Femtolasik using MEL 80 excimer laser with eye tracker. The histogram shows the distance of the points of maximum pachymetrical difference from the reference point of this technique (mm). SMILE eyes are represented by red columns and Femtolasik eyes with blue columns

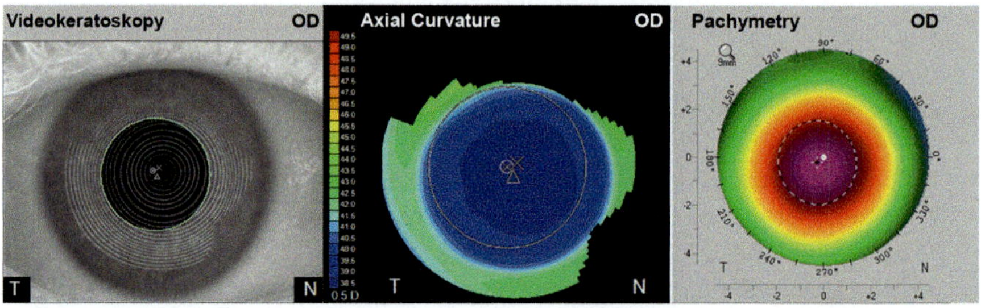

Fig. 15.3 Three examples of centration assessment. The first two images (videokeratoscopy and axial curvature map) derive from a placido-based corneal topography (Atlas, Carl Zeiss Meditec AG). The corneal vertex is depicted with an X, the pupil center (PC) with ⊗ and the corneal apex with ∇. The right hand image represents a postoperative Pentacam (Oculus Optikgeräte GmbH) pachymetry map. The PC is depicted with a + , the pupil edge with a white dotted circle and the corneal apex with a white dot. Note that the point identified as corneal apex by Pentacam is the same displacement in relation to the PC as the CV on Atlas image

blinking light during the docking process and after the suction has been applied. The "trick" of the first author of this chapter is to start the docking slightly away (usually superiorly) from the ideal position (which is the 1st Purkinje image the surgeon memorized) and encourage the patient to look at the blinking green light. Once it matches the memorized image, the suction button is pushed and the eye fixed. For the S size treatment cone, it is usually sufficient to have over 80% of applanation to initiate suction. In that way I am confident that the patient truly fixates the light and by coming from the slightly superior position, I can counteract the Bell's movement. If desired, this method can be further enhanced by printing the raw image from the topography (see left hand image on the Fig. 15.3) or IOL-Master 700 and place it upside-down next to the oculars of the microscope as a reference.

The tear film mark (TFM) method was described by Liu et al. in 2020 [18]. While the patient is in position 2 (under the laser) and focuses on a green blinking light, the bed is slowly raised to enlarge the tear film generated by the cone and cornea to approximately 80%. When the cornea contacts the cone, the flashing green dot is automatically adjusted according to the patient's refraction. The most important, but also the weakest aspect of this method, is that the patient must maintain focus on the green light. At this time, the contact point is the highest point of corneal morphology, which is approximately equivalent to the CV (Fig. 15.4).

The triple marking centration (TMC) method is a further development of the cyclotorsion compensation technique published by Ganesh et al. in 2017 [19]. We use Ganesh's technique in cases of preoperative astigmatism $\geq$ 1.5 D cyl. To avoid damage to the epithelium, we mark the horizontal axis at the slit lamp and extend the marks toward corneal center by applying a gentle touch with the spatula painted with infrared non-adsorbable ink (e.g., Viscot surgical skin marker 1436, Viscot Medical/USA) onto the cornea of the patient already on the table (Fig. 15.5). As

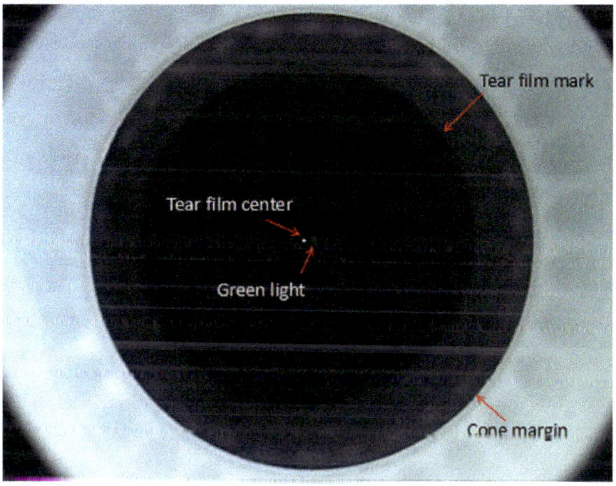

Fig. 15.4 Tear film mark centration method. At 80% applanation (approximately 7 mm diameter), the green light was modified to coincident with the tear film center (tear film mark was concentric with the margin of the cone). White dot = tear film center; green light = treatment center (courtesy of Dr Shengtao Liu, Shanghai)

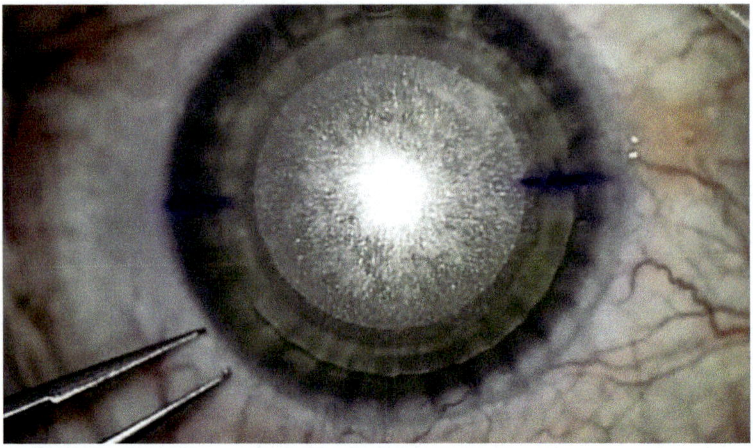

Fig. 15.5 A screenshot of the cornea with two horizontal marks. Note: the marks are just enough to be seen under applanation, but do not extend into the optical zone (seen as the bubble circle)

illustrated by Liang and Yan [15], the TMC marking method uses similarly two horizontal marking points instead of lines with a distance of 7 mm, which bisect the first Purkinje image. In addition, a point bisecting the first Purkinje image is also marked in the inferior aspect the cornea. Those three points correspond to the horizontal and vertical scale axes of the screen display to compensate for rotation. According to the authors, the TMC method has a better centration effect for patients with high astigmatism and decentration are smaller than in the TFM method. However, there are some disadvantages: corneal marks may be blurred by adjusting the cone, corneal marks seem to be difficult to identify in patients with a darker iris color, and excessive adjustment of the cone may lead to loss of suction.

For the sake of completeness, it should be mentioned that several corneal markers are available to mark the cornea preoperatively (e.g., Ganesh bubble marker, Epsilon Surgical/USA). They all must be used with caution and respect and—in our opinion—shell not intersect the optical 7mm zone since any minor indentation of the epithelium or ink not suitable for laser beam might decrease the quality of the femtocut.

15.3.2 Intraoperative Alignment in SMILE Pro with VisuMax 800 Femtosecond Laser

As stated above, the overall centration after SMILE is very good. However, occasionally either due to a poor compliance or a difficult anatomical situation, decentrations occur (Fig. 15.6). The incidence of decentration may decrease with the assisting tools. VisuMax 800 possesses such a tool called Centralign and is

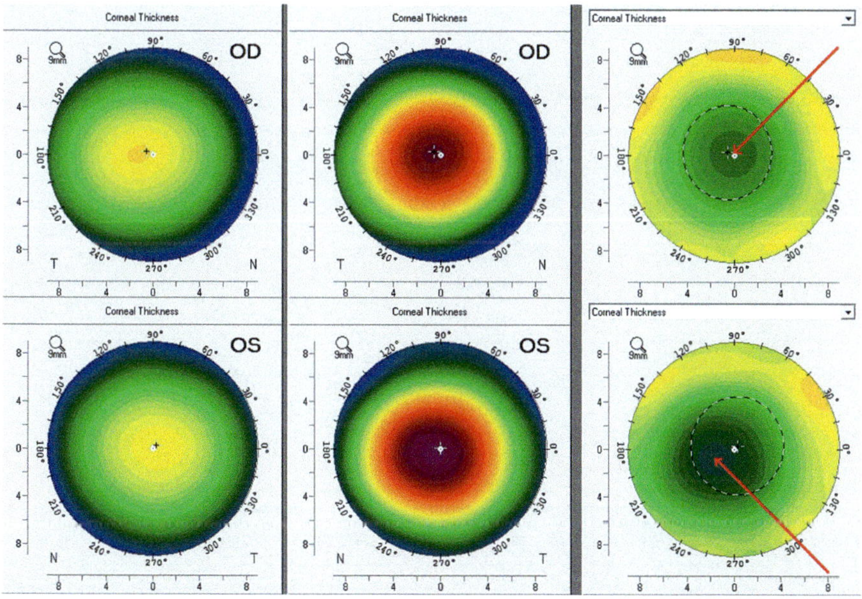

Fig. 15.6 An example of good (right eye) and poor (left eye) centration using differential pachymetry maps on Pentacam. The red arrow shows the point of the maximum pachymetrical difference. In the right, well centered eye the thickest point is 0.103mm from the apex while the left decentered eye has a distance of 0.863 mm

amended by a cyclotorsion assisting tool called Oculign. Figure 15.7a and b show the mode of employment of Centralign. Oculign simply shows horizontal lines on the laser's display. A simple joy stick rotation adjusts the axis to the corneal marks applied as described in the suction above. However, instead of an active rotation of the treatment cone as with SMILE surgery, the software in SMILE pro rotates the treatment zone. In the future, a full pupil recognition and registration using an IOL-Master 700 image will further automatize the process of centration.

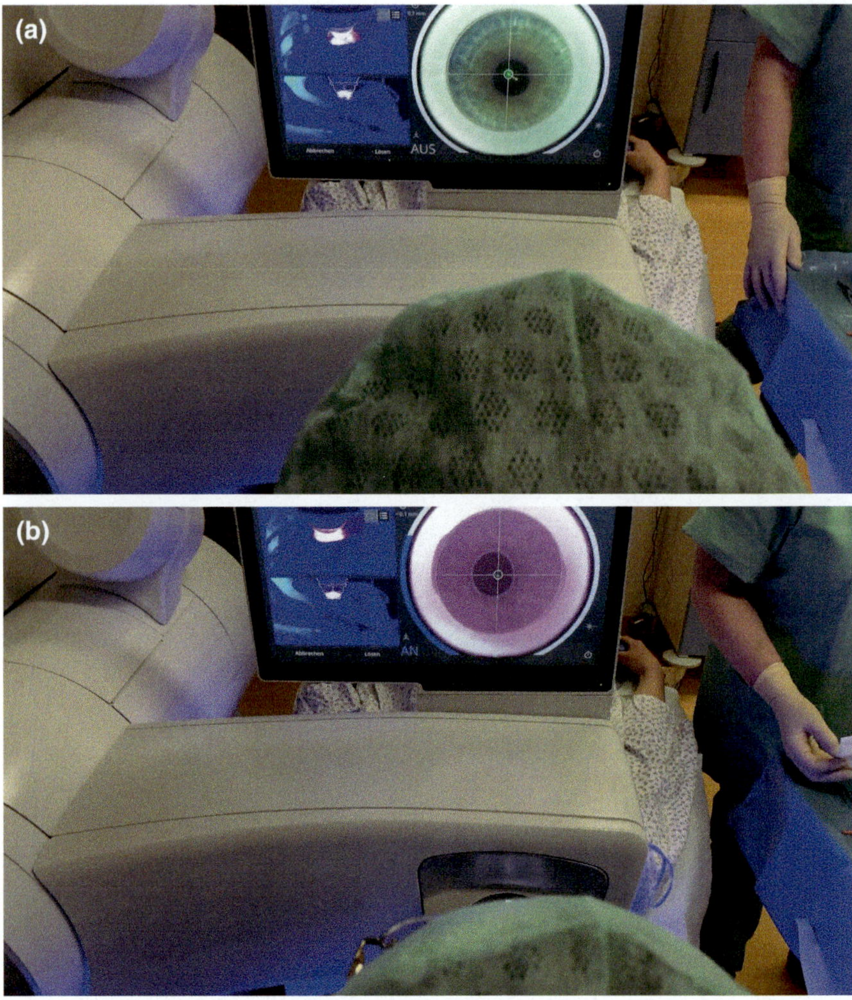

Fig. 15.7 Oculign centration assistant in action. a) Once the first applanation meniscus is formed the assisting system recognized the green dot and points in a "lolly-pop" fashion to the ideal point of centration in accordance to coordinates previously entered into laser's software. b) The infrared illumination eliminates any glare and makes it easier for the patient to look at the green blinking light. Once the perfect position has been achieved the suction is applied. Note the typical nasalization of the fixation (left eye)

References

1. Uozato H, Guyton DL. Centering corneal surgical procedures. Am J Ophthalmol. 1987;103:264–75.

2. Soler V, Benito A, Soler P, et al. A randomized comparison of pupil-centered versus vertex-centered ablation in LASIK correction of hyperopia. Am J Ophthalmol. 2011;152:591–9.
3. Pande M, Hillman JS. Optical zone centration in keratorefractive surgery: entrance pupil center, visual axis, coaxially sighted corneal reflex, or geometric corneal center? Ophthalmology. 1993;100:1230–7.
4. Reinstein DZ, Gobbe M, Archer TJ. Coaxially sighted corneal light reflex versus entrance pupil center centration of moderate to high hyperopic corneal ablations in eyes with small and large angle kappa. J Refract Surg. 2013;29(8):518–25.
5. Fay AM, Trokel SL, Myers JA. Pupil diameter and the principal ray. J Cataract Refract Surg. 1992;18(4):348–51.
6. Terrell J, Bechara SJ, Nesburn A, Waring GO, Macy J, Maloney RK. The effect of globe fixation on ablation zone centration in photorefractive keratectomy. Am J Ophthalmol. 1995;119(5):612–9.
7. Mulhern MG, Foley-Nolan A, O'Keefe M, Condon PI. Topographical analysis of ablation centration after excimer laser photorefractive keratectomy and laser in situ keratomileusis for high myopia. J Cataract Refract Surg. 1997;23(4):488–94.
8. Mrochen M, Kaemmerer M, Mierdel P, Seiler T. Increased higher-order optical aberrations after laser refractive surgery: a problem of subclinical decentration. J Cataract Refract Surg. 2001;27(3):362–9.
9. Park CY, Oh SY, Chuck RS. Measurement of angle kappa and centration in refractive surgery. Curr Opin Ophthalmol. 2012;23(4):269–75.
10. Tabernero J, Benito A, Alcon E, Artal P. Mechanism of compensation of aberrations in the human eye. J Opt Soc Am A Opt Image Sci Vis. 2007;24(10):3274–83.
11. Basmak H, Sahin A, Yildirim N, Papakostas TD, Kanellopoulos AJ. Measurement of angle kappa with synoptophore and Orbascan II in normal population. J Refract Surg. 2007;23(5):456–60.
12. Von Noorden G, Campos E. Examination of the patient II. In: Binocular vision and ocular motility-theory and management of strabismus. 6th ed. St. Louis: Mosby. 2002;168–173.
13. Scott WE, Mash AJ. Kappa angle measures of strabismic and nonstrabismic individuals. Arch Ophthalmol. 1973;89(1):18–20.
14. Lazaridis A, Droutsas K, Sekundo W. Topographic analysis of the centration of the treatment zone after SMILE for myopia and comparison to FS-LASIK: subjective versus objective alignment. J Refract Surg. 2014;30(10):680–6.
15. Liang C, Yan H. Methods of corneal vertex centration and evaluation of effective optical zone in small incision lenticule extraction. Ophthalmic Res. 2023;66(1):710–9.
16. Liu M, Sun Y, Wang D, Zhang T, Zhou Y, Zheng H. Decentration of optical zone center and its impact on visual outcomes following SMILE. Cornea. 2015;34:392–7.
17. Reinstein DZ, Pradhan KR, Carp GI, Archer TJ, Gobbe M, Sekundo W, Khan R, Citron K, Dhungana P. Small incision lenticule extraction for hyperopia: optical zone centration. J Refract Surg. 2017;33(3): 150156.
18. Liu S, Zhang X, You Z, Zhou X. Comparison of the distribution of lenticule decentration following SMILE by pupil center or tear film mark centration. JRS 2020;36(4):239–246.
19. Sri G, Brar S, Pawar A. Results of intraoperative manual cyclotorsion compensation for myopic astigmatism in patients undergoing small incision lenticule extraction (SMILE). J Refract Surg 2017;33(8):506–512.

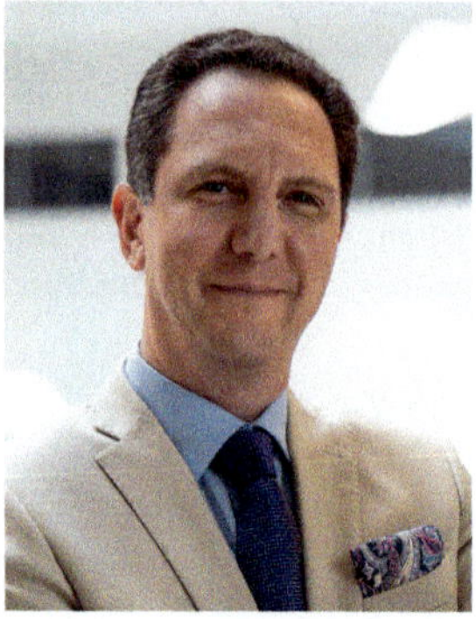

Walter Sekundo MD, PhD is Professor and Chairman, Department of Ophthalmology, Philipps University of Marburg, Germany. He studied Medicine in Frankfurt (Germany), New Orleans and Durham (US). He was a resident at the University of Bonn in Germany and a Fellow in Corneal and Refractive surgery at Moorfields Eyes Hospital and Ocular Pathology at the University of Glasgow in UK. He received his vitreoretinal training in Marburg and glaucoma training in Mainz (Germany). He also holds a degree of "Health Care Manager" from the Faculty of Economics in Marburg. Prof. Sekundo has published 200+ original papers, over 50 book chapters and edited the first international book on SMILE surgery. He gave countless presentations at national and international meetings. He is a reviewer for 21 Ophthalmic Journals and a Board Member of "Die Ophthalmologie". Prof. Sekundo is a busy surgeon with over 30,000 procedures in the anterior and posterior segment and has been repeatedly named as one of the 30 top refractive and cataract surgeons in Germany. Together with Marcus Blum he largely contributed to the development of KLEx. In fact, he was the first surgeon in the world who performed FLEx and SMILE. He received several prestigious prizes for the contribution to the field of ophthalmic surgery. In the last 25 years his research has been focused on corneal, cataract and refractive surgery.

The Refractive Predictability of SMILE with the VisuMax and VISUMAX 800

16

Stine Elkjaer Nielsen, Anders Ramlov Ivarsen, and Jesper Hjortdal

Abstract

This chapter explores the evolution of small incision lenticule extraction (SMILE) surgery, comparing refractive predictability of the VisuMax 500 and the VISUMAX 800 laser platform.

Keywords

Small incision lenticule extraction surgery (SMILE) • VisuMax • VISUMAX 800 • Refractive predictability • Femtosecond laser

16.1 Introduction

In 2006, the very first cases of a corneal laser refractive procedure using only femtosecond laser technology (ReLEx FLEX®) were presented by Dr. Sekundo and Dr. Blum at the meeting of the American Academy of Ophthalmology in Las Vegas. A few years later, the SMILE procedure was introduced. The advantages of the flap-less SMILE procedure compared to FS-LASIK were an expected reduction in eye dryness and a lower risk of epithelial ingrowth. It was clinically shown later that SMILE preserved the nerves better than LASIK [11]. Moreover SMILE of course had no risk of traumatic flap dislocation like LASIK. It was expected that SMILE surgery did not have the risk of corneal ectasia, however even in flap-less procedures such as SMILE, ectasia has been found to occur [7].

Since its introduction, SMILE surgery has been shown to be safe and accurate and is becoming increasingly popular. However, SMILE surgery has challenges, some of which are different from those of LASIK surgery: The docking time where

S. E. Nielsen (✉) · A. R. Ivarsen · J. Hjortdal
Department of Ophthalmology, Aarhus, Denmark
e-mail: stine.elkjaer.nielsen@auh.rm.dk

W. Sekundo and F. M. Wagner (eds.), *Femtosecond Laser Assisted Lenticule Extraction*,
https://doi.org/10.1007/978-3-031-60424-9_16

the patient must focus upto 30 s which is longer than in LASIK and suction loss during SMILE surgery occurs in up to 0.41% of treated eyes [20]. To have the full effect of the SMILE treatment and avoid higher-order aberrations, centration of the treatment zone is important [14] and some find the centration more challenging than in LASIK surgery where an eye tracker supports the surgeon. Cyclotorsion control has also been a challenge in SMILE surgery since cyclotorsion adjustment is done manually by rotating the contact glass after suction.

In 2021, the next generation FS laser "VISUMAX 800" became available. With VISUMAX 800, it is now possible to perform "SMILE Pro" which is expected to be of benefit for both surgeons and patients since it provides shorter operation time, better workflow, centration aid and cyclotorsion compensation.

This chapter will discuss the current data on predictability of the VisuMax and include new data on the VISUMAX 800. Challenging factors such as centration, docking and cyclotorsion will be described and suggestions to improve these will be reviewed.

16.2 Clinical Studies on Refractive Outcome After SMILE

Refractive surgery guidelines for reporting results of clinical studies have been available for more than two decades [51]. The standardized graphs make direct comparisons between studies easier and should therefore be used. Since the introduction of SMILE, a number of large clinical studies have been published, all showing very good predictability, efficacy, and safety, see Table 16.1 for an overview on studies with more than 200 eyes. In 2012, a study on SMILE was published by Hjortdal et al. [26]. It included 335 myopic patients (670 eyes) with an average preoperative refraction of −7.19 D (± 1.30 D) that were treated at Aarhus University Hospital and followed for three months postoperatively. The patients were myopic up to -10 D and had an astigmatism of up to −2 D. Postoperative results showed that in patients aimed for emmetropia, 80% achieved a spherical equivalent (SEQ) of ± 0.50 D and 94% of patients achieved a SEQ of ± 1.00 D. Uncorrected distance visual acuity (UDVA) was 20/25 or better in 84% of the treated patients. In general, patients were slightly undercorrected with a postoperative SEQ of -0.25 D ± 0.44 D. A multiple linear regression analysis showed that increasing patient age (0.1 D per decade) and steeper corneal curvature (0.04 D per D) had a significant but small impact on the undercorrection. These results did not support the use of nomogram adjustments, which will be discussed later in this chapter. In 2016 Pradhan et al. published a large study on 1396 eyes. Patients had a preoperative SEQ of −5.8 D. Postoperatively, 95% of patients had an uncorrected visual acuity (UCVA) of 20/20 or better. No patients lost 2 lines or more. Since then, a number of studies have confirmed the good results, with follow-up times of three to five years [15, 27, 35]. In low myopic patients with a SEQ of −2.6 D ± 0.54 D, SMILE has been shown to be precise with patients achieving a postoperative SEQ of −0.05 ± 0.36 D [12], 96% had a

UCVA of > 20/20 at 12 months follow-up. A large review on astigmatism correction in SMILE and LASIK including 1985 eyes showed that SMILE provides effective and predictable results and generally have equivalent outcomes regarding astigmatism, although there is a tendency toward undercorrection of cylinder in SMILE compared to LASIK [9]. However, patients with large astigmatisms have been shown to have a higher (16% per diopter) residual astigmatism compared to patients with low astigmatism (13% per diopter) [17].

In summary, VisuMax has showed good predictability and safety, but there is still room for improvement especially regarding the surgical technique.

In 2023, [13]published the first study on SMILE pro/VISUMAX 800 and visual outcomes in patients with myopia (SEQ -4.7 ± 1.9 D) and astigmatism (range 0.0 to −4.0 D). They showed very good clinical outcomes on safety and efficacy, that were not significantly different from reported data on VisuMax in the same clinical setting. They found that 91% of patients that were aimed for emmetropia had a postoperative UCVA > 20/20 and 86% had a postoperative SEQ within ± 0.50D while 100% had SEQ within ± 1.00D.

16.3 New Data on VISUMAX 800 and VisuMax

We included 40 patients (80 eyes) for bilateral SMILE treatment on VisuMax and 20 patients (40 eyes) for bilateral SMILE Pro treatment on VISUMAX 800. Patients were followed for 3 months. Mean age in both groups was 38 years (range 23–54). The patients were myopes or had myopic astigmatism and there were no differences between groups in any preoperative parameter (Table 16.2).

A 40–60° incision was performed at the 12 o'clock position, and through this, the lenticule was mobilized with a blunt spatula and removed with a forceps. The lenticule diameter was between 6.1 to 6.6 mm, cap diameter was 7.3 mm. Lenticule thickness was 52–141 μm and lenticule side cut 15 μm. Cap thickness was 120 μm in all patients. After removal of the lenticule, the stromal pocket was flushed with saline. Postoperatively, all patients were treated with tobramycin and dexamethasone four times daily for 1 week and two times daily for one week. If needed, patients also used over the counter lubricating eye drops. After three months, patients had a clinical examination including automated keratometry, Pentacam HR, slit lamp examination, manifest refraction and determination of uncorrected and corrected visual acuity by a specialized optometrist.

The achieved and attempted SEQ refraction was highly correlated in both the VISUMAX 800 and the VisuMax group (R^2 = 0.98 and 0.93, Fig. 16.1B)). The postoperative SEQ refraction in patients aimed for emmetropia was −0.1 D (±0.3 D) in the VISUMAX 800 group and −0.5 D ± 0.6 D in the VisuMax group ($p < 0.05$).

In eyes targeted for emmetropia, 89% in the VisuMax group and 100% the VISUMAX 800 group achieved an UCVA of ≤ 0,10 (logMAR), respectively. Three months after surgery, all patients had a corrected distance visual acuity (CDVA) of ≤ 0,10 (logMAR) in both the VisuMax and VISUMAX 800 group. Eyes treated

Table 16.1 Studies on refractive outcomes after SMILE in myopic patients, studies with sample size of more than 200 eyes are included

Study	Follow-up time	No eyes	Preop SEQ (mean ± SD)	Postop SEQ (mean ± SD)	Postop.SEQ within 0.50 D	Postop.SEQ within ± 1.00 D (%)	UCVA > 20/20 (%)	Lost 2 or more lines CDVA (%)
Hjortdal [26]	3 months	670	−7.19 ± 1.30	−0.25 ± 0.44	80%	94	61	2.4
Kim [6]	6 months	447	−6.75 ± 1.65	−0.21 ± 0.37	86.1	97.9	79.8	0.3
Pradhan [16]	3 months	1396	−5.78 ± 1.81	−0.28 ± 0.29	80	99	95	0
Hansen [5]	3 months	722	−6.43 ± 1.59	−0.06 ± 0.01	88	98	58	1.6
FDA (2016)	1 year	310	−4.76 ± 2.20	+ 0.02 ± 0.30	94%	99.7	89.4	0
Taneri [3]	3 months	206	−5.47 ± 2.37	−0.07 ± 0.38	87%	99	75	2.6
Dishler [4]	12 months	357	−5.39 D ± 2.30	−0.01 ± 0.24D	95.3%	100	89	0

Table 16.2 Demographic data

	VisuMax	VISUMAX 800	$P=$
Number of patients	40 (80 eyes)	20 (40 eyes)	
Age (years)	37.8 ± 7.4 (range 23–52)	38.1 ± 8.9 (range 25—54)	NS
Gender (female/male)	26/14	12/8	NS
Sphere (D)	−6.84 ± 1.8 (−11.5 to + 0.5)	−6.72 ± 1.1 (−8.25 to − 2.25)	NS
Cylinder (D)	−1.15 ± 1.1 (0 to -4.25)	−0.79 ± 0.74 (0 to −3)	NS
Keratometry (D)	44.0 ± 1.6 (40.9–49.3)	44.5 ± 1.7 (40.9–48.4)	NS
Spherical equivalent refraction (D)	−7.4 ± 1.5 (−12.1 to − 1.5)	−7.1 ± 1.1 (−9.00 to − 2.25)	NS
Central corneal thickness (μm)	541 ± 3 (491–615)	549 ± 3 (501–609)	NS

with the VISUMAX 800 laser had an improvement in CDVA from −0.08 to − 0.12 (logMAR) ($p < 0.01$). A similar improvement was seen in the VisuMax group, from −0.04 to −0.07 (logMAR) ($p < 0.01$). The change in CDVA was the same in the two groups. As seen in Fig .16.1D, no patient lost 2 lines in any of the groups.

Both lasers performed well in the treatment of astigmatism (Fig. 16.1F); however, VISUMAX 800 treated patients tended to have a better outcome. Thus, in the VisuMax group, 61% had a postoperative cylinder ≤ 0.50D, as compared to 78% in the VISUMAX 800 group. In the VISUMAX 800 group all patients had a postoperative cylinder of less than 1.00 D in contrast to 95% of patients in the VisuMax group (Fig. 16.1F).

There we no complications in any of the groups and we did not see suction loss in any of our patients.

The refractive results obtained in our and other SMILE studies are in general good. However, in the current small study, the VisuMax operated patients were undercorrected in terms of SEQ when compared to VISUMAX 800 patients. Optimizing predictability is always relevant, and in the rest of this chapter, we will discuss factors affecting the predictability, some of which are possible to affect whereas some are not.

16.4 Factors Affecting Predictability

16.4.1 Variations in Subjective Refraction

Preoperative manifest refraction is a critical component when planning keratorefractive surgery. The goal is to establish the sphere and cylinder correction that will result in maximal uncorrected visual acuity for the specific eye. It is difficult to accomplish perfection since variations in subjective refraction always occur [14]. The repeatability for manifest refraction has been investigated in a study by Nielsen et al. [18]. They examined patients before and after SMILE surgery

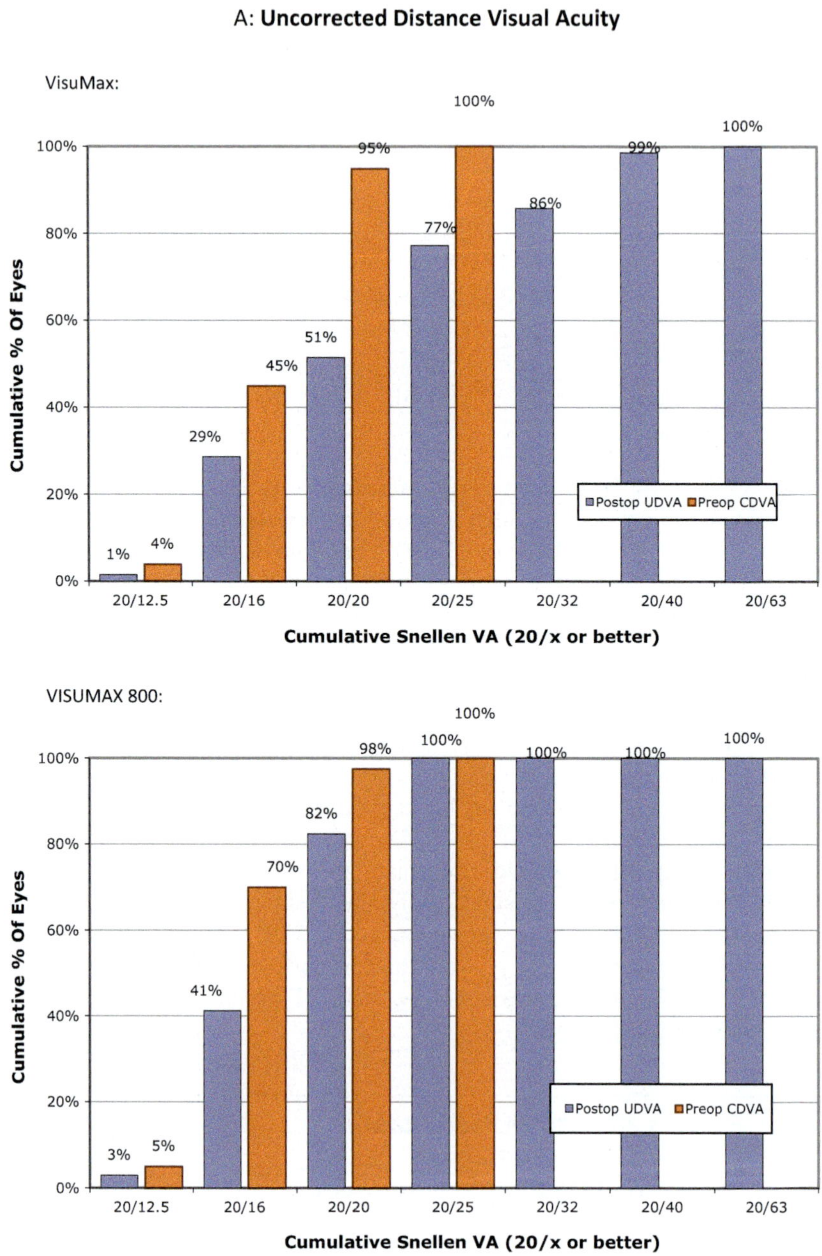

Fig. 16.1 A: Uncorrected distance visual acuity preoperatively and 3 months after SMILE surgery B: Attempted versus achieved change in refraction 3 months postoperatively after SMILE surgery C: Spherical equivalent refraction accuracy, results 3 months postoperatively. D: Postoperative changes in corrected distance visual acuity after SMILE surgery. E: Postoperative uncorrected distance visual acuity versus preoperative corrected distance visual acuity. F: Pre- and postoperative refractive astigmatism

B: Spherical Equivalent Refraction Attempted vs Achieved

VisuMax:

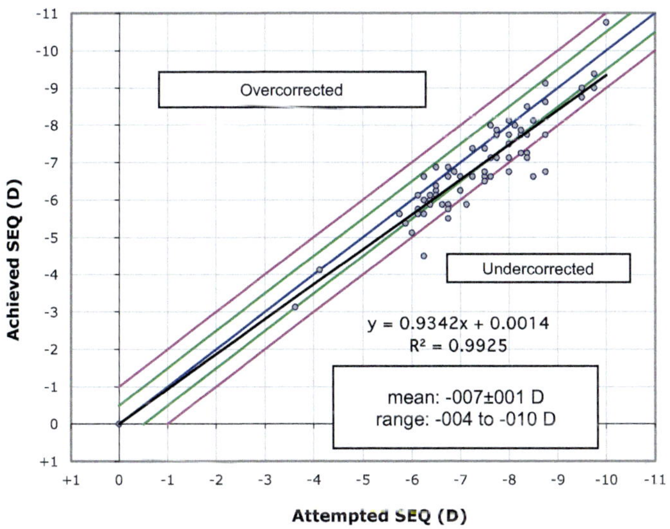

VISUMAX 800:

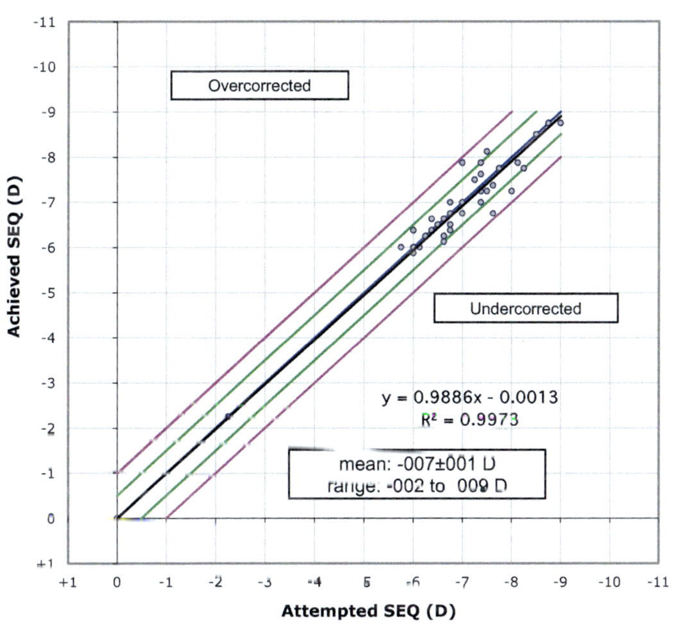

Fig. 16.1 (continued)

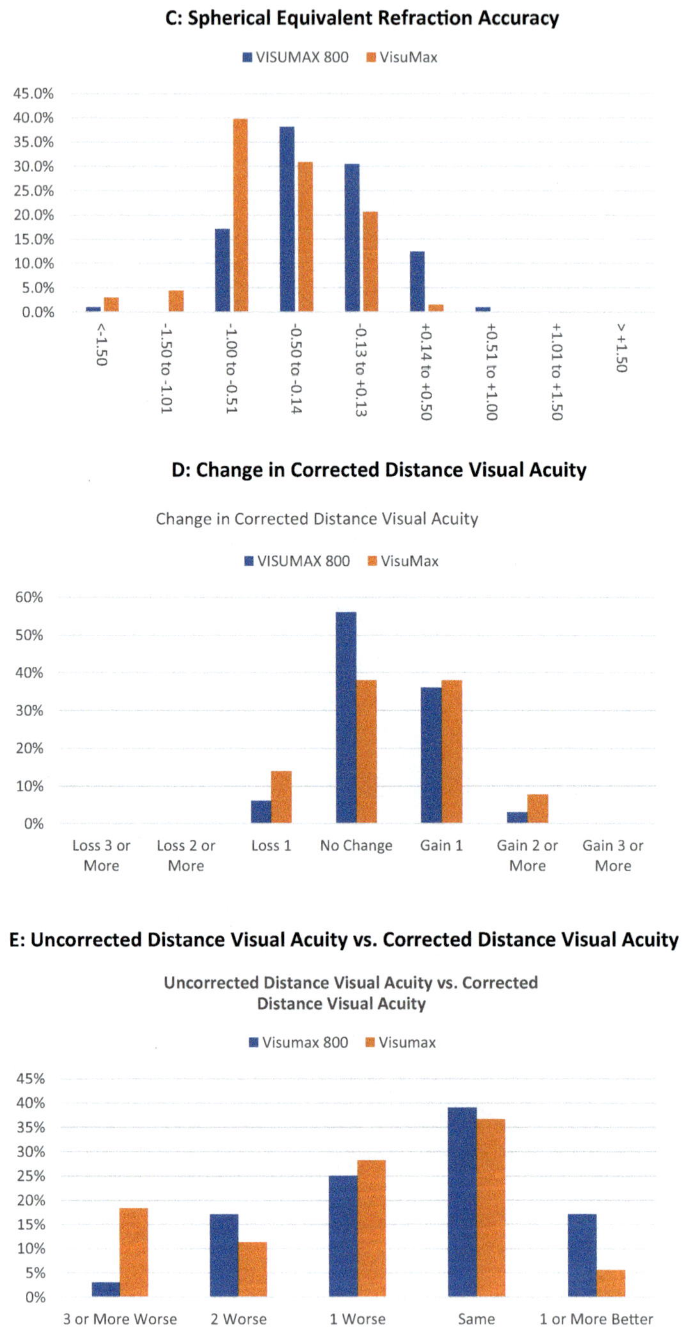

Fig. 16.1 (continued)

F: Refractive Astigmatism

VisuMax:

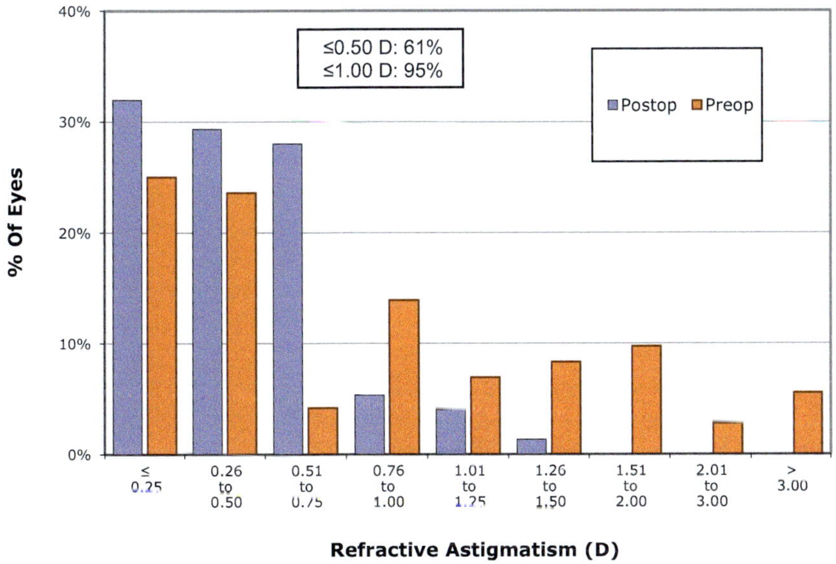

VISUMAX 800:

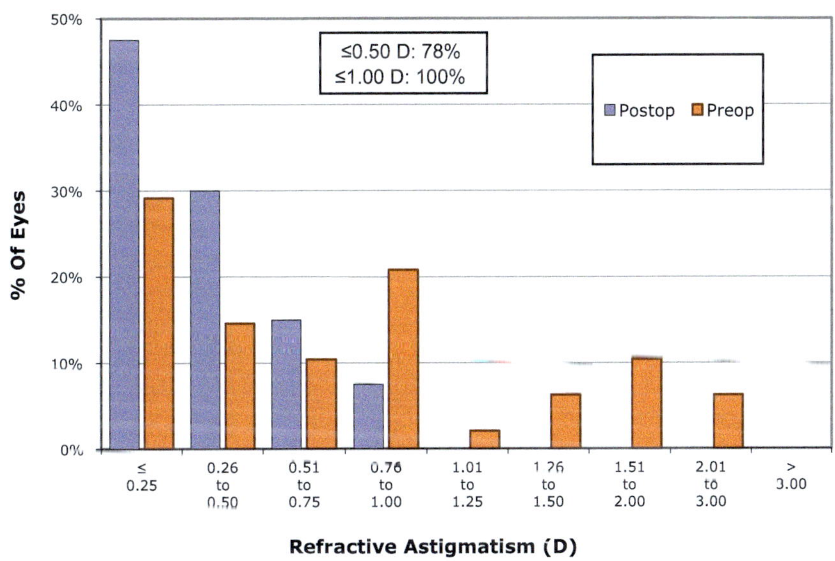

Fig. 16.1 (continued)

and found a variation in refraction of ± 0.15 D, others have reported a preoperative mean interobserver dioptric power difference of 0.21 D (range 0.15–0.32) [12]. Moreover, the study by Nielsen et al. found that small cylinders increase the uncertainty of the cylinder axis. The variation in subjective refraction can be due to intraobserver variation, defined as the difference in refraction when the patient is examined by the same observer repeatedly. In contrast, interobserver repeatability is the difference between two observers in the same clinical setting. Interobserver repeatability can be improved in a setting with experienced trained optometrists [18].

Even with a perfect laser cut, the standard deviation on the refractive outcome can never be more precise than the combined standard deviation of preoperative and postoperative subjective refraction, resulting in an expected standard deviation of approximately 0.2 D. Repeated measurement of manifest refractions pre- and postoperatively will provide a better estimate of the real manifest refraction. Further on, refraction in cycloplegia is recommended.

Preoperatively, it is of outmost importance to ensure a smooth and stable corneal surface. Pre-existing dry eye disease is a contraindication for refractive surgery, but also minor dryness can affect the refraction and the predictability of the surgery. Patients should not be pregnant or breastfeeding since this may also affect the refraction. Contact lens wear should be discontinued before preoperative assessment for refractive surgery. However, there is significant variation in guidelines: Studies have shown that the corneal biomechanics are being affected differently in each individual, and most clinics advice 2–14 days for discontinuation of soft lenses and more than 2 weeks for rigid gas permeable lenses [23].

16.4.2 Centration of the Treatment Zone

To obtain the full effect of the treatment and minimize the amount of induced higher-order aberrations postoperatively, centration of the treatment zone is of importance especially in hypermetropic patients, but also in myopic and patients with astigmatism [14]. A recent study in myopic patients (He 2022) showed that SMILE surgery resulted in larger decentration of the optical zone when compared with LASIK, but there was no effect on objective and subjective visual symptoms. Despite these divagating results, especially in myopic patients, centration should be as optimal as possible. Many approaches to improve centration have been described, such as coaxial corneal light reflection and the "tear film method" where patients focus on the green dot and then adjusting contact to 80% between eye and contact glass, this technique relies on the patients' cooperation and ability to focus on the light [57] (for details see Chap. 15). Some also print reference maps with corneal topography relative to pupil center and then adjust for the difference during the SMILE procedure. With the VISUMAX 800 it is by "Centralign" now possible to optimize centration. Preoperative measures of cornea vertex position relative to the pupil center can be established with the IOL master. Before treatment, this information is entered into the VISUMAX 800 and by this the centration is adjusted by visual overlay on the screen of the video microscope. This helps the surgeon to adjust the treatment to the corneal vertex.

16.4.3 Cyclotorsion Adjustment

In patients with larger astigmatism, many surgeons prefer to adjust for cyclotorsion.

A mean cyclotorsion of 5 degrees [43] has been shown to occur in myopic astigmatic patients during SMILE. A randomized contralateral study on the effect of cyclotorsion control did, however, not find that cyclotorsion compensation improved the visual and refractive outcomes [44]. A prospective study found that manual correction of cyclotorsion in SMILE is possible and safe with good visual outcomes [43], however, in the VisuMax, cyclotorsion adjustment needs to be done manually by rotating the contact glass after suction and some find this troublesome.

The VISUMAX 800 features a new system, "Oculign®", for cyclotorsion management. It allows quick and precise digital rotation of the laser pattern simply by rotation of the joystick after docking. In our study on VISUMAX 800, we marked the cornea with dye at 0 and 180 degrees when the patient was upright, but only if the patient has a preoperative cylinder > 2D. The VISUMAX 800 integrates with the IOL master, and in later software updates, it is expected that the cyclotorsion adjustment can be fully automatized by iris image without the use of corneal dye marks. In our small study (described above), we found a tendency of less postoperative residual cylinder in the VISUMAX 800 treated group compared to VisuMax, however numbers were small (Fig. 16.1F).

16.4.4 Use of Nomograms

To date, there is some variation in the use of nomograms among SMILE surgeons. Only few and mostly retrospective studies have been published on this subject.

A bivariate analysis on factors affecting the predictability has previously been performed from a large study on 670 SMILE operated eyes [26]. This showed that increasing age was associated with a small undercorrection and the same with corneal curvature, however, the effects were small. Ninety-five percent of the variation in the SEQ prediction error could not be explained in their study, why nomograms appeared to be of little relevance in that particular setting (high myopic patients, standard flap size). However, in other settings, i.e., thicker caps, it has been found that undercorrection is an important issue [25] which can be addressed by nomograms. Another study [29] confirmed a significant correlation between cap thickness and undercorrection.

In the present small cohort study on patients that were aimed for emmetropia, we found the VisuMax patients to be slightly undercorrected. Thus, only 53% had a SEQ within ± 0.50 D, whereas 93% was within ± 1.00 D, Fig. 16.1C. However, our group of patients was rather old, and it has previously been shown that especially the older patients with large refractive errors are at risk of undercorrection [22, 26], potentially providing an explanation for the observed undercorrection.

A retrospective study on SMILE [30] showed that the use of nomogram corrections based on the preoperative SEQ, reduced the variance in postoperative SEQ compared to not using a nomogram. The patients were myopic up to –8D with a fixed cap thickness of 120 μm and all operated by the same surgeon. By using the nomogram, 86% of the patients were postoperatively within ± 0.50 D and 98% within ± 1.00 D, as compared to 70% and 96% in patients operated without the use of nomogram. However, three months postoperatively the UDVA was not statistically different between the two groups, being − 0.064 ± 0.065 logMAR in the standard group and − 0.08 ± 0.06 logMAR in the nomogram group.

The VISUMAX 800 integrates with Forum Viewer and gives the opportunity of personalized nomograms using the Visulyze software. Based on previous results on the patients' manifest refraction, the surgeon can have a personalized nomogram developed. If nomograms are used, it is of importance that it is regularly updated as operation techniques and surgeons might change over time [19].

16.4.5 Variations in the Laser Cut in SMILE Surgery

VISUMAX 800 operates with the same wavelength and is general very similar to VisuMax but due to an increased laser frequency of 2 kHz instead of 500 Hz it is significantly faster. Thus, VISUMAX 800 has a shorter cutting time of approximately 10 s compared to 25–30 s with the VisuMax. This theoretically reduces the risk of suction loss which is a rare but feared complication in SMILE surgery. Studies have shown an incidence of suction loss of 0.17% [21] to 0.41% [20].

There are some well-described technical limitations on accuracy in the femtosecond laser cut that may affect the refractive precision [40]. The short pulse of the laser means minimal thermal damage to the surrounding tissue. At the laser focus point, the laser intensity increases above a critical level, thereby forming a small plasma bubble which stretches and mechanically separates the surrounding tissue. The accuracy of the laser cut is defined by the zone of interaction between the stroma and the focused laser beam in the axial and lateral direction. The axial point of interaction fluctuates statistically around the focus position within a range that is approximately given by the Rayleigh length (Fig. 16.2).

The wavelength of the VisuMax femtosecond laser is 1043 nm and its lateral focus diameter (beam waist) is about 3 μm, the novel VISUMAX 800 operates with the same wavelength and beam waist but with higher laser frequency (2 MHz). The beam waist is the result of the optical system in the femtosecond laser system, and from this, the Rayleigh length can be calculated to approximately 3 μm. So, the axial position of the individual points of interaction is controlled by the optical system with a certain accuracy but may vary within a range of up to 3 μm. If the Rayleigh length can be optimized further, even higher axial precision of individual points of interaction can be obtained. However, one should keep in mind that the cut surface is formed by millions of such points of interaction.

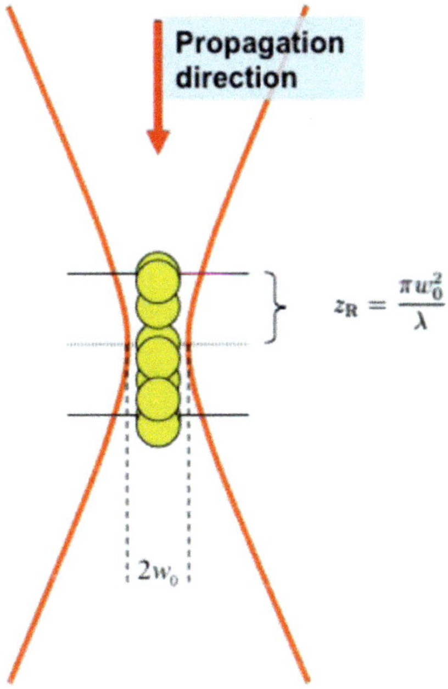

Fig. 16.2 Actual point of focus of the femtosecond laser is associated with some degree of imprecision and is characterized by the Rayleigh length (z_R). The Rayleigh length is dependent on the wavelength (λ) and the beam waist (w_0). (Courtesy: Dirk Mühlhoff, Carl Zeiss Meditec AG, Jena, Germany)

Thus, the accuracy of the surface geometry does not directly depend on the positional accuracy of individual interaction points, and the Rayleigh length is thus only one of several influencing technical parameters. Laser settings (spot distance and pulse energy) should be adjusted by the surgeon so that the laser cut is precise and predicable.

16.4.5.1 Cap Cutting

The anterior cut of the lenticule is in theory planar to the corneal surface and the cap thickness is preoperatively defined by the surgeon. In SMILE, it is the posterior cut of the lenticule that defines the programmed refractive correction. Cap thickness is known to play a role for the refractive effect in SMILE, as lenticule removal in the deeper corneal layers cause less flattening effect of the anterior corneal curvature. Damgaard and others [29] have found a significant undercorrection when using thick caps and some surgeons plan for overcorrection when performing SMILE with a thick cap (see Chap. 11 for details).

The biomechanical changes after SMILE surgery are not yet precisely understood. When the lenticule is removed, the collagen fibrils in the cap will be somewhat relaxed as the arc length of the corneal surface becomes smaller. Over time, the healing response in the cornea and fibril remodeling may compensate for this. On the other hand, a relatively thick cap has been suggested to preserve the tensile strength of the anterior stroma [24], but ex vivo studies have found only a minor insignificant difference in biomechanical strength with cap thickness of 160 microns versus 110 microns [25]. Choosing a thicker cap is suggested to better preserve the subbasal nerve plexus and gives better opportunities for retreatments.

Newer possibilities for assessing the corneal strength and risk of postoperative ectasia are now available, an example is Corvis ST II [52] that might add further knowledge on the impact of SMILE on corneal biomechanics.

Despite a predefined planned cap thickness the actual thickness may be slightly different. A variation in thickness between 2 and 11 microns has been shown [8, 10, 37]. Variations in cap thickness can influence the refractive reproducibility if there is a systematic error from the center to the periphery. If the cap thickness is higher than intended in the periphery, a larger refractive effect will be achieved, and vice versa, while scattered variations will have no systematic effect.

16.4.5.2 Lenticule Cutting

It is known that the attempted lenticule removal and the actual amount of removed stromal tissue is not exactly the same. In 2014, Reinstein et al. [13] published a study on changes in stromal thickness preoperatively and three months after SMILE surgery in high myopic patients. Stromal changes were measured with Artemis high-frequency ultrasound and compared to the VisuMax read-out lenticule thickness. The study showed that the Artemis measured lenticule was measured to be 8.2 (±8) μm thinner than planned, a finding that was later confirmed by others although the mismatch did not affect the refractive outcome [39]. The difference between observed and expected lenticule thickness may partly be due to Artemis measurement errors since the properties of the tissue change after surgery.

A prospective randomized contralateral eye study of myopic patients undergoing either ReLEx Flex or SMILE, investigated changes in stromal thickness [41, 42]. Central corneal thickness (CCT) was measured by optical low-coherence reflectometry before and 6 months after surgery. The net reduction in CCT was compared to the VisuMax read-out lenticule thickness. The results showed a net reduction in CCT of 22.9 μm ± 6.6 less than expected in the FLEX operated eyes and 21.5 μm ± 6.4 less than expected in the SMILE operated eyes. Correlation analyses showed, however, no significant relation between the error in refractive outcome and error in lenticule thickness.

16.4.6 Changes in Epithelium After Refractive Treatment

Changes in epithelial thickness after SMILE affect the primary outcome and refractive stability. In excimer laser surgery (PRK/LASIK) for high myopia, long-term studies have shown a substantial thickening of the central epithelium of up to 10 μm when correcting for up to −7D [47]. Others have shown that the epithelial hyperplasia is dependent of the magnitude of the refractive correction [28]. The thickening is a result of the epithelium smoothening the surface, compensating for the stromal loss, and the degree of thickening is possibly determined by the degree of attempted correction and the size of the optical zone. After SMILE, the change in epithelial thickness is somewhat smaller than after excimer laser surgery but varies consistently between eyes (mean 6 μm, range −2 to 13 μm) [10]. Other studies have confirmed that the epithelial change in SMILE is smaller than in

LASIK [50] and remodeling appears to stabilize more rapidly following SMILE than FS-LASIK [49]. A randomized study on LASIK versus SMILE found, however, no difference between epithelial thickness and remodeling after the two types of surgery [33]. Overall, the interindividual variations in epithelial hyperplasia may contribute to the refractive predictability and postoperative refractive changes after SMILE.

16.5 Discussion

SMILE surgery in myopic patients has been shown to have good refractive outcomes in several clinical studies and results on safety, efficacy and predictability have been shown to be comparable to LASIK [1, 2, 9, 44] as described in detail in the following Chap. 17. In this chapter, we have described various components affecting the refractive predictability and outcomes in SMILE surgery. Some of the variation is not possible to affect but obviously focus should be on the adjustable factors to minimize the risk of refractive surprises. Standardized protocols for patient evaluation and experienced optometrists at the pre- and postoperative visits are crucial. The surgeon performing the operation should be well trained and in SMILE a particular focus on centration of the treatment zone is important.

Regarding refractive predictability, we found that the VISUMAX 800 had refractive outcome on myopia that was superior to VisuMax. In the VISUMAX 800 group, the postoperative SEQ was −0.1 (±0.3) D. Our results in the present smaller study on VisuMax showed that patients were a bit undercorrected with a postoperative SEQ of -0.5 ± 0.6 D, this in contrast to our previously reported large study on 670 eyes where we had a SEQ of -0.25 ± 0.44 D [26]. In 2018, we changed our original VisuMax laser, which was then 10 years old, to a new VisuMax laser. During the COVID-19 pandemic, our refractive surgery activity was closed down for almost one year. Although we continuously perform quality control, the current more detailed comparison illustrates the need for a nomogram adjustment when we use our VisuMax laser, whereas this is not needed for the VISUMAX 800 laser used in our small study. Cylinder correction in VISUMAX 800 was satisfying, 78% had a postoperative cylinder $\leq$ 0.50D which is similar to previously reported results when performing SMILE on VisuMax. The safety was good with no patients losing 2 lines or more in any of the groups.

VISUMAX 800 offers shorter operation time and better workflow in the operating room [48]. Moreover, VISUMAX 800 has been proposed to reduce the risk of suction loss due to the shorter suction time. In the present study we experienced no suction loss, and less experienced surgeons may benefit from the shorter suction time. Furthermore, the patients typically appreciate the shorter total operation time.

In this chapter, we confirm that the both the VisuMax and the new VISUMAX 800 deliver safe and predictable results in SMILE surgery.

References

1. Yao L, Zhang M, Wang D, Zhao Q, Wang S, Bai H. Small Incision lenticule extraction (SMILE) and laser in situ keratomileusis (LASIK) used to treat myopia and myopic astigmatism: a systematic review and meta-analysis of randomized clinical trials. Semin Ophthalmol. 2023;38(3):283–293.
2. Tian H, Gao W, Xu C, Wang Y. Clinical outcomes and higher order aberrations of wavefront-guided LASIK versus SMILE for correction of myopia: a systemic review and meta-analysis Acta Ophthalmol 2023;101(6):606–618. https://doi.org/10.1111/aos.15638. Epub 2023 Feb 1.
3. Taneri S, Kießler S, Rost S, Schultz T, Dick B. Small-incision lenticule extraction for the correction of myopic astigmatism. J Cataract Refract Surg. 2019;45(1):62–71.
4. Dishler JG, Slade S, Seifert S, Schallhorn SC. Small-incision lenticule extraction (SMILE) for the correction of myopia with astigmatism: outcomes of the United States food and drug administration premarket approval clinical trial. Clinical Trial Ophthalmol. 2020;127(8):1020–1034.
5. Hansen RS, Lyhne N, Grauslund J, Vestergaard AH. Small-incision lenticule extraction (SMILE): outcomes of 722 eyes treated for myopia and myopic astigmatism. Graefes Arch Clin Exp Ophthalmol. 2016;254(2):399–405.
6. Kim JR, Hwang HB, Mun SJ, Chung YT, Kim HS. Efficacy, predictability, and safety of small incision lenticule extraction: 6-months prospective cohort study BMC Ophthalmol. 2014;3:14:117.
7. Brar S, Roopashree CR, Ganesh S. Incidence of ectasia after SMILE from a high-volume refractive surgery center in India. J Refract Surg. 2021;37(12):800–808. https://doi.org/10.3928/1081597X-20210812-03. Epub 2021 Dec 1.
8. Reinstein DZ, Archer TJ, Gobbe M. Accuracy and reproducibility of cap thickness in small incision lenticule extraction. J Refract Surg. 2013;29(12):810–5.
9. Song J, Cao H, Chen X, Chao X, Zhang J, Wu G, Wang Y. Small incision lenticule extraction (SMILE) versus laser assisted stromal in situ keratomileusis (LASIK) for astigmatism corrections: a systematic review and meta-analysis. Rev Am J Ophthalmol. 2023;247:181–99.
10. Vestergaard AH, Grauslund J, Ivarsen AR, Hjortdal JØ. Central corneal sublayer pachymetry and biomechanical properties after refractive femtosecond lenticule extraction. J Refract Surg. 2014;30(2):102–8.
11. Vestergaard AH, Grønbech KT, Grauslund J, Ivarsen AR, Hjortdal JØ. Subbasal nerve morphology, corneal sensation, and tear film evaluation after refractive femtosecond laser lenticule extraction. Graefes Arch Clin Exp Ophthalmo. 2013;251(11):2591–600.
12. Reinstein DZ, Carp GI, Archer TJ, Gobbe M. Outcomes of small incision lenticule extraction (SMILE) in low myopia. Refract Surg. 2014;30(12):812–8.
13. Reinstein DZ, Yap TE, Carp GI, Archer TJ, Gobbe M. London vision clinic optometric group reproducibility of manifest refraction between surgeons and optometrists in a clinical refractive surgery practice. J Cataract Refract Surg. 2014;40(3):450–9.
14. Liu M, Sun Y, Wang D, Zhang T, Zhou Y, Zheng H. Decentration of optical zone center and its impact on visual outcomes following SMILE. Cornea. 2015;34(4):392–7.
15. Han T, Zheng K, Chen Y, Gao Y, He L, Zhou X. Four-year observation of predictability and stability of small incision lenticule extraction. BMC Ophthalmoly. 2016;16(1):149.
16. Pradhan KR, Reinstein DZ , Carp GI , Archer TJ , Gobbe M , Dhungana P. Quality control outcomes analysis of small-incision lenticule extraction for myopia by a novice surgeon at the first refractive surgery unit in Nepal during the first 2 years of operation. J Cataract Refract Surgery. 2016;42(2):267–74.
17. Ivarsen A, Hjortdal J. Correction of myopic astigmatism with small incision lenticule extraction. J Refract Surg. 2014;30(4):240–7.
18. Nielsen R, Christiansen MK, Kristensen MS, Møller C, Hedegaard C, Aagaard N, Sejersen H, Hjortdal J, Ivarsen A. Reproducibility of subjective refraction before and after small incision lenticule extraction (SMILE) for myopia. Acta Ophthalmol. 2020;98(1):e130–e131.

19. Gailitis RP. Comparison of LASIK outcomes with the Alcon LADARVision4000 and the VISX STAR S2 excimer lasers using optimized nomograms. Refract Surg. 2005;21(6):683–90.
20. Liu M, Wang J, Zhong W, Wang D, Zhou Y, Liu Q. Impact of suction loss during small incision lenticule extraction (SMILE). Refract Surg. 2016;32(10):686–92.
21. Pradhan KR, Reinstein DZ, Carp GI, Archer TJ, Gobbe M, Dhungana P. Quality control outcomes analysis of small-incision lenticule extraction for myopia by a novice surgeon at the first refractive surgery unit in Nepal during the first 2 years of operation. J Cataract Refract Surg. 2016;42(2):267–74.
22. Feltham M, Wolfe R. Some variables to consider to avoid the need for LASIK surgical enhancements. Optom 2000;83(2):76–81.
23. Goudie C, Tatham A, Davies R, Sifton A, Wright M. The effect of the timing of the cessation of contact lens use on the results of biometry. Eye (Lond). 2018;32(6):1048–1054.
24. Lv X, Zhang F, Song Y, Zhai C, Guo N, Lai L, Xu Y. Corneal biomechanical characteristics following small incision lenticule extraction for myopia and astigmatism with 3 different cap thicknesses. BMC Ophthalmology. 2023;23(Article number: 42).
25. Damgaard IB, Ivarsen A, Hjortdal J. Refractive correction and biomechanical strength following SMILE with a 110 or 160-μm cap thickness, evaluated ex vivo by inflation test. Invest Ophthalmol Vis Sci. 2018;59(5):1836–43.
26. Hjortdal JØ, Vestergaard AH, Ivarsen A, Ragunathan S, Asp S. Predictors for the outcome of small-incision lenticule extraction for Myopia. J Refract Surg. 2012;28(12):865–71.
27. Pedersen IB, Ivarsen A, Hjortdal J. Changes in astigmatism, densitometry, and aberrations after SMILE for low to high myopic astigmatism: a 12-month prospective study. Refract Surg. 2017;33(1):11–7.
28. Luft N, Ring MH, Dirisamer M, Mursch-Edlmayr AS, Kreutzer TC, Pretzl J, Bolz M, Priglinger SG. Corneal epithelial remodeling induced by small incision lenticule extraction (SMILE). Invest Ophthalmol Vis Sci. 2016;57(9):176–83.
29. Güell JL, Verdaguer P, Mateu-Figueras G, Elies D, Gris O, Husseiny MAE, Manero F, Morral MJ. SMILE procedures with four different cap thicknesses for the correction of myopia and myopic astigmatism. Refract Surg. 2015;31(9):580–5.
30. Liang G, Chen X, Zha X, Zhang F. A nomogram to improve predictability of small-incision lenticule extraction surgery. Med Sci Monit. 2017;30(23):5168–75.
31. He S, Luo Y, Chen P, Ye Y, Zheng H , Lan M, Zhuang J, Yu K. Prospective, randomized, contralateral eye comparison of functional optical zone, and visual quality after SMILE and FS-LASIK for high myopi. Transl Vis Sci Technol;11(2):13. https://doi.org/10.1167/tvst.11.2.13
32. Han T, Zheng K, Chen Y, Gao Y, He L, Zhou X. Four-year observation of predictability and stability of small incision lenticule extraction. BMC Ophthalmol. 2016;16(1):149.
33. Kanellopoulos AJ. Comparison of Corneal epithelial remodeling over 2 years in LASIK versus SMILE: a contralateral eye study. Cornea. 2019;38(3):290–6.
34. US Food and drug administration 2016: VisuMax femtosecond laser system for refractive correcetion. 2016;13.
35. Blum M, Täubig K, Gruhn C, Sekundo W, Kunert KS. Five-year results of small incision lenticule extraction (ReLEx SMILE). Br J Ophthalmol. 2016;100(9):1192–5.
36. Lv X, Zhang F, Song Y, Zhai C, Guo N, Lai L, Xu Y. Corneal biomechanical characteristics following small incision lenticule extraction for myopia and astigmatism with 3 different cap thicknesses. BMC Ophthalmol. 2023;23(1).42. https://doi.org/10.1186/s12886-023-02786-8
37. Zhao J, Yao P, Li M, Chen Z, Shen Y, Zhao Z, Zhou Z, Zhou X (2013) The morphology of corneal cap and its relation to refractive outcomes in femtosecond laser small incision lenticule extraction (SMILE) with anterior segment optical coherence tomography observation .PLoS One 2013;8(8):e70208.
38. Reinstein DZ, Archer TJ, Gobbe M. Lenticule thickness readout for small incision lenticule extraction compared to artemis three-dimensional very high-frequency digital ultrasound stromal measurements. J Refract Surg. 2014;30(5):304–9.

39. Luft N, Priglinger SG, Ring MH, Mayer WJ, Mursch-Edlmayr AS, Kreutzer TC, Bolz M, Dirisamer M. Stromal remodeling and lenticule thickness accuracy in small-incision lenticule extraction: one-year results. J Cataract Refract Surg. 2017;43(6):812–818.
40. Sarayba MA, Ignacio TS, Binder PS, Dan B. Tran comparative study. Comparative study of stromal bed quality by using mechanical, IntraLase femtosecond laser 15 and 30-kHz microkeratomes. Cornea 2007;26(4):446–51.
41. Heichel J, Blum M, Duncker GIW, Sietmann R, Kunert KS. Surface quality of porcine corneal lenticules after femtosecond lenticule extraction. Ophthalmic Res. 2011;46(2):107–12.
42. Ang M, Chaurasia SS, Angunawela RI, Poh R, Riau A, Tan D, Mehta JS. Femtosecond lenticule extraction (FLEx): clinical results, interface evaluation, and intraocular pressure variation. Invest Ophthalmol Vis Sci. 2012;53(3):1414–21.
43. Ganesh S, Brar S, Pawar A. Results of intraoperative manual cyclotorsion compensation for myopic astigmatism in patients undergoing small incision lenticule extraction (SMILE). J Refract Surg. 2017;33(8):506–12.
44. Xu J, Liu F, Liu M, Yang X, Weng S, Lin L, Lin H, Xie Y, Liu Q. Effect of Cyclotorsion Compensation With a Novel Technique in Small Incision Lenticule Extraction Surgery for the Correction of Myopic Astigmatism. J Refract Surg. 2019 May 1;35(5):301-308. doi: 10.3928/1081597X-20190402-01. Erratum in: J Refract Surg. 2020;36(4):280. https://doi.org/10.3928/1081597X-20200225-01. PMID: 31059579.
45. Reinstein DZ, Archer TJ, Potter JG, Gupta R, Wiltfang R. Refractive and visual outcomes of SMILE for compound myopic astigmatism with the VISUMAX 800. J Refract Surg. 2023;39(5):294–301.
46. Ivarsen A, Hjortdal J. Seven-year changes in corneal power and aberrations after PRK or LASIK. Invest Ophthalmol Vis Sci. 2012;53(10):6011–6.
47. Brar S, Ganesh S, Bhargav S. Comparison of intraoperative time taken for docking, lenticule dissection, and overall workflow for SMILE performed with the VisuMax 800 versus the VisuMax 500 femtosecond laser. J Refract Surg. 2023;39(9):648.
48. Ryu I, Kim BJ, Lee J, Kim SW. Comparison of corneal epithelial remodeling after femtosecond laser-assisted LASIK and small incision lenticule extraction (SMILE). J Refract Surg. 2017;33(4):250–6.
49. Wang Y, Zhanf ZF, Qian YF, Luo BG, Li C, Yang XL. Comparison of corneal epithelial remodeling after small incision lenticule extraction and femtosecond laser-assisted LASIKZhonhua Yan Ke. 2020;56(2):93−102.
50. Waring GO. Standard graphs for reporting refractive surgery. Refract Surg. 2000;16(4):459–66.
51. Liu M, Li N, Chen T, Tian G, Lin Y, Gao H, Shi W. Comparison of corneal biomechanics treated with femtosecond laser-assisted in situ keratomileusis and small-incision lenticule extraction by new corneal biomechanical parameters of Corvis ST II, Cornea 2022, Online ahead of print.
52. Liang C, Yan H. Methods of corneal vertex centration and evaluation of effective optical zone in small incision lenticule extraction. Ophthalmic Res. 2023.
53. Song J, Cao H, Chen X, Zhao X, Zhang J, Wu G, Wang Y. Small incision lenticule extraction (SMILE) versus laser assisted stromal in situ keratomileusis (LASIK) for astigmatism corrections: a systematic review and meta-analysis review. Am J Ophthalmol. 2023;247:181–199.
54. Reinstein DZ, Yap TE, Carp GI, Archer TJ, Gobbe M. Reproducibility of manifest refraction between surgeons and optometrists in a clinical refractive surgery practice. J Cataract Refract Surg 2014;40(3):450–9.
55. Aygun BT, Cankaya KI, Agca A, et al. Five-year outcomes of small-incision lenticule extraction versus femtosecond laser-assisted laser in situ keratomileusis: a contralateral eye study. J Cataract Refract Surg. 2020;46(3):403–9.

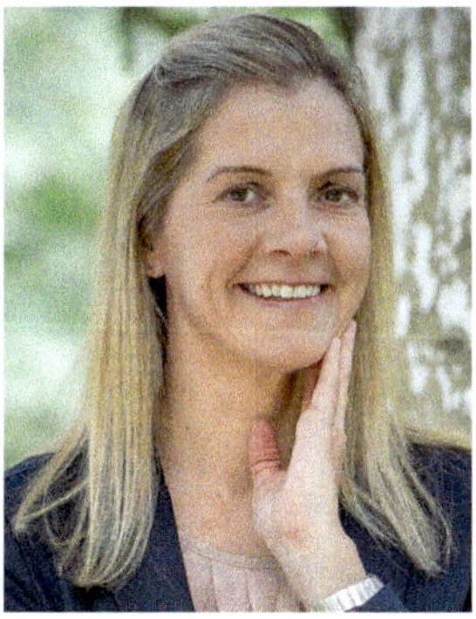

Stine Elkjær Nielsen is a consultant and assistant professor within the cornea and refractive section in the Department of Ophthalmology in Aarhus, Denmark. She received her Ph.D. in 2011. After this she started her ophthalmology residency training at the Department of Ophthalmology in Aarhus, Denmark and finished training in 2016. She started performing SMILE procedures in 2016. Stine Elkjær Nielsen has published 20 scientific papers. Her clinical, surgical and research activity focuses on cataract, corneal refractive surgery, keratoplasty, keratoconus and corneal wound healing .

Comparison of Results Between SMILE, Femtolasik and Surface Ablation for Myopia

17

B. Tülü Aygün, Kİ Çankaya, A. Ağca, Y. Yıldırım, B. Kepez Yıldız, M. E. Sucu, N. Kandemir Beşek, and A. Demirok

Abstract

Various factors impact the visual and refractive outcomes of refractive surgery. In our effort to minimize patient-related variables, we conducted a five-year postoperative study focusing on individuals who underwent SMILE (Small Incision Lenticule Extraction) in one eye and FS-LASIK (Femtosecond Laser-Assisted Laser Keratomileusis) in the contralateral eye. The refractive outcomes were found similar between the groups at 5 years postoperatively, along with corneal high-order aberrations. Extensive literature examines the comparative results of SMILE, LASIK, and PRK, all of which have demonstrated efficacy, safety, and predictability in addressing myopia. Notably, SMILE appears to offer potential advantages, particularly concerning corneal high-order aberrations and dry eye symptoms.

17.1 Introduction

Corneal refractive surgery has been an integral part of our clinical practice for an extended duration. Nevertheless, over the past decade, the introduction of Small Incision Lenticule Extraction (SMILE) surgery has significantly broadened our treatment options. This development has prompted ophthalmological societies to embark on comprehensive research endeavors aimed at delineating the similarities

In the loving memory of our mentor and guide Prof. Dr. Ahmet Demirok

B. Tülü Aygün (✉) · K. Çankaya · A. Ağca · Y. Yıldırım · B. Kepez Yıldız · M. E. Sucu · N. K. Beşek · A. Demirok
Istanbul Medipol University, Istanbul, Türkiye
e-mail: beriltulu@gmail.com

W. Sekundo and F. M. Wagner (eds.), *Femtosecond Laser Assisted Lenticule Extraction*,
https://doi.org/10.1007/978-3-031-60424-9_17

and disparities between various procedures, including Surface Ablation (Photoreactive Refractive Keratotomy [PRK]), Femtosecond Laser-Assisted Laser in Situ Keratomileusis (FS-LASIK), and SMILE.

Given the inherent procedural distinctions among these surgical modalities, divergence in outcomes pertaining to visual acuity, refractive correction, complications, and patient-reported subjective symptoms can be anticipated. However, a substantial body of literature shows that they are all safe and effective in the treatment of myopia and myopic astigmatism. In pursuit of a more comprehensive understanding of long-term outcomes and to minimize the impact of uncontrolled variables, we conducted an investigational study aimed at comparing the long-term results of SMILE and FS-LASIK for the correction of myopia and myopic astigmatism in contralateral eyes of the same patients.

17.1.1 Patients and Methods

We included patients with a spherical error less than −10 diopters (D) and cylindrical error less than −5 D, with healthy and regular corneal topography, and mesopic pupil diameter less than 6,5 mm. Patients underwent a full ophthalmological evaluation preoperatively. Uncorrected (UDVA) and corrected (CDVA) distance visual acuities, and subjective and objective refractive errors were noted. Full manifest refractions were used for the surgical correction.

All patients received first SMILE in one eye, and then corneal flap for FS-LASIK was created in the other eye. Then the patients were relocated to the excimer laser platform for the ablation. All surgeries were performed by the same experienced surgeon (A.D.). The laser used for this study was VisuMax 500. The settings and parameters of both procedures were set the same for every eye. All patients received the same topical treatment for both eyes. The parameters of both of the procedures are described in the original article [1].

The follow-up period of our study was 5 years postoperatively. We also planned visits at 1st and 3rd year. We recorded manifest refraction, UDVA, CDVA, and corneal topography data including total HOAs (high order aberrations), spherical aberrations, coma and trefoil aberrations at the 6.0 mm diameter central corneal zone. Any reported complaints, and complications were also noted. The statistical analysis was performed using Wilcoxon signed-rank test to compare preoperative and postoperative data within each procedure as well as between the procedures.

Twenty-four patients were enrolled into the study, which received FS LASIK for one eye and SMILE on the other eye. After losing 2 patients in the follow-up, the study was completed at 5 years postoperatively with 22 patients. The preoperative characteristics of the patients can be seen in Table 17.1. No statistical difference was found in any of the characteristics. We compared the efficacy, safety, predictability, stability and induced corneal HOAs at 5 years following surgery between the two procedures on contralateral eyes.

Table 17.1 Preoperative patient characteristics

	SMILE (n = 24)		FS-LASIK (n = 24)		*P* value
	Mean±SD	Range	Mean±SD	Range	
Spherical equivalent (D)	−4.81 ± 1.44	−1.50 to −7.00	−4.19 ± 1.67	−1.25 to −6.50	0.21
Astigmatism (D)	−0.48 ± 0.29	−0.25 to −1.25	−0.64 ± 0.35	0.00 to −1.50	0.11
Average keratometry (D)	43.72 ± 1.33	42 to 46	43.64 ± 1.40	42 to 46	0.94
Thinnest corneal thickness (μm)	554.91 ± 27.06	509 to 586	553.45 ± 26.49	506 to 587	0.86

SMILE: Small incision lenticule extraction, FS-LASIK: Femtosecond laser assisted laser in situ keratomileusis, SD: standard deviation

17.1.2 Our Results

The efficacy was evaluated as the improvement in the UDVA, compared to the preoperative CDVA, and no statistically significant difference was found between the surgeries (p = 0.572). In Fig. 17.1 the cumulative visual acuities for SMILE and FS-LASIK are shown. The efficacy index was 0.95 and 0.96 for SMILE and FS LASIK, respectively.

In terms of safety, none of the eyes in either of groups has lost more than 2 lines of CDVA. The mean CDVA was found to be not statistically different between the groups of SMILE and FS LASIK (p = 0.389), which can be seen as the change in the lines in Fig. 17.2. The safety index was 1.01 and 1.03 for SMILE and FS LASIK, respectively.

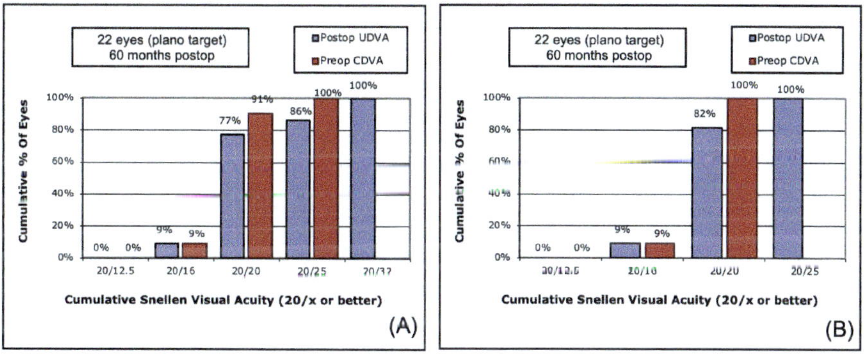

Fig. 17.1 The cumulative visual acuities for SMILE (A) and FS-LASIK (B) after 5 years

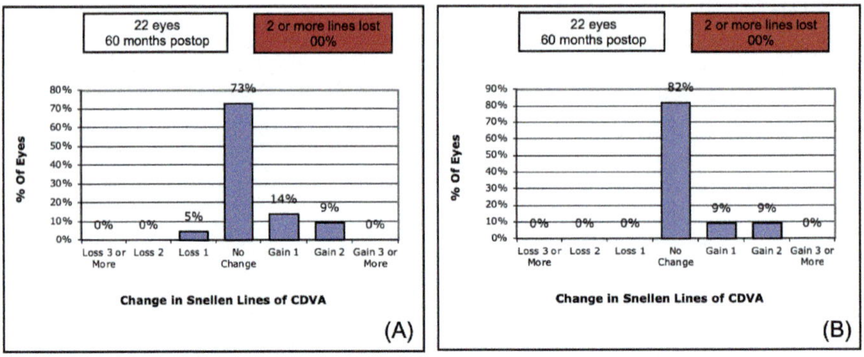

Fig. 17.2 Gain and loss of Snellen lines in SMILE (A) and FS-LASIK (B) after 5 years

The predictability was also similarly high in both groups as seen in Fig. 17.3, showing the attempted versus achieved SE refraction of under- and overcorrected eyes. Figure 17.4 demonstrates that in SMILE group, 91%, and in FS-LASIK group 95% of eyes were within ± 0.5 D in terms of attempted spherical equivalent (SE) refraction; and all eyes were in the range of ± 1.0 D in both groups at 5 years postoperatively. Since astigmatism correction is also an important matter of subject, it was also separately evaluated as represented in Fig. 17.5. In both SMILE and FS LASIK groups, 91% of eyes had astigmatism ≤ 0.5 D, and all of eyes had ≤ 1.0 D.

The difference between intended and achieved SE correction were interpreted as the stability of the procedures, and the course of SE over time was summarized in Fig. 17.6. No statistically significant difference ($p = 0.157$, 0.459 and 0.174 respectively) was observed at any of the time points (1, 3, and 5 years postoperatively).

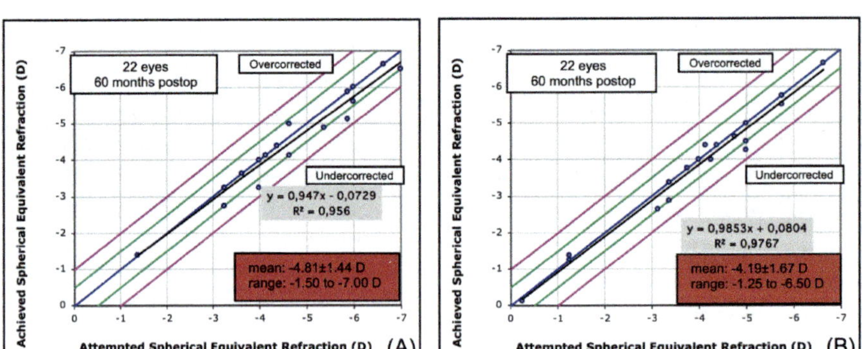

Fig. 17.3 Predictability of refractive treatment in SMILE (A) versus FS-LASIK (B)

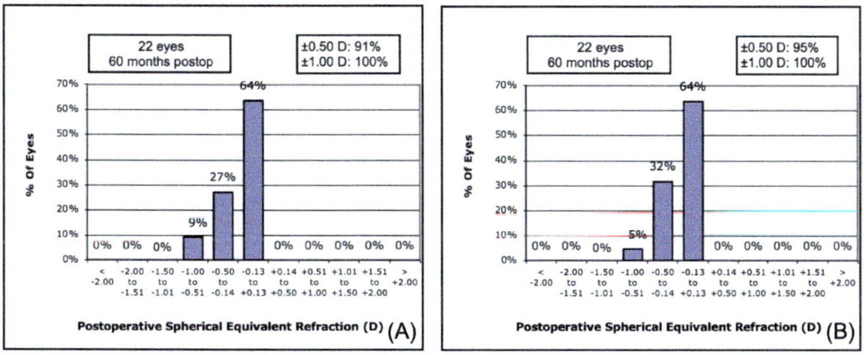

Fig. 17.4 Accuracy of the refractive treatment shown as a spherical equivalent (SE) in SMILE (A) versus FS-LASIK (B)

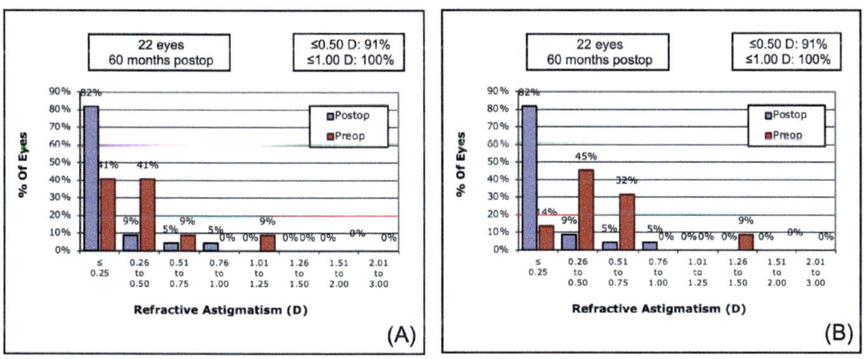

Fig. 17.5 Accuracy of astigmatism correction after 5 years shown as remaining refractive astigmatism in SMILE (A) versus FS-LASIK (B)

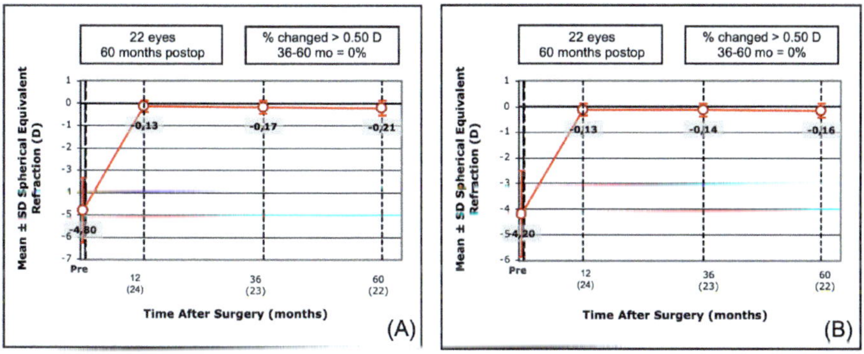

Fig. 17.6 Stability of the achieved spherical equivalent (SE) correction over the period up to 5 years in SMILE (A) versus FS-LASIK (B)

We found that total HOAs, spherical aberrations, and comatic aberrations were increased statistically significant from baseline to 5 years following surgery within both groups separately ($p < 0.001$), but no difference was detected in terms of trefoil aberrations. Most importantly, no significant difference was observed between the groups of FS LASIK and SMILE.

17.2 Discussion

Since the introduction of SMILE in corneal refractive surgery, the outcomes of itself and also the comparison of its results to the other refractive surgeries, mainly LASIK and surface ablation (PRK) has been an important issue. In order to enlighten the subject, many studies have been performed, especially in the last years, comparing refractive, visual, biomechanical and quality of life outcomes. As one of the first long term *intraindividual* studies observing the results of contralateral LASIK and SMILE, we have investigated the efficacy, safety, predictability, stability and corneal HOAs.

Our study yielded comparable and good results between LASIK and SMILE on contralateral eyes in 5 years, in terms of efficacy, safety, predictability and stability [1]. Similarly, other studies in the literature on contralateral eyes showed no significant change between these two procedures. In their prospective and randomized study, Chiang et al. reported that there was no difference in visual outcomes between SMILE and LASIK in contralateral eyes, and both results were excellent [2]. In their study, Ang. et al. also did not find any difference between LASIK and SMILE in contralateral eyes at 3 and 12 months [3]. In contrast, Kanellopoulos et al. published their results in contralateral SMILE and LASIK eyes first 3 months followed by 12 months postoperatively [3, 4]. They reported LASIK to show better results than SMILE, however at 12 months SMILE showed a notable improvement. This can be interpreted as a sign of slower visual rehabilitation in SMILE, compared to LASIK, which always should be considered while discussing results and counselling patients. In fact, visual rehabilitation after SMILE depends on both, laser settings and dissection techniques alike as described in detail in Chaps. 5, 6 and 10 of this book. Contralateral studies enable to obtain more accurate results by avoiding variables such as immune reaction, environmental factors and patient adherence. However, other studies comparing SMILE and LASIK, not including contralaterally treated eyes, also showed similar results between these two procedures [6–8].

PRK is a long-standing procedure with effective results in the treatment of myopia and myopic astigmatism. Through the vast number of surgeries and studies performed, the late visual and refractive recovery and patient discomfort at the early postoperative time are well known.

In an earlier study conducted in our clinic, Yildirim et al. demonstrated that visual and refractive outcomes of PRK at 12-month postoperatively were similar to SMILE [9]. In their study on a large population comparing PRK, LASIK and SMILE, Sia et al. demonstrated that at 1 month postoperatively the visual and refractive outcomes in PRK group are less favorable than in SMILE group, but at 3 months, both groups achieved similarly good results [10]. Lin et al. came to the same conclusion when reported a significant difference in terms of safety and efficacy at 1 week postoperatively favoring SMILE against PRK, while this difference disappeared at 6 months postoperatively with both SMILE and PRK achieving similar results [11].

Corneal high order aberrations are also an inevitable part of the evaluation of corneal refractive surgery. In our study, we have found that in 6 mm diameter zone, total HOAs, spherical and comatic aberrations increased significantly in both LASIK and SMILE groups at 5-year, however the difference between the groups was not statistically significant at any of the time points. The tendency in the literature also shows that the induction of HOAs is less or at least similar in SMILE, in comparison to PRK and LASIK. Miraftab et al. published their results comparing all three surgeries at postoperative 12 months [12]. Total corneal-HOA, spheric aberration and coma aberration were all found to be lower in SMILE group than femto-LASIK and PRK group at 6 mm zone in eyes with moderate myopia. In their study comparing SMILE and FS-LASIK, Kim and Chung reported the induction of total HOAs and spherical aberrations after both surgeries [13]. However, it was significantly higher in FS-LASIK group than in SMILE group ($P < 0.001$ and $= 0.034$ respectively). In their study comparing SMILE and PRK, Zhang et al. reported a significant increase in total HOA, spherical aberration and coma after PRK in comparison to SMILE at 6 months after surgery [14]. Yet, in another study by Wang et al., PRK group had higher spherical aberrations, but lower coma aberrations than SMILE group [15]. They discussed that it could be the result of asymmetric side cut, angle of the laser or the decentration due to lack of pupil tracking system.

It should be kept in mind that technically SMILE is more surgeon dependent than PRK or FS-LASIK. The centration during the suction using VisuMax 500.

VisuMax 500 laser, and the manipulation during the removal of the lenticule may change the end refractive results. This is why only the patients who underwent SMILE by the same experienced surgeon were included in our study. Fortunately, the experience of surgeons performing SMILE has been steadily increasing. The decentration has the greatest impact on coma aberrations. Nevertheless, even in the absence of an active eye-tracker as with the VisuMax 500 (in contrast to VisuMax 800) the self-centration by the patient usually yields better results than eye tracker driven excimer lasers as shown by Lazaridis et al. as early as 2014 and discussed in Chap. 15 of this book [16]. Kim and Chung, along with many investigators in the literature, confirmed the decentration in SMILE to be less than in FS-LASIK [13]. He et al. also showed that SMILE achieved better results in terms of corneal HOA than FS-LASIK, and discussed that SMILE cap exhibited better uniformity and symmetry than the FS-LASIK flap [17]. These results can explain why there is not a unity in the findings of the literature, however, with a careful technique and good compliance, the induction of coma aberrations can be minimized in SMILE. The introduction of new devices for lenticule extraction with centration and cyclorotation assistance might further improve the outcomes (see Chaps. 6 and 15).

The corneal response to the refractive surgery is also a very important part of evaluating the long-term success. Epithelial hyperplasia occurring after the corneal ablation may cause regression in refractive outcomes and also corneal aberrations, more specifically spheric aberrations. SMILE has been known to cause less epithelial damage and less corneal remodeling than other surgeries, and thus hyperplasia, which is especially principal for maintaining effective optical zone (EOZ) [18, 19]. In their study, Hou et al. reported that the both FS-LASIK and SMILE resulted obviously in smaller EOZ; however, SMILE showed less reduction in EOZ than FS-LASIK [20]. This would be a good explanation, why spherical aberration is seen less in SMILE than in FS-LASIK, since a larger optical zone would result in a further away transition zone from the center, and thus less spherical aberrations [12]. Similarly, Zhang et al. found that postoperative EOZ was larger following SMILE than PRK, which may explain the higher aberrations reported after PRK [14]. Iversen et al. studied the epithelial and stromal changes after PRK and LASIK, and concluded that both surgeries induce epithelial thickness; which continues for one week in LASIK, but for 1 year in PRK [21]. The limited epithelial hyperplasia and larger EOZ could be possible reasons to expect less aberrations after SMILE.

One of the limitations of our study was the lack of questioning the quality of vision of patients and the evaluation of dry eye. It has been suggested in the literature that PRK and FS-LASIK cause more dry eye than SMILE [18]. In the studies by Lin et al. and Zhang et al. despite the discomfort at the early postoperative period, the final quality of vision after SMILE and PRK have been found similar [11, 14]. On the other hand, Wang et al. reported that subjective quality of life was better in SMILE group than in PRK group at 3 months postoperatively [15]. Ganesh and Gupta confirmed that in patients, who received SMILE, the presence of dry eye was seen less than patients who received FS-LASIK, which was evaluated by Schirmer and TBUT tests [22]. They also performed a subjective questionnaire for pain, watering and prickling and glare, which showed higher complaint scores in LASIK compared to SMILE. However, in the study of Ma und Manche despite a greater corneal denervation in LASIK, there was no statistically significant difference in self-reported dry eye symptoms evaluated with OSDI score between LASIK and SMILE [23]. One has to keep in mind that currently SMILE in US has to be executed via a 4 mm incision compared to the 2 mm incision used in other countries, though. Despite some contradictory results in the literature the majority of published research indicates that SMILE causes less ocular surface problems than PRK, and especially less than FS-LASIK. This in turn may affect the subjective quality of life of patients and induce less corneal, especially spherical aberrations [22, 24].

17.3 Conclusion

In our study the refractive outcomes of intraindividual comparison between SMILE and FS-LASIK were found to be similar at 5 years postoperatively, along with corneal high-order aberrations. Extensive literature search on comparative results of SMILE, LASIK, and PRK demonstrates similar efficacy, safety, and predictability in addressing myopia. Notably, SMILE appears to offer potential advantages, particularly concerning corneal high-order aberrations and dry eye symptoms.

References

1. Tülü Aygün B, Cankaya KI, Agca A, et al. Five-year outcomes of small-incision lenticule extraction vs femtosecond laser-assisted laser in situ keratomileusis: a contralateral eye study. J Cataract Refract Surg. 2020;46(3):403–9.
2. Chiang B, Valerio GS, Manche EE. Prospective, randomized contralateral eye comparison of wavefront-guided laser in situ keratomileusis and small incision lenticule extraction refractive surgeries. Am J Ophthalmol. 2022;237:211–20.
3. Ang M, Farook M, Htoon HM, et al. Randomized clinical trial comparing femtosecond LASIK and small-incision lenticule extraction. Ophthalmology. 2020;127(6):724–30.
4. Kanellopoulos AJ. Topography-guided LASIK versus small incision lenticule extraction (SMILE) for myopia and myopic astigmatism: a randomized, prospective, contralateral eye study. J Refract Surg. 2017;1;33(5):306–312.
5. Kanellopoulos AJ. Topography-guided LASIK versus small incision lenticule extraction: long-term refractive and quality of vision outcomes. Ophthalmology. 2018;125(10):1658–9.
6. Lin F, Xu Y, Yang Y. Comparison of the visual results after SMILE and femtosecond laser-assisted LASIK for myopia. J Refract Surg. 2014;30(4):248–54.
7. Han T, Xu Y, Han X, et al. Three-year outcomes of small incision lenticule extraction (SMILE) and femtosecond laser-assisted laser in situ keratomileusis (FS-LASIK) for myopia and myopic astigmatism. Br J Ophthalmol. 2019;103(4):565–8.
8. Li M, Li M, Chen Y, et al. Five-year results of small incision lenticule extraction (SMILE) and femtosecond laser LASIK (FS-LASIK) for myopia. Acta Ophthalmol. 2019;97(3):e373–80.
9. Yildirim Y, Olcucu O, Alagoz C, et al. Visual and refractive outcomes of photorefractive keratectomy and small incision lenticule extraction (SMILE) for myopia. J Refract Surg. 2016;32(9):604–10.
10. Sia RK, Ryan DS, Beydoun H, et al. Visual outcomes after SMILE from the first-year experience at a U.S. military refractive surgery center and comparison with PRK and LASIK outcomes. J Cataract Refract Surg. 2020;46(7):995–1002.
11. Lin M, Zhou H, Hu Z, et al. Comparison of small incision lenticule extraction and transepithelial photorefractive keratectomy in terms of visual quality in myopia patients. Acta Ophthalmol. 2021;99(8):e1289–96.
12. Miraftab M, Hashemi H, Aghamirsalim M, et al. Matched comparison of corneal higher order aberrations induced by SMILE to femtosecond assisted LASIK and to PRK in correcting moderate and high myopia: 3.00 versus 6.00 mm. BMC Ophthalmol. 2021;15;21(1):216.
13. Kim BK, Chung YT. Comparison of changes in corneal thickness and curvature after myopia correction between SMILE and FS-LASIK. J Refract Surg. 2023;39(1):15–22.
14. Zhang R, Zhang Y, Yuan Y, et al. Comparison of objective and subjective visual quality after flapless laser vision correction for mild to moderate myopia: SMILE versus PRK. Graefes Arch Clin Exp Ophthalmol. 2023;261(6):1731–41.

15. Wang LX, Wang XL, Tang J, et al. A 3-month comparison study of subjective and objective visual quality of small incision lenticule extraction and transepithelial photorefractive keratectomy in patients with low and moderate myopia. Int J Ophthalmol. 2023;18;16(4):608–615.
16. Lazaridis A, Droutsas K, Sekundo W. Topographic analysis of the centration of the treatment zone after SMILE for myopia and comparison to FS-LASIK: subjective versus objective alignment. J Refract Surg. 2014;30(10):680–6.
17. He X, He Q, Yuan M, et al. Evaluation of morphological features: femtosecond-LASIK flap versus SMILE cap, and the effects on corneal higher-order aberrations. Graefes Arch Clin Exp Ophthalmol. 2022;260(12):3993–4003.
18. Murueta-Goyena A, Cañadas P. Visual outcomes and management after corneal refractive surgery: a review. J Optom. 2018;11(2):121–9.
19. Ryu IH, Kim BJ, Lee JH, et al. Comparison of corneal epithelial remodeling after femtosecond laser-assisted LASIK and small incision lenticule extraction (SMILE). J Refract Surg. 2017;1;33(4):250–256.
20. Hou J, Wang Y, Lei Y, et al. Comparison of effective optical zone after small-incision lenticule extraction and femtosecond laser-assisted laser in situ keratomileusis for myopia. J Cataract Refract Surg. 2018;44(10):1179–85.
21. Ivarsen A, Fledelius W, Hjortdal JØ. Three-year changes in epithelial and stromal thickness after PRK or LASIK for high myopia. Invest Ophthalmol Vis Sci. 2009;50(5):2061–6.
22. Ganesh S, Gupta R. Comparison of visual and refractive outcomes following femtosecond laser- assisted lasik with smile in patients with myopia or myopic astigmatism. J Refract Surg. 2014;30(9):590–6.
23. Ma KK, Manche EE. Corneal sensitivity and patient-reported dry eye symptoms in a prospective randomized contralateral-eye trial comparing laser in situ keratomileusis and small incision lenticule extraction. Am J Ophthalmol. 2022;241:248–53.
24. Kobashi H, Kamiya K, Shimizu K. Dry eye after small incision lenticule extraction and femtosecond laser-assisted LASIK: meta-analysis. Cornea. 2017;36(1):85–91.

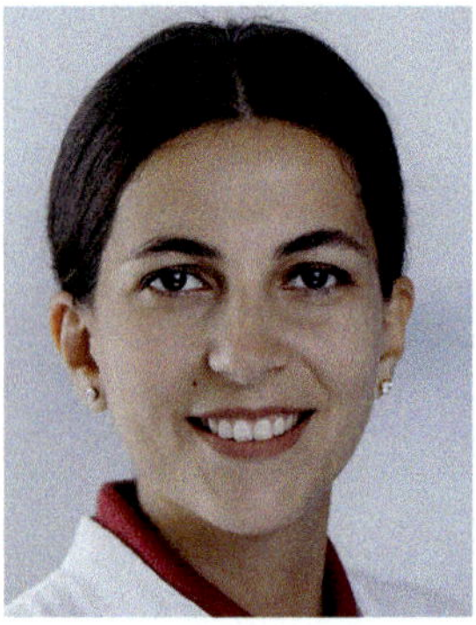

Beril Tülü Aygün is an Ophthalmologist at Medizentrum Eckert in Karlsruhe, Germany. She studied Medicine at Istanbul University, Cerrahpasa Medical Faculty, and attended an observership in Ophthalmology at Charité Universitätsmedizin Berlin. She completed her residency in Ophthalmology at Beyoglu Eye Hospital of the University of Health Sciences in Istanbul, where she gained significant experience in refractive and cataract surgeries, as well as treating keratoconus patients. Notably, she worked with the team that first performed SMILE surgery in Turkey.

Dr. Tülü Aygün continued her career in Germany at Augenklinik Rendsburg, where she served as a senior physician and specialist. She holds two international titles in ophthalmology, FEBO and FICO. Her research focuses on refractive surgery, keratoconus, and corneal diseases. She has published numerous articles in prestigious international and national journals, received awards for her contributions, presented at international conferences, and contributed to several book chapters.

18 Intraocular Lens Selection and Biometry for Cataract Surgery After SMILE

Nikolaus Luft

Abstract

This chapter explores the challenges and solutions in intraocular lens (IOL) power calculations for cataract surgery after small incision lenticule extraction (SMILE) surgery providing recommendations for better calculation.

Keywords

Small incision lenticule extraction surgery (SMILE) • Cataract surgery • Intraocular lens (IOL) power calculation • Keratorefractive surgery • Posterior corneal curvature • Total keratometry (TK)

18.1 Introduction

Internationally released in 2011, more than 10 million SMILE surgeries have been performed worldwide by the end of 2024. In light of the rising popularity of the SMILE technique as well as of aging demography, the number of patients with prior SMILE treatment requiring cataract surgery is expected to increase significantly in the foreseeable future. Hence, cataract surgeons will inevitably be challenged by accurate intraocular lens (IOL) power calculations in this patient group that typically values spectacle independence highly.

N. Luft (✉)
Maximilians-University of Munich, München, Germany
e-mail: nikolaus.luft@med.uni-muenchen.de

W. Sekundo and F. M. Wagner (eds.), *Femtosecond Laser Assisted Lenticule Extraction*,
https://doi.org/10.1007/978-3-031-60424-9_18

18.2 Pitfalls of IOL Power Calculation After Keratorefractive Surgery

There are three major sources of error in calculating IOL power after any kind of keratorefractive surgery [1]. The first and foremost pitfall is the so-called *keratometric index error*. Traditionally, keratometry devices measure the corneal radii only for the anterior corneal surface with the posterior corneal curvature radii being empirically estimated based on the assumption that the ratio between the anterior and posterior corneal curvature ("A/P ratio") is uniform, which is not the case after keratorefractive surgery. Hence, measuring not only the anterior but also the posterior corneal curvature radii to calculate total corneal power might help to minimalize the margin of error in IOL power calculation in eyes with previous keratorefractive surgery. The second error (*formula error*) arises from the fact that some standard IOL power calculation formulae tend to predict a more anterior effective lens position after keratorefractive surgery. Thirdly, corneal power at the corneal vertex that had been artificially altered (e.g. flattened after myopic correction) by keratorefractive surgery is overestimated from keratometry measurements as these are typically performed not centrally but paracentrally (*instrument error*). All three errors concordantly predispose to an underestimation of the required IOL power and, therefore, give rise to dissatisfying hyperopic residual refractive errors after IOL implantation in eyes with prior myopic keratorefractive surgery.

A plethora of IOL power calculation methods and formulae has been developed in an effort to circumvent these errors and to accurately predict IOL power after keratorefractive surgery irrespective of the availability of preoperative clinical or refractive data [2]. A selection of these formulae is accessible in the American Society of Cataract and Refractive Surgeons (ASCRS) post-keratorefractive surgery IOL power online calculator (https://iolcalc.ascrs.org; last accessed October 5, 2023). However, all of the included formulae (e.g., Masket formula, Barrett True-K formula) are empirically optimized for post-Excimer laser ablation [photorefractive keratectomy (PRK) and laser in situ keratomileusis (LASIK)] eyes and do not account for the unique corneal wavefront changes introduced by SMILE. It is well known that the anterior corneal surface after SMILE is steeper near the corneal vertex but flatter in the corneal periphery compared with femtosecond-LASIK, thereby better preserving the physiological (low positive) corneal asphericity [3]. Hence, these formulae may not be unconditionally applicable to cataractous post-SMILE eyes as described in a recent case report of cataract surgery with multifocal IOL implantation after SMILE with an undesired refractive outcome[4].

As SMILE is a relatively young technique compared to PRK or LASIK, clinical data from cataract surgeries of post-SMILE eyes is sparse. In the peer-reviewed literature, only two case reports of cataract surgeries after SMILE [4, 5] as well as one case series [6] are available. Hence, up until today, lack of sufficient clinical data hampers the empirical optimization of existing IOL power calculation formulae for post-SMILE eyes as well as the development of novel SMILE-specific formulae.

18.3 Theoretical Studies of IOL Power Calculation After SMILE

As highlighted above, precise measurements of both the anterior and posterior corneal surface might benefit IOL power calculation accuracy in post-SMILE eyes. For instance, total corneal refractive power (TCRP) as measured with dynamic Scheimpflug imaging (Pentacam HR; Oculus Optikgeräte GmbH, Wetzlar, Germany) combines measurements of both corneal surfaces. TCRP is calculated based on Snell law of refraction and, hence, represents a corneal ray-tracing approach. In two theoretical studies (not involving actual cataract surgery) of eyes undergoing SMILE, TCRP of the central 4.0 mm zone has been proposed as a promising measure of the true corneal power change induced by SMILE [7, 8]. Nevertheless, Scheimpflug imaging offers subpar reliability for corneal curvature measurements as compared with optical coherence tomography (OCT) in corneas with previous keratorefractive surgery [9].

As a more modern indicator of total corneal power, total keratometry (TK) was realized in the IOLMaster 700 biometry system (Carl Zeiss Meditec AG, Jena, Germany). TK involves telecentric 3-zone keratometry for measurements of the anterior corneal radii and, simultaneously, swept-source OCT to directly measure the posterior corneal surface radii and corneal pachymetry [10]. Of note, TK-based IOL power calculation was shown to be advantageous over standard keratometry not only in eyes with treatment-naive corneas but especially in eyes with previous PRK and LASIK [10, 11]. In a recent theoretical study (not involving actual cataract surgery) of 40 eyes undergoing SMILE by Lischke et al. TK outperformed TCRP as a measure of the total corneal refractive power change elicited by SMILE [12].

A further approach incorporating direct measurements of both corneal surfaces into IOL power calculation is the ray tracing method [13]. Ray tracing represents an attractive alternative to post-keratorefractive surgery IOL power calculation formulae, which are commonly based on empirical optimization using "fudge factors" or "correction coefficients." Unlike conventional methods, which approximate corneal power using keratometry readings or corneal topography, ray tracing technology takes a more sophisticated approach. It simulates the path of light rays as they pass through the entire optical system of the eye, including the altered cornea. As a purely physical approach, ray tracing abolishes any empirical optimization and does not require any preoperative clinical or refractive history. Hence, this technique cannot be flawed by refractive changes (e.g., index myopia due to a cataractous lens) as it is the issue with formulae that incorporate preoperative clinical history. Ray tracing is available as an adjunct software on several Scheimpflug- or OCT-based corneal tomography platforms.

With respect to the ray tracing method's performance in post-SMILE eyes, comparative analyses with empirical IOL calculation formulae were conducted in multiple theoretical studies. For instance, Lazaridis et al. [14] used an arithmetic model including virtual IOL implantation to assess the prediction errors (PEs) of ray tracing and conventional IOL power calculation formulae. In their analysis, ray tracing achieved the smallest theoretical PE of − 0.06 ± 0.40 D translating into a theoretical accuracy of 82% of eyes within ± 0.50 Diopters (D) from target refraction. In addition, ray tracing yielded the lowest PE variance (as an indicator of the consistency of the IOL power calculation) of all investigated formulae. A further study from the same group [15] employed the identical theoretical methodology to compare ray tracing with TK-based IOL calculation formulae in 98 post-SMILE eyes. Ray tracing and the Haigis TK formula showed the highest theoretical ± 0.50 D accuracies of 79% and 73%, respectively. The widely popular Haigis-L formula, which is optimized for eyes after PRK and LASIK, seemed to produce an overestimation of IOL power theoretically entailing myopic refractive surprises after SMILE. Luft et al. [16] made similar observations for post-SMILE eyes in their theoretical comparative study between ray tracing and a range of empirical formular available in the ASCRS online calculator.

18.4 Clinical Studies of IOL Power Calculation After SMILE

The first clinical case report of bilateral cataract surgery after SMILE in a 54-year-old patient was published in the year 2019 by Ganesh et al. [5] The authors did not use TK-dedicated formulae as these were not available during the surgical planning of their case. Instead, K-readings were simply substituted with TK-readings in the Barrett Universal II formula. Despite these methodological limitations and the high level of myopia previously treated with SMILE (−9.75 D and −10.25 D, respectively), the reported refractive result was surprisingly accurate with a manifest refractive error of + 0.25 D binocularly. Of note, however, an IOL with a diffractive multifocal optic was implanted in both eyes, which can deteriorate the accuracy of postoperative subjective refraction itself.

Interestingly, the second case report of monocular cataract surgery in a former low myopic (−2.00 D) 49-year-old patient by Li et al. also involved implantation of a diffractive multifocal IOL. [4] In their case report, the ray tracing method yielded the smallest PE of all examined formulae. Unfortunately, a multi-formula averaging method was used, which led to an undesired myopic outcome of −1.50 D (spherical equivalent).

In the worldwide first clinical case series of 11 post-SMILE eyes undergoing cataract surgery that were gathered in Germany and Austria, Lischke et al. [6] compared ray tracing with a range of empirically optimized formulae available in the ASCRS post-keratorefractive surgery IOL power online calculator. Ray tracing yielded the smallest absolute PE (0.40 D) and the largest fraction of eyes within ± 0.50 D (82%) and ± 1.00 D (91%) from target refraction. The second-best formula was the Scheimpflug tomography-based Potvin-Hill formula with a mean absolute error of 0.66 D and ± 0.50/ ± 1.00 D accuracies of 45%/73%, respectively. The next best keratometry-based formulae were the Masket (PE -0.25 ± 0.98 D) and Barrett True-K (−0.44 ± 1.13 D) formula with ± 0.50/ ± 1.00 D accuracies of 36%/63% and 27%/73%, respectively. Of note, the accuracy of the Barrett True-K formula was non-inferior when preoperative refractive data were not entered but estimated (Barrett True-K no history formula). On average, the ASCRS online formulae uniformly overestimated the required IOL power (theoretically resulting in myopic refractive surprises) with the Shammas and Haigis-L formula resulting in the largest IOL power overestimation with mean PEs of − 0.96 ± 1.14 D and − 0.81 ± 1.28 D.

Building on the aforementioned theoretical utility of TK-based formulae for IOL power calculation after SMILE, our group gathered the first clinical case series comparing a range of TK-based formulae (Haigis TK, Barrett TK Universal II, Barrett True-K with TK, EVO TK) with ray tracing (unpublished data). In the six included eyes, ray tracing yielded the smallest arithmetic PE (+0.01 ± 0.07 D) and mean absolute PE (0.25 D) of all formulae (Figs. 18.1 and 18.2) as well as the largest fraction of eyes within ± 0.50 D from target refraction (83%). The Haigis TK and Barrett TK Universal II showed slightly inferior ± 0.50D accuracies of 67% and 50%, respectively (Fig. 18.3). Of note, all investigated TK-fomulae as well as ray tracing yielded ± 1.00 D accuracies of 100%. On average, the TK-based formulae showed a small propensity toward underestimating the required IOL power by approximately + 0.10 D to + 0.50 D. Surprisingly, the latest TK-based IOL power calculation formula, the Emmetropia Verifying Optical formula with TK (EVO TK), resulted in the largest arithmetic PE (+0.52 ± 0.27 D) and the smallest fraction of eyes (33%) within ± 0.50 D from target refraction.

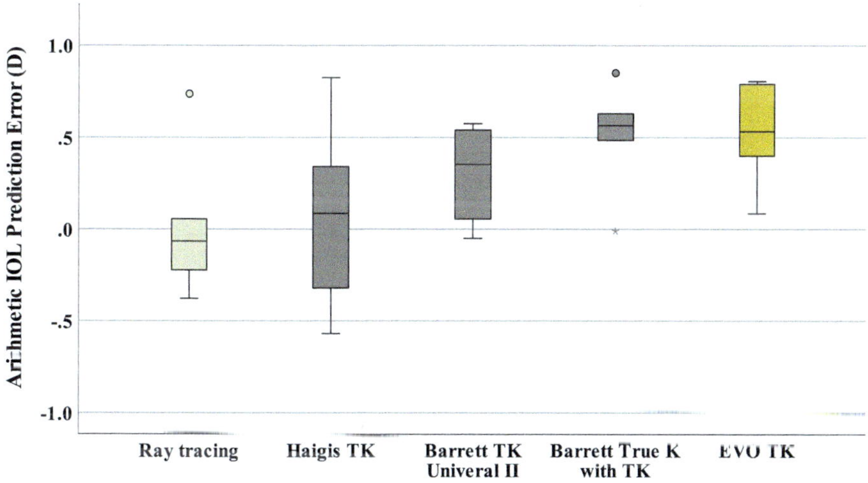

Fig. 18.1 Arithmetic IOL power prediction errors ranked by mean

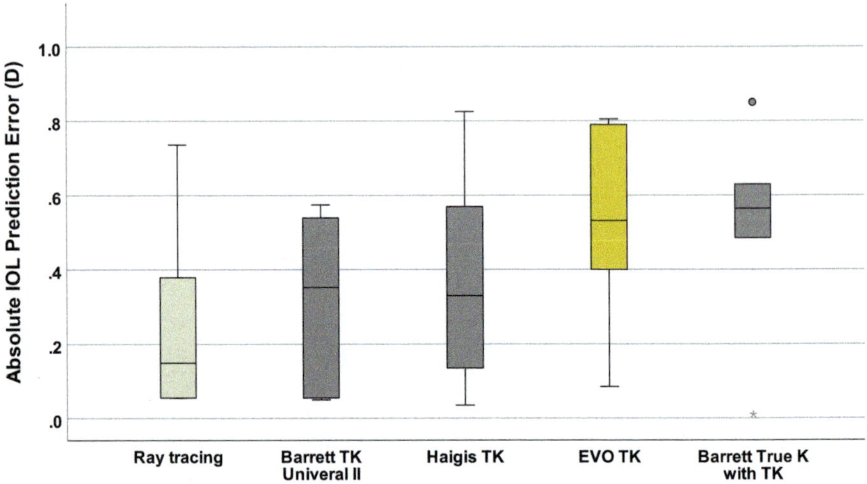

Fig. 18.2 Absolute IOL power prediction errors ranked by mean

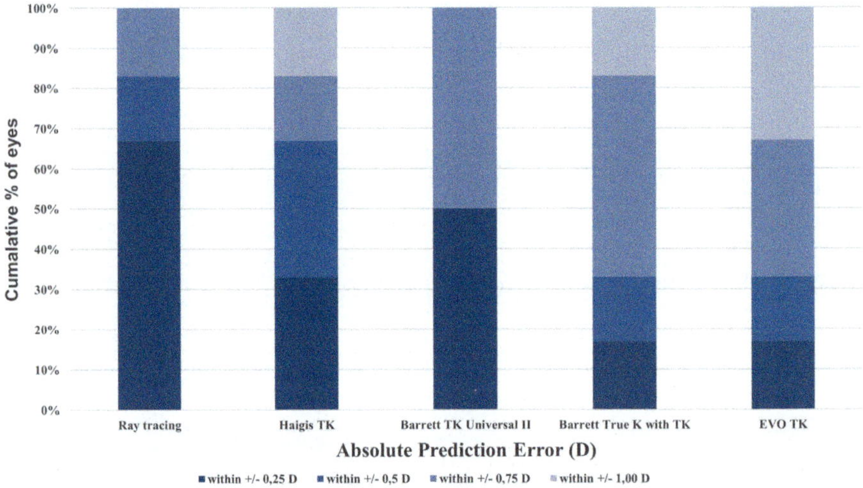

Fig. 18.3 Stacked histogram analysis comparing the percentage of eyes within given absolute prediction error ranges ranked by the proportion of eyes within ± 0.50 D in descending order

18.5 Recommended IOL Power Calculation Methods After SMILE

Reflecting on the current body of evidence, implementation of posterior corneal curvature measurements into IOL power calculation after SMILE is recommended to ascertain precise predictions. Scheimpflug- or OCT-based ray tracing approaches as well as TK-based formulae (in particular Haigis TK and Barrett TK Universal II) are readily available, do not require any pre-SMILE refractive data and show the highest potential to minimize refractive surprises [6, 12, 15]. Ideally, these formulae should be interpreted in a comparative manner whereby TK-based formulae may show a small propensity toward underestimating the required IOL power of approximately + 0.10 to + 0.50 D at the spectacle plane. If only Scheimpflug tomography is available, the Potvin-Hill formula may be preferred [6, 16]. If only traditional keratometry is available, the Barrett True-K (with and without clinical history) formulae as well as the Masket formula may be used bearing in mind a small tendency to overestimating the required IOL power of approx. −0.25 to − 0.50 D at the spectacle plane [6]. The latter four formulae are available in the ASCRS online calculator.

18.6 Recommendations for IOL-Type Selection

In patients who had previously undergone SMILE and are now candidates for cataract surgery, selecting the most suitable type of IOL is a multifaceted and highly individualized decision. Careful consideration of multiple factors such as astigmatism correction, topographic optical zone size of the SMILE treatment, pupil size, the corneal aberrometric profile (higher order aberrations, HOAs) as well as patient expectations is prudent. In the peer-reviewed literature, mainly monofocal or monofocal-toric IOLs implantations have been reported after SMILE [6], and only one case of a binocular trifocal IOL implantation after SMILE has been reported [5]. In their case, the high myopic prior SMILE treatment (−9.75 D and −10.25 D, respectively) resulted in a typical hyper-oblate corneal aberrometric profile with markedly elevated (positive) corneal spherical aberration (SA) of + 0.68 μm and + 0.53 μm, respectively. Remarkably, the patient achieved excellent binocular unaided distance (20/20), near (N6) and intermediate (logMAR −0.1) vision accompanied by "acceptable, minimal haloes at night." However, contrast sensitivity testing was not performed in their study.

In the author's experience, a majority of previously myopic SMILE patients will achieve highly satisfactory spectacle independence for distance and intermediate tasks and satisfactory spectacle independence for near with a SA optimized mini-monovision approach. Thereby, the total corneal wavefront aberrometry over a 6.00 mm zone (centered on the corneal vertex) is examined using a dedicated tomography system and the SA ($Z^4{}_0$) polynomial is extracted. Today's rich variety of monofocal (or "monofocal plus") IOLs allows tailoring of the IOL-induced SA to the individual patient's corneal asphericity profile with the aim to arrive at a positive ocular SA level of approximately + 0.30 to + 0.40 μm (typically in post-myopic keratorefractive corneas). This level of SA level is generally well tolerated [17] and provides enhanced depth of focus and near vision adding to the mini-monovision approach [18]. In post-hyperopic keratorefractive surgery eyes, typically, negative corneal SA will be present and the target level would be approximately −0.40 μm to −0.30 μm of ocular SA.

Post-SMILE patients with large topographic optical zones and low levels of corneal HOAs may be the most suitable candidates for the implantation of more complex IOL optics (e.g., trifocal IOLs). In the author's experience, a polypseudophakic approach—i.e., implantation of a monofocal IOL in the capsular bag and of dedicated supplementary multifocal IOL in the ciliary sulcus—may be preferrable. This approach enables reversible multifocality [19, 20] with on-par visual outcomes as compared with a standard in-the-bag multifocal IOL [21, 22]. In light of the increased variability of IOL power calculation accuracy in post-SMILE eyes, an easily exchangeable sulcus-based supplementary IOL in case of residual refractive error seems attractive [23]. Moreover, reversible multifocality may be prudent due to remaining concerns regarding intensified dysphotopsia (haloes) in post-keratorefractive surgery eyes [24].

18.7 Conclusion

In conclusion, the increasing prevalence of small incision lenticule extraction (SMILE) as a myopia correction technique is expected to lead to a growing number of patients requiring cataract surgery after SMILE in the coming years. Accurate IOL power calculation in these patient cohort is paramount to meet their typically elevated expectations for continued spectacle independence. While challenges and limitations exist, both theoretical and clinical studies have provided valuable insights into IOL power calculation methods, highlighting the importance of posterior corneal curvature measurements and suggesting the superiority of ray tracing and TK-based formulae, such as the Barrett TK Universal II. Additionally, individualized IOL selection should consider factors like corneal aberrometry, optical zone size and patient expectations, with a preference for monofocal IOLs with an individualized mini-monovision approach in most cases. More complex IOL optics may be reserved for patients with large topographic optical zones and low corneal HOA profiles.

References

1. Hoffer KJ. Intraocular lens power calculation after previous laser refractive surgery. J Cataract Refract Surg. 2009;35(4):759–65. https://doi.org/10.1016/j.jcrs.2009.01.005.
2. Savini G, Barboni P, Carbonelli M, Ducoli P, Hoffer KJ. Intraocular lens power calculation after myopic excimer laser surgery: selecting the best method using available clinical data. J Cataract Refract Surg. 2015;41(9):1880–8. https://doi.org/10.1016/j.jcrs.2015.10.026.
3. Gyldenkerne A, Ivarsen A, Hjortdal J. Comparison of corneal shape changes and aberrations induced By FS-LASIK and SMILE for myopia. J Refract Surg. 2015;31(4):223–9. https://doi.org/10.3928/1081597x-20150303-01.
4. Li X, Li S, Li L, Liu C, Li Q. Myopic outcome after intraocular lens implantation in a patient who previously had small-incision lenticule extraction. JCRS Online Case Reports. 2022;10(2): e00071. https://doi.org/10.1097/j.jcro.0000000000000071.

5. Ganesh S, Brar S, Sriprakash K. Post-small incision lenticule extraction phacoemulsification with multifocal IOL implantation: a case report. Indian J Ophthalmol. 2019;67(8):1353–6. https://doi.org/10.4103/ijo.IJO_2069_18.
6. Lischke R, Sekundo W, Wiltfang R, Bechmann M, Kreutzer TC, Priglinger SG, et al. IOL power calculations and cataract surgery in eyes with previous small incision lenticule extraction. J Clin Med. 2022;11(15). https://doi.org/10.3390/jcm11154418
7. Pan C, Tan W, Hua Y, Lei X. Comprehensive evaluation of total corneal refractive power by ray tracing in predicting corneal power in eyes after small incision lenticule extraction. PLoS ONE. 2019;14(6): e0217478. https://doi.org/10.1371/journal.pone.0217478.
8. Qian Y, Liu Y, Zhou X, Naidu RK. Comparison of corneal power and astigmatism between simulated keratometry, true net power, and total corneal refractive power before and after SMILE surgery. J Ophthalmol. 2017;2017:9659481. https://doi.org/10.1155/2017/9659481.
9. Chan TCY, Biswas S, Yu M, Jhanji V. Longitudinal evaluation of cornea with swept-source optical coherence tomography and scheimpflug imaging before and after lasik. Medicine (Baltimore). 2015;94(30): e1219. https://doi.org/10.1097/md.0000000000001219.
10. Fabian E, Wehner W. Prediction accuracy of total keratometry compared to standard keratometry using different intraocular lens power formulas. J Refract Surg. 2019;35(6):362–8. https://doi.org/10.3928/1081597x-20190422-02.
11. Wang L, Spektor T, de Souza RG, Koch DD. Evaluation of total keratometry and its accuracy for intraocular lens power calculation in eyes after corneal refractive surgery. J Cataract Refract Surg. 2019;45(10):1416–21. https://doi.org/10.1016/j.jcrs.2019.05.020.
12. Lischke R, Mayer WJ, Feucht N, Siedlecki J, Wiltfang R, Kook D, et al. Total keratometry for determination of true corneal power after myopic small-incision lenticule extraction. J Cataract Refract Surg. 2021;47(10):1285–9. https://doi.org/10.1097/j.jcrs.0000000000000630.
13. Preussner PR, Wahl J, Lahdo H, Dick B, Findl O. Ray tracing for intraocular lens calculation. J Cataract Refract Surg. 2002;28(8):1412–9. https://doi.org/10.1016/s0886-3350(01)01346-3.
14. Lazaridis A, Schraml F, Preußner PR, Sekundo W. Predictability of intraocular lens power calculation after small-incision lenticule extraction for myopia. J Cataract Refract Surg. 2021;47(3):304–10. https://doi.org/10.1097/j.jcrs.0000000000000405.
15. Meziane Elotmani A, Messerschmidt-Roth A, Nehme A, Müller HH, Sekundo W. Comparison of intraocular lens power calculation formulas with and without total keratometry and ray tracing in patients with previous myopic SMILE. J Cataract Refract Surg. 2023;49(5):467–73. https://doi.org/10.1097/j.jcrs.0000000000001139.
16. Luft N, Siedlecki J, Schworm B, Kreutzer TC, Mayer WJ, Priglinger SG, et al. Intraocular lens power calculation after small incision lenticule extraction. Sci Rep. 2020;10(1):5982. https://doi.org/10.1038/s41598-020-63118-0.
17. Reinstein DZ, Archer TJ, Couch D, Schroeder E, Wottke M. A new night vision disturbances parameter and contrast sensitivity as indicators of success in wavefront-guided enhancement. J Refract Surg. 2005;21(5):S535–40. https://doi.org/10.3928/1081-597x-20050901-23.
18. Rocha KM, Vabre L, Chateau N, Krueger RR. Expanding depth of focus by modifying higher-order aberrations induced by an adaptive optics visual simulator. J Cataract Refract Surg. 2009;35(11):1885–92. https://doi.org/10.1016/j.jcrs.2009.05.059.
19. Baur ID, Labuz G, Yildirim TM, Auffarth GU, Khoramnia R. Reversible multifocality achieved through polypseudophakia. Klin Monbl Augenheilkd. 2023;240(8):981–8. https://doi.org/10.1055/a-2079-1692.
20. Feldhaus L, Mayer WJ, Siedlecki J, Schworm B, Dirisamer M, Priglinger SG, et al. Myopic multifocal duet implantation for the correction of presbyopia and myopia. Ophthalmologie. 2023;120(7):759–62. https://doi.org/10.1007/s00347-022-01692-6.
21. Harrisberg BP, Chua AW, Chua MJ, Taher A. Comparison of primary duet lens procedures: in the-bag monofocal with sulcus multifocal, and standard single multifocal lens for cataract surgery. Clin Ophthalmol. 2023;17:273–82. https://doi.org/10.2147/opth.S396472.
22. Łabuz G, Auffarth GU, Knorz MC, Son HS, Yildirim TM, Khoramnia R. Trifocality achieved through polypseudophakia: optical quality and light loss compared with a single trifocal

intraocular lens. J Refract Surg. 2020;36(9):570–7. https://doi.org/10.3928/1081597x-20200715-01.

23. Baur ID, Auffarth GU, Yildirim TM, Mayer CS, Khoramnia R. Reversibility of the duet procedure: bilateral exchange of a supplementary trifocal sulcus-fixated intraocular lens for correction of a postoperative refractive error. Am J Ophthalmol Case Rep. 2020;20: 100957. https://doi.org/10.1016/j.ajoc.2020.100957.
24. Moshirfar M, Thomson AC, Thomson RJ, Martheswaran T, McCabe SE. Use of presbyopia-correcting intraocular lenses in patients with prior corneal refractive surgery. Curr Opin Ophthalmol. 2021;32(1):45–53. https://doi.org/10.1097/icu.0000000000000722.

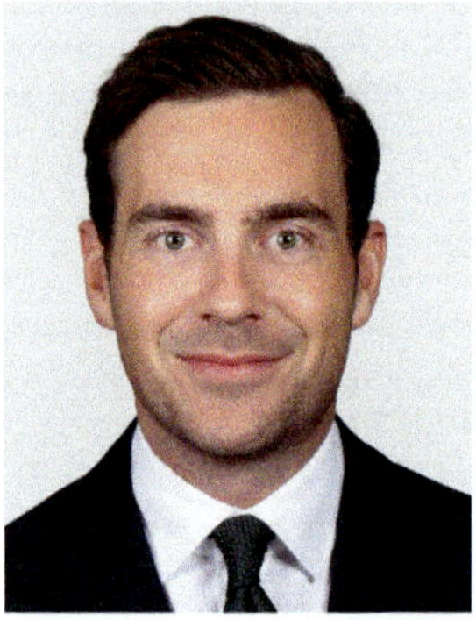

Nikolaus Luft Nikolaus Luft, MD, PhD, FEBO, FWCRS, is a Professor and Consultant Ophthalmologist at the Department of Ophthalmology, Ludwig-Maximilians-University in Munich, Germany. He began his scientific career with a research fellowship at the Vienna Institute for Research in Ocular Surgery (VIROS) after completing his medical degree at the Medical University of Vienna. Concurrently, he pursued a PhD-degree in Applied Medical Science at the same university, researching Laser Speckle Flowgraphy (LSFG), a novel non-invasive ocular perfusion quantification method. He was a resident at the Kepler University Clinic in Linz (Austria) and Ludwig-Maximilians-University in Munich. Dr. Luft was awarded the Highest Overall EBOD Score Award of 651 contestants from 28 countries at the 2018 European Board of Ophthalmology Diploma Examination in Paris (France). He acquired his venia docendi in 2020 focusing on optimizing the safety and efficiency of corneal refractive and lens surgery before being appointed Professor of Ophthalmology by the Ludwig-Maximilians-University in 2024. Dr. Luft has received several research awards, including the Best Poster Award from the American Academy of Ophthalmology. In 2022, he was elected to the board of the Cornea Section of the German Ophthalmological Society (DOG) and in 2023, he was nominated as a Fellow of the World College of Refractive Surgery & Visual Sciences (FWCRS) for his contributions to refractive surgery. Dr. Luft is a versatile ophthalmic surgeon covering therapeutic and refractive corneal surgery, corneal transplantation and complex lens surgery at the Ludwig-Maximilians-University and his private practices in Austria (Auge Laser Chirurgie, Linz & Vienna).

Keratectasia Prevention, Recognition, and Treatment

19

Felix Mathias Wagner and Walter Sekundo

Abstract

This chapter reviews the critical aspects of corneal thinning and protrusions, encompassing both natural occurrences like keratoconus and surgically induced conditions such as post Laser Vision Correction ectasia and provide the reader with practical tools for assessment.

Keywords

Small Incision Lenticule Extraction (SMILE) • Laser-Assisted In Situ Keratomileusis (LASIK) • Keratectasia • Keratoconus • Post-Laser-Assisted In Situ Keratomileusis (LASIK) ectasia • Corneal thinning • Refractive surgery complications

19.1 Introduction

Keratectasia, encompassing both naturally occurring and surgically induced corneal thinning and protrusions, presents a critical concern in the domain of ophthalmology, particularly within the realm of refractive surgery. Keratoconus, a naturally occurring form, is characterized by a progressive thinning and steepening of the cornea. On the contrary, iatrogenic keratectasia, often referred to as post-LASIK ectasia, arises due to a compromise in the biomechanical integrity of the cornea following refractive laser surgeries [1]. The similarities

F. M. Wagner (✉)
Department of Ophthalmology, University Medical Center of the Johannes Gutenberg University, Mainz, Germany
e-mail: felix.wagner@unimedizin-mainz.de

W. Sekundo
Department of Ophthalmology, Philipps University of Marburg, Marburg, Germany

W. Sekundo and F. M. Wagner (eds.), *Femtosecond Laser Assisted Lenticule Extraction*,
https://doi.org/10.1007/978-3-031-60424-9_19

between keratoconus and post-LASIK ectasia extend to their diagnosis and treatment paradigms, making an understanding of keratoconus essential in addressing iatrogenic keratectasia.

The advent of refractive laser surgery in the early 1990s ushered in a new era of vision correction. However, it also highlighted the need for a deeper understanding of ectatic disorders, given the devastating complications like keratectasia that could ensue post-surgery [2, 3]. Identifying eyes with a higher propensity toward biomechanical decompensation and iatrogenic ectasia after refractive surgical interventions became pivotal [4–8]. Thus, screening for potential keratectasia risk turned into an integral part of the preoperative phase of elective refractive procedures [5, 9].

The application of advanced imaging techniques has significantly contributed to the early detection of subclinical stages of keratectasia, allowing for timely intervention to control disease progression [2]. The comprehensive understanding of the etiology of keratectasia, including genetic factors, enzymatic anomalies, and mechanical factors such as eye rubbing, along with advancements in surgical techniques, facilitates a holistic approach for the prevention, early detection, and treatment of iatrogenic keratectasia.

19.2 Causes

19.2.1 Clinical Factors

Classic risk factors for the development of keratectasia include atopy, especially when associated with chronic allergies and ocular itchiness, often accompanying abnormal eye rubbing [10]. Apart from eye rubbing, atopy itself is significant in the pathogenesis of keratectasia due to its intrinsic predisposition toward Type 1 immune and allergic reactions [11].

Other allergic conditions posing risks include hay fever, asthma, eczema, and vernal keratoconjunctivitis. Eye inflammation should be managed in patients with the latter to reduce the tendency to rub the eyes. Hormonal changes, for example thyroid afflictions and pregnancy are also implicated [12].

The Two-Hit Hypothesis suggests that iatrogenic ectasia can arise due to inadequate corneal thickness or pre-existing subclinical or clinical keratoconus, exacerbated by further weakening after refractive laser surgery, analogous to the mechanical stress from frequent eye rubbing seen in cases of keratoconus [3, 13–16]. Eye rubbing is considered by some as the essential 'sine qua non' component of keratoconus development. According to this perspective, neither keratoconus nor keratectasia are elusive genetic conditions, but direct outcomes of consistent mechanical trauma [17, 18]. While some may question the centrality of the 'sine qua non' concept, it's clear that there is an inherent corneal vulnerability to biomechanical decompensation [19]. It's also established that occasional eye rubbing doesn't affect the biomechanics of standard corneas, but can intensify keratectasia in those already at risk [20]. Moreover, investigations involving human corneal stromal cell lines reveal that the mechanical stretch from rubbing activates protease gene expression. This highlights that eye rubbing not only impacts biomechanical integrity but also triggers significant biochemical responses in corneal stromal cells [21].

Thinner-than-planned postoperative stromal beds, excessively thick flaps, and signs of subclinical keratoconus not detected before surgery are risk factors for keratectasia. While these are significant, iatrogenic keratectasia can also emerge in different situations, and the choice of refractive surgery holds considerable importance. Specifically, the incidence rates of post-refractive ectasia in eyes without prior risk factors stand at 20 per 100,000 for post-PRK, 90 for post-LASIK, and 11 for post-SMILE [2, 22].

19.2.2 Biomechanical Stability

The cornea is composed of approximately 200 collagen lamellae, containing collagen fibers crucial for maintaining corneal shape [23, 24]. The lamellar intertwining and natural corneal cross-linking ensure its biomechanical strength, with the anterior third of the cornea being the strongest [25]. Tensile strength in the corneal lamellae decreases after incision and does not contribute to the overall resistance of the cornea to intraocular pressure. Due to the orientation of the lamellae, a vertical incision causes a greater reduction in biomechanical stability than an incision parallel to the corneal surface [26]. Both SMILE and LASIK separate parallel lamellae over a large area. However, SMILE preserves most of the anterior lamellae integrity since vertical cuts are minimal. As a result, corneal biomechanical stability is better preserved in SMILE compared to LASIK. Theoretical and mathematical descriptions of these biomechanical relationships by Reinstein and Sinha [27, 28] were confirmed through experiments on cadaver eyes by the research groups of Sekundo and Hafezi. A 1.5-fold greater instability in corneas after LASIK compared to SMILE, with no discernible difference between PRK and SMILE was found [29, 30].

19.2.3 Cellular and Molecular Biology Factors

Corneal thinning in keratoconus results from collagen degradation [14, 31]. Altered enzyme activities and oxidative stress have been proposed for keratoconus pathogenesis and associated keratectasia. Specifically, keratoconic corneas, when compared to normal ones, have shown elevated matrix metalloproteinase levels with reduced tissue inhibitors of metalloproteinases [14, 32–37]. Tears from keratoconus patients also contain elevated inflammatory mediators like Interleukin-6 and TNF-alpha [38, 39]. Such mediators might induce keratocyte apoptosis and decreased keratocyte cell density. This suggests a likely inflammatory component either directly or indirectly associated with the pathogenesis and progression of this form of keratectasia [40]. Tears from post-LASIK and post-SMILE ectasia patients also show elevated pro-inflammatory cellular and biomolecular markers, suggesting a similar enhanced inflammatory role in biomechanical corneal changes [41–43].

19.3 Examination Techniques

Three-dimensional corneal tomography is mainly used for analyzing the cornea. While topography accurately captures the anterior curvature of the cornea, tomography is able to represent the overall shape of the cornea, allowing for the creation of a stereographic model of the cornea, facilitating analysis of both the anterior and posterior aspects of the cornea, as well as pachymetry mapping. With the portrayal of elevations of the anterior and posterior corneal surfaces and pachymetric imaging, the sensitivity and specificity in detecting keratectasia have been notably enhanced in comparison to traditional topography (Fig. 19.1) [44–46].

Advancements like single-layer tomography allow the creation of epithelial thickness maps using high-frequency ultrasound or OCT, which can further refine risk scores [47–49]. Because the epithelium may initially mask the ectatic area by focal hypoplasia, epithelial thickness maps can be helpful in detecting early stages of ectatic disease (Fig. 19.2).

Another approach involves measuring corneal biomechanics. This entails analyzing corneal deformation caused by an air pulse, utilizing either an electro-optical infrared system (Ocular Response Analyzer, Reichert Ophthalmic Instruments, Buffalo, NY, USA) or a high-speed Scheimpflug camera (Corvis ST, Oculus, Wetzlar, Germany). However, these devices differ in their measurement parameters. While the Ocular Response Analyzer primarily determines viscoelastic parameters like corneal hysteresis, the Corvis ST more accurately identifies the elastic properties of the cornea. Studies have demonstrated the efficacy of both

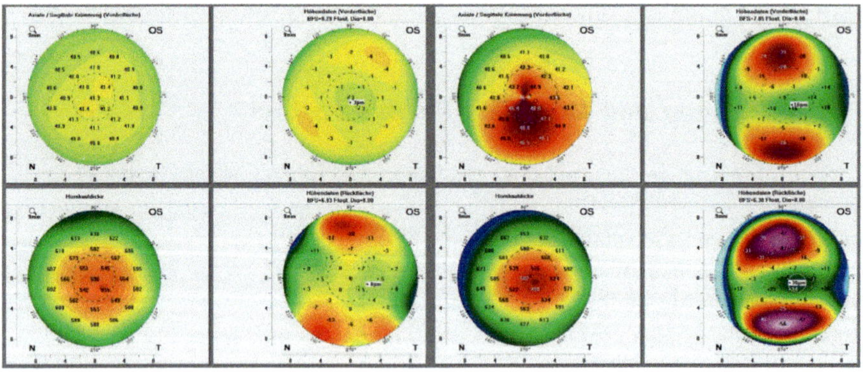

Fig. 19.1 Pentacam 4 map refractive: Left: normal corneal tomography, Right: Typical keratoconus with inferior steepening (upper left quadrant) and elevation more on the posterior than the anterior surface (upper and lower right quadrant)

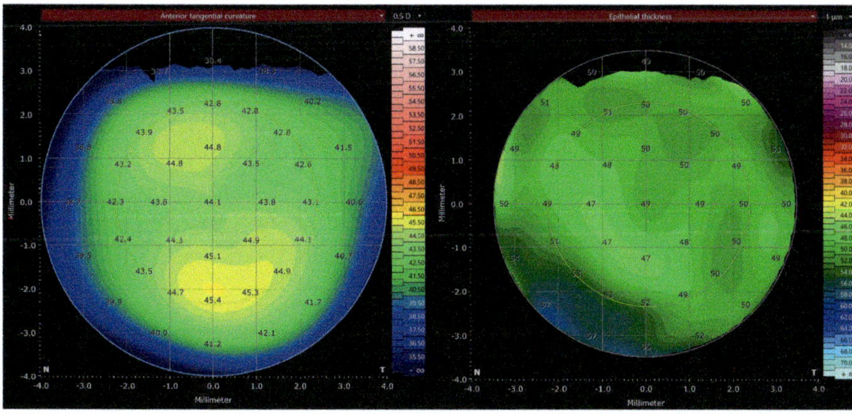

Fig. 19.2 Anterion (Heidelberg Engineering): On the left, only a slight abnormality is visible in the anterior corneal curvature map, while on the right, the epithelial thickness map shows corresponding epithelial thinning at the same location, indicating early signs of ectasia.Courtesy of Dr. Damien Gatinel.

devices in detecting clinical keratoconus [50]. However, when it comes to detecting early ectasia, the Corvis ST provides better predictive capabilities [51]. A disadvantage of these two methods is that they assess biomechanics only globally across the cornea.

Biomechanical changes can precede observable morphological alterations in the cornea [52] and that these variations within an individual cornea are locally heterogeneous [53]. Therefore, a more thorough approach is to map the biomechanical characteristics of the cornea with high spatial resolution. This is the objective of elastography, an imaging method designed to depict the biomechanical properties of soft tissues.

Currently, the most advanced approach to optical elastography is Brillouin light scattering microscopy. This technique, grounded on Brillouin spectroscopy, enables 3-dimensional measurements of the longitudinal P-wave M-modulus in tissues, with a high sensitivity and spatial resolution, by measuring the interaction between incident light and acoustic phonons in a medium [54, 55]. It enables a non-contact, three-dimensional estimation of the Brillouin shift, which indicates the corneal biomechanical state [56, 57]. Recent developments have incorporated 3-D motion tracking, which improves the capability to detect subtle biomechanical alterations, improving diagnosis of subclinical keratoconus with a sensitivity and specificity of 1.0 under study conditions [58]. However, since the data acquisition with current Brillouin spectroscopy devices is time consuming when compared with tomography or OCT machines its implementation in the clinical routine is still very low.

19.4 Risk Assessment

Several independent and device-dependent indices and scores exist to evaluate the presence of ectasia in the cornea and the likelihood of iatrogenic keratectasia developing post-laser surgery. Traditional risk indicators include the following:

- Elevated central refractive power (K) (> 47.20 diopters [D])
- Inferior steepening, especially when combined with abnormal posterior elevation or unusual inferior thinning
- Superior flattening
- Asymmetry in the difference of inferior to superior corneal refractive power ($I - S$) ($I - S > 1.2$)
- Skewness of radial axis (SRAX) > 21°.

From the traditional risk indicators, the Rabinowitz–McDonnell Index is derived: $K > 47.20$ D and $I - S > 1.2$ and SRAX > 21°. With these conditions present, 98% of eyes with an already conical cornea can be identified [59]. Other notable scores include the "Ectasia Risk Score System" (ERSS) (Table 19.1) by Randleman [15] and the "Percentage of Tissue Alteration" (PTA) (s. Table 19.2). The ERSS scale assists in preoperatively identifying high-risk patients using a cumulative point system. PTA considers the central corneal thickness and laser ablation to identify patients who, despite having normal topography, have a risk of keratectasia. A PTA score of more than 40% at the time of surgery is associated with the development of ectasia in eyes with regular preoperative topography, with an odds ratio of 22.03 [60]. The PTA formula was originally developed for LASIK surgery but has been adapted for PRK and SMILE. Furthermore, a more comprehensive formula for SMILE-PTA ($\mathrm{mPTA_{SMILE}}$) is available, which considers the ratio of the length of the incision to the total circumference of the cap.

$$\mathrm{mPTA_{SMILE}} = 100 \times [(S/L) \times \text{cap thickness} + \text{lenticule thickness}]/\text{central corneal thickness},$$

where S/L represents the ratio between the length of the SMILE incision and the total circumference of the cap. A $\mathrm{mPTA_{SMILE}}$ value of more than 20% is considered as high risk [3].

Calculation example $\mathrm{mPTA_{SMILE}}$
with a cap diameter of 7.5 mm, a cap circumference of 23.6 mm, an incision size of 2.5 mm, a cornea of 500 μm, and a cap and lenticule thickness of 120 μm each
-> $\mathrm{mPTA_{SMILE}}$ becomes 26.5%
-> High Risk.

Table 19.1 ERSS

Parameters	Points				
	4	3	2	1	**0**
Topography	Abnormal topography	Inferior steepening/ SRAX		ABT	Normal/SBT
RSD	<240 μ	240–259 μ	260–279 μ	280–299 μ	≥ 300 μ
Age		18–21 years	22–25 years	26–29 years	≥ 30 years
PP	<450 μ	451–480 μ	481–510 μ		≥ 510 μ
MRSE	> −14 D	> −12 to 14 D	> −10 to 12 D	> −8 to 10 D	≤ −8D
0–2 points	Low risk		**→ Perform laser surgery**		
3 points	Moderate risk		**→ Laser procedure should only be performed with special caution**		
4 points	High risk		**→ Do not recommend laser surgery**		

SRAX oblique radial axis, *ABT* asymmetrical bowtie, *SBT* symmetrical bowtie (sand clock shape), *RSD* residual thickness, *PP* preoperative pachymetry, *MRSE* preoperative manifest refraction as spherical equivalent

Table 19.2 PTA scores for PRK, LASIK, and SMILE

$PTA_{LASIK} = 100 \times$ (flap thickness + depth of ablation)/central corneal thickness
$PTA_{PRK} = 100 \times$ (epithelial thickness + depth of ablation)/central corneal thickness
$PTA_{SMILE} = 100 \times$ (cap thickness + lenticule thickness)/central corneal thickness
$PTA \geq 40\% \rightarrow$ increased risk of ectasia
$mPTA_{SMILE} = 100 \times$ [(S/L) × cap thickness + lenticule thickness]/central corneal thickness
$mPTA_{SMILE} \geq 20\% \rightarrow$ increased risk of ectasia

Device-specific indices include the "Screening Corneal Objective Risk of Ectasia" (SCORE) based on Orbscan measurements (Bausch & Lomb; Rochester, USA), also available on the ANTERION (Heidelberg Engineering, Heidelberg, Germany), keratoconus screening of the Galilei Dual-Scheimpflug Analyzer (Ziemer; Port, Switzerland), and the "Belin-Ambrósio Enhanced Ectasia Display" (BAD) of the Pentacam (Oculus, Wetzlar, Germany). Other indices, combining tomographic data from the Scheimpflug-based Pentacam (Oculus, Wetzlar, Germany) and biomechanical data from the Corvis-ST Tonometer (Oculus, Wetzlar, Germany) such as the Tomographic Biomechanical Index (TBI) and the Corvis Biomechanical Index (CBI) of Corvis, surpassed metrics like BAD in detecting preclinical keratoconus (Fig. 19.3) [4, 61–63]. However, indices like CBI and TBI, while highly sensitive and specific in detecting ectatic corneas, were not designed to detect

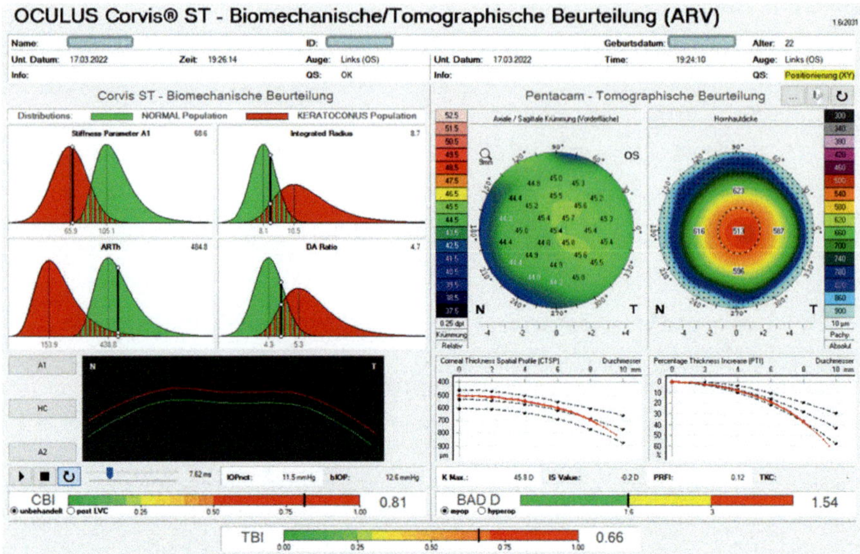

Fig. 19.3 Corvis ST/Pentacam: CBI correctly identified subclinical keratoconus (left score) in the BAD it was incorrectly classified as normal (≤ 1.6) (right score) despite beginning SRAX in the axial/sagittal curvature

post-refractive laser surgery ectasia. To distinguishes stable eyes after laser correction from eyes with post-laser ectasia the Corvis biomechanical index-laser vision correction (CBI-LVC) is available [64].

19.5 Therapy

Treatment of keratectasia varies based on the severity of the condition. Specialized contact lenses, like rigid gas permeable and scleral lenses, are commonly used for early stages of the disease [65]. However, while contact lenses offer improved vision quality, they don't halt disease progression. Improper fitting of hard lenses could even pose a risk for disease progression.

The primary treatment option for progressing ectasias is corneal cross-linking (CXL) [66]. CXL has proven effective in halting the progression of ectasia by increasing corneal biomechanical stability [67, 68]. Notably, the prospective, randomized, controlled multicenter study that led to the FDA's approval of CXL for iatrogenic ectasia demonstrated improvements in maximal refractive power and both uncorrected and corrected vision with an excellent safety profile [69]. Modifications to the original technique, such as using hypoosmolar riboflavin or adjusting UVA energy for thinner corneas (Sub400-Protocol), broaden the range of applicability [70, 71]. Since the corneal epithelium acts as a barrier to riboflavin diffusion, the standard method remains to remove the epithelium [72].

CXL has been effectively combined with other surgical techniques for iatrogenic keratectasia treatment, such as topography-guided PRK (Athens protocol) [73]. and intracorneal ring segment (ICRS) implantation [74]. Initially designed for myopia treatment, ICRS became a popular keratectasia treatment [75]. The procedure involves introducing PMMA segments into the stroma to achieve central cornea flattening, consequently reducing higher-order aberrations and improving visual acuity in ectasia cases that are mild to moderate [76, 77]. A new evolving technique proposed by Soosan Jacobs and coworkers is the implantation of corneal allogenic intrastromal ring segments (CAIRS). Because the allogenic material has extremely low risk of cheese-wiring through the host's cornea the implantation of CAIRS is carried out at the depth of 250μm instead of 400μm as for ICRS. It can therefore be successfully utilized in thinner corneas [78] either post CXL or combined with CXL [79]. The introduction of dryed and sterilized stromal tissue with 2 years shelf-life time (KeraNatural®) might further promote this technique. Phakic and pseudophakic intraocular lenses, particularly pinhole-based lenses, are also utilized for keratectasia treatment, especially for correcting high refractive errors [80].

Another promising approach is the implantation of lenticules for tissue addition within the corneal stroma using femtosecond lasers. Implantation of stromal lenticules into SMILE-like pockets shows improved vision with low inflammatory reaction (see Chap. 20).

References

1. Binder PS. Ectasia after laser in situ keratomileusis. J Cataract Refract Surg. 2003;29(12):2419–29. https://doi.org/10.1016/j.jcrs.2003.10.012.
2. Binder PS. Analysis of ectasia after laser in situ keratomileusis: risk factors. J Cataract Refract Surg. 2007;33(9):1530–8. https://doi.org/10.1016/j.jcrs.2007.04.043.
3. Moshirfar M, Albarracin JC, Desautels JD, Birdsong OC, Linn SH, Hoopes PC Sr. Ectasia following small-incision lenticule extraction (SMILE): a review of the literature. Clin Ophthalmol. 2017;11:1683–8. https://doi.org/10.2147/opth.S147011.
4. Ambrósio R Jr, Lopes BT, Faria-Correia F, Salomão MQ, Bühren J, Roberts CJ, et al. Integration of Scheimpflug-based corneal tomography and biomechanical assessments for enhancing ectasia detection. J Refract Surg. 2017;33(7):434–43. https://doi.org/10.3928/1081597x-20170426-02.
5. Ambrósio R Jr, Randleman JB. Screening for ectasia risk: what are we screening for and how should we screen for it? J Refract Surg. 2013;29(4):230–2. https://doi.org/10.3928/1081597x-20130318-01.
6. Ambrósio R Jr. Post-LASIK Ectasia: twenty years of a conundrum. Semin Ophthalmol. 2019;34(2):66–8. https://doi.org/10.1080/08820538.2019.1569075.
7. Binder PS, Lindstrom RL, Stulting RD, Donnenfeld E, Wu H, McDonnell P, et al. Keratoconus and corneal ectasia after LASIK. J Cataract Refract Surg. 2005;31(11):2035–8. https://doi.org/10.1016/j.jcrs.2005.12.002.
8. Seiler T, Quurke AW. Iatrogenic keratectasia after LASIK in a case of forme fruste keratoconus. J Cataract Refract Surg. 1998;24(7):1007–9. https://doi.org/10.1016/s0886-3350(98)80057-6.

9. Ambrósio R Jr, Valbon BF, Faria-Correia F, Ramos I, Luz A. Scheimpflug imaging for laser refractive surgery. Curr Opin Ophthalmol. 2013;24(4):310–20. https://doi.org/10.1097/ICU.0b013e3283622a94.
10. McMonnies CW. Mechanisms of rubbing-related corneal trauma in keratoconus. Cornea. 2009;28(6):607–15. https://doi.org/10.1097/ICO.0b013e318198384f.
11. Edwards M, McGhee CN, Dean S. The genetics of keratoconus. Clin Exp Ophthalmol. 2001;29(6):345–51. https://doi.org/10.1046/j.1442-9071.2001.d01-16.x.
12. Jani D, McKelvie J, Misra SL. Progressive corneal ectatic disease in pregnancy. Clin Exp Optom. 2021;104(8):815–25. https://doi.org/10.1080/08164622.2021.1924627.
13. Espandar L, Meyer J. Keratoconus: overview and update on treatment. Middle East Afr J Ophthalmol. 2010;17(1):15–20. https://doi.org/10.4103/0974-9233.61212.
14. Sugar J, Macsai MS. What causes keratoconus? Cornea. 2012;31(6):716–9. https://doi.org/10.1097/ICO.0b013e31823f8c72.
15. Randleman JB, Trattler WB, Stulting RD. Validation of the Ectasia risk score system for preoperative laser in situ keratomileusis screening. Am J Ophthalmol. 2008;145(5):813–8. https://doi.org/10.1016/j.ajo.2007.12.033.
16. Binder PS, Trattler WB. Evaluation of a risk factor scoring system for corneal ectasia after LASIK in eyes with normal topography. J Refract Surg. 2010;26(4):241–50. https://doi.org/10.3928/1081597x-20100212-02.
17. Gatinel D. Eye rubbing, a Sine Qua non for keratoconus? Int J Kerat Ect Cor Dis. 2016;5(1):6–12. https://doi.org/10.5005/jp-journals-10025-1114.
18. Moran S, Gomez L, Zuber K, Gatinel D. A case-control study of keratoconus risk factors. Cornea. 2020;39(6):697–701. https://doi.org/10.1097/ico.0000000000002283.
19. McGhee CN, Kim BZ, Wilson PJ. Contemporary treatment paradigms in keratoconus. Cornea. 2015;34(Suppl 10):S16-23. https://doi.org/10.1097/ico.0000000000000504.
20. Torres-Netto EA, Abdshahzadeh H, Abrishamchi R, Hafezi NL, Hillen M, Ambrósio R Jr, et al. The impact of repetitive and prolonged eye rubbing on corneal biomechanics. J Refract Surg. 2022;38(9):610–6. https://doi.org/10.3928/1081597x-20220715-03.
21. Dou S, Wang Q, Zhang B, Wei C, Wang H, Liu T, et al. Single-cell atlas of keratoconus corneas revealed aberrant transcriptional signatures and implicated mechanical stretch as a trigger for keratoconus pathogenesis. Cell Discov. 2022;8(1):66. https://doi.org/10.1038/s41421-022-00397-z.
22. Moshirfar M, Tukan AN, Bundogji N, Liu HY, McCabe SE, Ronquillo YC, et al. Ectasia after corneal refractive surgery: a systematic review. Ophthalmol Ther. 2021;10(4):753–76. https://doi.org/10.1007/s40123-021-00383-w.
23. Aghamohammadzadeh H, Newton RH, Meek KM. X-ray scattering used to map the preferred collagen orientation in the human cornea and limbus. Structure. 2004;12(2):249–56. https://doi.org/10.1016/j.str.2004.01.002.
24. Bergmanson JP, Horne J, Doughty MJ, Garcia M, Gondo M. Assessment of the number of lamellae in the central region of the normal human corneal stroma at the resolution of the transmission electron microscope. Eye Contact Lens. 2005;31(6):281–7. https://doi.org/10.1097/01.icl.0000165280.94927.0d.
25. Randleman JB, Dawson DG, Grossniklaus HE, McCarey BE, Edelhauser HF. Depth-dependent cohesive tensile strength in human donor corneas: implications for refractive surgery. J Refract Surg. 2008;24(1):S85–9. https://doi.org/10.3928/1081597x-20080101-15.
26. Knox Cartwright NE, Tyrer JR, Jaycock PD, Marshall J. Effects of variation in depth and side cut angulations in LASIK and thin-flap LASIK using a femtosecond laser: a biomechanical study. J Refract Surg. 2012;28(6):419–25. https://doi.org/10.3928/1081597x-20120518-07.
27. Reinstein DZ, Archer TJ, Randleman JB. Mathematical model to compare the relative tensile strength of the cornea after PRK, LASIK, and small incision lenticule extraction. J Refract Surg. 2013;29(7):454–60. https://doi.org/10.3928/1081597x-20130617-03.
28. Sinha Roy A, Dupps WJ Jr, Roberts CJ. Comparison of biomechanical effects of small-incision lenticule extraction and laser in situ keratomileusis: finite-element analysis. J Cataract Refract Surg. 2014;40(6):971–80. https://doi.org/10.1016/j.jcrs.2013.08.065.

29. Spiru B, Torres-Netto EA, Kling S, Lazaridis A, Hafezi F, Sekundo W. Biomechanical properties of human cornea tested by two-dimensional extensiometry ex vivo in fellow eyes: PRK versus SMILE. J Refract Surg. 2019;35(8):501–5. https://doi.org/10.3928/1081597x-20190730-02.
30. Spiru B, Kling S, Hafezi F, Sekundo W. Biomechanical properties of human cornea tested by two-dimensional extensiometry ex vivo in fellow eyes: femtosecond laser-assisted LASIK versus SMILE. J Refract Surg. 2018;34(6):419–23. https://doi.org/10.3928/1081597x-20180402-05.
31. Critchfield JW, Calandra AJ, Nesburn AB, Kenney MC. Keratoconus: I. biochemical studies. Exp Eye Res. 1988;46(6):953–63. https://doi.org/10.1016/s0014-4835(88)80047-2.
32. Atilano SR, Coskun P, Chwa M, Jordan N, Reddy V, Le K, et al. Accumulation of mitochondrial DNA damage in keratoconus corneas. Invest Ophthalmol Vis Sci. 2005;46(4):1256–63. https://doi.org/10.1167/iovs.04-1395.
33. Arnal E, Peris-Martínez C, Menezo JL, Johnsen-Soriano S, Romero FJ. Oxidative stress in keratoconus? Invest Ophthalmol Vis Sci. 2011;52(12):8592–7. https://doi.org/10.1167/iovs.11-7732.
34. Balasubramanian SA, Pye DC, Willcox MD. Are proteinases the reason for keratoconus? Curr Eye Res. 2010;35(3):185–91. https://doi.org/10.3109/02713680903477824.
35. Chwa M, Atilano SR, Hertzog D, Zheng H, Langberg J, Kim DW, et al. Hypersensitive response to oxidative stress in keratoconus corneal fibroblasts. Invest Ophthalmol Vis Sci. 2008;49(10):4361–9. https://doi.org/10.1167/iovs.08-1969.
36. Kenney MC, Chwa M, Atilano SR, Tran A, Carballo M, Saghizadeh M, et al. Increased levels of catalase and cathepsin V/L2 but decreased TIMP 1 in keratoconus corneas: evidence that oxidative stress plays a role in this disorder. Invest Ophthalmol Vis Sci. 2005;46(3):823–32. https://doi.org/10.1167/iovs.04-0549.
37. Smith VA, Matthews FJ, Majid MA, Cook SD. Keratoconus: matrix metalloproteinase-2 activation and TIMP modulation. Biochim Biophys Acta. 2006;1762(4):431–9. https://doi.org/10.1016/j.bbadis.2006.01.010.
38. Lema I, Durán JA. Inflammatory molecules in the tears of patients with keratoconus. Ophthalmology. 2005;112(4):654–9. https://doi.org/10.1016/j.ophtha.2004.11.050.
39. Lema I, Sobrino T, Durán JA, Brea D, Díez-Feijoo E. Subclinical keratoconus and inflammatory molecules from tears. Br J Ophthalmol. 2009;93(6):820–4. https://doi.org/10.1136/bjo.2008.144253.
40. Matthews FJ, Cook SD, Majid MA, Dick AD, Smith VA. Changes in the balance of the tissue inhibitor of matrix metalloproteinases (TIMPs)-1 and -3 may promote keratocyte apoptosis in keratoconus. Exp Eye Res. 2007;84(6):1125–34. https://doi.org/10.1016/j.exer.2007.02.013.
41. Elmohamady MN, Abdelghaffar W, Salem TI. Tear martix metalloproteinase-9 and tissue inhibitor of metalloproteinase-1 in post-Lasik Ectasia. Int Ophthalmol. 2019;39(3):631–7. https://doi.org/10.1007/s10792-018-0861-y.
42. Pahuja NK, Shetty R, Deshmukh R, Sharma A, Nuijts R, Jhanji V, et al. In vivo confocal microscopy and tear cytokine analysis in post-LASIK ectasia. Br J Ophthalmol. 2017;101(12):1604–10. https://doi.org/10.1136/bjophthalmol-2016-309142.
43. Shetty R, Kumar NR, Khamar P, Francis M, Sethu S, Randleman JB, et al. Bilaterally asymmetric corneal ectasia following SMILE with asymmetrically reduced stromal molecular markers. J Refract Surg. 2019;35(1):6–14. https://doi.org/10.3928/1081597x-20181128-01.
44. Belin MW, Ambrósio R. Scheimpflug imaging for keratoconus and ectatic disease. Indian J Ophthalmol. 2013;61(8):401–6. https://doi.org/10.4103/0301-4738.116059.
45. Li Y, Meisler DM, Tang M, Lu AT, Thakrar V, Reiser BJ, et al. Keratoconus diagnosis with optical coherence tomography pachymetry mapping. Ophthalmology. 2008;115(12):2159–66. https://doi.org/10.1016/j.ophtha.2008.08.004.
46. Ambrósio R Jr, Caiado AL, Guerra FP, Louzada R, Sinha RA, Luz A, et al. Novel pachymetric parameters based on corneal tomography for diagnosing keratoconus. J Refract Surg. 2011;27(10):753–8. https://doi.org/10.3928/1081597x-20110721-01.

47. Li Y, Tan O, Brass R, Weiss JL, Huang D. Corneal epithelial thickness mapping by Fourier-domain optical coherence tomography in normal and keratoconic eyes. Ophthalmology. 2012;119(12):2425–33. https://doi.org/10.1016/j.ophtha.2012.06.023.
48. Li Y, Chamberlain W, Tan O, Brass R, Weiss JL, Huang D. Subclinical keratoconus detection by pattern analysis of corneal and epithelial thickness maps with optical coherence tomography. J Cataract Refract Surg. 2016;42(2):284–95. https://doi.org/10.1016/j.jcrs.2015.09.021.
49. Reinstein DZ, Archer TJ, Urs R, Gobbe M, RoyChoudhury A, Silverman RH. Detection of keratoconus in clinically and algorithmically topographically normal fellow eyes using epithelial thickness analysis. J Refract Surg. 2015;31(11):736–44. https://doi.org/10.3928/1081597x-20151021-02.
50. Herber R, Ramm L, Spoerl E, Raiskup F, Pillunat LE, Terai N. Assessment of corneal biomechanical parameters in healthy and keratoconic eyes using dynamic bidirectional applanation device and dynamic Scheimpflug analyzer. J Cataract Refract Surg. 2019;45(6):778–88. https://doi.org/10.1016/j.jcrs.2018.12.015.
51. Herber R, Hasanli A, Lenk J, Vinciguerra R, Terai N, Pillunat LE, et al. Evaluation of corneal biomechanical indices in distinguishing between normal, very asymmetric, and Bilateral Keratoconic eyes. J Refract Surg. 2022;38(6):364–72. https://doi.org/10.3928/1081597x-20220601-01.
52. Sinha Roy A, Shetty R, Kummelil MK. Keratoconus: a biomechanical perspective on loss of corneal stiffness. Indian J Ophthalmol. 2013;61(8):392–3. https://doi.org/10.4103/0301-4738.116057.
53. Scarcelli G, Besner S, Pineda R, Yun SH. Biomechanical characterization of keratoconus corneas ex vivo with Brillouin microscopy. Invest Ophthalmol Vis Sci. 2014;55(7):4490–5. https://doi.org/10.1167/iovs.14-14450.
54. Randall J, Vaughan JM. The measurement and interpretation of Brillouin scattering in the lens of the eye. Proc R Soc Lond B Biol Sci. 1982;214(1197):449–70. https://doi.org/10.1098/rspb.1982.0021.
55. Scarcelli G, Kling S, Quijano E, Pineda R, Marcos S, Yun SH. Brillouin microscopy of collagen crosslinking: noncontact depth-dependent analysis of corneal elastic modulus. Invest Ophthalmol Vis Sci. 2013;54(2):1418–25. https://doi.org/10.1167/iovs.12-11387.
56. Scarcelli G, Pineda R, Yun SH. Brillouin optical microscopy for corneal biomechanics. Invest Ophthalmol Vis Sci. 2012;53(1):185–90. https://doi.org/10.1167/iovs.11-8281.
57. Zhang J, Scarcelli G. Mapping mechanical properties of biological materials via an add-on Brillouin module to confocal microscopes. Nat Protoc. 2021;16(2):1251–75. https://doi.org/10.1038/s41596-020-00457-2.
58. Randleman JB, Zhang H, Asroui L, Tarib I, Dupps WJ Jr, Scarcelli G. Subclinical keratoconus detection and characterization using motion tracking brillouin microscopy. Ophthalmology. 2023. https://doi.org/10.1016/j.ophtha.2023.10.011.
59. Rabinowitz YS. Videokeratographic indices to aid in screening for keratoconus. J Refract Surg. 1995;11(5):371–9. https://doi.org/10.3928/1081-597x-19950901-14.
60. Santhiago MR, Wilson SE, Smadja D, Chamon W, Krueger RE, Randleman JB. Validation of the percent tissue altered as a risk factor for Ectasia after LASIK. Ophthalmology. 2019;126(6):908–9. https://doi.org/10.1016/j.ophtha.2019.01.018.
61. Kataria P, Padmanabhan P, Gopalakrishnan A, Padmanaban V, Mahadik S, Ambrósio R Jr. Accuracy of Scheimpflug-derived corneal biomechanical and tomographic indices for detecting subclinical and mild keratectasia in a South Asian population. J Cataract Refract Surg. 2019;45(3):328–36. https://doi.org/10.1016/j.jcrs.2018.10.030.
62. Ferreira-Mendes J, Lopes BT, Faria-Correia F, Salomão MQ, Rodrigues-Barros S, Ambrósio R Jr. Enhanced Ectasia detection using corneal tomography and biomechanics. Am J Ophthalmol. 2019;197:7–16. https://doi.org/10.1016/j.ajo.2018.08.054.
63. Chan TCY, Wang YM, Yu M, Jhanji V. Comparison of corneal tomography and a new combined tomographic biomechanical index in subclinical keratoconus. J Refract Surg. 2018;34(9):616–21. https://doi.org/10.3928/1081597x-20180705-02.

64. Vinciguerra R, Ambrósio R Jr, Elsheikh A, Hafezi F, Yong Kang DS, Kermani O, et al. Detection of postlaser vision correction ectasia with a new combined biomechanical index. J Cataract Refract Surg. 2021;47(10):1314–8. https://doi.org/10.1097/j.jcrs.0000000000000629.
65. Downie LE, Lindsay RG. Contact lens management of keratoconus. Clin Exp Optom. 2015;98(4):299–311. https://doi.org/10.1111/cxo.12300.
66. Wollensak G, Spoerl E, Seiler T. Riboflavin/ultraviolet-A–induced collagen crosslinking for the treatment of keratoconus. Am J Ophthalmol. 2003;135(5):620–7.
67. Yildirim A, Cakir H, Kara N, Uslu H, Gurler B, Ozgurhan EB, et al. Corneal collagen crosslinking for ectasia after laser in situ Keratomileusis: long-term results. J Cataract Refract Surg. 2014;40(10):1591–6.
68. Marino GK, Torricelli AA, Giacomin N, Santhiago MR, Espindola R, Netto MV. Accelerated corneal collagen cross-linking for postoperative LASIK ectasia: two-year outcomes. J Refract Surg. 2015;31(6):380–4.
69. Hersh PS, Stulting RD, Muller D, Durrie DS, Rajpal RKUS. Multicenter clinical trial of corneal collagen crosslinking for treatment of corneal ectasia after refractive surgery. Ophthalmology. 2017;124(10):1475–84. https://doi.org/10.1016/j.ophtha.2017.05.036.
70. Raiskup F, Spoerl E. Corneal cross-linking with hypo-osmolar riboflavin solution in thin keratoconic corneas. Am J Ophthalmol. 2011;152(1):28-32.e1. https://doi.org/10.1016/j.ajo.2011.01.016.
71. Cifariello F, Minicucci M, Di Renzo F, Di Taranto D, Coclite G, Zaccaria S, et al. Epi-off versus epi-on corneal collagen cross-linking in keratoconus patients: a comparative study through 2-year follow-up. J Ophthalmol. 2018;2018:4947983. https://doi.org/10.1155/2018/4947983.
72. Randleman JB, Khandelwal SS, Hafezi F. Corneal cross-linking. Surv Ophthalmol. 2015;60(6):509–23. https://doi.org/10.1016/j.survophthal.2015.04.002.
73. Kanellopoulos AJ, Binder PS. Management of corneal ectasia after LASIK with combined, same-day, topography-guided partial transepithelial PRK and collagen cross-linking: the athens protocol. J Refract Surg. 2011;27(5):323–31. https://doi.org/10.3928/1081597x-20101105-01.
74. Yildirim A, Uslu H, Kara N, Cakir H, Gurler B, Colak HN, et al. Same-day intrastromal corneal ring segment and collagen cross-linking for ectasia after laser in situ Keratomileusis: long-term results. Am J Ophthalmol. 2014;157(5):1070–6. https://doi.org/10.1016/j.ajo.2014.02.011.
75. Colin J, Cochener B, Savary G, Malet F. Correcting keratoconus with intracorneal rings. J Cataract Refract Surg. 2000;26(8):1117–22. https://doi.org/10.1016/s0886-3350(00)00451-x.
76. Israel M, Yousif MO, Osman NA, Nashed M, Abdelfattah NS. Keratoconus correction using a new model of intrastromal corneal ring segments. J Cataract Refract Surg. 2016;42(3):444–54. https://doi.org/10.1016/j.jcrs.2015.11.044.
77. Siganos D, Ferrara P, Chatzinikolas K, Bessis N, Papastergiou G. Ferrara intrastromal corneal rings for the correction of keratoconus. J Cataract Refract Surg. 2002;28(11):1947–51. https://doi.org/10.1016/s0886-3350(02)01495-5.
78. Bteich Y, Assaf JF, Mrad AA, Jacob S, Hafezi F, Awwad ST. Corneal allogenic intrastromal ring segments (CAIRS) for corneal ectasia: a comprehensive segmental tomography evaluation. J Refract Surg. 2023;39(11):767–76.
79. Jacob S, Patel SR, Agarwal A, Ramalingam A, SAijimol AI, Raj JM. Corneal allogenic intrastromal ring segments (CAIRS) combined with corneal cross-linking for keratoconus. J Refract Surg 2018;34(5):296–303
80. Emerah SH, Sabry MM, Saad HA, Ghobashy WA. Visual and refractive outcomes of posterior chamber phakic IOL in stable keratoconus. Int J Ophthalmol. 2019;12(5):840–3. https://doi.org/10.18240/ijo.2019.05.22.

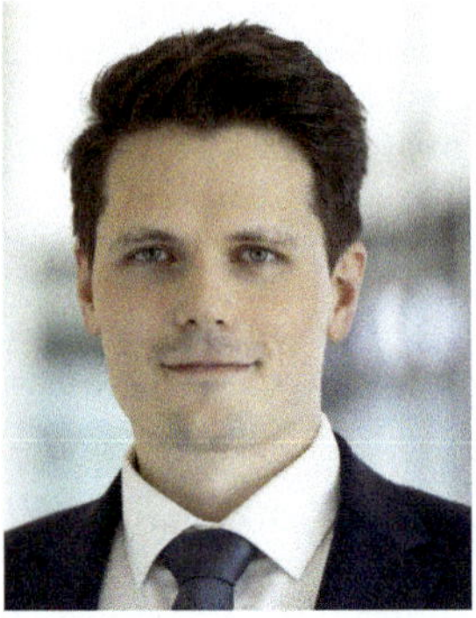

Felix Mathias Wagner is the head of Refractive Laser Surgery and a consultant at the Department of Ophthalmology, University Medical Center of the Johannes Gutenberg University Mainz, Germany. He studied medicine at the Ruperto Carola University Heidelberg and received his doctorate there in 2019. Dr. Wagner completed his residency in ophthalmology at the University Medical Center Mainz, where he became a board-certified ophthalmologist and a Fellow of the European Board of Ophthalmology (FEBO) in 2022. He pursued his clinical fellowship in refractive surgery under Professor Sekundo at the Philipps University of Marburg from 2021 to 2022. Dr. Wagner has published over 30 original research papers.

Part IV

Small Incision Lenticule Extraction (SMILE® and SMILE pro®): Novel Concepts in SMILE Surgery

20 Lenticule Implantation (Keratophakia) for Refractive and Therapeutic Purposes

Xingtao Zhou

20.1 Introduction: Definition and Overview of Keratophakia Surgery

Keratophakia surgery is performed as therapy for high hyperopia, aphakia, or keratoconus, which implants a fresh or preserved lenticule from small incision lenticule extraction into patients' corneal surface or stroma. Historically, the lenticule was carved as an 0.2-mm-thick and 6-mm-diameter lens. This lens was placed on the patients' cornea which underwent lamellar keratectomy and then sutured with the anterior lamellar cap [1, 2]. The implanted lenticule steepened the corneal anterior curvature of patients, improving the refractive power of the cornea of hyperopic patients [3]. Therefore, keratophakia is an additive procedure based on stromal tissue that restructures the recipient's corneal volume.

20.2 History of Keratophakia Surgery

The first technique adding more corneal tissue to reach refractive purposes was described by Barraquer in the 1950s and first attempted in the 1980s [4, 5]. Barraquer described the original technique where an anterior lamellar keratectomy was performed in a fresh or preserved cornea whose epithelium, Bowman's membrane, and a portion of stroma were eliminated to produce a stromal lenticule in a controlled way. Scientists in the 1980s preserved the lenticule in a freezing tissue culture medium or a freeze-drying environment [1, 6]. To change the shape of the cornea, the recipient's cornea also underwent an anterior lamellar keratectomy forming the keratectomy bed to contain the lenticule. The lamellar cap was

X. Zhou (✉)
ENT Hospital of Fudan University, Shanghai, China
e-mail: doctzhouxingtao@163.com

W. Sekundo and F. M. Wagner (eds.), *Femtosecond Laser Assisted Lenticule Extraction*,
https://doi.org/10.1007/978-3-031-60424-9_20

replaced and then sutured in place. The anterior corneal curvature and the refractive power of the patient's eye were increased due to the additional corneal tissue. It was assumed that this technique was capable of correcting up to + 20D of hyperopia [6].

In the era of the excimer laser, there are only a few peer-reviewed publications documenting results from stromal keratophakia in the long term. Troutman and colleagues attempted keratophakia in 32 cases whose ages ranged from 35 to 84 years old and took an average of 13 months (ranging from 3 to 23 months) for all patients [3]. In total, 10% of cases were aborted because of irregular resection of the lamellar disks. In total, 6.25% of patients evolved into wound dehiscence, requiring secondary ophthalmic surgery. In total, 6.25% of patients evolved into postoperative corneal edema. At the end of the follow-up visit, 84.6 and 38.5% of the patients had best corrected visual acuity (BCVA) over 20/40 and achieved ± 1.00 D of emmetropia, respectively. Compared to the preoperative development of + 1.56 D astigmatism refraction was observed on average. Friedlander and colleagues performed their first study on 14 patients and followed up for 13–35 months [7]. On average, the results demonstrated that patients developed + 1.41 D astigmatism, although 50% of them achieved stability of refraction (within ± 1.00 D of emmetropia). Between 1977 and 1981, they conducted a second study but failed to draw a better conclusion [8]. Taylor et al. followed up 10 patients (age between 36 and 93 years old) after surgery for 6 months at least [9, 10]. Two patients developed filamentary keratitis and one graft was decentered. From 10 patients treated, only 1 patient achieved a spherical equivalent of ± 1.00 D of emmetropia, 6 patients had BCVA ranging from 20/20 to 20/40. As in previous studies, this result was similar in that these patients suffered + 0.93 D astigmatism following the procedure. In a study published later, Villasenor described 23 patients (aged between 6 and 80 years old) with a follow-up period ranging from 12 to 38 months [11]. Eight patients had successively undergone cataract and keratophakia surgery. There, 62% of the patients obtained 20/40 or better BCVA at seven months without postoperative complications. Significantly, 75% of Villasenor's patients achieved ± 1.00D of emmetropia and only + 0.84 D relative to pre-operative astigmatism, which was the best performance among all related clinical studies.

In 2007, the generation of VisuMax® femtosecond lasers (fs-laser) (Carl Zeiss Meditec, Jena, Germany) established a new age of lamellar corneal refractive surgery and lenticule implantation surgery. The refractive correction procedure performed by fs-laser involves the intrastromal creation and removal of a refractive lenticule, after disassembly of the lenticular interfaces, through a miniature 2–3 mm corneal limbal incision, therefore avoiding the need for a flap [12–14]. This technique is called small incision lenticule Extraction (SMILE) and produces smoother lenticule surfaces without surface irregularities, insignificant attachments or tissue bridges and regular collagen arrangement of the lenticule tissue [15, 16]. The potential for application of such optimized lenticules to implement additive refractive surgery can have significant appeal to researchers by offering them the feasibility of being able to thicken the patients' cornea with better visual outcomes.

The first case exploiting a lenticule extracted via SMILE involved implantation as a treatment to correct high hyperopia. Pradhan et al. [17] published this allogeneic transplant research in Nepal in 2013 and referred to the procedure as endokeratophakia. At 1 year postoperatively, the spherical equivalent refraction had reduced by 5.25 D, and central corneal thickness (CCT) had increased by 121 mm with clear lenticule. Based on these promising results, implantation of intrastromal lenticule from SMILE could be further utilized to correct hyperopia without significant adverse effects. Following this, many researchers successfully reported the use of allogenic and autologous SMILE lenticules for the management of conditions such as high hyperopia, keratoconus, presbyopia, and sealing corneal defects [18–21]. In the technique of femtosecond intrastromal lenticule implantation, published by Ganesh et al. [18] in 2014, the cornea is made steeper by the addition of a SMILE lenticule of known thickness and power into a pocket created in the recipient's cornea using a femtosecond laser. The concept was subsequently adopted by various authors, who reported their results with certain modifications in the technique [19, 22]. Recently, Liu et al. [23] published their 2-year results with SMILE lenticule implantation and suggested that allogeneic lenticule transplantation may be a promising option for correcting moderate to high hyperopia.

Jacob et al. published their study in 2017 to describe PrEsbyopic Allogenic Refractive Lenticule (PEARL), a novel refractive surgical technique, for the treatment of presbyopia using SMILE lenticules. In this procedure, SMILE lenticules were implanted intrastromally to increase the radius of curvature of the central cornea and make it hyperprolate. This is performed effectively altering the refractive properties of the eye and enhancing near visual acuity. The near visual acuity of all eyes improved by three lines or more, with conservation of uncorrected distance visual acuity (20/20). The consequence indicated that all patients acquired clear vision at near, intermediate, or far distances without glasses, and lenticule implantation did not lead to any complications 6 months postoperatively. This study had one limitation that the follow-up period was short and lacked documentation of long-term complications (i.e., corneal haze). The use of allogenic tissue could increase bioavailability and decrease the risk of inflammation while maintaining the ability to be removed or adjusted [21].

In 2015, Ganesh and Brar undertook a study with six eyes with keratoconus of six subjects in which the patients underwent implantation of a donut-shaped stromal lenticule simultaneously with corneal collagen cross-linking. Lenticules were gained from SMILE procedures remedying myopia. They reported a mean increase in CCT of 18.3 ± 7.3 μm, no loss of lines in CDVA, no haze, and no infection 6 months postoperatively [20].

In 2017, lenticule implantation as a treatment for laser-assisted in situ keratomileusis (LASIK)-induced ectasia was first attempted in China. Three patients involved in this study developed progressive post-LASIK ectasia with central corneal thickness < 400 μm. Researchers obtained the donor lenticules from patients receiving SMILE earlier than implantation at the same day. The average central corneal thickness at 1 year postoperatively had been significantly thicker than that before surgery (446.67 ± 41.63 μm vs. 360 μm), and all the implanted lenticules were transparent with no indication of immune rejection or other complications [24].

20.3 Refractive Correction

20.3.1 Hyperopia Correction

Hyperopia is a common refractive error in which the light rays are focused at a theoretical point behind the retina when the accommodation is at rest. The prevalence of hyperopia varies with age and ethnic group [25, 26]. The pooled prevalence of hyperopia in adults is 36% in Asia, 40% in Europe, 47% in Africa, and 49% in America. At present, wearing spectacles is a commonly used method to correct hyperopia, but for those patients who desire to see without depending on spectacles, surgical management may be considered. Laser in situ keratomileusis (LASIK) is the most common procedure to correct hyperopia [27, 28]. However, the refractive predictability and stability of hyperopic-LASIK are poor, especially for high hyperopia correction, its application is limited by complications such as postoperative regression, induction of higher-order aberrations (HOAs) and so on [29, 30]. Similarly, poor stability was observed following the first hyperopic FLEx study, but improved to the level of Femtolasik with modified lenticule design (see Chap. 9). Hyperopic small incision lenticule extraction (SMILE) is a recently proposed procedure for the correction of hyperopia, in which the axial cornea is steepen by removing a concave lenticule from the stroma [31, 32]. However, so far only 12 months results were published for hyperopic and its long-term stability remains to be determined. Other treatment options include photorefractive keratectomy that delivers outcome inferior to lamellar procedures, and phakic intraocular lens implantation. Although the latter provides refractively stable outcomes, it has significant risks of intraocular surgery in eyes with shallow anterior chamber [33, 34]. While the refractive lens exchange (RLE) is a viable option for presbyopic hyperopes, it is not a justifiable option at younger age.

Stromal keratophakia is another treatment option for hyperopia correction which steepens the cornea by inserting a convex lenticule into the stroma [35]. Currently, stromal keratophakia has been demonstrated to be a safe, effective, and predictable surgical procedure to correct hyperopia. The procedure offers certain advantages, including the ability to restore stromal volume, reversibility, and low risk of regression. It may be a better alternative to hyperopic-LASIK or hyperopic-SMILE because the shape of the cornea becomes more natural after tissue addition than after tissue subtraction, and induces fewer HOAs. Moreover, stromal keratophakia may not cause midperipheral epithelial hyperplasia to compensate for the loss of stromal tissue, so it has an advantage in reducing refractive regression [18].

As stated above, stromal keratophakia was first proposed by Dr. Barraquer and then many scholars carried out clinical research followed it. However, due to the difficult lathing techniques and poor cutting accuracy of microkeratome, the cutting accuracy of lenticule and cornea was not consistent. In the summary of clinical results from six studies, only 31.9 ± 11.8% of the patients had best corrected visual acuity (BCVA) ≥ 20/40, and 41.1 ± 21.3% had refractive stability within ± 1.00D [35]. Among them, induced astigmatism was the most common, and the average postoperative astigmatism (2.45 ± 0.37D) was almost a twofold increase from preoperative astigmatism. Additionally, complications such as epithelial ingrowth, interface scarring, decentration, and even corneal perforation might occur.

With the development of femtosecond laser technology, especially the emergence of refractive lenticule extraction (ReLEx), accurately sculpting the corneal stromal lenticule and creating the corneal flap or stromal pocket become possible [36]. The application of femtosecond lasers has significantly helped revive this technology. SMILE has been widely used in myopia correction worldwide. As of 2023, 8 million SMILEs have been performed worldwide with more than a half in China. The byproduct of the procedure, a convex lenticule, could provide a wide range of lenticule sources for the application of femtosecond laser assisted stromal keratophakia in hyperopia correction.

Depending on the type of implantation, femtosecond laser-assisted stromal keratophakia can be divided into femtosecond laser-assisted lenticule intrastromal keratoplasty (FS-LIKE) [19, 37–40], small incision lenticule intrastromal keratoplasty (SMI-LIKE) [17, 41] and combined surgery [24, 42–45]. FS-LIKE uses femtosecond laser to create a corneal flap, which is lifted for lenticule implantation. This method is beneficial for centration, axial alignment and spread of the lenticule. It induces less astigmatism and HOAs, and increases the functional optical zone, thus achieving better refractive correction efficacy and predictability [40]. However, FS-LIKE also brings flap-related risks, including epithelial ingrowth and flap necrosis [38]. SMI-LIKE uses femtosecond laser to create an intrastromal pocket, and the lenticule is implanted through a small incision. This procedure could reduce many invasive injuries, including flap-related complications, reduction of corneal biomechanical strength as well as the sub-basal nerve plexus injury leasing to the postoperative dry eye symptoms [46]. The combined surgery includes femtosecond laser-assisted stromal keratophakia combined with SMILE, LASIK and intrastromal lenticule rotation (ISLR). At present, studies have reported that FS-LIKE, SMI-LIKE and combined surgery could achieve good refractive results for the correction of hyperopia.

SMI-LIKE

As reported above in 2013, Pradhan reported the first clinical case of SMI LIKE for correcting hyperopia they called "keyhole endokeratophakia" [17]. Their patient had high hyperopia due to aphakia (+ 12.00 − 1.50 × 155). She received a 10.50 D lenticule implantation. One year postoperatively, the spherical equivalent (SE) decreased by 5.25D, indicating a 50% under-correction. The authors attributed the postoperative under-correction and regression to the posterior surface bulge and epithelial remodeling caused by the thick lenticule implanted. In addition, the small optical zone (5.75 mm) induced less stromal volume addition. Therefore, it is challenging to achieve complete correction for aphakia with high hyperopia, and further parameters optimization are needed to improve the correction efficacy.

In another study performed by Ganesh et al., the effective index and safety index were 1.09 ± 0.31 and 1.18 ± 0.23, respectively, indicating that SMI-LIKE was safe and effective for correcting moderate hyperopia [18]. These authors called the procedure "Femtosecond intrastromal lenticule implantation = FILI [18]. Although the moderate hyperopia was mainly included in this study, an excessively implantation depth (160 μm) still affected the morphology of the posterior surface, resulting in 21% under-correction. In addition, only mild epithelial thinning was observed. The authors proposed that the epithelial thickness profile following hyperopic SMI-LIKE might be more favorable than after hyperopic LASIK.

In view of this, Liu et al. chose a shallow implantation depth (100 μm) to perform SMI-LIKE for correction of moderate to high hyperopia. At 2 years postoperatively, the refractive correction efficacy was 91%, and the mean prediction error (MPE) was − 0.45 ± 0.75 D, without posterior corneal surface change [41]. In addition, during the 2 years follow-up, the corneas remained transparent, without haze or rejection, and no significant change in corneal curvature and SE was observed, indicating that SMI-LIKE treatment for hyperopia showed good safety and stability.

FS-LIKE

Li et al. reported a case series of 10 patients, who had one myopic eye and one hyperopic eye. In this autologous lenticule implantation following FS-LIKE, the effective index and safety index were 1.11 ± 0.11 and 1.50 ± 0.46, respectively, which were significantly higher than other studies [16]. Notably, additional ablation was performed prior to the implantation to correct the expected residual refraction in 5 cases, which might improve the postoperative visual acuity. After these 5 cases were excluded, the indices of the remaining patients were 0.92 ± 0.36 and 1.10 ± 0.10, respectively. This was consistent with other studies [18]. There were no significant differences in the anterior and posterior corneal curvature from postoperative 1 month to 2 years, suggesting good stability.

Moshirfar et al. reported a case of FS-LIKE for correction of high hyperopia. The refraction decreased from preoperative + 6.00 − 1.00 × 40 to 0 − 1.25 × 71 [29]. However, the BCVA of the patient decreased by one line at 6 months postoperatively, which was suspected to be related to epithelial ingrowth. The author observed the epithelial ingrowth one month after surgery, and increased the application of topical prednisolone acetate. Two months after the FS-LIKE procedure, the patient underwent scraping of epithelial ingrowth, and the UDVA recovered to 20/25.

In two recent studies of FS-LIKE, authors have chosen a relatively shallow implantation depth (100–110 μm) and recommended lenticule diameter (6.5 mm). The results showed that the refractive correction efficacy was 96 and 102%, and the

MPE were only − 0.25 D and 0.14 D, respectively, suggesting good predictability [18, 19].

Combined Surgery

In the absence of lenticule banking, it is difficult to obtain a lenticule matching the appropriate refraction, since the lenticule refraction is predetermined by the refractive status of the donor patients undergoing SMILE. In addition, most patients with hyperopia are accompanied by astigmatism. It is rare to achieve a perfect match for both the sphere and the cylinder when choosing a determined myopic donor lenticule. Therefore, expected residual refraction could be taken into account during preoperative planning. In recent years, it has been reported that femtosecond laser assisted stromal keratophakia, combined with SMILE, LASIK, and ISLR, could correct expected residual refraction.

Zhang et al. reported a case series of SMILE combined with SMI-LIKE for correcting hyperopia with astigmatism [24]. The hyperopic eye with astigmatism was first treated with SMILE to correct astigmatism, then a lenticule was extracted from a donor myopic eye and subsequently implanted into the hyperopic eye with astigmatism. One year postoperatively, the SE decreased from 7.42 ± 3.12 D to − 0.75 ± 0.79 D, and refractive astigmatism reduced from + 1.95 ± 1.04 D to − 0.65 ± 0.63 D. 94.7% of treated eyes had no change or increase in BCVA, UDVA, and UNVA postoperatively were obviously better than those before surgery. During 1-year follow-up, there was no significant difference in SE, astigmatism, corneal curvature and central corneal thickness (CCT), indicating good stability for correcting hyperopia with astigmatism.

Sun et al. reported 5 cases, which underwent LASIK combined with FS-LIKE to correct hyperopia with astigmatism [19]. The hyperopic eye with astigmatism first underwent LASIK to correct the expected residual refraction, then the autologous lenticules extracted from contralateral eye was implanted under a 110 μm flap. There was no significant difference in the SE from postoperative 1 month to 1 year, suggesting good stability. However, the MPE and the refractive correction efficacy were 1.13 ± 3.18 D and 140%, respectively.

Toric lenticule implantation could be another treatment option for hyperopia with astigmatism. Lazaridis et al. reported a case of iatrogenic hyperopia and high astigmatism after LASIK (+ 6.50 − 9.00 × 84) [42]. A toric lenticule (− 4.00 − 4.25 × 14), obtained from a myopic donor eye, was implanted by Walter Sekundo beneath the original LASIK flap at 140 μm, aiming to reduce the refractive errors. The postoperative refraction showed a reduction of astigmatism but a stronger myopization compared to preoperative calculations (− 6.50 − 4.00 × 70). The authors attributed the unexpected refraction to the prior LASIK ablation, implantation under the LASIK flap, and epithelial remodeling. The refraction remained stable and the implanted lenticule was barely discernible after 10 years (Sekundo W, personal communication), confirming a long-lasting effect (Fig. 20.1).

Stodulka et al. describe a case of intrastromal toric lenticule rotation (ISRL) to correct high astigmatism in an amblyopic eye (+ 2.00 − 5.00 × 10) [43]. The postoperative astigmatism changed to 0.00 D, but a postoperative myopic shift was

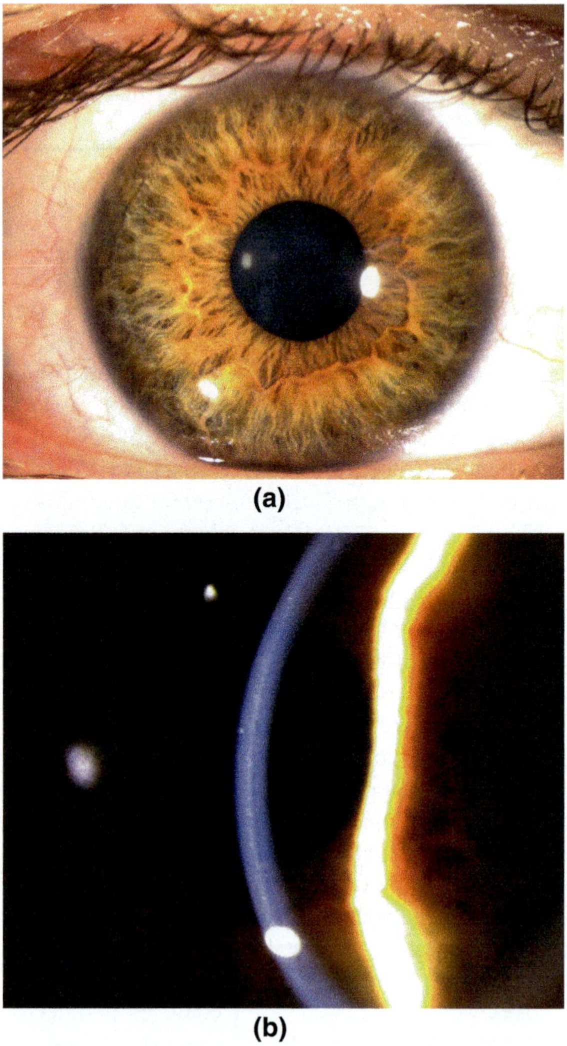

Fig. 20.1 Slit lamp appearance of an transplanted allogenic toric lenticule after 10 years. **a** Front view shows an unremarkable cornea; **b** One can hardly see the anterior and posterior surface of the lenticule at oblique illumination (courtesy of Prof. Sekundo)

also observed (see Chap. 23 for details). His first clinical case followed en ex-vivo study by Damgaard et al. who demonstrated ISLR to be feasible and precise for the management of regular astigmatism up to 10.00 D in human donor corneas [44]. The correction index (CI) and angle of error (AE) were 1.14 ± 0.25 and $-0.80° \pm 4.61°$, respectively, in the 5.00 D group, and were 9.57 ± 1.10 D and $2.75° \pm 3.60°$, respectively, in the 10.00 D group. Liu et al. reported the first use of toric lenticule implantation with the triple marking method to correct hyperopia and astigmatism following SMI-LIKE [45]. The results showed that astigmatism decreased from -2.15 ± 1.10 D to -0.70 ± 0.21 D at 6 months postoperatively.

The author attributed the unexpected astigmatism to the SIA, mismatch of donor lenticule refraction, and axial misalignment.

Although the feasibility, safety, and efficacy have been demonstrated in animal and clinical studies, the nomograms need to be refined further to achieve better predictability and stability. For the treatment of hyperopia, the refractive predictability after implantation depends not only on the thickness and diameter of the implanted lenticule, but also on the implantation depth, centration and axial alignment, as well as corneal remodeling. Therefore, we recommend FS-LIKE to correct moderate to high hyperopia, with a conventional lenticule diameter and a shallower implantation depth. Currently, the concentric centration method and triple marking method demonstrated accurate centration, axial alignment, and effectively correct hyperopia and astigmatism. In future, the application of image-guided systems in lenticule centration might be a direction to control the SIA. Next investigation should be focused on the lenticule preservation and lenticule customization, which may enrich the supply for a wider application. We believe that it is wise and necessary to promote the concept of the "recycling" of SMILE lenticule.

20.3.2 Presbyopia Correction

Presbyopia is a common age-related vision condition which causes difficulty in focusing on close objects and typically becomes noticeable around the age of 40 and progressively worsens with age. It was estimated that approximately 2 billion people worldwide were affected by presbyopia [47]. Presbyopia manifests when the natural age-related decline in the eye's focusing ability progresses to a stage where, even with optimal distance vision correction, the clarity of near vision becomes inadequate to meet an individual's needs [48]. While presbyopia cannot be permanently cured, there are several treatment options available to help manage the condition and improve near vision. The common treatments for presbyopia included spectacle lenses (bifocals, trifocals, and progressive addition lenses), contact lenses (monovision and multifocal contact lenses), surgical approaches (corneal inlays, laser refractive surgery, intraocular lenses implantation, corneal collagen shrinkage and scleral expansion), pharmacological treatment, and electro-stimulation [48].

Among all the treatments, corneal inlay, which related to small implantable devices placed in the cornea, have emerged as an exciting option [47, 49, 50]. By creating a hyper-prolate region featuring elevated central corneal power, increasing the depth of focus, or by adding refractive power to focus on the near objects, corneal inlay could enhance the uncorrected near and intermediate vision while still maintaining distance acuity [51]. However, most of the layers, such as shape-changing corneal inlay (Raindrop), small-aperture corneal inlay (KAMRA), and the refractive corneal inlay (Flexivue), are composed of synthetic materials and could cause host response leading to corneal haze [52, 53]. On the contrary, keratophakia yields good efficacy and safety in the correction of presbyopia with less immune response [21, 54]. By implanting small incision lenticule extraction (SMILE) derived lenticule into the recipient's corneal stromal, keratophakia reshapes the curvature and introduces multifocality which enabling individuals to simultaneously focus on objects at different distances [35].

Liu et al. initially reported the feasibility of biological corneal inlay for the correction of presbyopia in macaque. They showed that all the autogeneic, decellularized xenogeneic and xenogeneic SMILE-derived lenticule significantly increased the simulated keratometric value and corneal anterior surface elevation. Additionally, autogeneic and decellularized lenticules showed good biocompatibility with no rejection occurred at 6 months postoperatively [55]. Nowadays, there are two types of allograft corneal inlays for presbyopic subjects, including presbyopic TransForm™ corneal allograft (TCA) and PrEsbyopic allogenic refractive lenticule (PEARL) [21, 54]. The TCA, derived from eye bank, undergoes electron beam (e-beam) sterilization process and shaping by excimer laser. The final shape of 2–3.5 mm diameter and 15–25 microns central thickness enable the subject to experience enhanced vision for both near and intermediate distances, while also maintaining distance vision through the peripheral entry of light around the TCA. Kilic et al. evaluated the visual outcomes of 12 eyes for the correction of presbyopia by TCA implantation with a 6 months follow-up [54]. They implanted a TCA lenticule with target add power of 2.5 D in the non-dominant eye and found that the uncorrected near visual acuity (UCNVA) significantly increased from 0.52 ± 0.14 to 0.10 ± 0.06 LogMAR postoperatively with a myopic shift of spherical equivalent refraction from $+ 0.25 \pm 0.29$ D to $- 0.11 \pm 0.28$ D. PEARL was created by a SMILE derived lenticule centrally trephined to a diameter of 1 mm. The surgeon then implanted the PEARL inlay into the corneal stroma beneath a 120 μm femtosecond laser-produced cap, aligned with the coaxially sighted light reflex. Jacob et al. evaluated the visual outcomes of 4 presbyopic subjects after PEARL inlay implantation [21]. They found that one subject had an improved UCNVA from J8 to J2 and the other three subjects had an improved UCNVA from J5, J6, and J7, respectively, to J2. Additionally, the immediate and distance vision were not affected in all four eyes.

Keratophakia is not an exempt from complications, such as graft dislocation, induced astigmatism, and corneal rejection. The centration of lenticule implantation during the procedure may still be challenging in some cases as the pupil is a dynamic aperture. Additionally, we are still conducting researches on how to customize the lenticular diopter based on the unique refractive needs of presbyopic subjects. It is worth noting that advanced surgical techniques, such as femtosecond laser-assisted keratophakia, hold the potential for improving visual outcomes. Lim et al. initially evaluated the feasibility of laser in-situ keratomileusis (LASIK) after lenticule implantation in rabbits [56]. They found that eyes that underwent SMILE and subsequent SMILE-derived lenticule re-implantation with additional LASIK shared similar tissue responses with eyes that underwent solely LASIK.

In conclusion, keratophakia offers a unique approach to addressing presbyopia by modifying the cornea's curvature with less inflammatory response. Despite challenges, ongoing research, technological advancements, and refined surgical techniques may establish keratophakia as a viable treatment option for presbyopia, contributing to improved quality of life for affected individuals.

20.4 Post-LASIK Ectasia and Keratoconus Treatment

Many recent studies have shed light on the reuse of SMILE-derived lenticules for corneal ectasia diseases management. This section overviews recent applications of SMILE corneal stromal lenticules in treating corneal ectasia diseases.

The corneal ectasia diseases comprise a group of disorders characterized by progressive corneal thinning and subsequent bulging [57]. The phenotypic variations include keratoglobus, pellucid marginal degeneration (PMD), and the widely recognized keratoconus (KC), characterized by bilateral, asymmetrical, and progressive corneal steepening, leading to irregular astigmatism, and visual impairment [58]. Additionally, post-LASIK ectasia has emerged as a significant concern following refractive surgeries [59]. The underlying etiology of post-LASIK ectasia remains unclear, but the cornea's biomechanical weakening following the corneal tissue's ablation might contribute to postoperative corneal ectasia. The risk factors included preoperative abnormal corneal topography, low residual stromal bed thickness [60], young age, low preoperative corneal thickness, and high myopia, as evaluated by the Ectasia Risk Score System reported by Randleman et al. [61].

The current aim of treatment is to prevent progression, improve refractive status and aberrations, and restore the normal prolate shape of the cornea. Contemporary approaches for managing corneal ectasia involve contact lens use, intracorneal ring segments, corneal collagen cross-linking, and in severe cases, penetrating keratoplasty, depending on the severity and progression of keratoconus. For mild keratoconus, spectacles can be an option for astigmatism under 2.5D if the patient is satisfied with the visual acuity. Contact lenses, especially rigid gas permeable contact lenses may be fitted for mild and moderate KC, usually providing a better visual acuity than spectacles. Corneal crosslinking aims to keep and restore corneal volume, biomechanical stability, and structural rigidity to prevent further progression facilitated by riboflavin. However, severe cases often need corneal transplantation, which is constrained by donor scarcity and risk of rejection. Addressing these challenges, additive corneal surgery emerges as a potential solution to enhance visual acuity and increase corneal biomechanical stability, particularly for progressive cases and individuals intolerant to contact lenses.

In 1992 Merlyn et al. reported 5 patients who underwent epikeratoplasty for keratoconus, but the postoperative outcomes showed poor visual acuity and interface scarring [62].

Our own report involved an 18-year-old keratoconus patient undergoing epikeratophakia using SMILE-derived lenticule transplantation. The procedure involved corneal regularization through transepithelial phototherapeutic keratectomy, followed by lenticule transplantation from a myopic astigmatism donor to the central cornea. Accelerated transepithelial CXL was conducted a month later. Over a 3-year follow-up, the patient exhibited no complications, with notable improvements in corneal thickness and visual acuity [63]. Anterior segment optical coherence tomography revealed a well-attached lenticule with a demarcation line. The corneal thickness increased from 365 to 470 μm (Fig. 20.2).

Following epikeratoplasty for keratoconus, investigations into the viability and effectiveness of endokeratophakia utilizing lenticules were conducted. A 29-year-old individual with post-LASIK ectasia underwent allogenic corneal lenticule implantation, resulting in significant corneal flattening, reduced posterior elevation, and increased central corneal thickness [64]. Notably, the demarcation line of the lenticule became indistinct but seamlessly integrated with the surrounding tissue. Substantial improvements in refraction were observed, with a notable

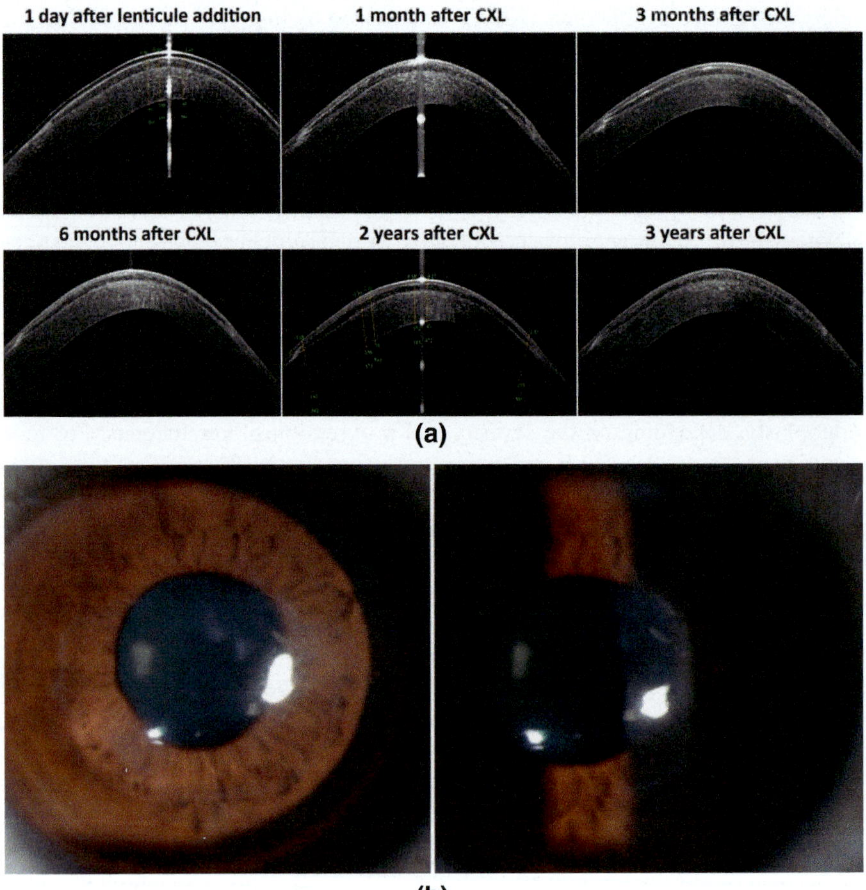

Fig. 20.2 **a** Anterior segment optical coherence tomography images after small-incision lenticule extraction lenticule addition and after CXL (corneal cross-linking). **b** Slit lamp image of the cornea 3 years after epikeratophakia

increase from $-13.50/-6.00 \times 10^\circ$ to $-3.25/-1.50 \times 10^\circ$, leading to a corrected distance visual acuity of 20/40. A 30-month follow-up study, combining lenticule addition with corneal cross-linking, demonstrated sustained enhancements in visual acuity and stable corneal parameters. Another study focusing on femtosecond intrastromal lenticular implantation (FILI) showed increased corneal thickness, reduced spherical equivalent (SE), and improved uncorrected visual acuity, particularly in patients intolerant to contact lenses [20]. However, optimal outcomes were predominantly observed in mild to moderate keratoconus cases, as late-stage conditions did not exhibit satisfactory results. Furthermore, Mastropasqua et al. explored the insertion of negative meniscus-shaped stromal lenticules into the intrastromal pocket of ten patients with stage III and IV stable keratoconus [65]. Remarkable enhancements in uncorrected and corrected distance visual acuity were noted, accompanied by decreased anterior mean curvatures and anterior Q values. Additionally, both central and mid-peripheral corneal thickness increased significantly postoperatively [66]. Variations in the central corneal thickness, corneal thinnest point, and central epithelial thickness were found 1 and 6 months after stromal lenticule addition keratoplasty for keratoconus, with regional variations like the outer annular area increased and the inner annular area decreased, which remained unchanged 6 months postoperatively.

To investigate the predominant structural changes following the implantation, an in-depth analysis was conducted utilizing In Vivo Confocal Microscopy (IVCM) [67]. Activated keratocytes were observed near the lenticule in the first 6 months, and elongated, deformed keratocyte nuclei were found in the implanted lenticules in the first year. The anterior and posterior interfaces showed a decrease in keratocytes and the presence of small particles. Recipient keratocytes repopulated the lenticules, and the keratocytes in the lenticules gradually returned to their normal morphology. Evident corneal nerve regeneration was also observed in the transplanted lenticular graft. Nakamura et al. examined histopathological and immunohistochemical changes in lenticules and host corneal buttons from patients who underwent epikeratoplasty for keratoconus. Alpha1-PI and alpha2M immunostaining was lower in the lenticules, host, and keratoconus specimens compared to normal corneas [68].

Additional potential advantages of the technique are that cornea with a thin stroma (with the thinnest pachymetry below the recommended values for CXL) might become treatable after lenticule addition and that the need for keratoplasty might be delayed or avoided, which was also described in the previous case. Crosslinking typically requires a minimum corneal thickness of at least 400 μm post-epithelial removal to adhere to safety protocol guidelines [69]. Sachdev et al. introduced a technique involving the placement of a stromal lenticule with a central thickness of 80–100 μm over the host cornea after epithelial debridement, followed by routine collagen cross-linking [70]. Postoperative observations revealed a discernible demarcation line at 6 months, demonstrating increased rigidity and collagen fiber thickness, indicating cross-linking effectiveness.

Customized SMILE-derived stromal lenticules were also reported for treating advanced keratoconus [71]. 22 lenticules were customized into a simple necklace or necklace-with-ring based on corneal thickness and topography. The authors implanted them into 9.5 mm corneal lamellar pockets. The successful implantations significantly improved corrected distance visual acuity with no complications reported, along with a mean enhancement of 100.4 μm in corneal thickness at the thinnest point. The cornea remained transparent 1 year postoperatively.

A comparative analysis between small-incision femtosecond laser-assisted intracorneal concave lenticule implantation (SFII) and penetrating keratoplasty (PKP) was conducted in progressive keratoconus [72]. Both procedures exhibited improved visual acuity, stable corneal curvature, and central corneal thickness 24 months postoperatively. Notably, SFII showcased more prominent corneal biomechanical changes with fewer dendritic and inflammatory cells compared to PKP, indicating a reduced risk of graft-versus-host disease.

The recent findings suggest that lenticule reuse offers multiple potential applications in treating corneal ectasia and keratoconus. Its increasing corneal thickness, enhancing visual acuity, and fostering corneal stability underlines its promise as a feasible and effective treatment. Further research and long-term observations are warranted to validate its role as a promising intervention for ocular ectasia diseases.

20.5 Treatment for Corneal Perforation and Other Applications in Corneal Diseases

Corneal perforation, which leads to severe complications such as endophthalmitis, iris–corneal touch, hypotony with choroidal detachment, atrophy of eyeball and subsequent permanent visual loss. Therefore, it is urgently needed to restore the tectonic integrity of the globe to prevent these complications. Penetrating keratoplasty can later be performed in an adequate clinical setting [73]. A large number of studies have focused on conventional tissue adhesive, conjunctival flaps [74], and amniotic membrane techniques for corneal perforation closure [75]. However, these techniques are not suitable because the patient invariably requires a secondary permanent procedure in the form of a lamellar or full-thickness corneal graft, which are risky and associated with a high rate of immunological rejection and subsequent graft failure.

With the development of SMILE, corneal lenticule provides a new option for the treatment of corneal perforation. Recent reports show that corneal lenticule can be also applied to restore the corneal perforation or defects. Recently, Wu et al. reported that they used a SMILE lenticule with an extra amniotic membrane patch overlaid on the lenticule grafts to seal corneal perforation in 6 patients [76]. Although sutures provide stable fixation and the amniotic membrane would accelerate the healing process under lenticule grafts, they increase the surgical time, cause irregular astigmatism, and patient discomfort. Hence, Bhandari et al. published a case series in which the lenticule was secured to the recipient eye using fibrin glue [77]. Even though the use of fibrin glue would decrease irregular astigmatism, the process is complex and time-consuming, and the fresh lenticule may undergo severe rejection in this case series. Cross-stitch was used for the lenticule when the defect needed 1 patch only, while 2 overlapped lenticules were used in the surgery to make sure they are strong enough to cover the perforation. In 2 lenticules there is no need to suture the inner lenticule. We think, it reduces the irregular astigmatism and saves time. This technique has been applied to all kinds of corneal micro-perforation or defects including corneal dermoid tumor, corneal inert ulcer, virus keratitis, and fungal keratitis. In all cases, the procedure was successful and the patch graft was well accepted by the host cornea.

Song et al. [78] presented the three successful applications of the SMILE-extracted stromal lenticule in an Ahmed-valve-tube-exposure and bullous keratopathy patient without complications. Wan et al. [79] reported a novel technique to treat superficial limbal dermoid by using the corneal intrastromal lenticules, and no immune rejection or perforation was detected at follow-up. Liu et al. [80] further utilized the fibrin glue instead of traditional sutures to treat corneal dermoid. This technique was also considered to be safe and feasible. He et al. [81] performed lamellar keratoplasty using a SMILE-derived lenticule for the treatment of Mooren's ulcer coexisting with a pterygium. The patient was stable with no complications or recurrence at 1 year postoperatively. Therefore, a SMILE-derived corneal lenticule, with its biocompatibility, ease of handling, and low cost, is a useful patch graft for various ocular diseases.

In conclusion, the finding demonstrates that SMILE-generated corneal lenticule is a safe, effective, and inexpensive alternative graft for corneal perforation or defects. However, this technique is limited, for example, the diameter of SMILE-generated corneal lenticule is usually 6.5 mm, which means that the management may not be a suitable choice for very large corneal perforation or defects. Although the 17 cases were successfully repaired through this method, longer follow-up periods are required to substantiate the success of this novel method and its long-term effects on corneal stabilization.

20.6 Lenticule Preservation and Lenticule Banking

In recent years, many studies have reported that SMILE lenticules can be used in the treatment of hyperopia, presbyopia and other ocular diseases, but most of these studies used fresh lenticules tissue, which to some extent is a limitation of its application, and it is of great research significance to know how to preserve these lenticules for reuse. This section provides an overview of new advances in SMILE corneal stromal lenticules preservation technology.

The SMILE procedure involves the creation of corneal stromal lenticules with two scans at different depths in the corneal stroma using a femtosecond laser and an edgewise cut, which is separated and removed to correct the refractive error [82]. These removed lenticules are routinely discarded postoperatively. With the rise of SMILE surgery, a large number of corneal stromal lenticules have been produced, which can be reused for transplantation [19, 83], but most of the previous studies have used fresh lenticules, which has limited the application and popularization of the lenticules. The lack of corneal donors and the mismatch between the demand for surgical volume are becoming more and more obvious, which makes it necessary to expand the application of corneal stromal lenticules. Fresh corneal stromal lenticules transplantation is usually performed immediately after the SMILE lenticules are removed, and a variety of infectious agents can be transmitted through corneal transplantation, therefore, before allograft transplantation, the donor needs to be screened for HIV, hepatitis B virus, and other infectious indicators with the appropriate serologic testing, and it usually takes 1–3 days to get the results. If the matching lenticules donor has an infectious disease, in this case, the doctor needs more time to find an additional lenticules donor that matches the recipient, in addition, the lenticules donor and the recipient need to be scheduled for surgery on the same day, all of which increases the difficulty of promoting the clinical application of fresh lenticules.

One of the main challenges in the reuse of corneal stromal lenticules is preservation, especially in some less developed countries and regions. In general, the entire clinical workflow of tissue organ donation should include qualified acquisition, preservation, and transportation in order to ensure the quality and success of transplantation. Once the stromal lenticules are removed from the cornea, damage due to hypoxia and dehydration can destroy the original morphology and microstructure of the lenticules. Corneal stromal lenticules have a collagenous lamellar structure, with a large number of collagen fibers in each lamella, and flat and elongated stromal cells in the narrow gaps between the lamellae, and the regular arrangement of the collagen fibers is a key factor in maintaining the transparency of the lenticules. Irregular collagen fiber structure has been reported to affect corneal transparency. Therefore, preserving the integrity of the lenticules and maintaining its activity are essential for preserving corneal stromal lenticules.

According to the duration of corneal tissue preservation, it can be categorized into short, medium and long-term preservation [18, 84, 85]. The preservation time for short-term preservation is usually less than 2 days, and the most commonly used preservation fluids for medium-term preservation are M-K fluid, K-SOK, GSM, Dexsol, and Optisol-GS, among which Optisol corneal medium-term preservation fluid has become the most commonly used corneal preservation fluid since it was proposed by Lindstrom et al. at the beginning of the 1990s [86, 87]. In contrast, Optisol can only preserve corneal cells for 14 days [88, 89]. In addition to Optisol-GS, the routinely applied anhydrous glycerol and color-changing silica gel are inactive methods of corneal tissue preservation. Long-term preservation refers to the preservation of corneas in liquid nitrogen, which has the advantage of flexibility in use but requires liquid nitrogen storage equipment, a complex process, and high technical difficulty [90–92].

At present, relevant studies mainly focus on the short and medium-term preservation of SMILE lenticules. Liu discussed the preservation methods of corneal stromal lenticules before re-implantation [93]. Corneal stromal lenticules derived from SMILE were stored in phosphate buffer salt solution, DMEM (Dulbecco's modified eagle's medium), Optisol-GS and anhydrous glycerol, under 8 different conditions for 48 h. The results showed that lenticules preserved by various methods at 4 °C or room temperature showed good transparency, collagen structural integrity and low immunogenicity, suggesting that lenticules could be preserved by relatively simple methods without the need for specialized and expensive laboratory equipment for at least 48 h before transport to large facilities for long-term storage. Liang et al. stored the lenticules in anhydrous glycerin, silica gel and Optisol GS liquid at 4 °C, respectively, and observed them under light microscope and transmission electron microscope after 1, 3, 7, and 14 days of storage. The results showed that the anhydrous glycerin and silica gel groups showed more obvious histological changes than the Optisol-GS group. It showed obvious edema of collagen fibers, interlayer cavitation bubbles. Moreover, the cell structure changes of Optisol-GS group were slower than those of the other two groups, and clear cell structure was still visible at 14 days [5]. Xia et al. explored three different preservation methods, including anhydrous glycerin, silicone oil, and silica gel, in which the lenticules was stored at different temperatures (including room temperature, 4, − 20, and − 80 °C) for 4 h, 3 days, and 4 weeks, and the lenticules transmittance in the silica gel remained unchanged, while the other two groups showed significantly lower transmittance. Ultrastructural study of preserved corneal stromal lenticules showed that there was partial edema and the collagen fiber density decreased in the glycerol group. Corneal stromal cells showed necrosis and apoptosis in all groups [94].

For long-term storage of corneal stromal lenticules, deep cryopreservation under aseptic conditions is preferred. Deep cryopreservation minimizes the degradation of collagen tissue and the death of corneal stromal cells, thus maintaining the structure of the corneal stromal scaffolds, the protein content, and the transparency. There have been numerous studies on the long-term deep cryopreservation of corneal stromal lenticules. Glycerol, as a classical preservation medium, is a common osmotic cryoprotectant used for the preservation of corneal stromal lenticules under deep cryopreservation conditions, and it has good antibacterial and antimicrobial properties. Glycerol method is one of the common methods for long-term corneal preservation, which greatly reduces the economic cost due to its dehydrating and anti-microbial properties that can maintain the structure of corneal collagen fibers for a long period of time, removing the biogenicity. The molecular structure of glycerol contains three hydroxyl structures, so it has good water solubility and hygroscopicity, and it can be tightly bound to water molecules inside the cell through the cell membrane, thus preventing the formation of ice crystals of water molecules inside and outside the cell during the freezing process, and glycerol has been widely used in the preservation of tendons, skin, and strains of bacteria, etc. [95–98], but it is prone to cause edema of the tissues after thawing [95, 97, 99]. In a study exploring the optimal conditions for long-term preservation of corneal stromal lenticules, Liu et al. preserved corneal stromal lenticules by placing them in glycerol at − 80 °C for 4 weeks, and showed that glycerol-preserved lenticules displayed a collagen fiber structure similar to that of the fresh lenticules [93]. Shang et al. classified the 132 corneal stromal lenticules removed from SMILE into a fresh group, a pure glycerol − 78 °C preservation group, and 0.1% SDS decellularization group, and performed immunohistochemistry, Western blot, transmission electron microscopy observation, and nanoindentation detection. He found that fresh corneal stromal lenticules taken out during SMILE expressed HLA-class I and HLA-class II antigens. There was a risk of graft rejection for immediate reuse, while preservation in pure glycerol at − 78 °C was an ideal method to reduce the expression of antigens [100]. Xia et al. explored the effects of different temperatures (including room temperature, 4, − 20, and − 80 °C) and auxiliary dehydrating material, silica gel, on glycerol-preserved SMILE lenticules, and concluded that − 80 °C glycerol with or without silica gel conditions maintained similar transparency as fresh lenticules, while the immunogenicity of the lenticules was reduced [94, 101].

How to standardize the transfer, preservation, transportation and use of the lenticules needs requires further investigations with more comprehensive and in-depth research. This will lead to a broader application, bringing light and hope to more patients with corneal disease.

References

1. Friedlander MH, Rich LF, Werblin TP, Kaufman HE, Granet N. Keratophakia using preserved lenticules. Ophthalmology. 1980;87:687–92. https://doi.org/10.1016/s0161-6420(80)35186-5.
2. Troutman RC, Swinger C. Refractive keratoplasty: keratophakia and keratomileusis. Trans Am Ophthalmol Soc. 1978;76:329–39.
3. Troutman RC, Swinger C, Goldstein M. Keratophakia update. Ophthalmology. 1981;88:36–8. https://doi.org/10.1016/s0161-6420(81)35087-8.
4. Barraquer JI. Method for cutting lamellar grafts in frozen cornea. New orientation for refractive surgery. Arch Soc Am Oftalmol Optom. 1958;1:271–286.
5. Barraquer JI. Basis of refractive keratoplasty–1967. Refract Corneal Surg. 1989;5:179–93.
6. Maguen E, Pinhas S, Verity SM, Nesburn AB. Keratophakia with lyophilized cornea lathed at room temperature: new techniques and experimental surgical results. Ophthalmic Surg. 1983;14:759–62.
7. Swinger CA, Barraquer JI. Keratophakia and keratomileusis–clinical results. Ophthalmology. 1981;88:709–15. https://doi.org/10.1016/s0161-6420(81)34958-6.
8. Friedlander MH, Werblin TP, Kaufman HE, Granet NS. Clinical results of keratophakia and keratomileusis. Ophthalmology. 1981;88:716–20. https://doi.org/10.1016/s0161-6420(81)34957-4.
9. Friedlander MH, Safir A, McDonald MB, Kaufman HE, Granet N. Update on keratophakia. Ophthalmology. 1983;90:365–8. https://doi.org/10.1016/s0161-6420(83)34561-9.
10. Taylor DM, Stern AL, Romanchuk KG. Keratophakia: clinical evaluation. Trans Am Ophthalmol Soc. 1981;79:47–63.
11. Taylor DM, Stern AL, Romanchuk KG, Keilson LR. Keratophakia. Clinical evaluation. Ophthalmology. 1981;88:1141–50.
12. Villaseãor, RA Keratophakia. Long-term results. Ophthalmology. 1983;90:673–5. https://doi.org/10.1016/s0161-6420(83)34515-2
13. Sekundo W, Kunert KS, Blum M. Small incision corneal refractive surgery using the small incision lenticule extraction (SMILE) procedure for the correction of myopia and myopic

astigmatism: results of a 6 month prospective study. Br J Ophthalmol. 2011;95:335–9. https://doi.org/10.1136/bjo.2009.174284.

14. Shah R, Shah S, Sengupta S. Results of small incision lenticule extraction: All-in-one femtosecond laser refractive surgery. J Cataract Refract Surg. 2011;37:127–37. https://doi.org/10.1016/j.jcrs.2010.07.033.
15. Hjortdal J, Vestergaard AH, Ivarsen A, Ragunathan S, Asp S. Predictors for the outcome of small-incision lenticule extraction for Myopia. J Refract Surg. 2012;28:865–71. https://doi.org/10.3928/1081597x-20121115-01.
16. Ziebarth NM, Lorenzo MA, Chow J, Cabot F, Spooner GJ, Dishler J, Hjortdal J, Yoo SH. Surface quality of human corneal lenticules after SMILE assessed using environmental scanning electron microscopy. J Refract Surg. 2014;30:388–93. https://doi.org/10.3928/1081597x-20140513-01.
17. Riau AK, Angunawela RI, Chaurasia SS, Tan DT, Mehta JS. Effect of different femtosecond laser-firing patterns on collagen disruption during refractive lenticule extraction. J Cataract Refract Surg. 2012;38:1467–75. https://doi.org/10.1016/j.jcrs.2012.03.037.
18. Pradhan KR, Reinstein DZ, Carp GI, Archer TJ, Gobbe M, Gurung R. Femtosecond laser-assisted keyhole endokeratophakia: correction of hyperopia by implantation of an allogeneic lenticule obtained by SMILE from a myopic donor. J Refract Surg. 2013;29:777–82. https://doi.org/10.3928/1081597x-20131021-07.
19. Ganesh S, Brar S, Rao PA. Cryopreservation of extracted corneal lenticules after small incision lenticule extraction for potential use in human subjects. Cornea. 2014;33:1355–62. https://doi.org/10.1097/ico.0000000000000276.
20. Sun L, Yao P, Li M, Shen Y, Zhao J, Zhou X. The safety and predictability of implanting autologous lenticule obtained by SMILE for hyperopia. J Refract Surg. 2015;31:374–9. https://doi.org/10.3928/1081597x-20150521-03.
21. Ganesh S, Brar S. Femtosecond intrastromal lenticular implantation combined with accelerated collagen cross-linking for the treatment of keratoconus-initial clinical result in 6 eyes. Cornea. 2015;34:1331–9. https://doi.org/10.1097/ico.0000000000000539.
22. Jacob S, Kumar DA, Agarwal A, Agarwal A, Aravind R, Saijimol AI. Preliminary evidence of successful near vision enhancement with a new technique: PrEsbyopic Allogenic Refractive Lenticule (PEARL) corneal inlay using a SMILE Lenticule. J Refract Surg. 2017;33:224–9. https://doi.org/10.3928/1081597x-20170111-03.
23. Moshirfar M, Shah TJ, Masud M, Fanning T, Linn SH, Ronquillo Y, Hoopes PCS. A modified small-incision lenticule intrastromal keratoplasty (sLIKE) for the correction of high hyperopia: a description of a new surgical technique and comparison to lenticule intrastromal keratoplasty (LIKE). Med Hypothesis Discov Innov Ophthalmol. 2018;7:48–56.
24. Liu S, Wei R, Choi J, Li M, Zhou X. Visual outcomes after implantation of allogenic lenticule in a 100-μm pocket for moderate to high hyperopia: 2-year results. J Refract Surg. 2021;37:734–40. https://doi.org/10.3928/1081597x-20210730-02.
25. Jiang Y, Li Y, Yang S, Lu TC. Tuck-in Lamellar keratoplasty with an lenticule obtained by small incision lenticule extraction for treatment of Post-LASIK Ectasia. Sci Rep. 2017;7:17806. https://doi.org/10.1038/s41598-017-18201-4.
26. Hashemi H, Fotouhi A, Yekta A, Pakzad R, Ostadimoghaddam H, Khabazkhoob M. Global and regional estimates of prevalence of refractive errors: Systematic review and meta-analysis. J Curr Ophthalmol. 2018;30:3–22. https://doi.org/10.1016/j.joco.2017.08.009
27. Hyman L. Myopic and hyperopic refractive error in adults: an overview. Ophthalmic Epidemiol. 2007;14:192–7. https://doi.org/10.1080/09286580701535517.
28. Llorente L, Barbero S, Merayo J, Marcos S. Total and corneal optical aberrations induced by laser in situ keratomileusis for hyperopia. J Refract Surg. 2004;20:203–16. https://doi.org/10.3928/1081-597x-20040501-03.
29. Zadok D, Maskaleris G, Montes M, Shah S, Garcia V, Chayet A. Hyperopic laser in situ keratomileusis with the Nidek EC-5000 excimer laser. Ophthalmology. 2000;107:1132–7. https://doi.org/10.1016/s0161-6420(00)00097-x.

30. Moshirfar M, Desautels JD, Walker BD, Murri MS, Birdsong OC, Hoopes PCS. Mechanisms of optical regression following corneal laser refractive surgery: epithelial and stromal responses. Med Hypothesis Discov Innov Ophthalmol. 2018;7:1–9.
31. Reinstein DZ, Carp GI, Archer TJ, Buick T, Gobbe M, Rowe EL, Jukic M, Brandon E, Moore J, Moore T. LASIK for the correction of high hyperopic astigmatism with epithelial thickness monitoring. J Refract Surg. 2017;33:314–21. https://doi.org/10.3928/1081597x-20170111-04.
32. Reinstein DZ, Pradhan KR, Carp GI, Archer TJ, Day AC, Sekundo W, Dhungana P. Small incision lenticule extraction for hyperopia: 3-month refractive and visual outcomes. J Refract Surg. 2019;35:24–30. https://doi.org/10.3928/1081597x-20181025-01.
33. Pradhan KR, Reinstein DZ, Carp GI, Archer TJ, Dhungana P. Small Incision Lenticule Extraction (SMILE) for hyperopia: 12-month refractive and visual outcomes. J Refract Surg. 2019;35:442–50. https://doi.org/10.3928/1081597x-20190529-01.
34. Benda F, Filipová L, Filipec M. Correction of moderate to high hyperopia with an implantable collamer lens: medium-term results. J Refract Surg. 2014;30:526–33. https://doi.org/10.3928/1081597x-20140711-05.
35. Bartels MC, Santana NT, Budo C, van Rij G, Mulder PG, Luyten GP. Toric phakic intraocular lens for the correction of hyperopia and astigmatism. J Cataract Refract Surg. 2006;32:243–9. https://doi.org/10.1016/j.jcrs.2005.12.083.
36. Riau AK, Liu YC, Yam GHF, Mehta JS. Stromal keratophakia: corneal inlay implantation. Prog Retin Eye Res. 2020;75:100780. https://doi.org/10.1016/j.preteyeres.2019.100780.
37. Moarefi MA, Bafna S, Wiley W. A review of presbyopia treatment with corneal inlays. Ophthalmol Ther. 2017;6:55–65. https://doi.org/10.1007/s40123-017-0085-7.
38. Li M, Li M, Sun L, Ni K, Zhou X. Predictive formula for refraction of autologous lenticule implantation for hyperopia correction. J Refract Surg. 2017;33:827–33. https://doi.org/10.3928/1081597x-20171016-01.
39. Moshirfar M, Hopping GC, Somani AN, Vaidyanathan U, Liu H, Barnes JR, Linn S, Ronquillo YC, Hoopes PC. Human allograft refractive lenticular implantation for high hyperopic correction. J Cataract Refract Surg. 2020;46:305–11. https://doi.org/10.1097/j.jcrs.0000000000000011.
40. Wu J, Xiong L, Wang Z, Reinstein DZ, Vida RS, Archer TJ. Correction of moderate to high hyperopia with implantation of an allogeneic refractive lenticule. J Refract Surg. 2020;36:772–9. https://doi.org/10.3928/1081597x-20200826-01.
41. Liu S, Zhang X, Yu L, Li M, Zhou X. Comparison of optical zone decentration following FS-LIKE and SMI-LIKE for correcting hyperopia. J Refract Surg. 2022;38:184–90. https://doi.org/10.3928/1081597x-20211213-03.
42. Zhang J, Zhou Y. Small incision lenticule extraction (SMILE) combined with allogeneic intrastromal lenticule inlay for hyperopia with astigmatism. PLoS ONE. 2021;16:e0257667. https://doi.org/10.1371/journal.pone.0257667.
43. Lazaridis A, Reinstein DZ, Archer TJ, Schulze S, Sekundo W. Refractive lenticule transplantation for correction of iatrogenic hyperopia and high astigmatism after LASIK. J Refract Surg. 2016;32:780–6. https://doi.org/10.3928/1081597x-20160726-01.
44. Stodulka P, Hjortdal J, Slovak M. Intrastromal lenticule rotation for the treatment of high astigmatism. J Refract Surg. 2020;36:415–8. https://doi.org/10.3928/1081597x-20200506-02.
45. Damgaard IB, Ivarsen A, Hjortdal J. Intrastromal lenticule rotation for treatment of astigmatism up to 10.00 diopters ex vivo in human corneas. J Refract Surg. 2019;35:451–458. https://doi.org/10.3928/1081597x-20190618-02
46. Liu S, Zhang X, Zhou X. Toric lenticule implantation for correction of hyperopia and astigmatism following small incision lenticule intrastromal Keratoplasty with the triple marking method. J Refract Surg. 2022;38:82–8. https://doi.org/10.3928/1081597x-20211117-01.
47. Shah R. History and results; indications and contraindications of SMILE compared with LASIK. Asia Pac J Ophthalmol (Phila). 2019;8:371–6. https://doi.org/10.1097/01.APO.0000580132.98159.fa.

48. Lindstrom RL, Macrae SM, Pepose JS, Hoopes PC Sr. Corneal inlays for presbyopia correction. Curr Opin Ophthalmol. 2013;24:281–7. https://doi.org/10.1097/ICU.0b013e328362293e.
49. Wolffsohn JS, Davies LN. Presbyopia: effectiveness of correction strategies. Prog Retin Eye Res. 2019;68:124–43. https://doi.org/10.1016/j.preteyeres.2018.09.004.
50. Furlan WD, García-Delpech S, Udaondo P, Remón L, Ferrando V, Monsoriu JA. Diffractive corneal inlay for presbyopia. J Biophotonics. 2017;10:1110–4. https://doi.org/10.1002/jbio.201600320.
51. Tomita M, Kanamori T, Waring GOt, Yukawa S, Yamamoto T, Sekiya K, Tsuru T. Simultaneous corneal inlay implantation and laser in situ keratomileusis for presbyopia in patients with hyperopia, myopia, or emmetropia: six-month results, J Cataract Refract Surg. 2012; 38:495–506. https://doi.org/10.1016/j.jcrs.2011.10.033
52. Konstantopoulos A, Mehta JS. Surgical compensation of presbyopia with corneal inlays. Expert Rev Med Devices. 2015;12:341–52. https://doi.org/10.1586/17434440.2015.1007124.
53. Whitman J, Dougherty PJ, Parkhurst GD, Olkowski J, Slade SG, Hovanesian J, Chu R, Dishler J, Tran DB, Lehmann R, Carter H, Steinert RF, Koch DD. Treatment of presbyopia in emmetropes using a shape-changing corneal inlay: one-year clinical outcomes. Ophthalmology. 2016;123:466–75. https://doi.org/10.1016/j.ophtha.2015.11.011.
54. Fenner BJ, Liu YC, Koh SK, Gao Y, Deng L, Beuerman RW, Zhou L, Theng JTS, Mehta JS. Mediators of corneal haze following implantation of presbyopic corneal inlays. Invest Ophthalmol Vis Sci. 2019;60:868–76. https://doi.org/10.1167/iovs.18-25761.
55. Kiliç A, et al. Excimer laser shaped allograft corneal inlays for presbyopia: initial clinical results of a pilot study. J Clin Exp Ophthalmol. 2019;10. https://doi.org/10.4172/2155-9570.1000799
56. Liu YC, Teo EPW, Ang HP, Seah XY, Lwin NC, Yam GHF, Mehta JS. Biological corneal inlay for presbyopia derived from small incision lenticule extraction (SMILE). Sci Rep. 2018;8:1831. https://doi.org/10.1038/s41598-018-20267-7.
57. Lim CH, Riau AK, Lwin NC, Chaurasia SS, Tan DT, Mehta JS. LASIK following small incision lenticule extraction (SMILE) lenticule re-implantation: a feasibility study of a novel method for treatment of presbyopia. PLoS ONE. 2013;8:e83046. https://doi.org/10.1371/journal.pone.0083046.
58. Salomão MQ, Hofling-Lima AL, Gomes Esporcatte LP, Correa FF, Lopes B, Sena, Jr. N, Dawson DG, Ambrósio, Jr. R. Ectatic diseases. Exp Eye Res. 2021; 202:108347. https://doi.org/10.1016/j.exer.2020.108347
59. Santodomingo-Rubido J, Carracedo G, Suzaki A, Villa-Collar C, Vincent SJ, Wolffsohn JS. Keratoconus: an updated review. Cont Lens Anterior Eye. 2022;45:101559. https://doi.org/10.1016/j.clae.2021.101559.
60. Dawson DG, Randleman JB, Grossniklaus HE, O'Brien TP, Dubovy SR, Schmack I, Stulting RD, Edelhauser HF. Corneal ectasia after excimer laser keratorefractive surgery: histopathology, ultrastructure, and pathophysiology. Ophthalmology. 2008;115:2181-2191.e1. https://doi.org/10.1016/j.ophtha.2008.06.008.
61. Santhiago MR, Smadja D, Gomes BF, Mello GR, Monteiro ML, Wilson SE, Randleman JB. Association between the percent tissue altered and post-laser in situ keratomileusis ectasia in eyes with normal preoperative topography. Am J Ophthalmol. 2014;158:87-95.e1. https://doi.org/10.1016/j.ajo.2014.04.002.
62. Randleman JB, Woodward M, Lynn MJ, Stulting RD. Risk assessment for ectasia after corneal refractive surgery. Ophthalmology. 2008;115:37–50. https://doi.org/10.1016/j.ophtha.2007.03.073.
63. Rodrigues M, Nirankari V, Rajagopalan S, Jones K, Funderburgh J. Clinical and histopathologic changes in the host cornea after Epikeratoplasty for Keratoconus. Am J Ophthalmol. 1992;114:161–170. https://doi.org/10.1016/S0002-9394(14)73980-7
64. Zhao J, Sun L, Shen Y, Tian M, Yao P, Zhou X. Using donor lenticules obtained through SMILE for an Epikeratophakia technique combined with phototherapeutic keratectomy. J Refract Surg. 2016;32:840–5. https://doi.org/10.3928/1081597x-20160920-01.

65. Li M, Zhao F, Li M, Knorz MC, Zhou X. Treatment of corneal ectasia by implantation of an allogenic corneal lenticule. J Refract Surg. 2018;34:347–50. https://doi.org/10.3928/1081597x-20180323-01.
66. Mastropasqua L, Nubile M, Salgari N, Mastropasqua R. Femtosecond laser-assisted stromal lenticule addition keratoplasty for the treatment of advanced keratoconus: a preliminary study. J Refract Surg. 2018;34:36–44. https://doi.org/10.3928/1081597x-20171004-04.
67. Nubile M, Salgari N, Mehta JS, Calienno R, Erroi E, Bondì J, Lanzini M, Liu YC, Mastropasqua L. Epithelial and stromal remodelling following femtosecond laser-assisted stromal lenticule addition keratoplasty (SLAK) for keratoconus. Sci Rep. 2021;11:2293. https://doi.org/10.1038/s41598-021-81626-5.
68. Li M, Wei R, Yang W, Shang J, Fu D, Xia F, Choi J, Zhou X. Femtosecond laser-assisted allogenic lenticule implantation for corneal ectasia after LASIK: A 3-year in vivo confocal microscopic investigation. J Refract Surg. 1995;36(2020):714–22. https://doi.org/10.3928/1081597X-20200826-02.
69. Nakamura H, Riley F, Sakai H, Rademaker W, Yue BY, Edward DP. Histopathological and immunohistochemical studies of lenticules after epikeratoplasty for keratoconus. Br J Ophthalmol. 2005;89:841–6. https://doi.org/10.1136/bjo.2004.054684.
70. Kymionis GD, Portaliou DM, Diakonis VF, Kounis GA, Panagopoulou SI, Grentzelos MA. Corneal collagen cross-linking with riboflavin and ultraviolet-A irradiation in patients with thin corneas. Am J Ophthalmol. 2012;153:24–8. https://doi.org/10.1016/j.ajo.2011.05.036.
71. Sachdev MS, Gupta D, Sachdev G, Sachdev R. Tailored stromal expansion with a refractive lenticule for crosslinking the ultrathin cornea. J Cataract Refract Surg. 2015;41:918–23. https://doi.org/10.1016/j.jcrs.2015.04.007.
72. Doroodgar F, Jabbarvand M, Niazi S, Karimian F, Niazi F, Sanginabadi A, Ghoreishi M, Alinia C, Hashemi H, Alió JL. Customized stromal lenticule implantation for keratoconus. J Refract Surg. 2020;36:786–94. https://doi.org/10.3928/1081597x-20201005-01.
73. Jin H, He M, Liu H, Zhong X, Wu J, Liu L, Ding H, Zhang C, Zhong X. Small-incision femtosecond laser-assisted intracorneal concave lenticule implantation in patients with keratoconus. Cornea. 2019;38:446–53. https://doi.org/10.1097/ico.0000000000001877.
74. Jhanji V, Young AL, Mehta JS, Sharma N, Agarwal T, Vajpayee RB. Management of corneal perforation. Surv Ophthalmol. 2011;56:522–38. https://doi.org/10.1016/j.survophthal.2011.06.003.
75. Sandinha T, Zaher SS, Roberts F, Devlin HC, Dhillon B, Ramaesh K. Superior forniceal conjunctival advancement pedicles (SFCAP) in the management of acute and impending corneal perforations. Eye (Lond). 2006;20:84–9. https://doi.org/10.1038/sj.eye.6701814.
76. Fernandes M, Sridhar MS, Sangwan VS, Rao GN. Amniotic membrane transplantation for ocular surface reconstruction. Cornea. 2005;24:643–53. https://doi.org/10.1097/01.ico.0000151501.80952.c5.
77. Wu F, Jin X, Xu Y, Yang Y. Treatment of corneal perforation with lenticules from small incision lenticule extraction surgery: a preliminary study of 6 patients. Cornea. 2015;34:658–63. https://doi.org/10.1097/ico.0000000000000397.
78. Bhandari V, Ganesh S, Brar S, Pandey R. Application of the SMILE-derived glued lenticule patch graft in microperforations and partial-thickness corneal defects. Cornea. 2016;35:408–12. https://doi.org/10.1097/ico.0000000000000741.
79. Song YJ, Kim S, Yoon GJ. Case series: use of stromal lenticule as patch graft. Am J Ophthalmol Case Rep. 2018;12:79–82. https://doi.org/10.1016/j.ajoc.2018.09.009.
80. Wan Q, Tang J, Han Y, Ye H. Surgical treatment of corneal dermoid by using intrastromal lenticule obtained from small-incision lenticule extraction. Int Ophthalmol. 2020;40:43–9. https://doi.org/10.1007/s10792-019-01201-w.
81. Liu JL, Ji JY, Ye Q, Wei LQ, Zhong X, Jiang LZ, Zeng J. Treatment of corneal dermoid with lenticules from small incision lenticule extraction surgery: a surgery assisted by fibrin glue, Int J Ophthalmol. 2023;16:547–553. https://doi.org/10.18240/ijo.2023.04.08

82. He N, Song W, Gao Y. Treatment of Mooren's ulcer coexisting with a pterygium using an intrastromal lenticule obtained from small-incision lenticule extraction: case report and literature review. J Int Med Res. 2021;49:3000605211020246. https://doi.org/10.1177/03000605211020246.
83. Blum M, Lauer AS, Kunert KS, Sekundo W. 10-year results of small incision lenticule extraction. J Refract Surg. 2019;35:618–23. https://doi.org/10.3928/1081597x-20190826-02.
84. Zhao J, Zhao F, Huang J, Xu H, Chen Y, Zhou X. Two-year outcome of a patient treated with phototherapeutic keratectomy and autologous SMILE lenticule transplantation for flap-related complications following LASIK. J Refract Surg. 2018;34:281–5. https://doi.org/10.3928/1081597x-20180130-01.
85. Riau AK, Angunawela RI, Chaurasia SS, Lee WS, Tan DT, Mehta JS. Reversible femtosecond laser-assisted myopia correction: a non-human primate study of lenticule re-implantation after refractive lenticule extraction. PLoS ONE. 2013;8:e67058. https://doi.org/10.1371/journal.pone.0067058.
86. Liang G, Wang L, Pan Z, Zhang F. Comparison of the different preservative methods for refractive lenticules following SMILE. Curr Eye Res. 2019;44:832–9. https://doi.org/10.1080/02713683.2019.1597890.
87. Walkenbach RJ, Corwin JG, Ye GS. Corneal function after storage in commercial eye bank media. Invest Ophthalmol Vis Sci. 1991;32:1551–7.
88. Weckbach LS, Bloom HR, Wander AH, Staneck JL. Survival of Streptococcus pneumoniae in corneal storage media. Cornea. 1992;11:200–3.
89. Chang SW, Wang YH, Pang JH. The effects of epithelial viability on stromal keratocyte apoptosis in porcine corneas stored in Optisol-GS. Cornea. 2006;25:78–84. https://doi.org/10.1097/01.ico.0000160970.58330.09.
90. Komuro A, Hodge DO, Gores GJ, Bourne WM. Cell death during corneal storage at 4 degrees C. Invest Ophthalmol Vis Sci. 1999;40:2827–32.
91. Bandeira F, Yam GH, Liu YC, Devarajan K, Mehta JS. Three-dimensional neurite characterization of small incision lenticule extraction derived lenticules. Invest Ophthalmol Vis Sci. 2019;60:4408–15. https://doi.org/10.1167/iovs.19-27566.
92. Yang J, Cai N, Zhai H, Zhang J, Zhu Y, Zhang L. Natural zwitterionic betaine enables cells to survive ultrarapid cryopreservation. Sci Rep. 2016;6:37458. https://doi.org/10.1038/srep37458.
93. Rall WF, Fahy GM. Ice-free cryopreservation of mouse embryos at -196 degrees C by vitrification. Nature. 1985;313:573–5. https://doi.org/10.1038/313573a0.
94. Liu YC, Williams GP, George BL, Soh YQ, Seah XY, Peh GSL, Yam GHF, Mehta JS. Corneal lenticule storage before reimplantation. Mol Vis. 2017;23:753–64.
95. Xia F, Zhao J, Fu D, Qin B, Chen Z, Zhao Y, Shen Y, Hou J, Zhou X. Comparison of the effects of temperature and dehydration mode on glycerin-based approaches to SMILE-derived lenticule preservation. Cornea. 2022;41:470–7. https://doi.org/10.1097/ico.0000000000002846.
96. Saegeman VS, Ectors NL, Lismont D, Verduyckt B, Verhaegen J. Short- and long-term bacterial inhibiting effect of high concentrations of glycerol used in the preservation of skin allografts. Burns. 2008;34:205–11. https://doi.org/10.1016/j.burns.2007.02.009.
97. van Baare J, Ligtvoet EE, Middelkoop E. Microbiological evaluation of glycerolized cadaveric donor skin. Transplantation. 1998;65:966–70. https://doi.org/10.1097/00007890-199804150-00017.
98. Giovani AM, Croci AT, Oliveira CR, Filippi RZ, Santos LA, Maragni GG, Albhy TM. Comparative study of cryopreserved bone tissue and tissue preserved in a 98% glycerol solution. Clinics (Sao Paulo). 2006;61:565–70. https://doi.org/10.1590/s1807-59322006000600013.
99. Tomford WW. Bone allografts: past, present and future. Cell Tissue Bank. 2000;1:105–9. https://doi.org/10.1023/a:1010158731885.
100. Sumida S. Transfusion and transplantation of cryopreserved cells and tissues. Cell Tissue Bank. 2006;7:265–305. https://doi.org/10.1007/s10561-006-9005-0.

101. Shang Y, Li Y, Wang Z, Sun X, Zhang F. Risk evaluation of human corneal stromal lenticules from SMILE for reuse. J Refract Surg. 2021;37:32–40. https://doi.org/10.3928/1081597x-20201030-03.
102. Xia F, Zhao J, Fu D, Xu Y, Yao P, Li M, Aruma A, Zhou X. Optical transmittance and ultrastructure of SMILE-derived lenticules subjected to three different preservative methods. Exp Eye Res. 2020;201:108357. https://doi.org/10.1016/j.exer.2020.108357.

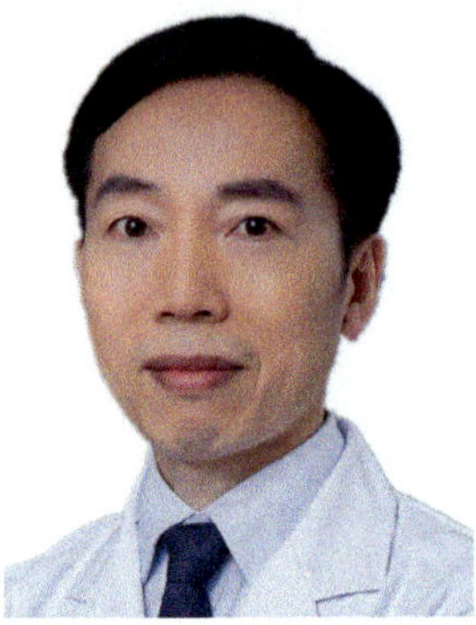

Prof. Xingtao Zhou, PhD is a distinguished chief ophthalmologist, post-doctor of ophthalmology, PhD supervisor, and professor of ophthalmology at EENT Hospital of Fudan University, China. He serves as the President of EENT Hospital and Director of the Shanghai Research Center of Ophthalmology and Optometry. He also holds the position of Deputy Head of the National Expert Group on Comprehensive Prevention and Control of Myopia in Children and Adolescents. Prof. Zhou is a section editor for APJO and a reviewer for prestigious journals such as The Lancet, Ophthalmology, AJO, JRS, JCRS, IOVS, BJO, etc. Renowned for his pioneering work in myopia prevention and laser treatment of refractive errors, Prof. Zhou has published over 200 SCI articles and holds more than 30 patents. He has been the principal investigator for 15 major research projects and edited 8 professional books. Notably, he performed the first SMILE procedure in China and has completed over 45,000 cases. He also performed the first case of TICL, epikeratophakia with SMILE lenticule. His innovative contributions to surgical equipment have earned him the National Invention Award and the National Science and Technology Progress Award. Prof. Zhou's dedication to public education is evident in his establishment of the Asian-Pacific ICL/TICL Education Center and the annual "Care for Myopia, Smile Symposium." His initiatives in myopia management span all age groups, from children to the elderly. His numerous accolades include the titles of Young and Middle-aged Experts with Outstanding Contributions to National Health, Outstanding Doctors of China, and Eye Health Hero, alongside multiple national and regional awards for science and technology progress.

Corneal Stromal Lenticule Rotation for High Astigmatism Correction

21

Pavel Stodulka and Walter Sekundo

21.1 Introduction

Lenticule rotation is a new method of high astigmatism correction utilizing corneal stromal lenticule rotation. The spherocylindrical lenticule is not extracted from the cornea like in SMILE surgery but left in situ and rotated 90° to compensate for the astigmatism.

Refractive surgery of high astigmatism is a challenging task. It can be performed by altering the corneal curvature, by intraocular procedure or a combination of both.

The **corneal** refractive surgeries can be classified into four basic categories: incisions, laser ablation and stromal lenticule extraction currently coined "Keratorefractive Lenticule Extraction" = KLEX, but for the majority of ophthalmologists known as SMILE, because of the long-standing record of this very first method of lenticule extraction and corneal inlay implantation (allograft, synthetic and modified xenograft).

The **intraocular** procedures are divided into two groups: toric phakic intraocular lens implantation and cataract surgery or refractive lens exchange with toric intraocular lens implantation.

A **combination** of corneal and intraocular surgeries can be phakic lens implantation or crystalline lens surgery typically combined **simultaneously** with one of

P. Stodulka (✉)
Gemini Eye Clinics, Zlín, Czech Republic
e-mail: stodulka@lasik.cz

W. Sekundo
Department of Ophthalmology, Philipps University of Marburg, Marburg, Germany

W. Sekundo and F. M. Wagner (eds.), *Femtosecond Laser Assisted Lenticule Extraction*,
https://doi.org/10.1007/978-3-031-60424-9_21

the astigmatic corneal incisions. Alternatively, the refractive outcome of intraocular surgery can be adjusted **post-surgery** using laser photorefractive keratectomy (PRK), laser in situ keratectomy (Lasik) or corneal lenticule extraction (KLEX).

The main challenges of **high astigmatism surgical correction** are precision and stability. By precision, it is meant astigmatism axis management and amount of astigmatism correction. Stability is concerned because corneas with high astigmatism are often less stable even without any surgery. Since high astigmatism laser surgical correction requires large incisions, large amount of laser tissue ablation or thick intrastromal lenticule extraction resulting in thin cornea and thin residual stromal thickness, these procedures may weaken the cornea and thus compromise long-term corneal stability.

21.2 Lenticule Rotation Inside of the Pocket

SMILE has been used for the management of myopia and myopic astigmatism for many years [1], and it was recently also investigated for hyperopia and hyperopic astigmatism [2, 3]. Hjortdal and his colleagues at the Aarhus University Hospital in Denmark introduced a theoretical innovative concept for high astigmatism correction based on corneal stromal lenticule rotation [4] and verified this concept on ex vivo human corneas for high astigmatism correction up to 10 cylindrical diopters.

The spherocylindrical lenticule created by a femtosecond laser (Fig. 21.1) is not extracted like in KLEX surgery but rather rotated by 90° within the corneal stromal pocket and left in situ.

This astigmatic lenticule rotation results in tissue addition in steep meridian at the periphery of optical zone and tissue subtraction in the flat meridian. The lenticule is shaped with a femtosecond laser with parameters set to approximately half

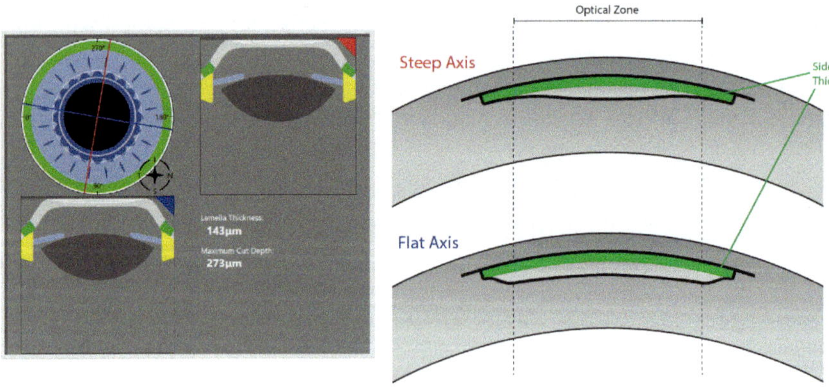

Fig. 21.1 Toric lenticule diagram

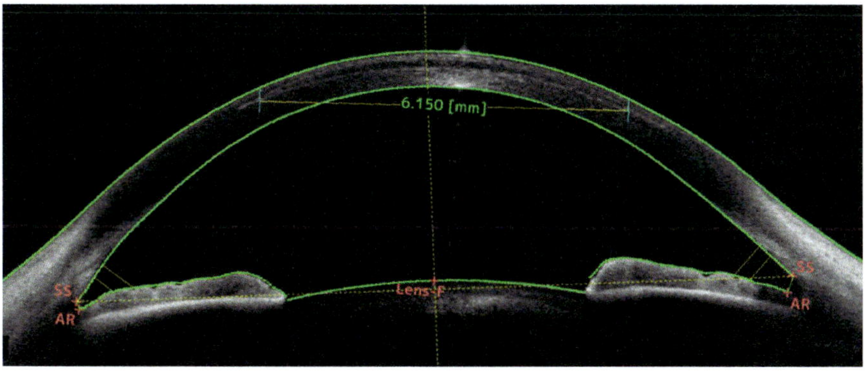

Fig. 21.2 Anterior segment OCT of cornea one week after lenticule rotation

of astigmatism intended to be corrected. Lenticule 90° rotation results in approximately half of the astigmatism corneal power decrease in the steep meridian and approximately half of the astigmatism corneal power increase in the flat meridian. The corneal curvature changes and astigmatism correction are caused by tissue redistribution. Since the lenticule is not extracted, there is no tissue removed, and therefore, the central corneal thickness is not reduced. Anterior segment OCT one week after lenticule rotation is shown in Fig. 21.2.

The impact on corneal stability should thus be significantly lower compared to conventional SMILE lenticule extraction surgery.

The lenticule can theoretically be later further rotated as a second procedure to finetune the refractive outcome of the first lenticule rotation. In addition, the lenticule can be either extracted achieving a partial correction or even rotated back if the patient is unhappy with the result. This makes the lenticule rotation a procedure open to adjustment or theoretically even reversal back to a preoperative state. Anyhow at our clinic, we typically adjust the refractive outcome of lenticule rotation by topoguided laser surface ablation (PRK) to correct the residual spherocylindrical refractive error and high-order aberrations as well which can result from uneven lenticule tissue distribution after its rotation.

Method

Corneal stromal lenticule rotation should be only performed on stable corneas with regular astigmatism with no signs of keratoconus or ectasia. Also, corneas thinner than 500 μm should be avoided.

The lenticule is created by a femtosecond laser with cap thickness of 110–160 μm. We have used typically 6.5-mm optical zone but the optimal optical zone diameter was not yet systematically determined. Since the lenticule rotation is a delicate and challenging maneuver, it is better to have a thicker lenticule which is easier to manipulate. Therefore, we used the maximal lenticule edge thickness allowed by a given femtosecond laser. With VisuMax 500 (Carl Zeiss Meditec AG, Germany) femtosecond laser, the maximal edge thickness was set to 30 μm. With

Z8 (Ziemer Ophthalmic Systems, Switzerland) femtosecond laser using therapeutic lamella application software option, we increased the side cut height and therefore the lenticule edge thickness as high as 100 μm. It is surgically easier to rotate the lenticule with thicker edge, and it is also easier to spread the lenticule as evenly as possible after its rotation. Originally for the first cases, we created two incisions by femtosecond laser to facilitate lenticule rotation. After these initial cases, we continued with only one incision which I consider suitable for lenticule rotation.

The incision at 90° was opened by spatula. Both anterior and posterior lenticule surfaces were separated from the stromal bed by a rounded-tip spatula. Following this, the lenticule and the cap were marked at 90° axis by two overlapping radial marks created by forceps stained from the inside with corneal marking ink. Then the lenticule edges were separated from corneal stroma all around lenticule circumference, and the lenticule was rotated by 90° so both radial marks were 90° apart. Finally, the lenticule was fully unfolded as evenly as possible by spatula and by gently pushing through the overlying cap.

Post-operatively patients typically applied our routine topical medication for SMILE surgery which is tobramycin and dexamethason combined drops (Tobradex®, Alcon) three times a day for two weeks. It was then typically prolonged twice a day for one week and then one time a day for one week followed by fluorometholon (Flucon®, Alcon) twice a day for two weeks and concluded one time a day for another two weeks. Artificial tears or autologous serum eye drops were used in case of eye dryness. No systematic medication was used.

We performed the corneal stromal lenticule rotation in 28 eyes of 20 patients (ten males and ten females). All surgeries were performed by a single surgeon (PS). The average age of the patients was 27.7 years, with a median of 27.5 years, ranging from 18 to 45 years. Among the 28 eyes, 20 were amblyopic, accounting for 71% of the eyes.

Results

Median of the preoperative uncorrected distance visual acuity UDVA was 0.77 (IQR: 0.7, 0.8) logMAR and corrected distance visual acuity CDVA 0.11 (0.0, 0.22) logMAR. Median of the absolute preop. cylinder was 4.5 (3.25, 5.0) D and spherical equivalent 0.38 (− 0.47, 0.84) D. Following the lenticule rotation, the cohort showed a decrease in absolute cylinder to 1.13 (0.5, 2.2) D resulting in an improvement in UDVA to 0.41 (0.29, 0.6) logMAR. There was a slight worsening of CDVA with median 0.18 (0.14, 0.3) logMAR and noticeable myopic shift—median spherical equivalent after rotation was − 1.38 (− 1.94, − 0.28) D. Distribution of spherical equivalent preop. and at three months is shown in Fig. 21.3, UDVA and CDVA at Figs. 21.4 and 21.5.

Additionally, after lenticule rotation, 13 eyes which are 46% underwent subsequent corneal laser **surface ablation by photorefractive keratectomy (PRK)** to correct the residual refractive error. The laser correction was performed three months to two years after the lenticule rotation. These eyes corrected by laser improved UDVA from median of 0.6 (0.51, 0.92) logMAR to 0.19 (0.1, 0.34) logMAR. CDVA was almost unchanged with median 0.14 (0.11, 0.18) logMAR

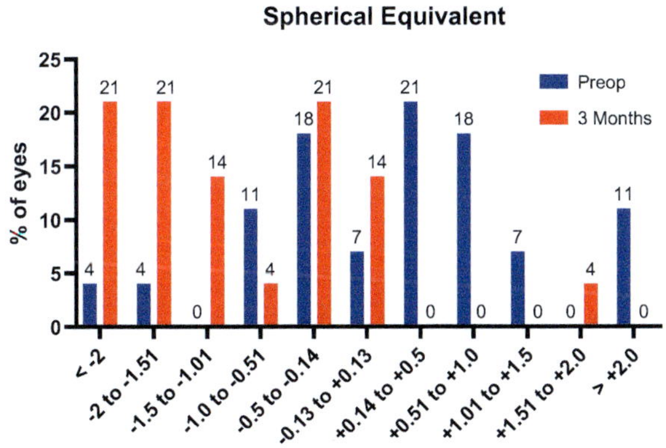

Fig. 21.3 Distribution of spherical equivalent after rotation

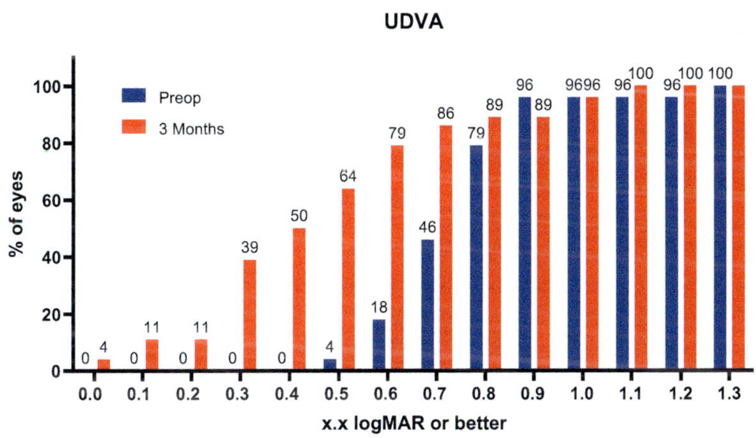

Fig. 21.4 Distribution of UDVA after rotation

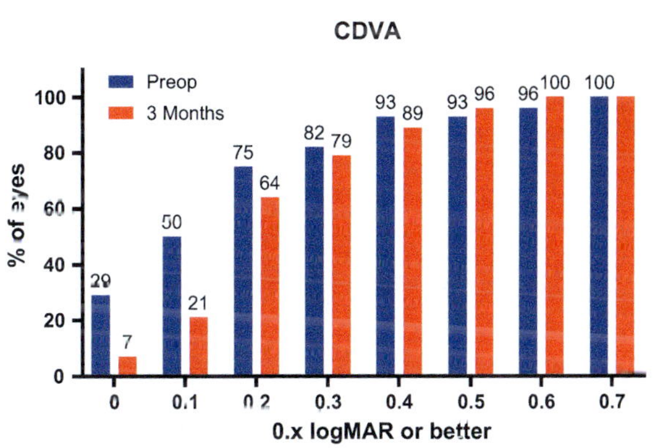

Fig. 21.5 Distribution of CDVA after rotation

Table 21.1 .

	Topoguided		Not topoguided	
	Before PRK	After PRK	Before PRK	After PRK
SE	– 1.88 (– 3.16, – 1.41)	0.0 (– 0.63, 0.41)	– 1.75 (– 2.31, – 1.09)	– 0.31 (– 0.97, – 0.06)
abs Cyl	1.63 (0.69, 3.0)	0.88 (0.0, 1.0)	1.25 (1.0, 1.94)	0.75 (0.5, 2.13)
UDVA	0.83 (0.58, 1.03)	0.19 (0.14, 0.31)	0.57 (0.2, 0.6)	0.21 (0.06, 0.38)
CDVA	0.17 (0.14, 0.27)	0.17 (0.14, 0.21)	0.11 (0.0, 0.13)	0.12 (0.0, 0.22)

before PRK and 0.17 (0.05, 0.2) logMAR 1–3 months after PRK. Median of the spherical equivalent of these cases corrected by PRK decreased from preoperative – 1.75 (– 2.66, – 1.34) D to – 0.25 (– 0.78, 0.28) D. The absolute preoperative cylinder 1.5 (1.0, 2.31) D decreased to 0.75 (0.5, 1.0) D.

Seven of these 13 eyes underwent topoguided PRK to correct also significant higher order aberrations. Difference between results in topoguided and not topoguided group is shown in Table 21.1.

Here are the **results of whole group** of patients after lenticule rotation and rotation followed by PRK. Median of spherical equivalent: – 0.31 (– 1.19 – 0.0) D, absolute cylinder: 0.75 (0.01–1.88) D, UDVA: 0.3 (0.11–0.49) logMAR and CDVA: 0.17 (0.09–0.3) logMAR (Figs. 21.6, 21.7, and 21.8).

I would like to share t**he world-first clinical case of SMILE lenticule rotation.**

A 31-year-old woman came was asked about the possibility to correct her high astigmatism by refractive surgery on her left, non-dominant, amblyopic eye with the refraction + 2.00 – 5.00 at 10°. Uncorrected distance visual acuity UDVA was 0.8 logMar and corrected distance visual acuity CDVA 0.7 logMAR. Her uncorrected near visual acuity UNVA was worse than Jaegar 13 (> 1.0 logMAR) and corrected near visual acuity CNVA Jaegar 13 (1.0 logMAR). The limited potential of refractive surgery to improve her vision because of amblyopia was explained to

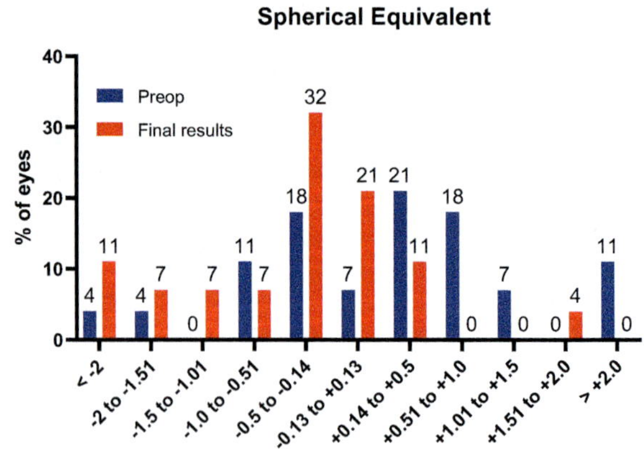

Fig. 21.6 Distribution of final spherical equivalent

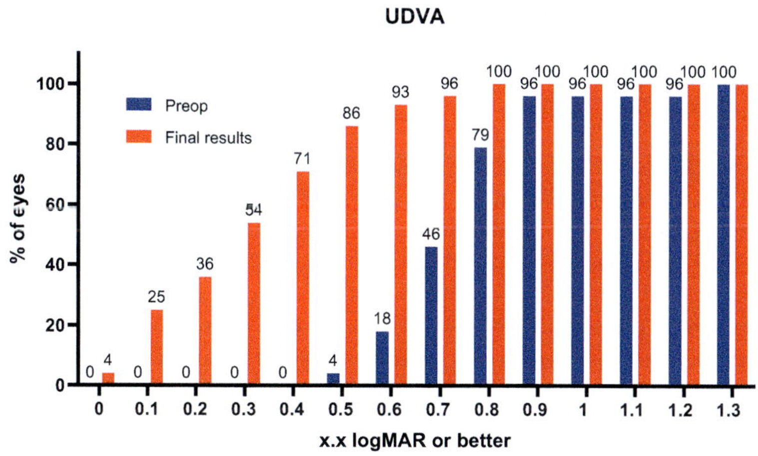

Fig. 21.7 Distribution of final UDVA

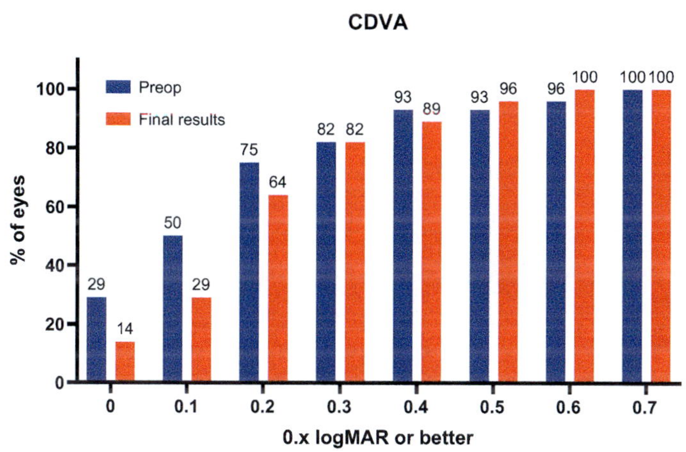

Fig. 21.8 Distribution of final CDVA

the patient. We decided to perform the first clinical case of corneal stromal lenticule rotation at this amblyopic eye to confirm we can clinically improve the shape of highly astigmatic cornea. The patient agreed with the procedure and signed the informed consent.

VisuMax 500 (Carl Zeiss Meditec AG, Germany) femtosecond laser system was used to create SMILE lenticule. The following parameters were set to the laser: refraction was set to − 3.00 − 3.00 at 10° as myopia with myopic astigmatism despite of patients mixed astigmatism to have thicker lenticule for easier manipulation during lenticule rotation, optical zone 6.5 mm, transition zone 0.1 mm, the minimum lenticule thickness of 30 μm and cap thickness of 130 μm with 7.0 mm in diameter. Two incisions 2.5 and 3.0 mm wide were created at 90° and 0° meridians, respectively. The second incision was created as a spare one to be used in case a surgeon needs extra access for easier lenticule manipulation but was not used.

One week after the surgery, the subjective astigmatism was 0 D. A significant myopic shift resulted in distance refraction − 4 D. Her UDVA stayed the same at 0.8 logMAR and CDVA improved to 0.5 logMAR. Keratometry astigmatism was 0.75 D. The patient noted slight uncorrected distance visual acuity UDVA improvement but a significant uncorrected UNVA reading improvement which was improved from preop. UNVA > 1.0 logMAR to 0.4 logMAR. Her preop. and one-week corneal topography is in Picture 3 (Figs. 21.9 and 21.10).

Her corneal incision, stromal pocket and lenticule edge are visible in Picture 4.

One month after surgery, subjective astigmatism remained 0 D. and distance spherical refraction − 3.75 D. Her UDVA and CDVA remained unchanged.

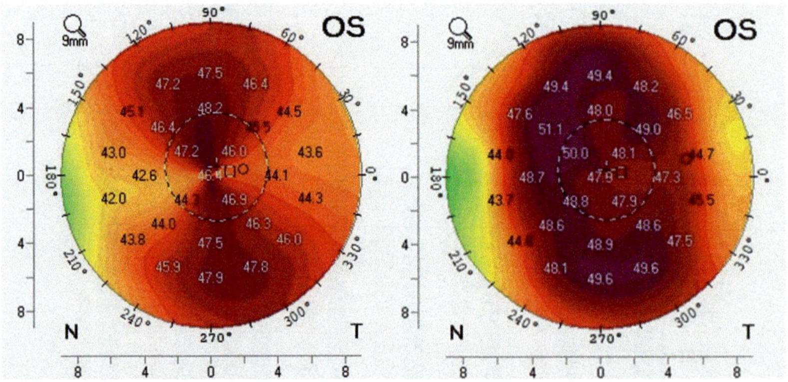

Fig. 21.9 Preoperative and one-week corneal topography

Fig. 21.10 Temporal incision, stromal pocket and lenticule edge

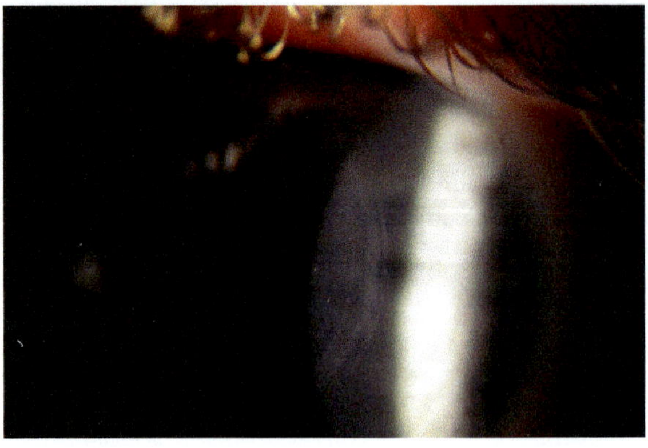

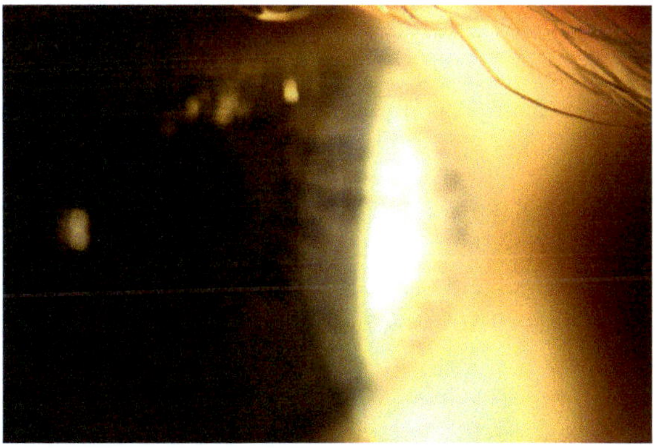

Fig. 21.11 Clear cornea with only temporal incision visible four years after surgery

Keratometry astigmatism was 0.25 D. Subjectively patient referred slight uncorrected distance visual acuity improvement but a significant uncorrected reading improvement and one-month UNVA achieved 0.3 logMAR.

One year post-op. of the subjective astigmatism remained 0 Dcyl. and distance spherical refraction is − 3.0 D. Her UDVA remained stable 0.8 logMAR and CDVA also remained stable 0.5 logMAR. For reading her UNVA is J5. The patient is subjectively very happy with especially with her near-reading vision. The one-year results confirm stability of lenticule rotation surgery.

Four-year follow-up shows stable refraction with subjective astigmatism 0 Dcyl. and distance spherical refraction − 3.5 D. Her UDVA remained stable 0.8 logMAR and CDVA is 0.6 logMAR. Her uncorrected reading UNVA is J6. The cornea remains clear as seen at Picture 5 (Fig. 21.11).

Central corneal thickness (CCT) slightly increased. Preoperative CCT was 520 μm and after the follow-up 532 and 535 μm at one week and one month, respectively, and 538 μm four years after surgery. The cornea remained clear throughout the follow-up period.

This was the world-first clinical case of astigmatism correction by corneal stromal lenticule rotation. We have published this case which despite of ambylopia demonstrated that the procedure is capable to correct both corneal and subjective astigmatism with a stable result [5].

Discussion

The **surgical manipulation** to rotate the lenticule is challenging. The lenticule was not taken out of the pocket at our reported series of surgeries, although it is possible to remove the lenticule and reinsert the lenticule in the desired 90° position as originally described by Hjortdal [4]. We have rotated the lenticule inside of the stromal pocket according to two radial marks. The advantage of this method over lenticule extraction and re-insertion is less manipulation and elimination of the risk to implant the lenticule upside down. We plan to treat several patients with the lenticule extraction followed by soaking the lenticule in hypotonic riboflavin solution to swollen it and irradiate it with 365 nm UV light to cross link it and then insert it back into the stromal pocket. Perhaps, the swollen lenticule will spread better inside of the stromal pocket.

We typically create **myopic lenticule** with − 3 to − 10 sphere to make it thicker in the center to facilitate its manipulation. Because we do not remove and only rotate this lenticule, the spherical component of the rotated lenticule does not change the refraction in theory. Therefore, we can create, e.g., myopic − 5 spherical diopters lenticule in case of hyperopic astigmatism and only the astigmatic component of the lenticule changes the refraction of this eye with hyperopic astigmatism. Anyhow because of myopic shift associated with rotated lenticule shrinkage, the hyperopic spherical equivalent of eyes with hyperopic astigmatism gets lower after this surgery.

Regarding the lenticule shape theoretically, the **hyperopic concave lenticule** used in clinical study to correct hyperopia by SMILE surgery might be a better option for lenticule rotation surgery as the thicker lenticule periphery of hyperopic lenticule could probably have better tendency to keep the lenticule shape and spread the lenticule evenly peripheral.

From the clinical results, we have learned that there is a **myopic shift** associated with this procedure. Myopic shift often brings uncorrected near visual acuity improvement and better uncorrected reading ability of patients after lenticule rotation. The amount of this myopic shift was mean − 1.6 D SE during our first series of procedures with lenticule edge thickness of 30 μm. By analyzing the corneal tomographies and surgical videos, I determined the centripetal lenticule tissue redistribution as a cause of this myopic shift. During lenticule manipulation, the lenticule diameter shrinks and its edges tend to be separated from pocket periphery. I tried to spread the lenticule as evenly as possible at the end of surgery but typically there is a gap between the lenticule periphery and the equator of stromal pocket created by laser. The astigmatic lenticule is oval and not circular. After 90° lenticule rotation, there is a narrower gap between the lenticule edge and the stromal pocket equator along the lenticule long axis and wider gap on the perpendicular axis. I asked the Ziemer laser manufacturer to provide a software with the possibility to create a longer side cut creating thicker lenticule edge. By more thorough lenticule spread and by cutting the thicker lenticules, the myopic shift was decreased to − 0.625 D SE at our first patient as shown in Tables 21.2 and 21.3. The subjective astigmatism of the eye of this 51-year-old lady decreased from 5 D cyl to 1.25 D cyl three-month post-op.

Table 21.2 Refraction

	Refraction		
	Sf	Cyl	Axis
Preop	4	− 5	180
1 week	2	− 2.5	20
1 month	1	− 2	20
3 months	1.5	− 1.25	25

Table 21.3 Refraction and distance visual acuities

	Preop.	1 week	1 month	3 months
dSE (D)	1.5	0.75	0	0.875
abs CYL (D)	5	2.5	2	1.25
UDVA (logMAR)	0.8	0.64	0.6	0.4
CDVA (logMAR)	0.1	0.4	0.44	0.2

I believe that there should be a **dedicated software** option for lenticule rotation surgery developed at femtosecond laser devices to enable optimal surgical planning and offer the possibility of thicker edge lenticule. Also, **cyclotorsion compensation** might increase the accuracy of outcome of lenticule rotation because the surgery corrects typically a very high astigmatism. The proper axis alignment is more important in case of higher astigmatism. Anyhow lenticule rotation and its manipulation inside of the corneal stromal pocket resulted not only in significant decrease of astigmatism but often also in **high-order aberrations**. High-order aberrations were created by uneven tissue distribution of rotated lenticule. In 13 eyes (46%) treated by lenticule rotation, the residual refractive error was corrected by corneal laser surface ablation PRK and 7 from them by topoguided PRK to correct also the high-order aberrations. The reason for high-order aberrations increases after lenticule rotation is an uneven spread of lenticule tissue.

Due to the described myopic shift, the lenticule rotation is suitable mainly for **high hyperopic astigmatism or for mixed astigmatism**. We do not use this method for myopic astigmatism. To my best knowledge, lenticule rotation is the only method of surgical correction of high hyperopic astigmatism on eyes of young patients with flat anterior chamber not suitable for toric phakic intraocular lens implantation.

21.3 Lenticule Rotation Under the Flap ("Open Sky Technique")

As mentioned above, lenticule rotation can also be executed using a flap technique instead of the pocket. In this technique, the initial SMILE procedure is programmed as Femtosecond Lenticule Extraction (FLEx). In fact, FLEx was the predecessor of SMILE [6]. As FLEx is not available any longer as a software option on VisuMax laser, one programs "SMILE" procedure with a very large entering incision virtually producing a flap. The 0–180° axis is marked prior to initiation of the suction and either the treatment cone (= contact glas) is manually adjusted to the marks with the VisuMax 500 or the adjustment is done using the joystick of the VisuMax 800 (see Fig. 8.1 in chapter 8). After completion of the laser scan, three marks (horizontal and vertical) are applied to the surface. Thereafter, the upper plane is dissected and the flap reflected. The three marks are transferred to the lenticule upper surface and a fourth eccentric mark is added.

The lower plane is dissected; the lenticule is rotated 90° and stretched with spear sponges till it becomes dry. Finally, the flap is reflected (Fig. 21.12 shows the individual steps).

The advantages of the flap-based technique are its easiness compared to in-pocket technique. Moreover, concomitant spherical error can be simultaneously corrected by excimer ablation (own data, manuscript in preparation). Similarly to the in-pocket technique, there is a myopisation of – 0.75 to – 1.0 D (according to the second author own data as well as to Dr. Taneri's presentation, ESCRS annual symposium, Vienna 2021) and a loss of 1 to 2 lines of CDVA can occur, albeit we also treated eyes with plano results and no loss of CDVA.

The disadvantages of this technique are similar to the comparison between Femtolasik and KLEX: poorer biomechanics and more dry eye issues.

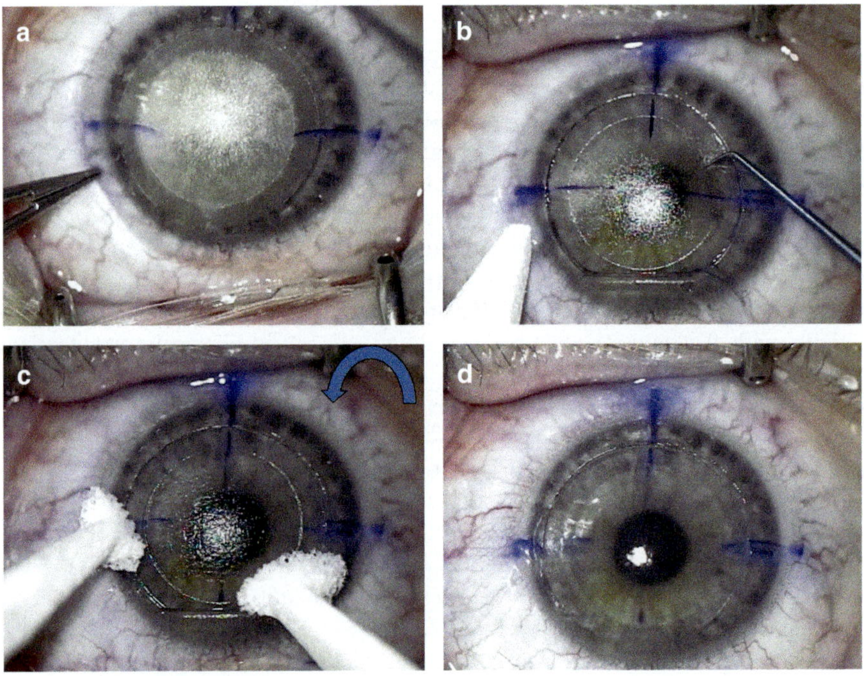

Fig. 21.12 Open sky technique for lenticule rotation for + 4.0 – 6.0 @5°. A FLEx procedure with 7-mm lenticule and 8.7-mm flap is performed (a). After the flap lift, the marks are extended onto the lenticule surface (b). Lenticule is dissected, turned anti-clockwise 3 clock hours, aligned with the marks and stretched with sponges (d). Thereafter, the flap is folded back using copious irrigation and ironed according to the marks. The post-op refraction after one year was + 0.25 – 0.5 @ 3°. The post-op UDVA was 1.0 similarly to preop CDVA

21.4 Conclusions

The series of world-first clinical cases operated by corneal stromal **lenticule rotation** shows that this method **can correct high astigmatism**. The procedure is associated with a myopic shift and often induces high-order aberration. Both residual refractive error and high-order aberrations can be further corrected by topoguided PRK. The long-term results seem to be stable, but some loss of CDVA is not uncommon. More data acquired on more eyes with longer follow-up are required, and the surgery itself deserves further refinement to reduce myopic shift and high-order aberrations induction.

Lenticule rotation is another surgical method in the armamentarium of refractive surgeon and is intended for astigmatism typically higher than four diopters.

References

1. Reinstein DZ, Archer TJ, Gobbe M. Small incision lenticule extraction (SMILE) history, fundamentals of a new refractive surgery technique and clinical outcomes. Eye Vis. 2014. https://doi.org/10.1186/s40662-014-0003-1.
2. Reinstein DZ, Pradhan KR, Carp GI, et al. Small incision lenticule extraction for hyperopia: 3-month refractive and visual outcomes. J Refract Surg. 2019;35(1):24–30. https://doi.org/10.3928/1081597X-20181025-01.
3. Pradhan KR, Reinstein DZ, Carp GI, Archer TJ, Dhungana P. Small incision lenticule extraction (SMILE) for hyperopia: 12-month refractive and visual outcomes. J Refract Surg. 2019. https://doi.org/10.3928/1081597X-20190529-01.
4. Damgaard IB, Ivarsen A, Hjortdal J. Intrastromal lenticule rotation for treatment of astigmatism up to 10.00 diopters ex vivo in human corneas. J Refract Surg. 2019;35(7):451–458. https://doi.org/10.3928/1081597X-20190618-02
5. Stodulka P, Hjortdal J, Slovak M. Intrastromal lenticule rotation for the treatment of high astigmatism. J Refract Surg. 2020. https://doi.org/10.3928/1081597X-20200506-02.
6. Sekundo W, Kunert K, Russmann C, Gille A, Bissmann W, Stobrawa G, Sticker M, Bischoff M, Blum M. First efficacy and safety study of femtosecond lenticule extraction for the correction of myopia: six-month results. J Cataract Refract Surg. 2008;34(9):1513–20. https://doi.org/10.1016/j.jcrs.2008.05.033.

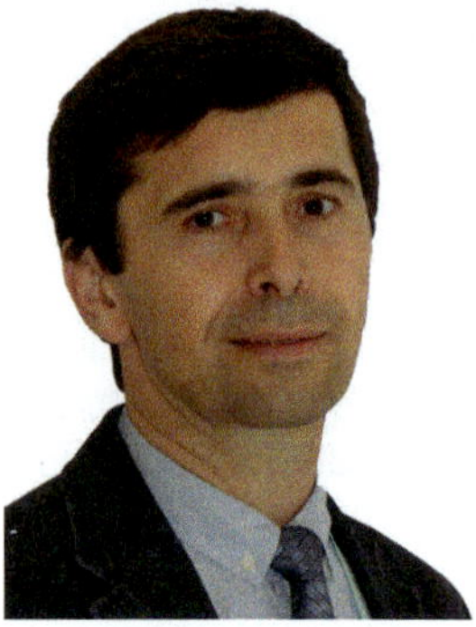

Pavel Stodulka Founder, chief surgeon and CEO of Gemini Eye Clinics in the Czech Republic and Vienna with 350 employees performing over 40 000 surgeries annually. In 2022 he founded corneal eye bank. AECOS Europe President (2022–2024) and ESCRS council member (2017–2025). He teaches ophthalmology at Charles University in Prague and gave over 1000 presentations worldwide and holds several patents regarding ophthalmic devices. The world firsts: presbyopic diffractive phakic IOL implantation (2014). Co-inventor of CAPSULaser and performed world first CAPSULaser capsulotomy (2015) and received the 1st price in innovative category for CAPSULaser video at ESCRS meeting in Copenhagen (2016). World first hydrophobic trifocal FineVision IOL (2016) implantation and EDOF LuxSmart IOL (2021) implantation. He designed presbyopic bio-synthetic collagen corneal inlay and performed its world first implantation (2018). He performed the world first femtomatrix laser cataract surgery (2019) and the presbyopic SMILE (2023). Surgeon dedicated to innovations performed the first in his country lasik (1994), MICS (2001), femtolasik (2006), DMEK (2006), FLACS femtocataract (2012) and many other surgeries. High volume surgeon with over 50,000 surgeries. He received several honors including Emilio Campos Medal Lecture for innovations from Italian Ophthalmology Society (2022) and the reward from a president of the Czech Republic for services to the state (2022).

SMILE in Special Cases

22

Moones Abdalla, Osama Ibrahim, and Walter Sekundo

Abstract

This chapter explores the application of small incision lenticule extraction (SMILE) in unique scenarios, emphasizing two specific cases: Combined small incision lenticule extraction (SMILE) and cross-linking (CXL) termed 'SMILE XTRA' and SMILE for post-penetrating keratoplasty (PKP) myopia and astigmatism.

Keywords

Small incision lenticule extraction (SMILE) • SMILE XTRA • Cross-linking (CXL)

As mentioned earlier in this book, SMILE has shown great efficacy and accuracy in normal corneas, having its unique and special advantages over any other refractive techniques, being flapless and less invasive. Furthermore, the ability to tailor and center the procedure as required within the cornea, together with better biomechanical stability [1], made SMILE a reasonable technique to deal with special cases which will be discussed in this chapter.

Financial Disclosure:The authors are consultants for Carl Zeiss Meditec AG

M. Abdalla · O. Ibrahim
Roayah Vision Correction Center, Alexandria University, Alexandria, Egypt

W. Sekundo (✉)
Department of Ophthalmology, Philipps University of Marburg, Marburg, Germany
e-mail: sekundo@med.uni marburg.de

W. Sekundo and F. M. Wagner (eds.), *Femtosecond Laser Assisted Lenticule Extraction*,
https://doi.org/10.1007/978-3-031-60424-9_22

22.1 Combined SMILE and Cross-Linking (CXL) = SMILE XTRA

Moones Abdalla, Ahmad Ei Massry, Assem Zahran, Eman Ei Maghraby, Osama Ibrahim and Walter Sekundo

Theoretically, SMILE has biomechanical advantages over LASIK because it does not involve the creation of a flap and leaves the stroma over the lenticule almost untouched, making it a procedure with minimal alterations of corneal biomechanics [2, 3]. This fact is explained in detail in Chapter 14 [1].

In SMILE, the refractive stromal tissue removal takes place in deeper stroma, leaving the stronger anterior stroma intact, thus leaving the cornea with greater tensile strength than LASIK for any given refractive correction [4, 5]. Based on Randleman's data, the model predicted that the post-operative tensile strength after SMILE was approximately 10% higher than PRK and 25% higher than LASIK [5]. Experimental work on the biomechanical properties of human corneas after Fs-LASIK and SMILE showed that the e-modulus for the SMILE group was actually 47% higher in stress–strain measurements than the LASIK group [6].

We anticipated that combining SMILE with intrastromal collagen cross-linking (CXL) would enhance the safety, predictability, and stability compared to using SMILE alone, especially in cases where conventional laser vision correction is not preferred due to suspicious topography or thin corneas. Moreover, we hypothesized that integrating CXL with SMILE in eyes diagnosed with forme fruste keratoconus (FFKC) or early keratoconus could reinforce the cornea, thereby halting the progression of the ectatic disease, while also addressing patient desires for improved unaided vision.

This prospective study included 34 eyes of 18 patients suffering from myopic astigmatism, with topography not suitable for LASIK or diagnosis of FFKC. In addition to stable refraction and topographic findings for at least 1 year, CDVA > 0.7 (Snellen decimal), central corneal thickness > 460 μm, and patient age > 21 years.

SMILE was performed using VisuMax® 500 kHz laser (Carl Zeiss Meditec AG, Germany). All cases had a 100 μm cap and a minimum of 250 μm of residual stromal bed. Intra-pocket injection of isotonic riboflavin three times with a 5 min interval was followed by 5 min of UV irradiation using 18 mW/cm^2. Biomechanical stability was assessed using the Corvis® ST (Oculus GmbH, Germany), measuring and correlating IOP and deformation amplitude.

Results

Mean patient age was 29.4 ± 5.63(22–35). Mean pre-operative refraction was -3.97 ± 1.87 D sphere (range-6.0 to -1.25) and -2.85 D cylinder (range -0.75 to -4.25). Mean post-operative spherical refraction was -0.14 ± 0.73 D (range -1.25 to $+ 1.5$), and mean astigmatism was -0.38 ± 0.45 D. 72% within ± 0.5 and 89% within ± 1.0 D at the end of the follow-up. The change in the mean UCVA is shown in Fig. 22.1. Delayed recovery of visual outcome was noticed due to haze, which was found to improve one to three months after surgery (Fig. 22.2).

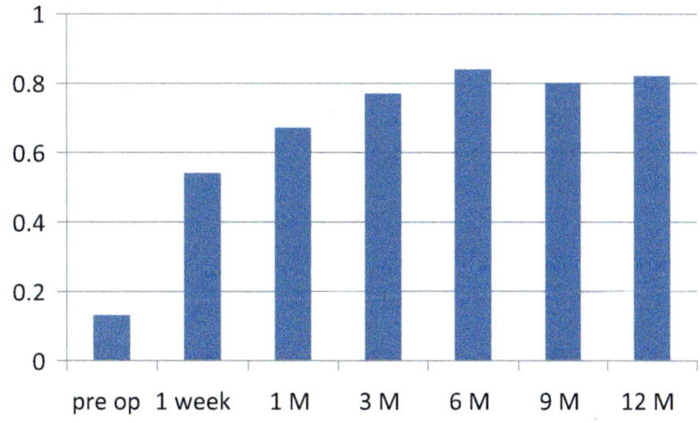

Fig. 22.1 Uncorrected visual acuity change (decimal) during the follow-up time

Topographic Changes

Example 1 See Fig. 22.2.

Example 2 For a 24-year-old male patient having −5 sphere and −1 cylinder with family history of keratoconus who was also considered to present contraindications for LASIK, SMILE and CXL were performed (Fig. 22.3).

Post-operatively, a further flattening was noticed, which we felt was due to the progressive effect of CXL and presumably resulting in more stability over time. This pattern of progressive flattening was observed in about 35% of cases.

Using Corvis® technology, mean deformation amplitude was 1.38 mm ± 0.29 pre-op. One month after surgery, the mean deformation amplitude decreased to 1.19 mm ± 0.29. No significant change over follow-up period occurred thereafter (for details see videos No 2 and No 3).

All cases treated so far showed topographic stability over the follow-up period up to 1 year. Figure 22.4 shows a Scheimpflug image of the cornea after combined SMILE and CXL.

After the herein reported study, several other investigators published their results using different protocols. Unfortunately, the vast majority of the studies published had a rather short follow-up period, which certainly is not sufficient to judge the mid- and long-term ectasia risk. A good exception is the paper by Brar et al. published in 2022 with a mean follow-up of 22 months (12–52 months) [7]. These authors compared SMILE XTRA with regular SMILE. Similarly, to our patients, they used additional CXL in borderline cases defined as such when

(1) Corneal thickness < 480 microns
(2) Residual bed thickness between 250 and 280 microns
(3) Refractive error > − 6.00D spherical equivalent (SE)
(4) Pentacam criteria: Belin Ambrosio display final D value > 1.65
(5) Corvis-ST criteria: Corvis Biomechanical Index (CBI) > 0.5 and Tomographic Biomechanical Index (TBI) > 0.29

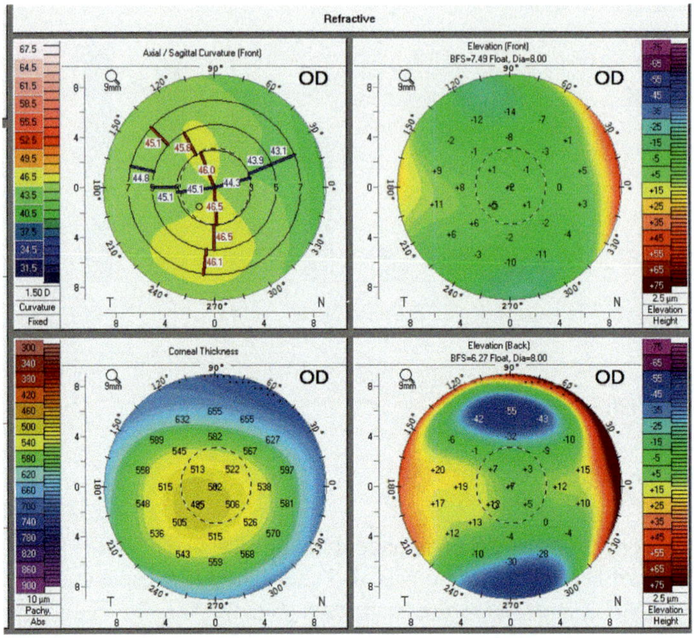

(a)

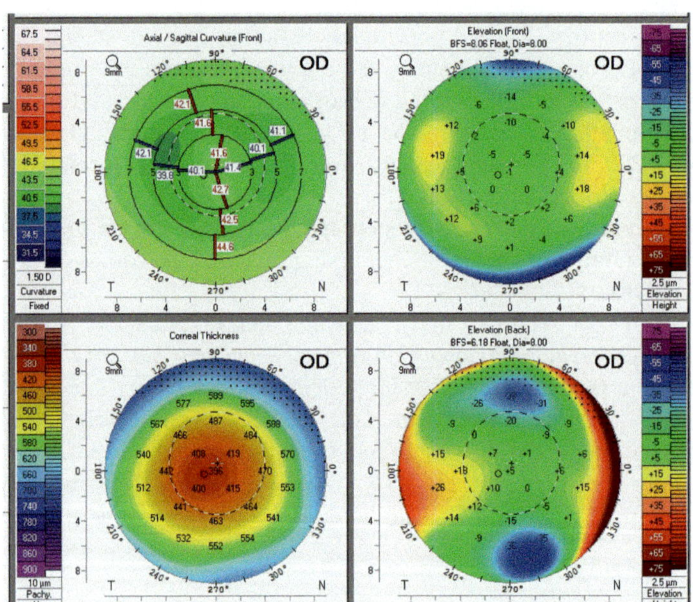

(b)

Fig. 22.2 a Pentacam® image of a 22-year-old male seeking refractive surgery showing thin cornea with infero-temporal steepening that was considered a contraindication to LASIK. Thus, a combined SMILE and CXL was performed. b Pentacam® of the same patient three months post-operatively showing topographic stability and no evidence of ectasia, which was noticed in all our cases

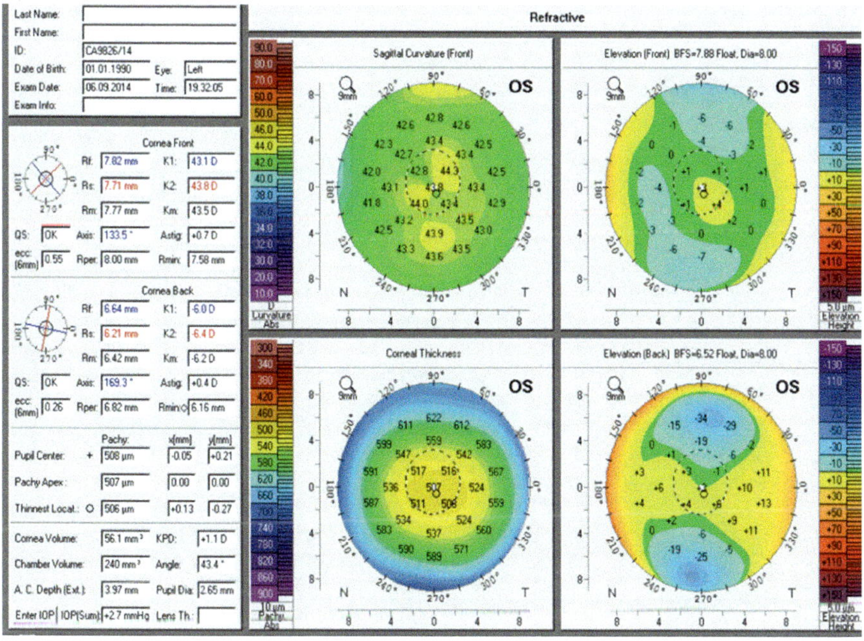

(a)

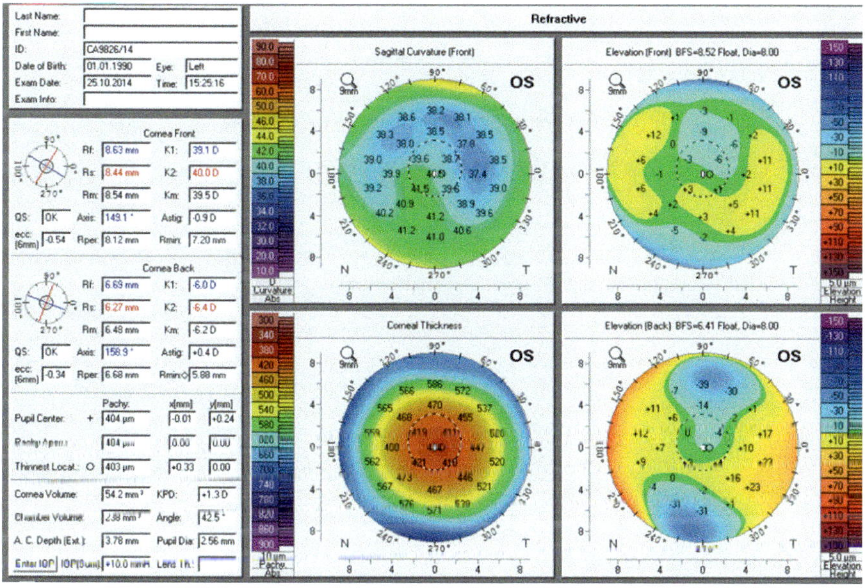

(b)

Fig. 22.3 a Irregular topography of the patient's left eye. Notably, the pachymetry map and the posterior float appear regular. b One month post-operative topography: Inferior steepening was noticed. c Three months after surgery, the anterior cornea is flatter and thinner

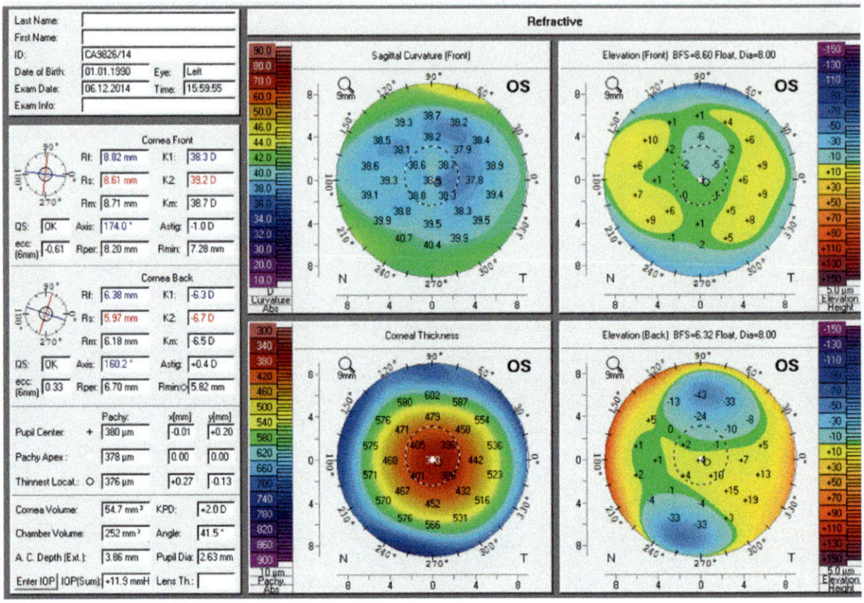

(c)

Fig. 22.3 (continued)

Fig. 22.4 Notice the CXL demarcation line in the cornea after combined SMILE and CXL

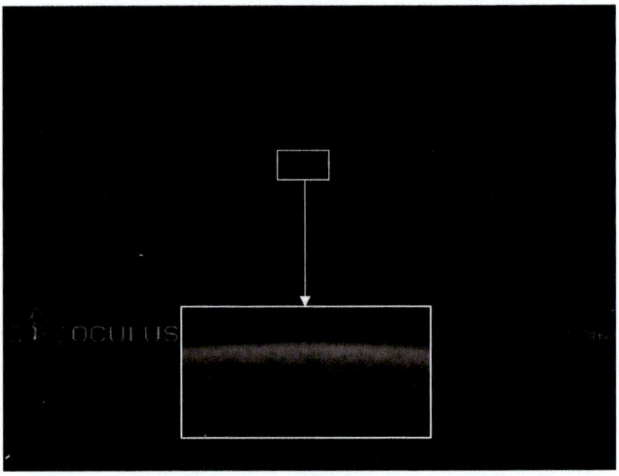

(6) Additional risk factors:
- Age < 30 years,
- Family history of keratoconus,
- History of eye rubbing.

They also used a different CXL protocol of 0.22% riboflavin in saline (Vibex XTRA, Avedro, Waltham, MA) or 0.23% riboflavin (Peschke L, Huenenberg, Switzerland) injected into the interface and allowed to diffuse for 60 s, followed by irrigation of the interface with balanced salt solution and UV-A irradiation through the cap using a power of 45 mW/cm^2 for 75 s, delivering a total energy 3.4 J/cm^2. There were no significant differences in the safety and efficacy index between the XTRA and standard SMILE groups. Moreover, with this high energy/short exposure accelerated protocol used, there was no hyperopic shift over the time. It is noteworthy that the same group analyzed a total of over 7000 eyes receiving SMILE or SMILE XTRA reporting an incidence of ectasia of 0.15%. Of these 10 eyes affected by ectasia, 8 had a borderline topography. Looking from this perspective, the incidence of ectasia in borderline cases was 0.8% with regular SMILE but 0% with SMILE XTRA. The only substantial side effect was a transient haze that would usually resolve on a prolonged course of topical steroids [8].

A recent review of SMILE XTRA (which also included the above-mentioned studies) as well as our study confirms the safety of the augmented procedure with a marginally lower safety index (0.96 versus 1.0) [9]. However, this statement applies to borderline cases only. In our opinion, keratoconus eyes are not suitable for SMILE surgery, even when combined with CXL.

22.2 SMILE for Post-Penetrating Keratoplasty Myopia and Astigmatism

Tamer Masoud, Moones Abdalla, Ibrahim Ahmed and Osama Ibrahim

Despite the high incidence of obtaining clear corneal grafts and improved surgical techniques, post-operative corneal toricity and high myopia after penetrating keratoplasty (PKP) are a major limitation of visual outcome. The incidence of high astigmatism following keratoplasty varies from 10 to 30% and is higher after PKP for keratoconus [10]. The unpredictable nature of corneal wound healing and the biomechanical response to surgery can lead to post-operative refractive surprises [11].

In LASIK for post-PKP errors, flap creation may induce astigmatism and higher-order aberrations [12, 13] because the flap itself is subject to shape changes induced by the vertical circumferential keratotomy of flap creation. This effect is magnified when the cut is through graft/host scar tissue. Furthermore, the risk of developing post-LASIK ectasia increases in patients with PKP for keratoconus, thick flaps, and deep laser ablation [14].

In SMILE, only a small vertical incision is made without the creation of a flap, minimizing trauma to the corneal surface if compared with other refractive laser procedures (PRK or LASIK) which helps to preserve the graft's healing scar, avoiding the more peripheral diseased cornea.

SMILE in post-PKP cases has the advantage of centration of the lenticule within the graft, avoiding cutting in the previous incision scar tissue giving better prediction of treatment results. Furthermore, patients with preexisting keratoconus could have a higher risk of recurrence of keratoconus if the flap cut is in the recipient cornea.

Our study was conducted with the following inclusion criteria:

- Clear central cornea,
- Corrected distance visual acuity (CDVA) of ≥ 0.5,
- Minimal corneal thickness not less than 500 μm,
- Maximum keratometric readings < 55 D,
- Spherical equivalent > −5 D,
- Stable graft for more than one year without any signs of rejection,
- All sutures should be removed at least three months before the procedure,
- Duration after PKP $\geq$ 18 months,
- Graft diameter more than 6 mm.

The 13 eyes of 13 patients with previous PKP and residual myopic astigmatism were enrolled in the study. Pentacam imaging and thickness measurements were within the acceptable range for laser vision correction. The procedure and its possible advantages and hazards were explained to the patients, and an informed consent was obtained from each of them. Pre-operatively, manifest refraction (MR), uncorrected distance visual acuity (UDVA), and corrected distance visual acuity (CDVA) were recorded. Intraoperatively, the cap and the lenticule diameters were calculated, so that they are centered within the graft. The other parameters (optical zone, transition zone and minimal thickness of the lenticule) were based on the degree of the refractive error, thinnest location of the graft, and the residual stromal depth under the cap. The same pre-operative measurements (MR, UDVA, and CDVA) were obtained and recorded post-operatively at one month, three months, and six months. Standard graphs for reporting refractive procedures were used [15].

Example of Treatment Parameters

The treatment zone is chosen to be 5.4 mm and the cap of 6.0 mm as shown in Fig. 22.5.

Surgical Procedure

The surgery is briefly summarized in Fig. 22.6a, b.

Results

Mean pre-operative refraction was −4.54 ± 1.46 D sphere (range −8.75 to −1.25) and -4.65 D cylinder (range −1.5 to −7.0), mean postoperative sphere was −0.56 ± 0.73 D (range −1.75 to + 1.5), and mean astigmatism was −0.98 ± 0.45 D. (up to −3.5). Figure 22.7a–c display the visual results.

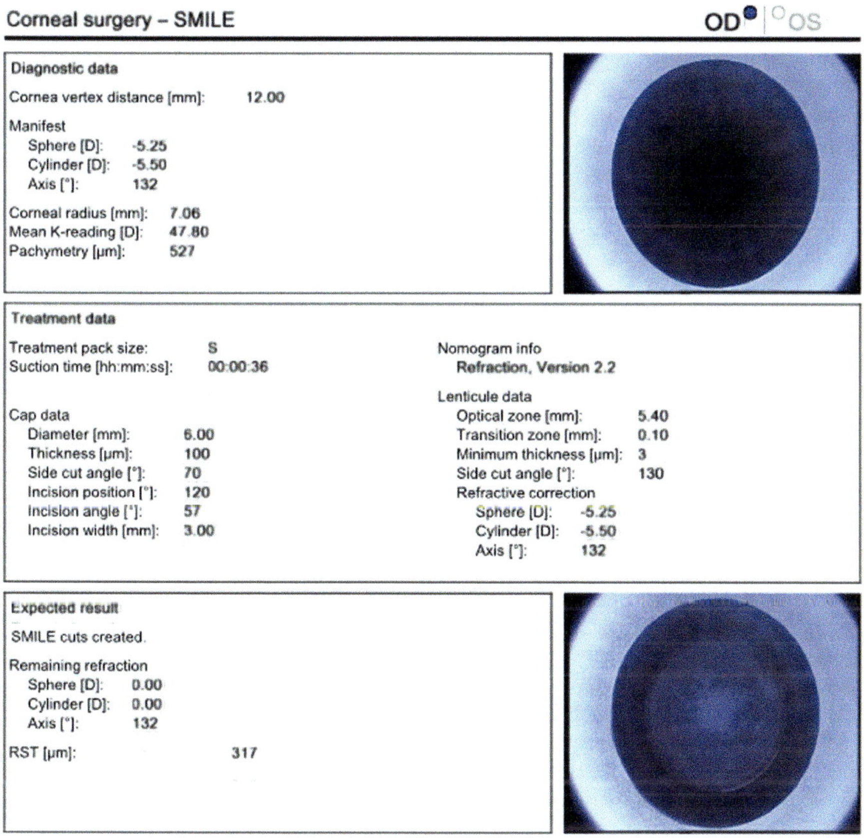

Fig. 22.5 Laser settings for SMILE after PKP

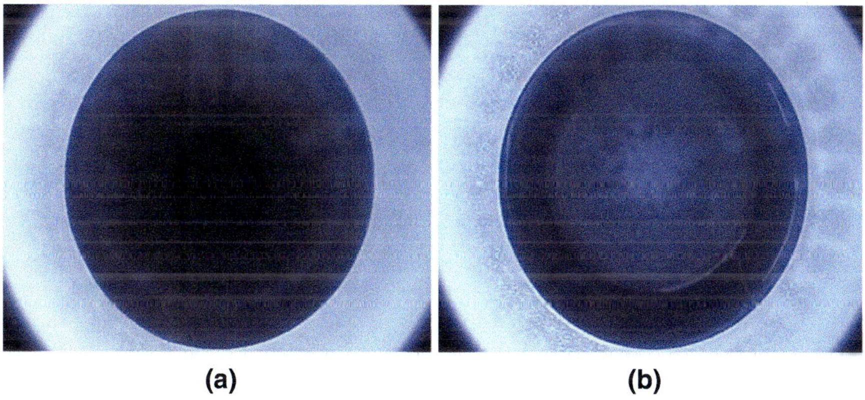

Fig. 22.6 a Post-PKP cornea is carefully applanated. The host-graft junction can be easily appreciated at this snapshot image. b Lenticule, the cap, and the opening incision are confined to the graft

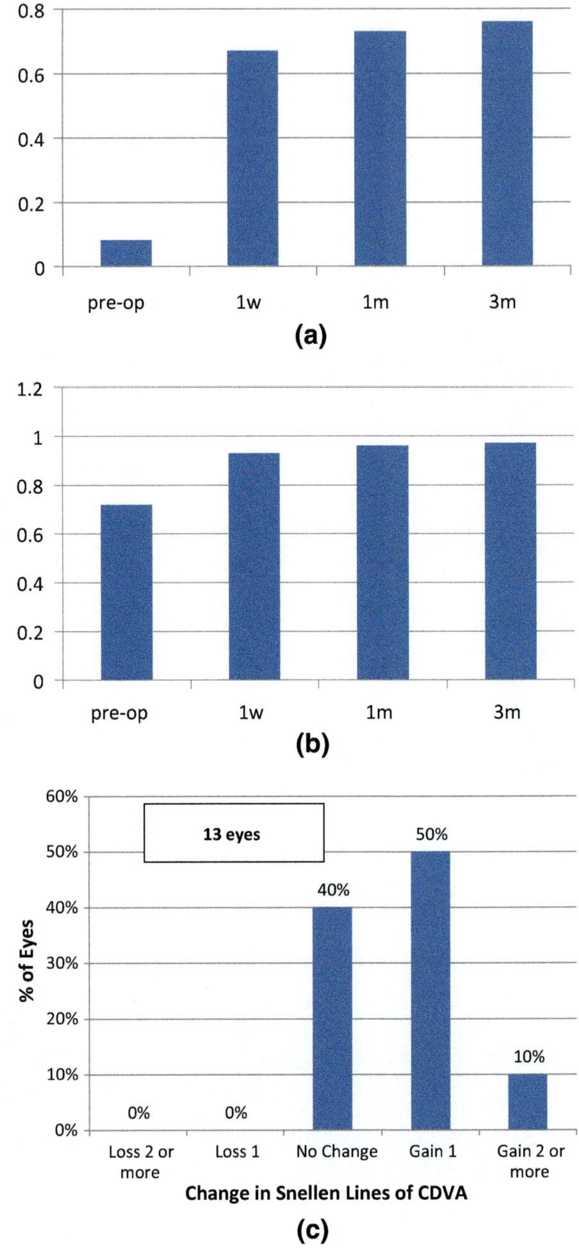

Fig. 22.7 a Mean UCVA over the follow-up period. b Mean CDVA over the follow-up period. c Safety parameters as a function of lost and gained visual acuity lines

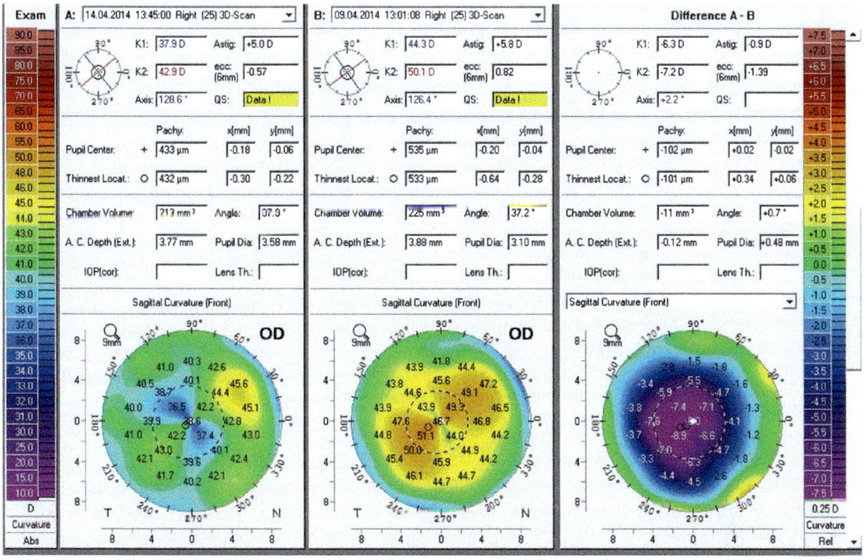

Fig. 22.8 Differential topography map of an uncomplicated case

It was noticed that post-operative topographic cylinder was almost double the number of manifest refraction in most cases. Figure 22.8 shows a differential map of an uncomplicated case.

One eye encountered buttonhole in the cap intra-operatively due to irregular topography. We observed that a cornea with an irregular bow tie pattern with steep and flat areas, acquired buttonhole in the flat area, so it is important to select regular topography to avoid complications and unpredictable results. A thicker cap of > 100 μm as used in this study might also contribute to a lesser risk of perforation.

In conclusion, SMILE procedure for the correction of post-keratoplasty myopia and astigmatism is a reproducible procedure with acceptable to good visual outcomes considering the severity of ametropia and astigmatism, in particular in these altered corneas. However, the parameters have to be modified and adjusted to the graft size. Irregular corneas should be avoided.

References

1. Reinstein DZ et al. Chapter 14 of this book.
2. Mastropaqua L et al. Chapter 3 of this book.
3. Reinstein DZ, Roberts C. Biomechanics of corneal refractive surgery. J Refract Surg. 2006;22:285.
4. Schmack I, Dawson DG, McCarey BE, et al. Cohesive tensile strength of human LASIK wounds with histologic, ultrastructural, and clinical correlations. J Refract Surg. 2005;21:433–45.

5. Randleman JB, Dawson DG, Grossniklaus HE, et al. Depth-dependent cohesive tensile strength in human donor corneas: implications for refractive surgery. J Refract Surg. 2008;24:85–9.
6. Spiru B, Torres-Netto EA, Kling S, Lazaridis A, Hafezi F, Sekundo W. Biomechanical properties of human cornea tested by two-dimensional extensiometry ex vivo in fellow eyes: PRK versus SMILE. J Refract Surg. 2019;35(8):501–5.
7. Brar S, Sriganesh S, Sute SS, Ganesh S. Comparison of long-term outcomes and refractive stability following SMILE versus SMILE combined with accelerated cross-linkung (SMILE XTRA). J Ophthalmol 2022; Article ID 4319785
8. Brar S, Roopashree CR, Ganesh S. Incidence of ectasia after SMILE from a high-volume refractive surgery center in India. J Refarct Surg. 2021;37:800–8.
9. Brar S, Gautam M, Suite SS, Ganesh S. Refarctive surgery with simulateneous collageb cross-linking for borderline corneas—a review of different techniques, their protocols and clinical outcomes. Ind J Ophthalmol. 2020;68(12):2744–56.
10. Troutman RC, Gaster RN. Surgical advances and results of keratoconus. Am J Ophthalmol. 1980;90:131–6.
11. Azar DT, Chang JH, Han KY, Wound healing after keratorefractive surgery: review of biological and optical considerations, Cornea 2012;31, supplement 1, pp. S9–S19.
12. Güell JL, Velasco F, Roberts C, et al. Corneal flap thickness and topography changes induced by flap creation during laser in situ keratomileusis. J Cataract Refract Surg. 2005;31:15–119.
13. Pallikaris IG, Kymionis GD, Panagopoulou SI, et al. Induced optical aberrations following formation of a laser in situ keratomileusis flap. J Cataract Refract Surg. 2001;28:1737–41.
14. Binder PS. Ectasia after laser in situ keratomileusis. J Cataract Refract Surg. 2003;29:2419–29.
15. Dupps WJ Jr, Kohnen T, Mamalis N, Rosen ES, Koch DD, Obstbaum SA. Standardized graphs and terms for refractive surgery results. J Cataract Refract Surg. 2011;37:1–3.

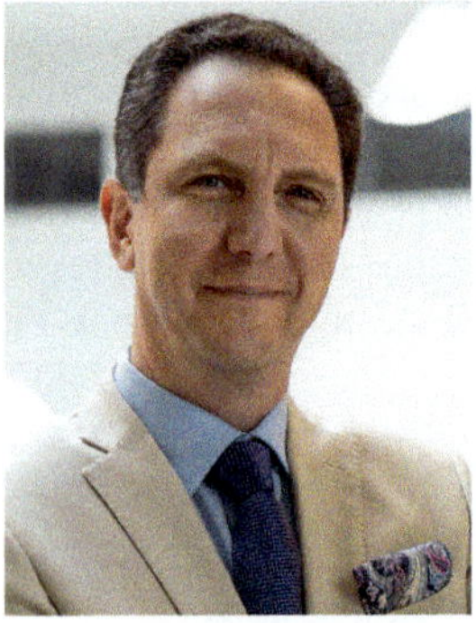

Walter Sekundo MD, PhD is Professor and Chairman, Department of Ophthalmology, Philipps University of Marburg, Germany. He studied Medicine in Frankfurt (Germany), New Orleans and Durham (US). He was a resident at the University of Bonn in Germany and a Fellow in Corneal and Refractive surgery at Moorfields Eyes Hospital and Ocular Pathology at the University of Glasgow in UK. He received his vitreoretinal training in Marburg and glaucoma training in Mainz (Germany). He also holds a degree of "Health Care Manager" from the Faculty of Economics in Marburg. Prof. Sekundo has published 200 + original papers, over 50 book chapters and edited the first international book on SMILE surgery. He gave countless presentations at national and international meetings. He is a reviewer for 21 Ophthalmic Journals and a Board Member of "*Die Ophthalmologie*". Prof. Sekundo is a busy surgeon with over 30,000 procedures in the anterior and posterior segment and has been repeatedly named as one of the 30 top refractive and cataract surgeons in Germany. Together with Marcus Blum he largely contributed to the development of KLEx. In fact, he was the first surgeon in the world who performed FLEx and SMILE. He received several prestigious prizes for the contribution to the field of ophthalmic surgery. In the last 25 years his research has been focused on corneal, cataract and refractive surgery.

Part V

Smart Sight®

Lenticule and Interface Properties and Geometries in SmartSight®

23

Kishore Raj Pradhan and Samuel Arba Mosquera

23.1 Introduction

It was back in 2007–2008 when SCHWIND eye-tech-solutions started a project to develop a femtosecond laser for refractive surgery [1]. Already at the time, it was obvious for SCHWIND to include a lenticule extraction as a treatment option of the system to be developed [2]. It took a long time since then, until FLEX[3] and, in particular, SMILE [4] (both by Carl Zeiss Meditec) became largely popular. And it took even longer, until SCHWIND made its own version of a lenticule extraction (coined SmartSight) performed by its own femtosecond laser system (the SCHWIND ATOS) a reality [5] (Fig. 23.1).

There is always a remaining question "is the effort for lenticules justified in terms of market penetration". Other issues like the treatment strategy, technical and legal issues can be sorted out. The confidence in the outcomes is brought by the clinical experience, but the market success of lenticule extraction remained unclear for quite a long time.

Bear in mind that SCHWIND has an excellent record in transepithelial ablations (TransPRK/SmartSurfACE) [6], in many regards comparable to lenticule extraction (SMILE) in terms of year of introduction, ramp for success, and number of treatments performed [7]. And this revived a surface ablation method that was essentially considered "out of the market".

SCHWIND's position and proposition is that lenticule extraction is a supplement, an alternative to and not a replacement for LASIK. SCHWIND refrains

K. R. Pradhan
KRP Matrika Eye Center, Kathmandu, Nepal

S. Arba Mosquera (✉)
SCHWIND eye-tech-solutions, Kleinostheim, Germany
e-mail: Samuel.Arba.Mosquera@eye-tech.net

W. Sekundo and F. M. Wagner (eds.), *Femtosecond Laser Assisted Lenticule Extraction*,
https://doi.org/10.1007/978-3-031-60424-9_23

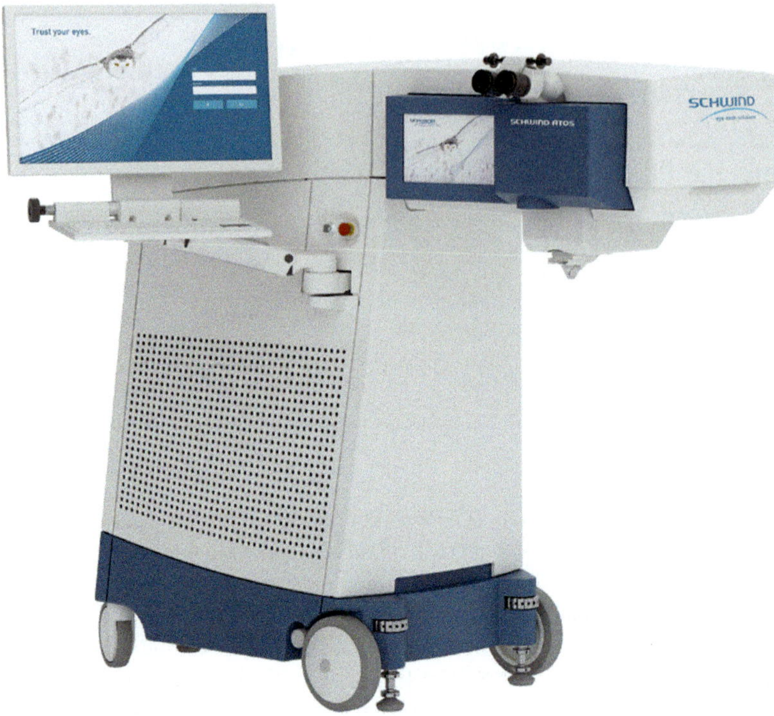

Fig. 23.1 SCHWIND ATOS femtosecond laser system

from pushing lenticule extraction on the grounds of promises to be better than LASIK (in terms of outcomes, biomechanics, dry eye, whatsoever). SCHWIND offers lenticule extraction in parallel to LASIK and TransPRK as one more tool in the armamentarium made available to the surgeon (Fig. 23.2).

23.2 Technical Data of SCHWIND ATOS

SCHWIND ATOS is a new development in femtosecond laser technology that enables the generation of LASIK flaps and lenticules for SmartSight lenticule extraction. It received the CE Mark in July 2020, early in the COVID-19 pandemic [5]. Since then, a steadily growing number of surgeons in and beyond Europe has performed SmartSight. So far, lenticule removal was reported to be performed without relevant intraoperative complications.

In a nutshell, the SCHWIND ATOS is engined by a regenerative amplified femtosecond laser source, delivering near IR pulses at around 1030 ± 50 nm, with a pulse duration of approximately 225 ± 70 fs, a repetition rate of up to around 4 MHz, and delivering a pulse energy in the range 75–135 nJ. The ATOS optical

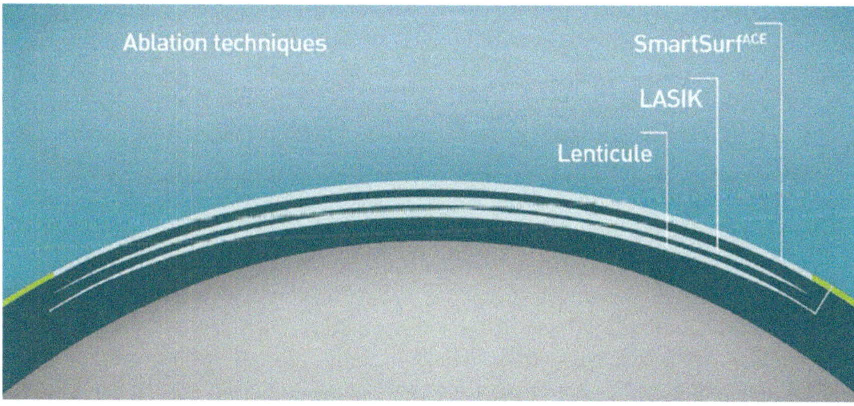

Fig. 23.2 Schematic representation of the treatment modalities offered by SCHWIND eye-tech-solutions. Please note that SmartSurf^{ACE} (transepithelial PRK) is placed through and direct underneath the epithelium, whereas LASIK and Lenticules are placed deeper at the anterior stroma

system includes a high numerical aperture (NA) and a short working distance leading to a very small spot in the focal plane.

The application occurs using a single-use disposable patient interface. This patient interface includes a plano-concave contact element. SCHWIND decided for a curved geometry of the contact element due to the theoretical advantages in IOP rise, and less folds at the posterior cornea. Technical/engineering considerations would always have led to a flat design for the contact element. The applied load onto the eye during applanation is low ~150 g (<250 g), along with an applied suction of ~250 mmHg (<300 mmHg), leading to a max IOP during treatment not going beyond 135–140 mmHg (barely above the systolic pressure) [8].

23.3 Principle of Operation

Due to the high NA of ATOS (along with the short pulse duration, and quasi-telecentric scanning optics), the threshold for laser-induced optical breakdown (LIOB) is reduced [9]. This reduced LIOB threshold enables ATOS to use lower pulse energies [10]. The reduced energies produce much smaller bubbles, thus many more bubbles contribute together to produce a cleavage plane [9]. But more bubbles require a higher repetition rate to keep the treatment time reasonable (in first approximation, Rep.Rate * Bubble area = area worked out per unit of time).

The advantage of a higher NA and smaller spots results in a smoother cut [11]. Low pulse energy concept provides better resolution and lower corneal reactions. The asymmetric spacing concept contributes to a more homogeneous cut for lower pulse energies and treatment dose [9]. SCHWIND ATOS works in the plasma-mediated ablation range [12], which is well below the photodisruption range [13] and slightly above the threshold for laser-induced optical breakdown [9]. It generates only low-density plasma [14] and pulses in the low-energy range, providing a gentle, tissue-friendly treatment. With ATOS, a typical setting would be 80 nJ 5.9 μm × 2.9 μm (~468 mJ/cm^2).

The low pulse energy (sub-100 nJ) of the ATOS provides better resolution and reduces corneal reactions, whereas the asymmetric spacings lead to more homogeneous cuts with less pulse energy.

The temporally and spatially scanned process eventually leads to a confluent (or coalescent) bubble (conforming a cleavage plane), enabling the separation of the tissue. There may be essential differences between the coalescence of one single, small bubble with another single, small bubble and the coalescence of one single, small bubble with a residual bubble layer which has already been accumulated by thousands of bubbles before. Every new single, small bubble contributes to the cutting of the cornea, but they may be governed by different underlying mechanisms. For instance, very different regimes have been observed for the interaction mechanisms of cavitation bubbles induced by spatially and temporally separated fs-laser pulses (at least for pulse energies well above the breakdown threshold). The repetition rate could play a crucial role. If the lifetime of the cavitation bubble (or the remaining gas bubble) is longer than the inverse of the pulse repetition rate (i.e., the interpulse time), the subsequent pulse may target the cavitation and will be distracted so that no breakdown can occur. Such effects can be inferred from previous works on the interaction mechanisms of cavitation bubbles induced by spatially and temporally separated fs-laser pulses (at least for pulse energies well above the breakdown threshold) [9].

The interplay between bubble size, spot spacing, and repetition rate is very complex. Recent work by Tinne et al. [15] showed that bubbles in water and 1% gelatin have lifetimes above 10 μs (for energies above 1 μJ and relative energies above 6× the threshold). In the same work, Tinne et al. [15] found in water that below 3.6× the threshold (≈500 nJ in their setup) no influence between the cavitation bubble oscillations was observed, and below 7.2 × the threshold (≈1000 nJ in their setup), an asymmetric bubble collapse can be observed. For the 2 and 5% gelatin an asymmetric bubble collapse was observable during the interaction oscillation for energies as high as 8.4× the threshold (≈1200 nJ in their setup) due to the decrease in maximum bubble radius and lifetime with increasing gelatin concentration [15], whereas the temporal overlap parameter was neglected for there was no influence on the interaction effects.

In fact, the repetition rate is crucial for intrastromal dissection in refractive surgery. The bubble remains within the cornea for a few microseconds (for low pulse energies slightly exceeding the breakdown threshold, only one expansion and collapse of the bubble occurs). So that below some 10 kHz repetition rate would probably not play a relevant role, whereas beyond some 100 kHz repetition rate (i.e., in the MHz regime) would probably play a crucial role and interactions with the bubble of the previous laser pulse have to be considered, which is additionally dependent on spot spacing and bubble size/laser energy.

In addition, closely neighboring pulses can strongly influence each other: A subsequent pulse may have to interact with material optically changed by the previous pulse, thus causing varying conditions for the laser–tissue interaction [15].

23.4 Lenticule Geometry of SmartSight

In general, the lenticule shape resembles very much (but it is not identical to) the equivalent aberration-free LASIK profiles of the AMARIS ablation design (besides the excimer spot's peripheral spreading compensation). The SmartSight profiles include a transition zone (TZ) (just like AMARIS LASIK profiles do) sharing many principles with the LASIK TZ, and the lenticule (encompassing optical zone (OZ) and TZ) tapers to zero at the outer edge of the TZ (just like AMARIS refractive profiles do). Comparing this to the three competitors (SMILE, CLEAR, and SILK), all showing a pedestal (minimum lenticule thickness) at the edge of the lenticule (outer edge of the TZ), SCHWIND seems to not need it, thus this pedestal tissue is saved (preserved).

The lenticule thickness calculated by ATOS in the SmartSight design is very close to the ablation depth for the equivalent of an aberration-free (AF) LASIK treatment in AMARIS (and similar to that of a correction based on the difference of two Cartesian ovals), and it lies between that of the standard Munnerlyn profile and its parabolic/paraxial approximation. This SmartSight profile design saves tissue also compared to the complete Munnerlyn equation (including TZ).

So, the geometry of the SmartSight lenticule is aspheric in nature, including a progressive refractive TZ, without pedestal.

Since there is no additional thickness added, there is a recurrent question for the case of low ametropia corrections. Once again, SCHWIND's vast experience with TransPRK is key in the specific recommendation for an optimal extraction in these cases. Ultimately, it is the same issue, how to get the tissue corrected in place. So the only recommendation is to enlarge the OZ as wide as possible/required. SCHWIND ATOS imposes as limit, that the maximum lenticule thickness (typically at or close to the center) has to exceed 25 μm for the treatment plan to be performed in ATOS (otherwise you cannot get it planned). Another limit is that the maximum OZ cannot exceed 8.0 mm. With these two conditions, lenticules barely below −1 D of myopia can be treated (Fig. 23.3).

Luckily, from the first clinical results, the deviations were minor [16], but even those deviations can be refined (as long as they show a systematic effect).

Another point of interest in the design of a lenticule is the depth/thickness and geometry of the anterior cap. In SmartSight, the anterior cap cut is overbent (i.e., becomes slightly thicker/deeper toward the periphery). This may serve as protective measure against slight decentrations (preventing cutting into the epithelium). Further, the anterior cap cut may become more anatomically natural, since both overall corneal thickness as well as epithelium thickness slightly grow toward the periphery [17].

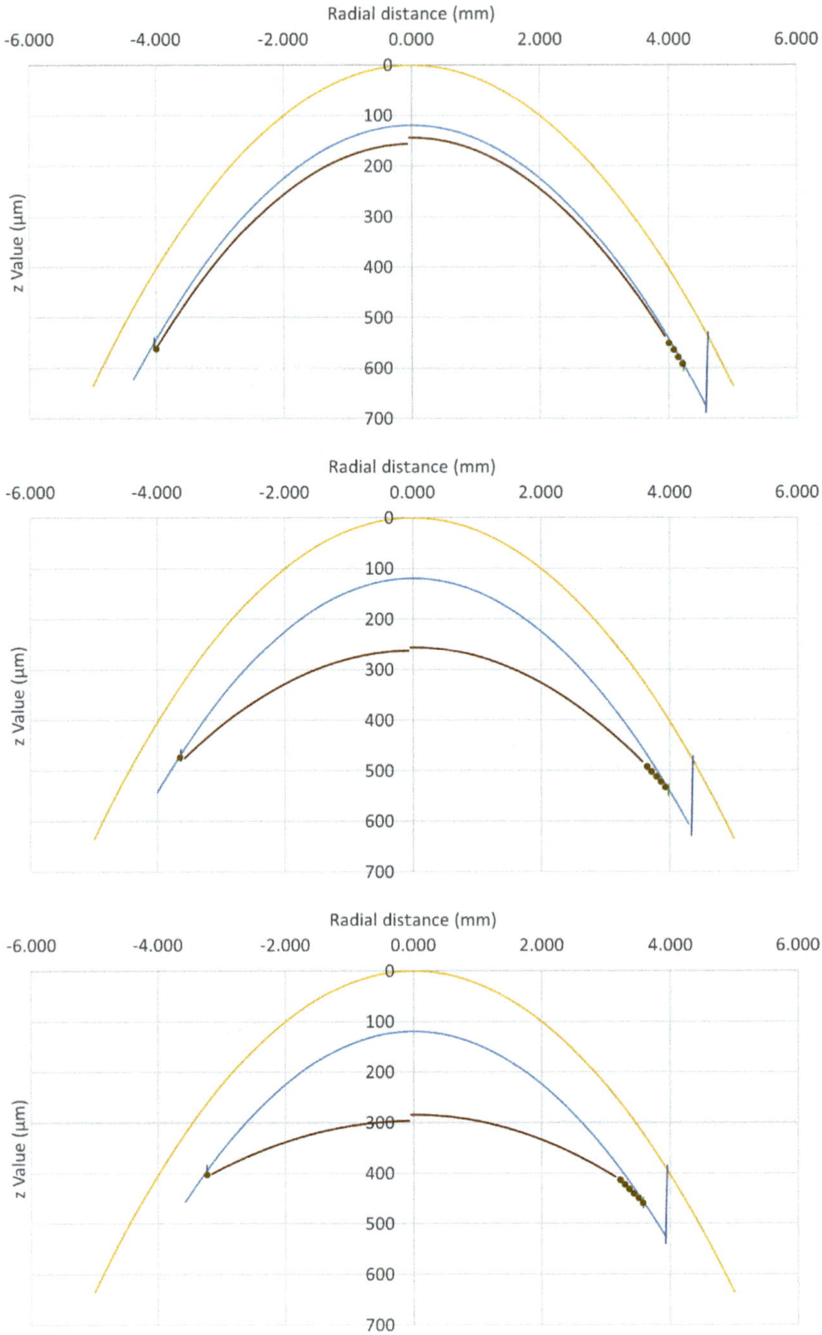

Radial distance (mm)
-6.000
-4.000
-2.000
0.000
2.000
4.000
6.000
0
100
200
300
400
500
600
700
z Value (µm)
Radial distance (mm)
-6.000
-4.000
-2.000
0.000
2.000
4.000
6.000
0
100
200
300
400
500
600
700
z Value (µm)
Radial distance (mm)
-6.000
-4.000
-2.000
0.000
2.000
4.000
6.000
0
100
200
300
400
500
600
700
z Value (µm)

◄**Fig. 23.3** Schematic comparison of three different lenticule geometries including a minimum-lenticule-thickness pedestal (left half-side, including a 15 μm pedestal) vs lenticule geometries including a refractive progressive TZ as offered by SCHWIND eye-tech-solutions. Please note that the maximum lenticule thickness is higher for the pedestal version (i.e., the SmartSight lenticules save tissue respect to a 15 μm pedestal version), whereas the refractive progressive TZ enlarges and softens the junction to the untreated cornea (i.e., providing a better transition between the fully corrected and the uncorrected regions of the cornea)

Treatment Ranges:

- Lenticule thickness: 25 to 165 μm
- CRST: > 275 μm

Treatment ranges for ATOS SmartSight lenticule treatment are summarized in the following Chap. 24.

The aim of the SmartSight aspheric profiles is to retain the preoperative HOAs (within OZ) after SmartSight, especially spherical aberration, coma, and trefoil shall remain essentially unchanged [10]. A further aim is to achieve an effective OZ equal (or at least comparable) to the planned OZ (thus the planned OZ is achieved) [18]. The planned OZ for SmartSight can be set freely between 5.5 and 8.0 mm diameter (+TZ of up to 0.8 mm outside of the OZ). Of course, as the lenticules get thicker (e.g., for higher corrections or larger optical zones), they are easier to extract, but less residual stroma is left behind. ATOS limits the maximum lenticule thickness to between 25 and 165 μm. Further, ATOS imposes a minimum 275 μm calculated residual stromal thickness (and we personally recommend the postoperative total corneal thickness to remain above 400 μm).

23.5 Potential Benefits of ATOS SmartSight

Since no minimum lenticule thickness is included in the profiles, this potentially reduces the overall thickness of the lenticules. Along with the progressive refractive TZ included in SmartSight, the epithelial remodeling is potentially reduced (which in fact may result in less regression and a true effective OZ) [19].

As for the scanning principle, the SmartSight treatment works from center to outside (centrifugally) for both cutting layers. This means that the most important part (center of the treatment providing the highest resolution in vision) is treated first (with both better patient compliance and less treatment induced disturbances).

The overbending of the cap may provide a protective measure against slight decentrations.

The compact ATOS system offers eye registration from diagnostic images (using an objective treatment offset) imported from SCHWIND diagnostic devices (SCHWIND SIRIUS, SCHWIND PERAMIS, SCHWIND SIRIUS + , and SCHWIND MS-39) [20], including a semi-automated eye-tracking guided centration (pupil recognition) [10], which shall correspond to a better positioning of the lenticule respect to the visual axis [21]. Actually, users may pre-offset the treatments at the planning stage to optimize the target position of the lenticule [20]. This along with the fully-automated cyclotorsion compensation incorporated in the system shall allow a better positioning of the lenticule respect to the meridional orientation (astigmatism axis) [22]. The eye-tracker guided centration and docking shall provide a robust, accurate, and precise alignment of the eye to the system [21].

The load onto the eye is kept to a reasonable minimum, achieved through a low applanation load (below 250 g) combined with a gentle suction (around 250 mmHg). The high rep rate (in the MHz regime) opens potential for faster treatments or better resolution.

The optical and scanning systems provide quasi-telecentric optics; this means that the same cutting quality is achieved for the whole cornea (over a cylindrical volume of 10 mm diameter and 1 mm depth).

23.6 Further Aspects and Future Outlook

Overall, there have been over 75,000 treatments performed with ATOS by the end of August 2024; approximately distributed with >45,000 SmartSight lenticules + >30,000 flaps. The detailed clinical results are all reported in Chap. 25.

In the future, the following advancements and features will be released for the SCHWIND ATOS:

- Optimized centration with an asymmetric transition zone concept (presented during ESCRS 2024 in Barcelona as part of the CenTrax feature);
- Inclusion of intrastromal corneal ring segment function (presented during ESCRS 2024 in Barcelona); and
- Inclusion of a keratoplasty function

Furthermore, treatment options such as custom lenticules for myopia, hyperopic lenticules, and presbyopia-correcting lenticules are being considered to broaden the ATOS application range in the future.

23.7 Conclusion

The SmartSight lenticule extraction procedure will continue to undergo enhancements with the SCHWIND ATOS. The innovative laser system incorporates properties of the successful and proven SCHWIND AMARIS technology.

The ATOS works in an optimized but minimum pulse energy range and spaces the laser pulses asymmetrically. Of the many advantages, the eye-tracking guided centration and static cyclotorsion control seem to be relevant for the clinical success of the lenticule extraction procedure (i.e., SmartSight in the SCHWIND nomenclature), paving the way for future customizations in lenticule profiles.

The concept for the SmartSight lenticule profiles was derived from the vast experience with the SCHWIND AMARIS and do not require any minimum thickness levels. The profiles incorporate a progressive refractive transition zone, possibly reducing the overall thickness of the lenticules and providing a true transition zone that causes less remodeling of the epithelium and less regression.

Both the current ATOS laser system and future developments can help surgeons stay on the cutting edge of laser vision correction.

References

1. Miclea M, Skrzypczak U, Faust S, Fankhauser F, Graener H, Seifert G. Nonlinear refractive index of porcine cornea studied by z-scan and self-focusing during femtosecond laser processing. Opt Express. 2010;18(4):3700–7. https://doi.org/10.1364/OE.18.003700. PMID: 20389380.
2. Miclea M, Skrzypczak U, Fankhauser F, Faust S, Graener H, Seifert G. Applanation-free femtosecond laser processing of the cornea. Biomed Opt Express. 2011;2(3):534–42. https://doi.org/10.1364/BOE.2.000534.PMID:21412459;PMCID:PMC3047359.
3. Sekundo W, Kunert K, Russmann C, Gille A, Bissmann W, Stobrawa G, Sticker M, Bischoff M, Blum M. First efficacy and safety study of femtosecond lenticule extraction for the correction of myopia: six-month results. J Cataract Refract Surg. 2008;34(9):1513–20. https://doi.org/10.1016/j.jcrs.2008.05.033.Erratum.In:JCataractRefractSurg.2008;34(11):1819. PMID: 18721712.
4. Blum M, Sekundo W. Femtosekunden-Lentikel-Extraktion (FLEx) [Femtosecond lenticule extraction (FLEx)]. Ophthalmologe. 2010;107(10):967–70. German. https://doi.org/10.1007/s00347-010-2222-8. PMID: 20694728.
5. https://eyewire.news/articles/schwind-receives-ce-mark-approval-for-the-schwind-atos-femtosecond/
6. Camellin M, Arba MS. Simultaneous aspheric wavefront-guided transepithelial photorefractive keratectomy and phototherapeutic keratectomy to correct aberrations and refractive errors after corneal surgery. J Cataract Refract Surg. 2010;36:1173–80.
7. CRSTG | Europe Edition | Broad Treatment Range With Latest Version of Trans-PRK (crstodayeurope.com)
8. Strohmaier C, Runge C, Seyeddain O, Emesz M, Nischler C, Dexl A, Grabner G, Reitsamer HA. Profiles of intraocular pressure in human donor eyes during femtosecond laser procedures–a comparative study. Invest Ophthalmol Vis Sci. 2013;54(1):522–8. https://doi.org/10.1167/iovs.12-11155. PMID: 23249707.
9. Arba-Mosquera S, Naubereit P, Sobutas S, Verma S. Analytical optimization of the cutting efficiency for generic cavitation bubbles. Biomed Opt Express. 2021;12:3819–35.
10. Gabric I, Bohaç M, Gabric K, Arba Mosquera S. First European results of a new refractive lenticular extraction procedure-SmartSight by SCHWIND eye-tech-solutions. Eye (Lond). 2023. https://doi.org/10.1038/s41433-023-02601-0. Epub ahead of print. PMID: 37277614.
11. Wang J, Schuele G, Palanker D. Finesse of transparent tissue cutting by ultrafast lasers at various wavelengths. J Biomed Opt. 2015;20(12): 125004. https://doi.org/10.1117/1.JBO.20.12.125004. PMID: 26720869.
12. Tsai PS, Blinder P, Migliori BJ, Neev J, Jin Y, Squier JA, Kleinfeld D. Plasma-mediated ablation: an optical tool for submicrometer surgery on neuronal and vascular systems. Curr Opin Biotechnol. 2009;20(1):90–9. https://doi.org/10.1016/j.copbio.2009.02.003. Epub 2009 Mar 5. PMID: 19269159; PMCID: PMC3123732.
13. Lubatschowski H, Maatz G, Heisterkamp A, Hetzel U, Drommer W, Welling H, Ertmer W. Application of ultrashort laser pulses XE "Ultrashort laser pulses" for intrastromal refractive

surgery. Graefes Arch Clin Exp Ophthalmol. 2000;238(1):33–9. https://doi.org/10.1007/s00 4170050006. PMID: 10664050.
14. Kuetemeyer K, Rezgui R, Lubatschowski H, Heisterkamp A. Influence of laser parameters and staining on femtosecond laser-based intracellular nanosurgery. Biomed Opt Express. 2010;1(2):587–97. https://doi.org/10.1364/BOE.1.000587.PMID:21258492;PMCID:PMC301 7989.
15. Tinne N, Lübking E, Lubatschowski H, Krüger A, Ripken T. The influence of a spatial and temporal pulse-overlap on the laser-tissue-interaction of modern ophthalmic laser systems. Biomed Tech (Berl). 2012;57 Suppl 1:/j/bmte.2012.57.issue-s1-P/bmt-2012–4115/bmt-2012–4115.xml. https://doi.org/10.1515/bmt-2012-4115. PMID: 23096345.
16. Pradhan KR, Arba Mosquera S. Twelve-month outcomes of a new refractive lenticular extraction procedure. J Optom. 2023;16(1):30–41. https://doi.org/10.1016/j.optom.2021.11.001. Epub 2021
17. Arba-Mosquera S, Awwad ST. Impact of the reference point for epithelial thickness measurements. J Refract Surg. 2020;36(3):200–20.
18. Camellin M, Arba MS. Aspheric optical zones: the effective optical zone with the SCHWIND AMARIS. J Refract Surg. 2011;27(2):135–46.
19. de Ortueta D, von Rüden D, Arba-Mosquera S. Refractive effect of epithelial remodelling in myopia after transepithelial photorefractive keratectomy. Vision. 2022;6(4):74. https://doi.org/10.3390/vision6040074.
20. de Ortueta D, Schreyger FD. Centration on the cornea vertex normal during hyperopic refractive photoablation using videokeratoscopy. J Refract Surg. 2007;23(2):198–200. https://doi.org/10.3928/1081-597X-20070201-13. PMID: 17326360.
21. Samuel AM, Victor D, Hamed H, Thomas M, Maren-Christina B. Automated method to determine Centration/Registration for Refractive Corneal Lenticule Extraction Treatments. Posterboard#: C0172. Abstract Number: 5327–C0172. ARVO2023, New Orleans
22. Aslanides IM, Toliou G, Padroni S, Arba Mosquera S, Kolli S. The effect of static cyclotorsion compensation on refractive and visual outcomes using the Schwind Amaris laser platform for the correction of high astigmatism. Contact lens & anterior eye: the journal of the British Contact Lens Association. 2011;34(3):114–20.

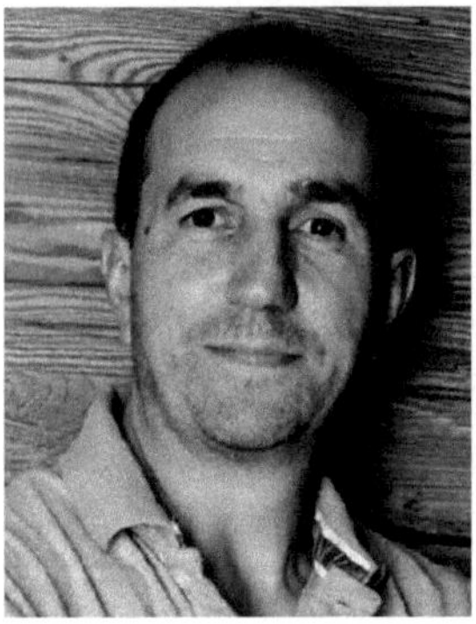

Samuel Arba Mosquera PhD is Senior Optical & Visual Scientist, Biomedical Engineering Office, SCHWIND eye-tech-solutions, Germany. He studied Physics in Santiago de Compostela (Spain). He further completed a Master's and Doctor's Degree in Sciences of Vision by the University of Valladolid in Spain. Dr. Arba Mosquera has published over 150 original papers, over 15 book chapters and is the inventor in over 100 patent applications. He gave countless presentations at national and international meetings. He is a reviewer for 21 Ophthalmic Journals. In the last 25 years his research has been focused on corneal and refractive surgery.

Unique Features of the ATOS Laser for Lenticule Extraction: Programming, Intraoperative Software Use, and Dissection Techniques

24

Ivan Gabric, Kishore Raj Pradhan, and Samuel Arba Mosquera

Abstract

This chapter delves into the distinctive attributes of the SCHWIND ATOS laser system for lenticule extraction, emphasizing programming, intraoperative software utilization, and dissection techniques.

Keywords

ATOS laser system • Lenticule extraction • Plasma-mediated ablation • Ultrashort laser pulses

24.1 Unique Features of the ATOS Laser for Lenticule Extraction

As described in the previous chapter, the ATOS system (SCHWIND eye-tech-solutions) benefits from the advantages of a high numerical aperture (NA) and small spots resulting in very smooth cuts [1]. SCHWIND ATOS works in the plasma-mediated ablation range [2], which is well below the photodisruption regime [3] and slightly above the threshold for laser-induced optical breakdown. It generates only low-density plasma [4] and pulses in the low-energy range. A

I. Gabric (✉)
IG Svjetlost Eye Clinic, Zagreb, Croatia
e-mail: ivan.gabric@svjetlost.hr

K. R. Pradhan
KRP Matrika Eye Center, Kathmandu, Nepal

S. Arba Mosquera
SCHWIND eye-tech solutions, Kleinostheim, Germany

W. Sekundo and F. M. Wagner (eds.), *Femtosecond Laser Assisted Lenticule Extraction*,
https://doi.org/10.1007/978-3-031-60424-9_24

typical all-round setting would be 85 nJ in 5.2 × 2.6 μm (~629 mJ/cm^2) or alternatively 80 nJ in 6.0 × 2.1 μm (~635 mJ/cm^2), with some surgeons routinely going as low as 80 nJ in 7.6 × 2.3 μm (~458 mJ/cm^2) without dissection issues. "Shall be modified to" typical all-round setting would be 80 nJ in 5.9 × 2.9 μm (~468 mJ/cm^2) or alternatively 75 nJ in 5.7 × 2.8 μm (~470 mJ/cm^2), with some surgeons routinely going as low as 75 nJ in 6.0 × 4.4 μm (~284 mJ/cm^2) without major dissection issues.

The low pulse energy (sub-100 nJ) of the ATOS is probably one of the responsible features for the excellent cutting resolution and minimal corneal reactions, whereas the asymmetric spacings (as in the examples above) lead to very homogeneous cuts with low pulse energies. The temporally and spatially scanned process eventually leads to a confluent (or coalescent) bubble (conforming a cleavage plane), enabling the separation of the tissue.

The lenticule shape and geometry is described in detail in Chapter 23.

SCHWIND ATOS imposes the limit that the maximum lenticule thickness (typically at or close to the center for myopic-like corrections) to exceed 25μm for the treatment plan to be performed in ATOS (otherwise you cannot get it planned). Another limit is the maximum OZ not to exceed 8.0mm diameter. With these conditions, barely below −1D of myopia can be treated. Anecdotal experiences with corrections as low as −0.75DS-0.25DC achieved excellent outcomes.

In the absence of the minimal lenticule thickness along with the progressive refractive transition zone included in SmartSight, the epithelial remodeling is potentially reduced [5].

As mentioned above in SmartSight, the anterior cap cut is overbent (i.e., becomes slightly thicker/deeper toward the periphery). This may serve as protective measure against slight decentrations and may become more anatomically natural, since both overall corneal thickness as well as epithelium becomes thicker toward the periphery [6] (of note, the SILK procedure with its bi-convex cutting design (upon flat applanation), essentially also represents an (even more aggressive) overbent (convex) anterior cut).

For the scanning principle as well as eye-tracker features of SCHWIND ATOS, the reader is referred to the previous chapter.

24.2 Programming of a Lenticule Creation Treatment

SCHWIND ATOS delivers ultrashort laser pulses in the near-infrared wavelength regime (i.e., non-visible). The delivered wavelength of 1030 ± 50 nm in SCHWIND ATOS has high transmission rate in eyes. The extremely short pulses deposit the lowest possible energy for a minimum collateral damage of the surrounding corneal tissue. Precisely tuned sequences of laser pulses are scanned within the corneal tissue creating μm-sized local dissections, collectively resulting in coalescent bubble layer(s), the so-called cleavage plane(s). Two separating bubble layers together with an incisional edge cut enable to dissect two cleavage planes and remove the created corneal lenticule.

The settings of the to be created cavitation bubbles, such as applied energy, spot distance, and track distance may be different for different systems, operators, or dissection techniques, and are usually determined upon installation with trained SCHWIND personnel, and further refined by operator's experience.

Settings may be based upon "symmetric spacings" (as intuitively expected by users to ideally generate a homogeneous pattern of bubbles), and these would approach 120 nJ in 4.2 × 4.2 μm (~680 mJ/cm^2) for the cleavage plane combined with 120 nJ in 4.0 × 1.5 μm (~2000 mJ/cm^2) for the edge cut. Or, these may benefit from asymmetric spacings and fully exploit the low-energy concept. This could be potentially approaching settings like 75 nJ in 2.0 × 5.0 μm (~750 mJ/cm^2) for the cleavage plane combined with 75 nJ in 2.0 × 1.5 μm (~2500 mJ/cm^2) for the edge cut, to provide a low-energy high-density carpet of bubbles. Yet, the most commonly used asymmetric spacings like 85 nJ in 5.2 × 2.6 μm (~629 mJ/ cm^2) for the cleavage plane combined with 90 nJ in 4.3 × 1.2 μm (~1744 mJ/cm^2) for the edge cut; which are currently swiftly evolving toward 80 nJ in 6.0 × 2.1 μm (~635 mJ/cm^2) for the cleavage plane combined with 85 nJ in 4.4 × 1.1 μm (~1756 mJ/cm^2) for the edge cut. "Shall be modified to" Settings may be based upon "symmetric spacings" (as intuitively expected by users to ideally generate a homogeneous pattern of bubbles), and these would approach 120 nJ in 4.7 × 4.7 μm (~543 mJ/cm^2) for the cleavage plane combined with 120 nJ in 4.7 × 1.3 μm (~1964 mJ/cm^2) for the edge cut. Or, these may benefit from asymmetric spacings and fully exploit the low-energy concept. This could be potentially approaching settings like 75 nJ in 2.0 × 6.0 μm (~625 mJ/cm^2) for the cleavage plane combined with 75 nJ in 2.0 × 1.5 μm (~2500 mJ/cm^2) for the edge cut, to provide a low-energy high-density carpet of bubbles. Yet, the most commonly used asymmetric spacings like 80 nJ in 5.9 × 2.9 μm (~468 mJ/cm^2) for the cleavage plane combined with 90 nJ in 4.3×1.2 μm (~1744 mJ/cm^2) for the edge cut; which are currently swiftly evolving toward 75 nJ in 5.7 × 2.8 μm (~470 mJ/cm^2) for the cleavage plane combined with 85 nJ in 4.4 × 1.1 μm (~1756 mJ/cm^2) for the edge cut.

In order to program a treatment plan, first you have to < Log in > to the ATOS system using your login credentials and start treatment process by pressing < Planning > . Treatment specific parameters can be changed in < Settings > . These are preset values and should be checked upon initialization.

The ATOS graphical user interface (GUI) guides you step by step through the entire process, starting with treatment planning, up to removing the lenticule (Fig. 24.1).

Patient demographics (ID, Last Name, First Name, Date of Birth, Gender) are required to plan a treatment. A treatment plan may include one or both eyes of a patient.

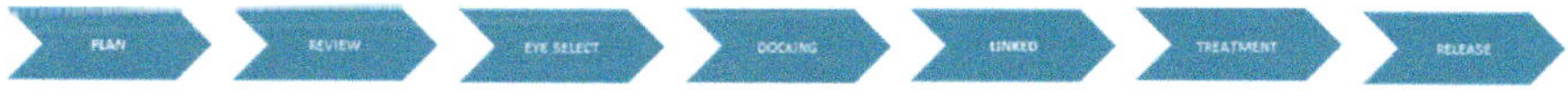

Fig. 24.1 Step-by-step guide of ATOS graphical user interface

Table 24.1 Programmable parameters of ATOS laser for SmartSight planning

Input Parameter for Lenticule	Unit	Minimum	Maximum	Step
Optical zone	mm	5.5	8.0	0.1
Cap thickness	μm	100	160	5
Incision Width	mm	2.0	5.0	0.1
Incision orientation	deg	0	360	1
Incision angle	deg	45	135	5
Cap diameter	mm	6.5	9.0	0.1
Vertex Distance	mm	0	24.0	0.5
Manifest Sphere	D	−12.00	0	0.25
Manifest Cylinder	D	−6.00	+ 6.00	0.25
Manifest Axis	deg	0	180	1
Target Sphere	D	−2.50	+ 1.50	0.25
Target Cylinder	D	−1.50	+ 1.50	0.25
Pupil Diameter	mm	2.0	8.0	0.1
Pupil Offset (r)	mm	0.01	0.70	0.01
Pupil Offset (angle)	deg	0	360	1
Pachymetry	μm	480	800	1
K1	D	35.0	48.0	0.1
K1 angle	deg	0	180	1
K2	D	35.0	48.0	0.1

The programmable parameters for the SmartSight are summarized in Table 24.1:

Of those, pupil and corneal data (along with the registration image) can be loaded from a diagnostic file (including SCHWIND SIRIUS, SCHWIND PERAMIS, SCHWIND MS-39, and SCHWIND SIRIUS +).

The GUI will show warning messages or information if any parameter needs additional attention and shall give hints for current settings. If one or more values are incorrect (e.g., out of range), you are asked to review the entries in the planning screen and you cannot proceed.

Further, after valid entry of all treatment parameters, the relevant ones are highlighted to be reviewed and checked for accuracy before treatment.

Patient data and treatments can be either pre-planned and loaded upon surgery day or configured on the fly just before treatment.

The recommendations for starting include: for the cap diameter (~8.5 mm), due to the use of a TZ (total lenticule diameter + 0.9 mm); thickness starting at 135 μm (or deeper 135–160 μm); 120 ° edge cut (or flatter 120–135 °); incision width: 3.0 mm (2.5–3.5 mm).

Start with those settings and deviate from them as experience and confidence are gained. OBLs seem to be the most questioned aspect, and there are many different parameters involved in the incidence of OBLs:

That is one of the reasons we suggest starting with not-so-thin caps (>135 μm), not-so-small caps (>8.0 mm), low pulse energy (80–85 nJ), wide asymmetric spacing (close to 6 × 2 μm Spot × Track distance).

Pay attention to the appearance of OBLs at the edge cut in the initial experiences.

Edge cut angle 90deg seems to be too steep for comfortably entering the edges. > 120 ° has been adopted for a softer entrance. Enlarging the cap diameter or reducing the lenticule size (i.e., OZ), in order to enlarge the clearance annulus, combined to ironing/massage shall facilitate having a larger untreated area (cap oversize) where the folds may be moved away.

24.3 Intraoperative Software Use

After validating all treatment entries (for both eyes), a new patient interface (PI) shall be inserted and OD or OS shall be selected for immediate surgery. After selection, you will proceed to < Docking > screen automatically once the PI checks are successfully completed.

After the patient is positioned on the bed, the cone (a disposable patient interface) is connected to the suction ports within the interface holder. The patient's eye is positioned under the cone and the patient instructed to fixate the light target.

Place the head (without stress for the patient) conveniently for exposing the cornea (a roll pillow may help at this aim). Drops of topical anesthetic shall be instilled in the upper and lower fornices. A sterile drape covering eye lashes shall be used to isolate the surgical field. A lid speculum shall be inserted to allow maximum exposure of the globe. The use of a hard lid speculum is strongly recommended, while a closed blade speculum may be of advantage. The lid speculum shall be opened wide, in order to move the tear lake away of the PI. The corneal surface shall be kept moist (not too dry, not to wet). To accomplish it, just before docking a wet microsponge (BSS) can be gently squeezed and passed over the corneal surface using 3 painting-like movements.

Long before the contact between PI and cornea, the eye-tracker recognizes the eye (both pupil boundaries as well as cyclotorsional position, respect to the diagnostic reference image). Pupil center is shown by a green cross, and the yellow cross represents the target position for the pupil center. Both crosses shall be overlapped (or as close as possible while the patient fixates the fixation light) using the patient bed. Remember that centration remains surgeon dependent (the eye-tracker only supports surgeon to optimize and speed up centration and docking). Patients shall be instructed to fixate on the fixation light to help centration [7].

To accomplish centration and docking of the eye to the system, an eye-tracker guided centration is used. A camera provides the operator with a coaxial view through the cone of the patient interface (Fig. 24.2). The operator is instructed to

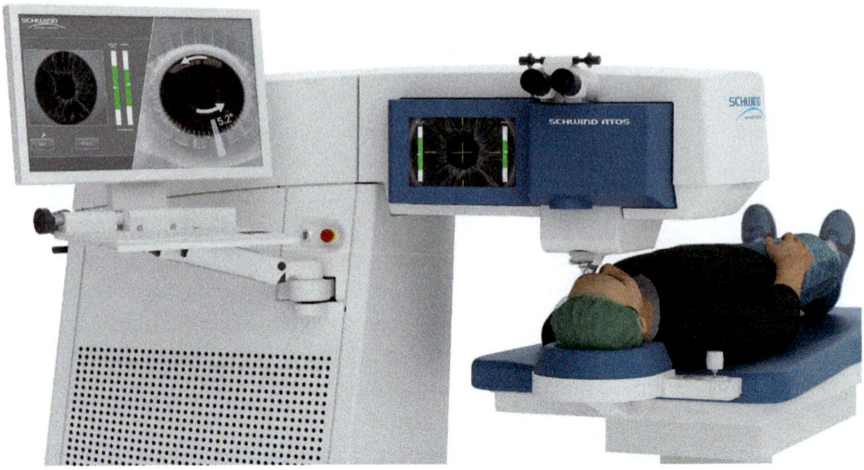

Fig. 24.2 Patient's positioning under ATOS

move the patient table and bring the pupil (detected by a video-based eye-tracker) coincident with the target pupil position (or as close as possible). Accurate alignment of the eye with the laser shall be achieved with an infrared eye-tracker with simultaneous limbus, pupil, and torsion tracking integrated into the laser system. The correction profile can be centered with respect to the corneal vertex determined by the topography (e.g., taking 70–100% of the pupil offset value [8] closely approximates the visual axis [9, 10]).

While lifting the patient into surgery position (establishing contact between the corneal surface and the lower curved surface of the PI), the lower half of the floating range shall be aimed and vacuum will be enabled and started.

Further recommendations from experience include a suggested vacuum level just above the minimum. The docking can be tricky in particular the patients' cheek may collide and interfere with the PI holder, thus making difficult to achieve stable vacuum. Liquid (tears) affects suction performance (speed of building vacuum, as well as stability of achieved vacuum).

Unlike other devices, at ATOS, the pressure onto the eye barely changes within the floating range. Thus, it does not help (much) to further move the bed up after entering the green region of the height sensor. The aim shall be to place the cornea in contact to the interface and place the height sensor **in the lower half of the green region. And then start vacuum**. If the eye (position sensor) is too high (e.g., in the upper green region), then **move down to the lower half of the green region. And then start vacuum**. (Vacuum level can be increased to provide a better suction/hold to the eye).

Make sure the cornea shows wide enough contact with the patient interface. Air bubbles and debris shall be avoided, since they may reduce the laser beam quality (and result in black spots within the treatment zone). By pressing < Start Vacuum > , the patient bed is blocked until laser application is finished.

The linking process is successful achieved upon:

Review that the float position is in the lower half of the green level and vacuum indication is stable.

Vacuum has reached the preset level, shown by green indication "vacuum good."

System gives status message if patient eye alignment is out of tolerance and if redocking is necessary.

Suction is applied, and it is confirmed that the pupil remains close to its target position; otherwise, a new docking shall be attempted. Further to that, the last valid laser videoframe of the eye-tracker is used for cyclotorsion control, and the torsional misalignment from the diagnostic image is determined and accounted for [11]. The treatment is applied, and the laser initiates after suction.

< START Treatment > on the surgery screen will proceed with treatment. Instruct the patient to stay still during laser application. Remember that breathing under a mask (or drape) may actually produce haze/fog in the optics before the laser starts.

During the phase before the laser starts to deliver pulses, there is a short period of time where the scanner is coming into position and spinning up. During this time if the surgeon is not satisfied with the vacuum or patient compliance, they can press < !ABORT Treatment! > button and reset the docking phase. From experience of the co-authors, most suction issues present before the laser pulses are delivered.

Two discs are visible during/after the laser application. The inner, more dense looking area indicates the region overlaid with posterior lenticule cut and anterior (cap) cut. The outer ring annulus represents the anterior (cap) cut. The incision can also be seen as a denser line at the outer rim of the anterior (cap) cut.

Both discs appear to be eccentric to each other, due to the oblique angle of the camera during treatment.

24.4 Dissection Techniques

Vacuum is automatically released once the laser treatment is completed. SCHWIND Patient Bed interlock switches off, and patient eye can be moved to observatory position (microscope view) for lenticular dissection and removal.

At the same time, the options to adjust < Illumination > and < Microscope > magnification are enabled at the secondary user interface (touchscreen close to the microscope).

To keep the eye still, the use of a forceps is strongly recommended (better than fixation rings). After opening the incision, keep the instrument ventrally in order to dissect the anterior cut first. Keep the instrument inside the incision to avoid epithelial migration during cleavage plane separation.

The recommended sequence can be summarized as follows:

Open incision using a hooked instrument and identify/separate anterior plane. Pay attention for light reflection at the surgical instruments. Crispier reflections suggest the instrument lies at the anterior lamellar interface, and duller reflections suggest the instrument lies at the posterior lamellar interface.

Identify/separate posterior plane. When entered the posterior lamellar interface correctly, the overall image quality is reduced in terms of sharpness and contrast.

Separate anterior lamellar plane first using a lenticule separator. Enter with a slight ventral pull. Separate anterior cut toward the edges using wide arc-segment swipes.

Entering the bed(s) from the edge cut is one of the reasons we suggest starting with not-so-steep edge cut angles (>120deg) facilitating a flatter access to the bed(s).

Long dissectors may not be good for maneuvering sharp edges. Instruments shall be a prolongation of the hand; they shall provide a feeling as to where the tip actually is (in all six degrees of freedom).

Dissecting the edge first (all around, there are different modifications of the technique), proved to be of help in different scenarios.

Enter posterior lamellar plane pushing the instrument dorsally. Separate posterior cut toward the edges using wide arc-segment swipes.

If you encounter difficulties entering the posterior interface, try to push at the edge of the lenticule in order to create folds which will give you "leverage" for advancing into the posterior lamellar interface.

For the posterior interface, do first the surface area and leave the edge for the end to avoid the lenticule folding over and making it more difficult in early stages of the learning curve.

Make sure to dissect both lamellar interfaces completely before any extraction attempt.

Massage the dissected lenticule in circular motions toward incision ("spoon" or wipe the lenticule out of the pocket). If required, drag the lenticule out using micro-forceps.

Finally, gently (but firmly) ironing/massage of the corneal cap in longitudinal straight movements toward the incision in order to spread the cap evenly and potentially decrease Bowman's wrinkles [12] has been tried in an attempt to preventing the folds to occur and seems to improve short-term outcomes. If you are not sure about any remaining tissue in the pocket, a check can be performed for any residual material or tears, and the easiest way is to spread the lenticule over the top of the cornea. If still unsure, triamcinolone can be inserted to the pocket to stain the potential remnants as described by Sachdev et al. [13]

References

1. Wang J, Schuele G, Palanker D. Finesse of transparent tissue cutting by ultrafast lasers at various wavelengths. J Biomed Opt. 2015;20(12): 125004. https://doi.org/10.1117/1.JBO.20.12.125004. PMID: 26720869.
2. Tsai PS, Blinder P, Migliori BJ, Neev J, Jin Y, Squier JA, Kleinfeld D. Plasma-mediated ablation: an optical tool for submicrometer surgery on neuronal and vascular systems. Curr Opin

Biotechnol. 2009;20(1):90 9. https://doi.org/10.1016/j.copbio.2009.02.003. Epub 2009 Mar 5. PMID: 19269159; PMCID: PMC3123732.
3. Lubatschowski H, Maatz G, Heisterkamp A, Hetzel U, Drommer W, Welling H, Ertmer W. Application of ultrashort laser pulses XE "Ultrashort laser pulses" for intrastromal refractive surgery. Graefes Arch Clin Exp Ophthalmol. 2000;238(1):33–9. https://doi.org/10.1007/s004170050006. PMID: 10664050.
4. Kuetemeyer K, Rezgui R, Lubatschowski H, Heisterkamp A. Influence of laser parameters and staining on femtosecond laser-based intracellular nanosurgery. Biomed Opt Express. 2010;1(2):587–597. https://doi.org/10.1364/BOE.1.000587. PMID: 21258492. PMCID: PMC3017989.
5. de Ortueta D, von Rüden D, Arba-Mosquera S. Refractive Effect of Epithelial Remodelling in Myopia after Transepithelial Photorefractive Keratectomy. Vision. 2022;6(4):74. https://doi.org/10.3390/vision6040074.
6. Arba-Mosquera S, Awwad ST. Impact of the reference point for Epithelial thickness measurements. J Refract Surg. 2020;36(3):200–20.
7. Kang DSY, Lee H, Reinstein DZ, Roberts CJ, Arba-Mosquera S, Archer TJ, Kim EK, Seo KY, Kim TI. Comparison of the distribution of Lenticule Decentration following SMILE by subjective patient fixation or triple marking centration. J Refract Surg. 2018;34(7):446–52.
8. Arba Mosquera S, Ewering T. New asymmetric centration strategy combining pupil and corneal vertex information for ablation procedures in refractive surgery: theoretical background. J Refract Surg. 2012;28(8):567–75.
9. De Ortueta D, ArbaMosquera S. Centration during hyperopic LASIK using the coaxial light reflex. J Refract Surg. 2007;23(1):11; author reply 11.
10. Arbelaez MC, Vidal C, Arba-Mosquera S. Clinical outcomes of corneal vertex versus central pupil references with aberration-free ablation strategies and LASIK. Invest Ophthalmol Vis Sci. 2008;49(12):5287–94.
11. Detection of and compensation for static cyclotorsion with an image-guided system in SMILE. Köse B. J Refract Surg. 2020;36(3):142–149. https://doi.org/10.3928/1081597X-20200210-01
12. Intra-operative cap repositioning in small incision Lenticule Extraction (SMILE) for enhanced visual recovery. Shetty R, Shroff R, Kaweri L, Jayadev C, Kummelil MK, Sinha Roy A. Curr Eye Res. 2016;41(12):1532–1538. https://doi.org/10.3109/02713683.2016.1168848. Epub 2016 Apr 4. PMID: 27044473.
13. Sachdev GS, Ramamurthy S, Dandapani R. Triamcinolone acetonide for remnant lenticule identification in small incision lenticule extraction. J Cataract Refract Surg. 2020;46(6):811–813. https://doi.org/10.1097/j.jcrs.0000000000000160

Clinical Results of SmartSight in Four Years Experience

25

Kishore Raj Pradhan, Victor Derhartunian, Ivan Gabric, and Samuel Arba Mosquera

Abstract

"This chapter provides a comprehensive overview of the clinical results and experiences with the SCHWIND ATOS femtosecond laser system, particularly focusing on SmartSight lenticule extraction."

Keywords

SCHWIND ATOS • SmartSight • Femtosecond laser technology • LASIK flaps • Lenticule extraction

25.1 Introduction

SCHWIND ATOS is a new development in femtosecond laser technology that enables the generation of LASIK flaps and lenticules for SmartSight lenticule extraction. It received the CE Mark in July 2020, early in the COVID-19 pandemic. Since then, a steadily growing number of surgeons in and beyond Europe has performed SmartSight. So far, lenticule removal was reported to be performed without relevant intraoperative complications.

K. R. Pradhan
KRP Matrika Eye Center, Kathmandu, Nepal

V. Derhartunian · I. Gabric
VD EYE-LASER Clinic Vienna/Zürich, Zürich, Switzerland

I. Gabric
IG Svjetlost Eye Clinic, Zagreb, Croatia

S. Arba Mosquera (✉)
SCHWIND eye-tech solutions, Kleinostheim, Germany
e-mail: Samuel.Arba.Mosquera@eye-tech.net

W. Sekundo and F. M. Wagner (eds.), *Femtosecond Laser Assisted Lenticule Extraction*,
https://doi.org/10.1007/978-3-031-60424-9_25

In a nutshell, the SCHWIND ATOS is engined by a regenerative amplified femtosecond laser source, delivering near IR pulses at around 1030 ± 50 nm, with a pulse duration of approximately 225 ± 70 fs, a repetition rate of up to around 4 MHz, and delivering a pulse energy in the range 75–135 nJ. The ATOS optical system includes a high numerical aperture (NA) and a short working distance leading to a very small spot in the focal plane.

Further details can be found in the two previous chapters on the basics of this relatively young technology. From the first clinical results, it was apparent that no major nomogram was required.

25.2 Clinical Experience

As per Sept 2024, there have been over 75,000 treatments performed with ATOS; distributed as > 45,000 SmartSight lenticules + > 30,000 flaps. SCHWIND's application team accompanies surgeons on their first days of treatment in the clinic to support ATOS users as best as possible. The feedback from the ever-growing SCHWIND ATOS user family is that "SmartSight is surprisingly easy to perform," the edges are very clean, but they can require attention to separate them cleanly in a single pass. Visual acuities on day 1 are good; on average, patients achieve UDVAs of 20/20 to 20/25 with a few exceptions of 20/32. Some even achieve 20/16.

We report here the collective experience of three different centers (accounting for six ATOS units) cumulating over 3000 SmartSight treatments in a four-year time span, which averages 250 SmartSight treatments per ATOS and year. These figures are constantly increasing every year.

25.2.1 Initial Experience with the SCHWIND ATOS and SmartSight Lenticule Extraction [1]

Small incision lenticule extraction is a commonly used technique for correction of refractive error (currently myopia and myopic astigmatism). It involves making a small incision in the peripheral cornea and cutting a lenticule in the stroma. Both the incision and lenticule are cut with a femtosecond laser. Once the ATOS device was available, the clinical authors of this chapter decided to adopt the new device able to perform SmartSight procedures. As usual, the initial aims were gaining confidence with the system and developing nomograms for the subsequent experiences (this is a continuous process). When we started using the system for refractive corrections, we were applying only spherical lenticules (without cylindrical component). Even if the patients showed a low-to-moderate astigmatism (typically below 0.75 D cylindrical error), the plan was based on the SEQ as spherical treatment. Further to that, to facilitate the lenticule extraction, we started with lenticule thicknesses above 85 μm (i.e., with spherical powers above −6 D of myopia).

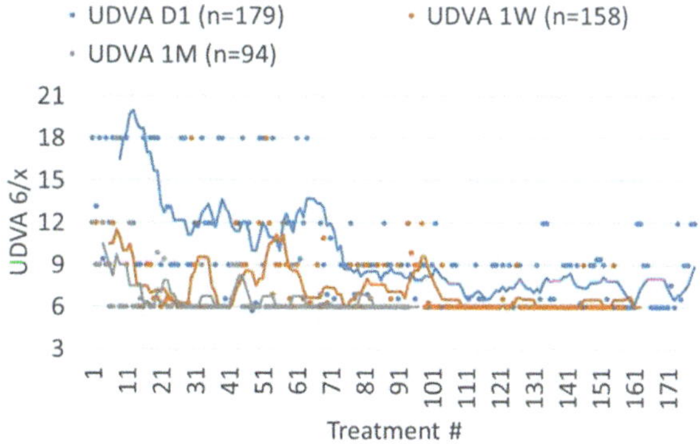

Fig. 25.1 Outcomes of UDVA. The first 16 treatments were performed without astigmatism correction, the next 52 treatments served for finding optimum laser settings and refinements in the technique, whereas the following 100 + treatments have been performed with the same settings and technique

Since the initial experiences were quickly encouraging, rather soon it was decided to incorporate astigmatism to the treatment spectrum (typically below 3 D cylindrical error) and treat lenticule thickness from 70 μm or more (maximum myopic meridian of −5 D or more). With those indications, the laser settings and the technique have been refined.

The first 16 treatments were performed without astigmatism correction, the next 52 treatments served to adjust optimum laser settings and refinements in the technique, whereas the last 700 + treatments have been performed using very similar settings and technique (Fig. 25.1).

As for the settings we are using now, they include spot/track distance: ~ 5.9/ ~ 2.9 μm; pulse energy: ~ 80 nJ; laser time: 34 s for SmartSight; total energy: < 500 mJ for SmartSight; avg. dose: 468 mJ/cm2; avg. laser power: < 45 mW.

During the last few months, all three surgical co-authors have begun to explore the bottom limit of the total energy dose to the corneal plane and it's relation to first post-op day (POD1) visual acuities. As a guide, they use the retro illumination feature of the SCHWIND PERAMIS (CSO Osiris-T). Although still not easy to quantify, there is a clear correlation between the apparent roughness of the retro illuminated image and the patients' perceived quality of vision. There are attempts to use this to optimize POD1 visual recovery versus just surgical experience on the device (Fig. 25.2).

In the gained experience, we have found that oversizing the cap by ~ 0.8 mm wider than the TZ provides sufficient room for surgical maneuvers and while keeping the cap diameter moderately narrow (8.0 mm to 8.8 mm). Although anecdotal experiences down to just 0.1 mm of oversize found no issues with extraction, a 0.5–0.9 mm cap oversize is safer for novice surgeons.

In order to preserve residual stromal thickness (RST), we recommend moderate OZs (~6.5 mm in our experience for corrections above −6D) combined with thin caps can be used to provide better quality of vision.

Since the cyclotorsion is acquired upon docking, when the epithelium is still intact, eye registration is improved compared to flap-based treatments with previous corneal manipulations.

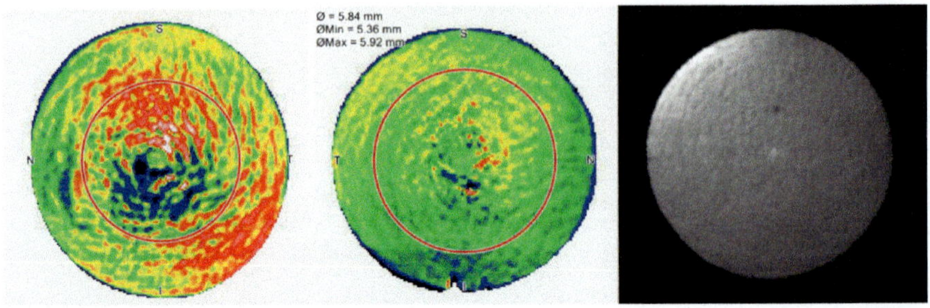

Fig. 25.2 Example of a POD1 patient after a high-energy dose extraction (Left: POD1 UDVA 20/25); patient after a medium dose extraction (Middle: POD1 UDVA 20/20); retro illuminated image after a low dose extraction (Right: POD1 UDVA 20/16)

The dissection was always easy (even in the presence of OBLs), and the appearance of the cut smooth. Surgeries went smoother and faster day by day. The final technique uses the incision half-way for the upper layer, and half-way for the lower layer. Followed by a dissection technique and wiping the lenticule out through the incision, a novel feature of the SmartSight lenticule is the fact that it has a zero-thickness edge, and a lack of pedestal ensures that the removal is usually without risk of retained lenticule fragments.

25.2.2 Outcomes of Myopic Astigmatism Correction [2]

We also studied a subset of eyes having a pre-operative manifest refractive astigmatism magnitude of 1.00 D or higher. For this subgroup of moderate astigmatism, the percentage of eyes achieving a post-operative refractive astigmatism of less than 0.50 D was 91% (401 eyes out of 443 treatments). The correlation between target-induced astigmatism and surgically induced astigmatism for manifest refraction was relatively good, but lower than for SEQ. Almost all eyes (92%) showed an angle of error between $-5°$ and $+ 5°$.

In all patients, lenticule removal was complete without relevant intraoperative complications. Pre-operatively, the patients had a CDVA below the normal range (mean: 0.00 ± 0.04 logMAR; range: -0.1 to $+ 0.3$ logMAR). This CDVA could be a characteristic specific to our patient population. In this subgroup, 1% of the eyes (four eyes) lost Snellen lines of CDVA at the 3 months post-operatively. At the three-month follow-up visit, 93% of the eyes had a UDVA of 6/6 or better. This is comparable to current LASIK and SMILE reports for lower amounts of astigmatism.

The scattergram of surgically induced astigmatism versus target-induced astigmatism showed a slight undercorrection. Our findings seem to challenge the notion of and concerns about the undercorrection of the astigmatic component in lenticule extraction procedures.[3] This challenge had been implied in previous reports

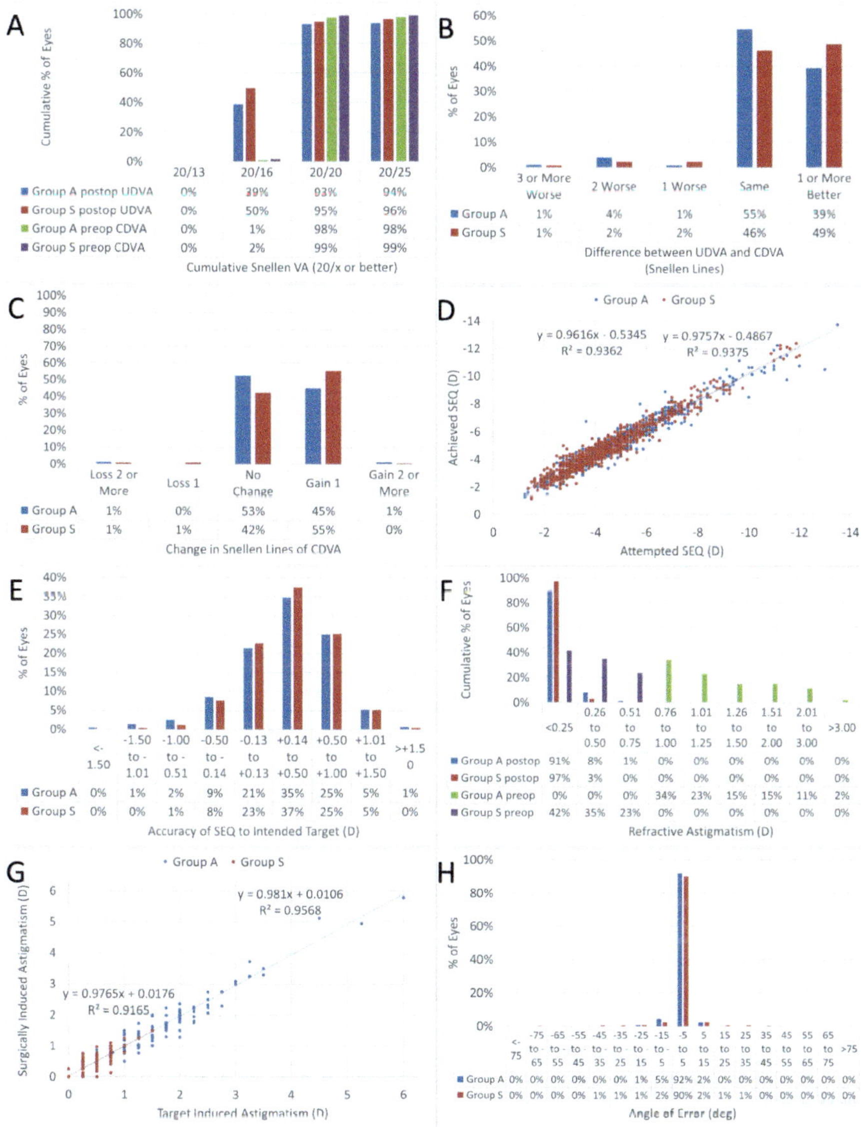

Fig. 25.3 Comparison of group A (with pre-operative astigmatism of 1D of higher) versus group S (mainly spherical, with pre-operative astigmatism below 1D)

[4], but cannot be confirmed in our results, in which residual astigmatism did not exceed 0.75 D, and 99% of the eyes had a residual astigmatism up to 0.50 D.

The change in manifest refractive astigmatism correlated well with the attempted values, suggesting that laser surgery could modify the corneal contour properly in moderately toric eyes. Therefore, it can be inferred that the planned goal of the treatment was met, even if patients were slightly undercorrected for refractive astigmatism. Patients may have been habituated to undercorrection of the cylinder in spectacles at the time of the pre-operative assessment, and thus accustomed to some residual astigmatism. This might have resulted in the treatment plans also being designed based on the "underrefracted" astigmatism. These results highlight the need for better ways to properly determine how much astigmatism should be incorporated into the treatment. It could be hypothesized, similar to hyperopic cases, not to overplan the treatment with the knowledge of a potential regression occurring post-operatively, but to instead push the refraction as much as possible. If so, then the cylinder correction chosen should be closest to the corneal toricity and compatible with best CDVA, analogous to the most positive SEQ compatible with best CDVA.[5] In this regard, it also can be noted that patients may not accept high cylinder at the spectacle plane but may more easily do so on the corneal plane.

Cyclotorsion compensation is reported to provide an advantage with astigmatic values greater than 1.00 D [6]. Because the treatments considered here included an astigmatic component of 1.00 D or greater, any cyclotorsion errors (i.e., uncompensated cyclotorsion movements or wrongly compensated cyclotorsion movements) would be expected to result in a measurable portion of astigmatism at a different axis, which should have been noticeable in the outcomes.

The outcomes reported here indirectly demonstrate proper placement of the correction profile in terms of both centration and cyclotorsion. We demonstrated that myopic astigmatism correction with SCHWIND ATOS SmartSight provided good results in terms of efficacy, safety, predictability, and visual outcomes in the first three months of follow-up. In addition, the outcomes showed good predictability for both SEQ and cylinder refraction. This finding is important and counters the accepted notion in the literature concerning undercorrections for sphere and cylinder in lenticule extraction, possibly because the treatment includes a transition zone and no lenticule side cut (thus no minimum lenticule thickness).

25.2.3 Actual Central Lenticule Thickness [7]

Laser refractive surgery aims to correct patients' refractive error by removing a portion of corneal tissue respective to the target correction. The Munnerlyn formula [8] is a simple closed form equation to determine the depth (thickness) of tissue to be removed, although alternative formulations (e.g., paraxial formulas, or aspheric profiles) may render more accurate results or better quality of the prescription to be corrected. Similarly, equations may need to be extended by incorporating the effects of, e.g., transition zones or high-order aberrations (HOA). The accuracy of corneal refractive procedures can be evaluated by the reduction of corneal thickness (rather stromal thickness) that aims to change corneal power by modulating the anterior corneal curvature [9].

In general, the lenticule shape resembles very much (but it is not identical to) the equivalent aberration-free LASIK profiles of the AMARIS ablation design (besides the excimer spot's peripheral spreading compensation). We described the SmartSight profiles in detail in Chap. 23.

In the present study, we assessed the predictability between the SCHWIND ATOS read-out and achieved lenticule thickness measured with MS-39 OCT at corneal vertex at different follow-up times.

The MS-39 combines the Placido corneal topography with high-resolution SD-OCT-based anterior segment tomography. This system achieves high-resolution imaging (axial: 3.6 μm; transversal: 35 μm) [10]. The MS-39 acquires one Placido top-view image and a sequence of 12 SD-OCT transversal field sections using 845-nm wavelength. Each 10-mm section is reconstructed from 600 A-scans and averaged five times. Corneal tomography is calculated from 31,232 measurement points on the anterior surface and 25,600 on the posterior surface.

Three repeated consecutive measurements were taken by the same experienced examiner (IG) according to the manufacturers' guidelines. Device was brought into focus, and the patient's eye was aligned along the visual axis with a central fixation light. The patients were instructed to blink completely just before each measurement, and no eye drops were applied before testing. Lenticule thickness was obtained by subtraction method (thickness of the pre-op cornea–thickness of the post-op cornea) and was measured on corneal vertex.

We included 130 eyes of 65 consecutive patients and found a lower reduction in CCT compared to laser read-out for all three follow-ups (Fig. 25.4).

The reduction in CCT is very similar at 3M versus 1M. The reduction in CCT is lowest at POD1. Taking the 1M and 3M data (essentially equivalent), one can see a best fit of $y = 0.94$ x -7 μm; i.e., a -6% and a -7 μm reduction. The difference reduction in CCT vs laser read-out cannot be at all explained from the SC, OZ, and TZ values; only the -7 μm remains statistically significant (isolated without any other explanator).

Laser refractive surgery aims to correct patients' refractive error by removing a portion of corneal tissue respective to the aimed correction. Thus, it would be logical to think that deviations in the lenticule thickness (amount of tissue removal) would determine refractive deviations in the final outcomes. On the other hand, removing too much tissue may result in unstable corneas post-op (at least for those

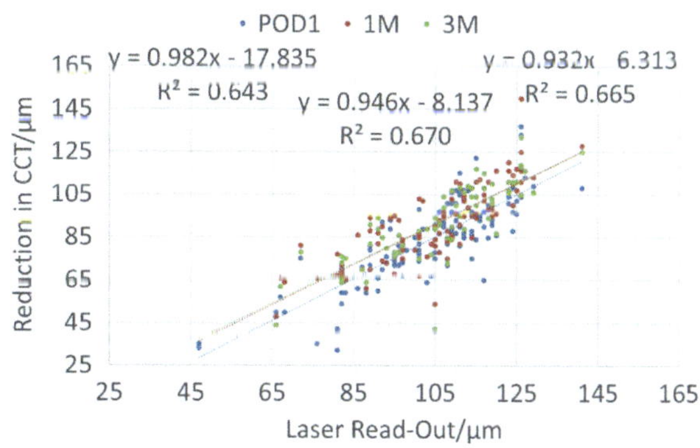

Fig. 25.4 Reduction in CCT vs laser read-out for three different follow-ups

corneas at risk). Both these aspects make essential to control and double-check the actual amount of tissue removal against the laser read-out.

For myopic corrections, measuring the reduction of central corneal thickness (as evaluated here) provides a reasonably accurate estimate of the thickness of the removed lenticule. In the presence of strong epithelial remodeling [11], the reduction in stromal thickness may have been a better predictor for the thickness of the removed lenticule. However, using the same laser as in our cohort, Pradhan et al. [12] reported minor changes in epithelial remodeling (of only 3 μm on average). On the other hand, using stromal thickness may be prone to more noise since the segmentation of the epithelium-Bowman interface is clearly more difficult than that of the air-tear film (or tear film-epithelium).

Results show a lower reduction in CCT compared to laser read-out for all three follow-ups. Essentially, the reduction in CCT is identical at 3M Versus 1M, likely indicating that the epi-remodeling processes are over already at 1M. The reduction in CCT is lowest at POD1 which may be indicative of both swelling processes and acute epi-remodeling ongoing (overshoot acute epithelial reaction).

According to the manufacturer, −5% are reduction by design, and the same strategy seems to have been used for the AMARIS system (same manufacturer) at least for the first seven years on the market, as well as for competing devices [13].

Clearing the −5% (from manufacturer) out, a best fit of y = 0.99 x −7 μm is obtained; i.e., a −1% combined with the same −7 μm reduction. Other groups assessed the accuracy and influence factors of predicting lenticule thickness in an alternative technique [14] (SMILE using the VisuMax system by CZM, Jena, Germany). In general, lenticule thickness was also always lower than laser read-out. However, opposite to our findings, refractive treatments were also undercorrected, correspondingly deviations in the lenticule thickness (amount of tissue removal) determine refractive deviations in the final outcomes. The extent of undersize in the thickness of the lenticules with the alternative technique was much higher than in this report, suggesting that may be the thickness deviations observed in this cohort may not be sufficiently large (despite being systematic) to be reflected in the residual post-operative refraction. Alternatively, the reduced lenticule thickness (while preserving the refractive correction) could be associated to a smaller than planned effective optical zone.

In conclusion, in this cohort of eyes, the reduction in CCT was stable from 1M follow-up. The stable reduction in CCT was −6% (−1% after accounting for design decisions) and −7 μm lower than the respective laser read-out. Findings are very predictable showing a certain level of the lenticules becoming slightly thinner than their respective laser read-outs.

25.2.4 Effective Optical Zone (EOZ)[15]

A further aim is to achieve an EOZ equal (or at least comparable) to the planned optical zone (OZ) [16]. The planned OZ for SmartSight can be set freely between 5.5 and 8.0 mm diameter (+TZ of up to 0.8 mm outside of the OZ). Of course, as the lenticules get thicker (e.g., for higher corrections or larger optical zones), they are easier to extract, but less residual stroma is left behind. ATOS limits the maximum lenticule thickness between 25 and 165 μm. Further, ATOS imposes a minimum 275 μm calculated residual stromal thickness (we personally also pay attention that the total corneal thickness after extraction remains above 400 μm).

Comparing not only the lenticule thickness read-out, but as introduced before also the size of the effective correction provides a comprehensive analysis of the effective vs planned corrections geometries, which may explain (to some extent) some clinical findings reported in the literature.

For this analysis of the effective optical zone, the evaluation is based on a different cohort of eyes (compared to the previous section), but they were also scanned using the SCHWIND MS-39 OCT.

We considered the pre-operative and one-month post-operative scans of 84 eyes from 47 patients treated with SmartSight using SCHWIND ATOS.

The difference in pre- versus post-operative scans provides the changes in topographical curvature (we analyzed tangential curvature in this case). With those differences, the EOZ was calculated by determining for each meridian (256 meridians, meaning 1.4° azimuthal resolution) the smallest radius for which a change of sign in the difference image occurred (cross-over through zero, i.e., end of the monotonically corrected region).

This way the boundary of the EOZ has been determined, without imposing any a priori size, shape, or centration. Both, the area of the free-form EOZ and the mean of all meridional lengths were considered to numerically calculate the size of the EOZ (Fig. 25.5).

Overall we obtained the following EOZs:

Pre-op SEQ	5.04D ± 1.72 [−2.0D to −8.88D]
Planned OZ	7.20mm ± 0.29 [6.5 mm to 7.50 mm]
EOZ-Ø	6.78 mm ± 0.46 [5.67 mm to 7.55 mm]
EOZ-Area	36.46mm2 ± 4.89 [25.26 mm^2 to 46.33 mm^2]

In this series, the larger the planned OZ is, the larger the EOZ-Area, showing a parabolic dependency. But also, we observed that the lower the correction to be treated, the larger the EOZ-Area and the EOZ-Ø (both roughly with a linear dependency). Of course, there is a "natural" tendency to use smaller optical zones (OZ) for higher corrections to balance tissue removal and to respect the residual stromal thickness (personal limit for RST = 300 μm).

The relative EOZ-Ø (EOZ− *Ø/planned OZ*) shows only a slight tendency to decrease with higher SEQ (Fig. 25.6).

Using univariate multilinear regression, a correlation EOZ-Ø = 0.981*planned OZ + 0.057*SEQ is obtained showing a 1.9% reduction in EOZ respect to planned OZ, and a secondary reduction of 57 μm in diameter per each diopter of correction.

The difference between EOZ and planned OZ shows a Gaussian distribution, with mean -0.43mm ± 0.34 EOZ-Ø smaller than planned OZ, i.e., the diameter of

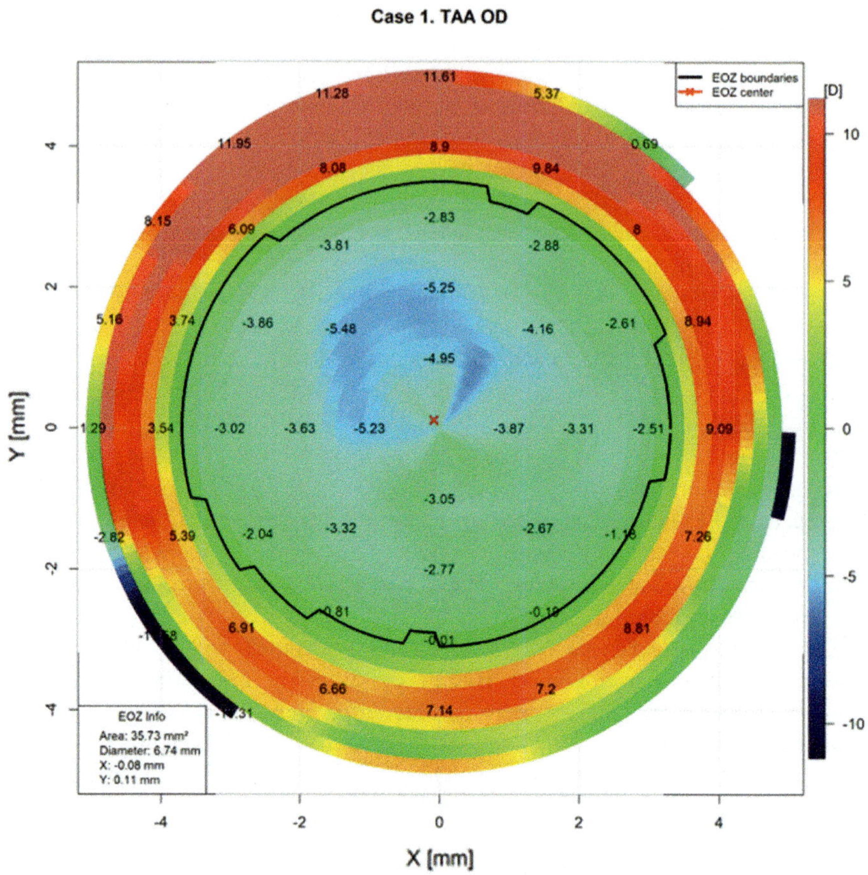

Fig. 25.5 Example of the method to determine the EOZ boundary in a meridional fashion

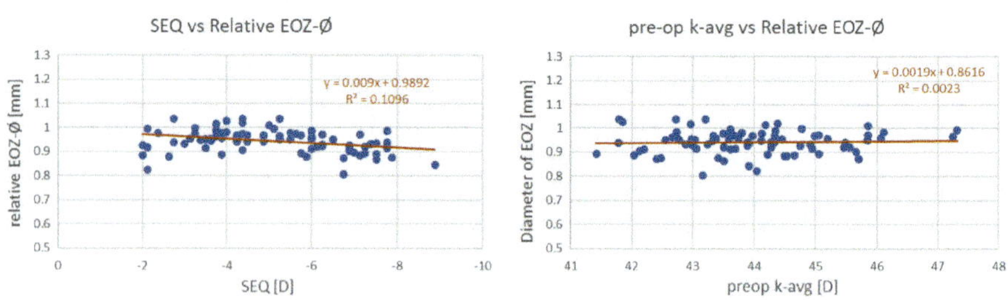

Fig. 25.6 Relative EOZ diameter (EOZ – *Ø/planned OZ*) versus correction power and corneal curvature

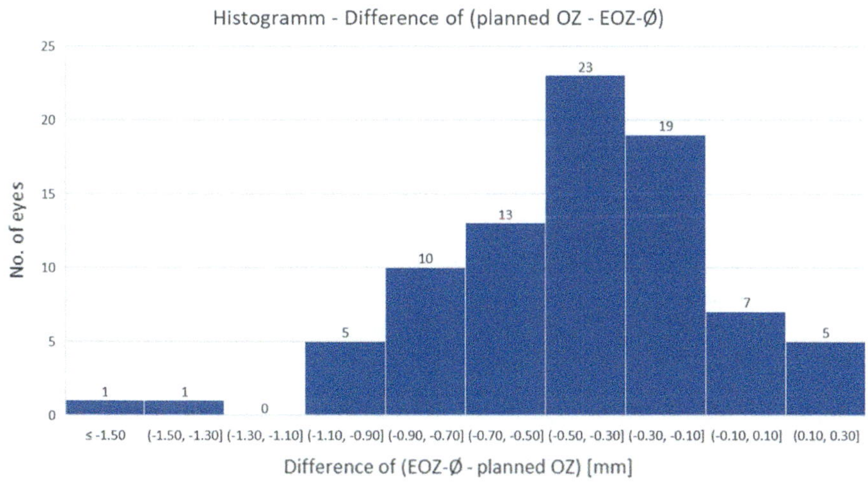

Fig. 25.7 Distribution of the difference between EOZ and planned OZ diameters

the effective optical zone EOZ was slightly smaller than the planned optical zone (Fig. 25.7).

This knowledge can be considered for treatment plannings in slightly enlarging the planned OZ by ~ + 3%. This information is especially helpful for patients with large pupil sizes and/or in high diopter treatments to avoid visual side effects under dark light conditions.

25.2.5 Centration of the Lenticule (Optical Zone) [17]

For a refractive treatment to be effective, it is important to center the optical correction at an adequate reference point, such as the corneal intersection of the visual axis. This ensures that the correction is applied in the correct location to improve vision [18].

However, if the actual correction is decentered with respect to this reference point, it can have a negative impact on visual performance. This can lead to problems such as coma (distorted vision), reduced contrast sensitivity, or reduced visual acuity[19]. Previous research has determined the permissible levels of decentration based on different optical measures [20].

To analyze the (de)centration of the lenticule, corneal measurements were performed with a Placido–Scheimpflug tomographer (SIRIUS, CSO, Italy) [21]. The dataset includes 101 eyes of 56 patients, 45 of them using bilateral data. To determine the actual centration, the difference between pre- and post-operative topographies has been calculated, and the "center of mass" (weighted average, and not merely the centroid) of this difference map is considered the actual centration of the achieved change. We used subtraction maps of pachymetry (related to the corneal change in morphology), as well as refractive equivalent power (related to the change of the optical properties of the cornea).

The XY plot for corneal thickness and corneal refractive equivalent power for all cases as well as the corresponding histogram (for corneal thickness and corneal refractive equivalent power) are shown as Fig. 25.8.

The centration of the lenticule can be determined with respect to various references, such as the pupil center, limbus center, visual axis, or corneal vertex normal. The method has been tested on a pilot cohort of clinical data and has been found to be effective. The different metrics provide complementary information about the geometry and optics of the lenticule. The X, Y plot of a specific metric for both eyes shows enantiomorphism (mirror symmetry) [22].

When a new method is presented, it is usually needed to prove that the results given by the method are reliable, or they agree with the experimental results. The best way is to provide experimental results to show which metric gives the best estimation of the centration. The discussion on different metrics to evaluate centration has been subject to debate in clinical papers, as it can be seen in the references.

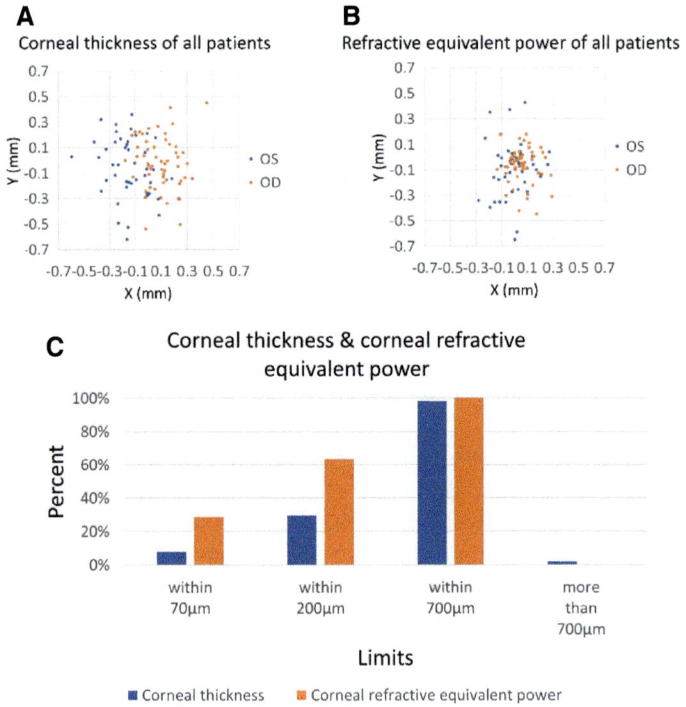

Fig. 25.8 X, Y plots for all treatments for the metrics a) corneal thickness, b) corneal refractive equivalent power, c) distribution of R for corneal thickness and corneal refractive equivalent power

Histograms showing the distribution of decentrations have been generated based on different optical metrics. The method has been compared to other methods for determining centration/decentration of corneal corrections, most of which require operator input or subjective judgment [23]. The evaluation of our pilot cohort (101 cases) shows that decentration remains within 200 μm in 30% of the cases for CT and 63% of the cases for REP.

Overall, the method provides a reliable and objective way to determine the centration of a lenticule of tissue extracted from a cornea. Theoretically, the same method can be easily used on pre- or post-surgery data to determine the most appropriate centration for a spectacle-like correction (sphere, cylinder, and axis), proxy for the visual axis [24].

25.2.6 Induction of Higher-Order Aberrations [25]

The aim of the SmartSight aspheric profiles is to retain the pre-operative HOAs (within OZ) after SmartSight, especially spherical aberration, coma, and trefoil shall remain essentially unchanged. The potential benefits of the SCHWIND ATOS are described in Chap. 23.

In the current study, examination included corneal and ocular aberrometry (MS-39 and Peramis, both CSO, Italy) for a 6 mm diameter. Root mean square (RMS) higher-order aberrations, coma, trefoil, and spherical aberrations were reported.

Ocular aberrations did not change from pre-operative to 3 M post-operative for coma or spherical aberration, whereas HOA-RMS increased by + 0.14±0.15 μm (range − 0.35 μm to + 0.40 μm). Corneal aberrations increased change from pre-operative to 3 M post-operative for coma by + 0.22±0.21 μm (range − 0.13 μm to + 1.08 μm), spherical aberration + 0.17±0.19 μm (range − 0.12 μm to + 0.85 μm), and HOA-RMS by + 0.32±0.26 μm (range − 0.03 μm to + 1.41 μm) (Fig. 25.9).

Corneal aberrations slightly increased after the treatment, but the change of ocular aberrations was very minor and nonsignificant. This may confirm the relatively neutral behavior in terms of aberrations reported from other refractive lenticule extraction techniques, as well as being indicative of adequate centration.

Aberrations were induced across a 6 mm corneal diameter, but ocular aberrations could only be measured through the pupil, so the actual values of analysis

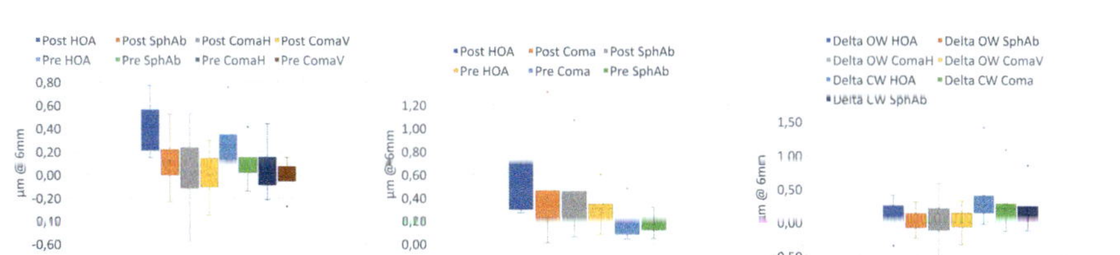

Fig. 25.9 Pre-operative, post-operative, and change in HOAs after SmartSight lenticule extraction

diameter were in the range of 5.4 ± 0.2 mm. SphAb was less positive when measured with ocular aberrations than for corneal aberrations. Post-operative corneal SphAb increased more than ocular SphAb. The RMS higher-order aberrations increased (both for corneal and ocular aberrations), with corneal aberrations showing systematically higher inductions HOA than the ocular counterparts. Corneal aberrometry revealed an induction of positive SphAb, associated with an increase in the RMS higher-order aberrations.

Alternative lenticule extraction techniques such as SMILE (Carl Zeiss Meditec) also induce certain levels of HOAs similar to this cohort[27]. This has also been previously reported for ablation-based procedures (to higher extent) and may be intrinsic to removing corneal tissue.

Although only three-month data were included in the study, longer follow-up of this patient cohort is available. In the up to 12 months follow-up, we did not observe any regression of the refractive outcome or necessity for additional enhancements due to regression (unpublished data). In the larger cohort of patients which includes more than 3000 eyes some initial undercorrections were observed (unpublished work of the same group of authors, surgeries and follow-up were performed during the period from 2020 to 2022).

25.3 Early Post-operative Outcomes [26]

The clinical success of lenticule extraction has been established in the literature as a safe and efficacious technique. Immediate and short-term visual recovery after lenticule extraction has not been commonly reported.

We investigated immediate and short-term (at post-operative day 1, (POD1)) visual recovery in myopic eyes (with or without astigmatism) treated with SmartSight procedure and compared the impact of low-energy asymmetric spacings versus high-energy symmetric spacings on the early (POD1) outcomes of SmartSight lenticule extraction for myopic astigmatism. All 1262 eyes completed day 1 follow-up. POD1 standard graphs for reporting astigmatism outcomes are presented (Fig. 25.10).

POD1 Outcomes

Overall, over 90% of the eyes reached UDVA of 20/20 or better at POD1, with almost 50% in 20/16 or better (Fig. 25.1A). Overall, 96% of the eyes achieved a UDVA at POD1 within a line from pre-operative CDVA baseline (Fig. 25.1B). Overall, over 50% of the eyes gained lines of CDVA at POD1; whereas less than 2% of eyes lost lines of CDVA (Fig. 25.1C). Scattergram of the SEq correction showed a ~ 0.5D overcorrection (Fig. 25.1D, with the overall predictability of 58% of the eyes within 0.75D of the attempted SEq at POD1 (Fig. 25.1E). Scattergram of the astigmatic correction showed no overcorrection or undercorrection (Fig. 25.1G), with the overall predictability of 97% of the eyes with less than 0.5D astigmatism at POD1 (Fig. 25.1F) and 90% of the eyes within 5deg of attempted astigmatic axis (Fig. 25.1H).

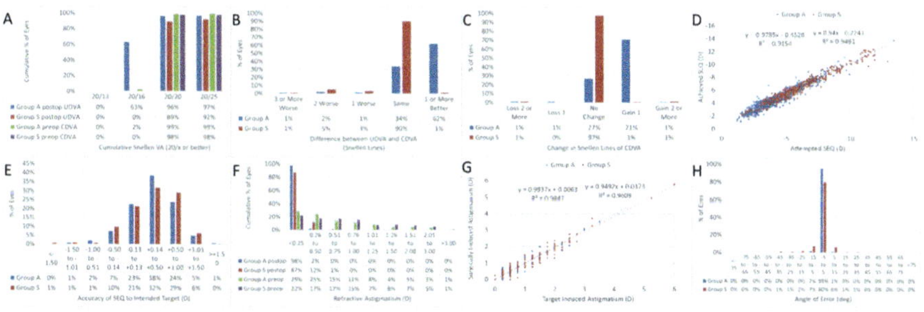

Fig. 25.10 Standard graphs for reporting astigmatism outcomes of refractive surgery at POD1 comparing 920 eyes consecutively treated using low-energy asymmetric spacings (Group A; Study group) versus 342 eyes consecutively treated using high-energy symmetric spacings (Group S; Controls). A) Cumulative Snellen visual acuity. B) Difference between achieved UDVA at POD1 and pre-operative CDVA baseline. C) Change in Snellen lines of CDVA. D) Scattergram of the SEq. E) Predictability of the SEq respect to the target. F) Predictability of the refractive astigmatism respect to the target. G) Scattergram of the astigmatic correction. H) Predictability of the refractive astigmatic axis respect to the target

Laser energy was -34 ± 1nJ lower for asymmetric treatments ($p < 0.0001$); spot distance was + 0.7 ± 0.1 μm larger ($p < 0.0001$); track distance was – 1.2 ± 0.1 μm shorter for asymmetric treatments ($p < 0.0001$).

Incision length was -0.2 ± 0.1 mm shorter for asymmetric treatments ($p < 0.0001$).

This changes apparently led in this cohort to a lower post-op Cyl (-0.10 ± 0.01D lower), along with a better UDVA at POD1 (+0.7 ± 0.1lines BETTER) for asymmetric treatments ($p < 0.0001$).

The post-operative outcomes were evaluated immediately after the surgery (at day 1, POD1) after myopic SmartSight treatment comparing the impact of low-energy asymmetric spacings versus high-energy symmetric spacings on the immediate/early (POD1) outcomes of SmartSight lenticule extraction for myopic astigmatism.

The positive impact of the change in laser settings is seen in terms of the quick recovery in visual acuity after the SmartSight treatments, with the achieved POD1 average UDVA being four optotypes better for the low-energy asymmetric spacings, with a higher proportion of eyes reaching the 20/20 and 20/16 levels of UDVA at POD1. The eyes treated with the low-energy asymmetric spacings performed slightly better in terms of astigmatic correction as well.

Donate and Thaëron [27] were the first to propose low-energy levels to enhance early visual recovery after lenticule extraction. In their study, spot and track distances remained symmetric (4.5μm for both), and pulse energy was reduced from 180 nJ down to 100nJ for the study group (with better early recovery). This simple measure actually reduced not only pulse energy but simultaneously treatment dose (from 0.9 J/cm^2 down to 0.5 J/cm^2) and laser average power. In our cohort, as well, not only pulse energy but simultaneously treatment dose (from 0.8 down to

0.7 J/cm^2) and laser average power (from 99 down to 61 mW) were also reduced, yet to a much lower extent.

Hamilton et al. [28] compared low-energy (LE) versus high-energy (HE) small incision lenticule extraction (SMILE) and femtosecond laser-assisted laser in situ keratomileusis (FS-LASIK) procedures in terms of uncorrected distance visual acuities (UDVAs) in the early post-operative period. The LE group achieved a highly statistically significant better UDVA at POD1 compared to the HE group in SMILE patients (−0.003 vs 0.141, $P < 0.0001$), whereas no significant difference in mean UDVA at POD1 was noted between the LE group and FS-LASIK group (−0.003 vs −0.011, $P = 0.498$).

Donate and Thaëron [29], and Ji et al. [30, 31] further confirmed the benefit of reducing energy levels, using pulse energies above 100nJ, and symmetric spacings (Spot distance = Track distance).

In ATOS, asymmetric treatments performed better for post-op UDVA and CDVA (+0.7 ± 0.1lines).

We shall acknowledge that the POD1 data does not necessarily lead to clinically meaningful differences later on. Thus, emphasizing the interest in longer-term data. Yet, the emphasis lies in the comparison between groups, and this comparison is irrespective of the stability or evolution of the outcomes. The observed differences at POD1 between these two groups tend to reduce for longer follow-ups, while maintaining some advantages for the asymmetric settings group. A similar behavior (with advantages only observed at the shorter-term follow-up) has also been reported for previous comparisons of low-energy settings of another lenticule extraction technique. This can be explained by longer-term improvements in vision for the higher energy settings [32].

Upon availability and due to the initial positive experience with low-energy asymmetric settings, it became the treatment of choice at our practice for SmartSight procedures. Currently, we are using low-energy asymmetric settings of 80 nJ in 5.9 × 2.9 μm distance (468 mJ/cm^2 and ~ 40 mW).

In order to analyze the early outcomes with SmartSight, we evaluated the visual recovery at POD1, because the maximum effect of the smoothness will be observable immediately after ablation, before epithelialization has begun. The best way to analyze if the low-energy asymmetric spacings improve the immediate postoperative visual results after SmartSight should be a comparative eye-paired study, in which one eye should be treated with high-energy symmetric spacings and the other eye of the same patient treated with low-energy asymmetric spacings.

In addition, it would be advisable to compare not only the immediate visual recovery, but also the epithelial remodeling in both groups, in order to analyze if the SmartSight offers the advantage of a reduced epithelial healing or whether difference between low-energy asymmetric settings and high-energy symmetric settings are observed.

It would be interesting to analyze if asymmetric spacings offer the advantage to induce lower HOAs, as compared to other lenticule extraction procedures (with symmetric settings) or using the same ATOS system and the same correction profile (i.e., SmartSight with symmetric spacings).

Very early visual recovery (at POD1) after SmartSight was rapid, providing excellent UDVA immediately after the surgery. We postulate that it is the advanced myopic ablation pattern of the low-energy asymmetric spacings used in the last group of SmartSight treatments that results in a smoother extraction and thus a more rapid visual recovery for patients.

25.3.1 Predictors of Visual Acuity Improvement and Supernormal Vision After SmartSight [15]

We have analyzed which parameters statistically affect the post-operative VA (UDVA and CDVA) respect to the pre-operative CDVA baseline. We determined the eyes with gains in post-op UDVA/CDVA vs pre-op CDVA and compared to eyes with no gains. Further, we determined the correlations between the difference in post-op UDVA/CDVA vs pre-op CDVA and the different parameters. Parameters were grouped in extrinsic (eye related) or intrinsic (laser related):

Extrinsic parameter	Correlation	T-test	Short version	Interpretation
DOB	*0.03844*	*0.00104*	The larger the better	Younger patients achieve more gains in VA
treatDate	*0.00000*	*0.00000*	The larger the better	Long-term learning curve
Seq	*0.00000*	*0.00000*	The larger the better	Reduction of the minification effects
Cyl	*0.00141*	*0.00072*	The larger the worse	Spherical corrections provide better optics
targetSph	*0.00493*	*0.00007*	The larger the better	Accommodation reflex in younger patients
Keratometry (D)	*0.01452*	*0.00106*	The larger the worse	Flatter corneas suffer less deformation under the PI
Epithelium (μm)	*0.00257*	*0.00008*	The larger the better	Better ocular surface pre-op?

Intrinsic parameter	Correlation	T-test	Short version	Interpretation
OZ (mm)	0.00960	*0.01317*	The larger the better	Larger OZ produces better optics
Cap thickness (μm)	*0.00000*	*0.00000*	The larger the better	???
Laser energy (nJ)	*0.00000*	*0.00000*	The larger the worse	Lower energies, smoother cuts
Spot Distance (μm)	*0.00000*	*0.00000*	The larger the better	Less cross-talks between spots

(continued)

(continued)

Intrinsic parameter	Correlation	T-test	Short version	Interpretation
Track distance (μm)	*0.00000*	*0.00000*	The larger the worse	Keeps a good pulse density
Dose	*0.00000*	*0.00000*	The larger the worse	Lower dose, less reactions
Power	*0.00000*	*0.00000*	The larger the worse	Lower power, less reactions
Asymmetry	*0.00000*	*0.00000*	The larger the better	Asymmetric spacings avoid cross-talks between spots

25.3.2 Long-Term Outcomes [12]

So far, over 1000 patients completed the one-year follow-up. All patients had a remaining corneal residual bed thickness of 290 μm or more. A complete dissection and removal of the lenticule was achieved in all cases without relevant intraoperative complications, and at post-operative day 1, all patients had a clear cornea.

At 12M, 93% of the eyes reached an UDVA of 20/20 or better, for all eyes UDVA remained within two lines of pre-operative CDVA, no eyes lost two lines of CDVA. At 12M, the scattergram showed an excellent refractive correction of the SEQ and refractive astigmatism, with 90% and 95% of the eyes within 0.5D from target for SEQ and refractive astigmatism, respectively. For 89% of the treatments, the axis of the refractive astigmatism was within 15deg from the plan.

Corneas in Nepal are rather small, and so are pupil sizes as well; thus, a smaller OZ (compared to other regions in the world) is usually adopted. Further, treatments were in general of moderate to high myopia, which are associated with smaller planned OZ as a measure to reduce tissue consumption (and respect RST of 275 μm, with total corneal thickness after extraction above 400 μm).

25.4 Conclusions

An advanced high-end lenticule generation strategy was successfully compared to more conventional lenticule generation strategies using the same novel femtosecond laser system (SCHWIND ATOS). This represents the next generation of lenticule extraction technology and a new tool for improving refractive and visual outcomes.

We postulate that the advanced myopic ablation pattern of the low-energy asymmetric spacings results in a smoother extraction and thus a more rapid visual recovery for patients.

References

1. Pradhan KR, Arba MS. Initial experience with the SCHWIND ATOS and SmartSight Lenticule extraction. J Clin Res Med. 2020;3(4):1–5.
2. Pradhan KR, Arba MS. Three-month outcomes of myopic astigmatism correction with Small Incision guided human-cornea Treatment. J Refract Surg. 2021;37(5):304–11.
3. Arba Mosquera S, Verma S. A review of clinical outcomes XE "Clinical outcomes" following SMILE for the treatment of astigmatism. Expert Rev Ophthalmol. 2020;15(6):321–30. https://doi.org/10.1080/17469899.2020.1810017.
4. Jun I, Kang DSY, Reinstein DZ, et al. Clinical outcomes of SMILE with a triple centration technique and corneal wavefront-guided transepithelial PRK in high astigmatism. J Refract Surg. 2018;34(3):156–63. https://doi.org/10.3928/1081597X-20180104-03.
5. Jun I, Kang DSY, Arba-Mosquera S, et al. Comparison of clinical outcomes between vector planning and manifest refraction planning in SMILE for myopic astigmatism. J Cataract Refract Surg. 2020;46(8):1149–58. https://doi.org/10.1097/j.jcrs.0000000000000100.
6. Aslanides IM, Toliou G, Padroni S, Arba Mosquera S, Kolli S. The effect of static cyclotorsion compensation on refractive and visual outcomes using the Schwind Amaris laser platform for the correction of high astigmatism. Cont Lens Anterior Eye. 2011;34(3):114–20. https://doi.org/10.1016/j.clae.2011.02.012.
7. Predictability of the achieved Lenticule thickness in smart sight Lenticule extraction for Myopia correction
8. Munnerlyn CR, Koons SJ, Marshall J. Photorefractive keratectomy: A technique for laser refractive surgery. J Cataract Refract Surg. 1988;14(1):46–52. Available from: https://journals.lww.com/jcrs/Fulltext/1988/01000/Photorefractive_keratectomy__A_technique_for_laser.6.aspx
9. Zisimopoulos A, Vingopoulos F, Kanellopoulos AJ. Comparison of planned versus achieved central stromal thickness reduction in LASIK versus SMILE: A contralateral eye study. J Refract Surg. 2021;37(7):454–9.
10. MS-39-CSO Italia. 2023. Available from: www.csoitalia.it/en/prodotto/info/63-ms-39-as-oct
11. Reinstein DZ, Archer TJ, Gobbe M. Lenticule thickness readout for small incision lenticule extraction compared to artemis three-dimensional very high-frequency digital ultrasound stromal measurements. J Refract Surg. 2014;30(5):304–9. https://doi.org/10.3928/1081597X-20140416-01. PMID: 24893355.
12. Pradhan KR, Arba Mosquera S. Twelve-month outcomes of a new refractive lenticular extraction procedure. J Optom. 2021:S1888–4296(21)00085–6. https://doi.org/10.1016/j.optom.2021.11.001. Epub ahead of print. PMID: 34949535.
13. Reinstein DZ, Archer TJ, Gobbe M. Corneal ablation depth readout of the MEL 80 excimer laser compared to Artemis three-dimensional very high-frequency digital ultrasound stromal measurements. J Refract Surg. 2010;26(12):949–59. https://doi.org/10.3928/1081597X-20100114-02. Epub 2010 Jan 15 PMID: 20128534.
14. Wang H, Zheng S, Tang S, Zhang X, Chen Y, Zhu Y. Investigation of accuracy and influence factors of predicting Lenticule thickness in small incision Lenticule extraction by machine learning models. J Pers Med. 2023;13(2):256. https://doi.org/10.3390/jpm13020256. PMID: 36836490; PMCID: PMC9959370.
15. ESCRS 2023
16. Camellin M, Arba MS. Aspheric optical zones: The effective optical zone with the SCHWIND AMARIS. J Refract Surg. 2011;27(2):135–46.
17. Haidari H, Derhartunian V, Arba-Mosquera S. Method to determine the centration of a Lenticule of tissue extracted from a cornea. Biomed Opt Express. 2023;14:4080–96.
18. Arba Mosquera S, Verma S, McAlinden C. Centration axis in refractive surgery. Eye Vis (Lond). 2015;2:4. https://doi.org/10.1186/s40662-015-0014-6. PMID: 26605360; PMCID: PMC46554554

19. Mrochen M, Kaemmerer M, Mierdel P, Seiler T. Increased higher-order optical aberrations after laser refractive surgery: a problem of subclinical decentration. J Cataract Refract Surg. 2001;27(3):362–9. https://doi.org/10.1016/s0886-3350(00)00806-3. PMID: 11255046.
20. Bueeler M, Mrochen M, Seiler T. Maximum permissible lateral decentration in aberration-sensing and wavefront-guided corneal ablation. J Cataract Refract Surg. 2003;29(2):257–63. https://doi.org/10.1016/s0886-3350(02)01638-3. PMID: 12648634.
21. Savini G, Barboni P, Carbonelli M, Hoffer KJ. Repeatability of automatic measurements by a new Scheimpflug camera combined with Placido topography. J Cataract Refract Surg. 2011;37(10):1809–16. https://doi.org/10.1016/j.jcrs.2011.04.033. PMID: 21852068.
22. Arbelaez MC, Vidal C, Arba-Mosquera S. Bilateral symmetry before and six months after aberration-free™ correction with the SCHWIND AMARIS TotalTech Laser: clinical outcomes. J Optom. 2010;3:20–8.
23. Kang DSY, Lee H, Reinstein DZ, Roberts CJ, Arba-Mosquera S, Archer TJ, Kim EK, Seo KY, Kim TI. Comparison of the distribution of Lenticule Decentration following SMILE by subjective patient fixation or triple marking centration. J Refract Surg. 2018;34(7):446–52.
24. Arba Mosquera S, De Ortueta D, Verma S. Corneal functional optical zone under monocular and binocular assessment. Eye and Vision 20185:3. https://doi.org/10.1186/s40662-018-0097-y
25. Gabric I, Bohac M, Gabric K, Arba Mosquera S. First European results of a new refractive lenticular extraction procedure-SmartSight by SCHWIND eye-tech-solutions. Eye (Lond). 2023. https://doi.org/10.1038/s41433-023-02601-0. Epub ahead of print. PMID: 37277614.
26. Pradhan KR, Arba Mosquera S. Comparing high and low energy outcomes on day one for SmartSight myopic-astigmatism treatments with the SCHWIND ATOS: a retrospective case series. BMC Ophthalmol. 2023;23(1):328. https://doi.org/10.1186/s12886-023-03076-z. PMID: 37464345; PMCID: PMC10354973.
27. Donate D, Thaëron R. SMILE with low energy levels: assessment of early visual and optical quality recovery. J Refract Surg. 2019;35(5):285–93. https://doi.org/10.3928/1081597X-20190416-01.
28. Hamilton DR, Chen AC, Khorrami R, Nutkiewicz M, Nejad M. Comparison of early visual outcomes after low-energy SMILE, high-energy SMILE, and LASIK for myopia and myopic astigmatism in the United States. J Cataract Refract Surg. 2021;47(1):18–26. https://doi.org/10.1097/j.jcrs.0000000000000368. PMID: 32769749.
29. Donate D, Thaëron R. Lower energy levels improve visual recovery in small incision Lenticule extraction (SMILE). J Refract Surg. 2016;32(9):636–42. https://doi.org/10.3928/1081597X-20160602-01.
30. Ji YW, Kim M, Kang DSY, Reinstein DZ, Archer TJ, Choi JY, Kim EK, Lee HK, Seo KY, Kim TI. Lower laser energy levels lead to better visual recovery after small-incision Lenticule extraction: prospective randomized clinical trial. Am J Ophthalmol. 2017;179:159–70. https://doi.org/10.1016/j.ajo.2017.05.005. Epub 2017 May 10 PMID: 28499707.
31. Ji YW, Kim M, Kang DSY, Reinstein DZ, Archer TJ, Choi JY, Kim EK, Lee HK, Seo KY, Kim TI. Effect of lowering laser energy on the surface roughness of human corneal Lenticules in SMILE. J Refract Surg. 2017;33(9):617–24.
32. Awwad ST, Btaiche Y. Visual outcomes with CLEAR Lenticule extraction: early results with the procedure were safe, efficient, and stable. Cat Refract Surg Today Global (Europe Edition) Jan/Feb 2023 Digital Suplement CLEAR Lenticue Extraction

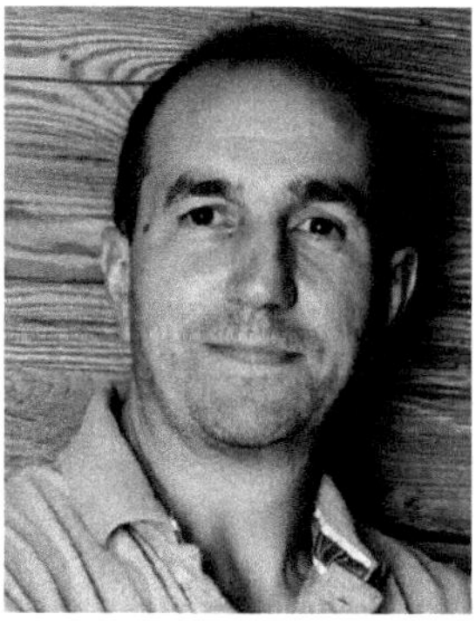

Samuel Arba Mosquera PhD is Senior Optical & Visual Scientist, Biomedical Engineering Office, SCHWIND eye-techsolutions,Germany. He studied Physics in Santiago de Compostela (Spain). He further completed a Master's and Doctor's Degree in Sciences of Vision by the University of Valladolid in Spain. Dr. Arba Mosquera has published over 150 original papers, over 15 book chapters and is the inventor in over 100 patent applications. He gave countless presentations at national and international meetings. He is a reviewer for 21 Ophthalmic Journals. In the last 25 years his research has been focused on corneal and refractive surgery.

Part VI

Corneal Lenticule Extraction for Advanced Refractive Correction (CLEAR®)

Lenticule and Interface Properties in CLEAR®

26

Christian Rathjen and Michael Steinlechner

26.1 The Ziemer Laser Systems

The FEMTO LDV Z8 and its newer version FEMTO Z8 NEO (Fig. 26.1) are compact portable laser systems designed for carrying out surgery on the anterior segment of the eye. A laser applicator is applied by the surgeon in an instrument style fashion (Fig. 26.2). This way neither the surgeon nor the patient has to move during surgery. Patient movements are compensated by an articulated arm. This flexible arrangement keeps the surgical area clear before and after the laser intervention and allows the surgeon to use a microscope and bed of his/her choice.

26.2 Scanning Scheme

To cut into the cornea and the lens of the eye, the Z8 applies a fast-scan-slow-scan scheme, where an optical micro-scan is performed through a movable lens with very high focusing power and consequently limited field of view [1].

In this scanning scheme, a fast-scan module repeatedly generates a so-called fast-scan line at high frequency, which consists of a tightly spaced sequence of laser spots that are used to dissect tissue. The fast-scan line can be compared to the cutting edge of a surgical blade, with the essential difference being that the fast-scan line has an adjustable width that can be set continuously from zero to about one millimetre while cutting.

C. Rathjen (✉)
PhD, Technology & Strategy, Ziemer Ophthalmic Systems AG, Port, Switzerland
e-mail: christian.rathjen@ziemergroup.com

M. Steinlechner
PhD, Technology & Strategy, Ziemer Ophthalmic Systems AG, Port, Switzerland
e-mail: michael.steinlechner@ziemergroup.com

W. Sekundo and F. M. Wagner (eds.), *Femtosecond Laser Assisted Lenticule Extraction*,
https://doi.org/10.1007/978-3-031-60424-9_26

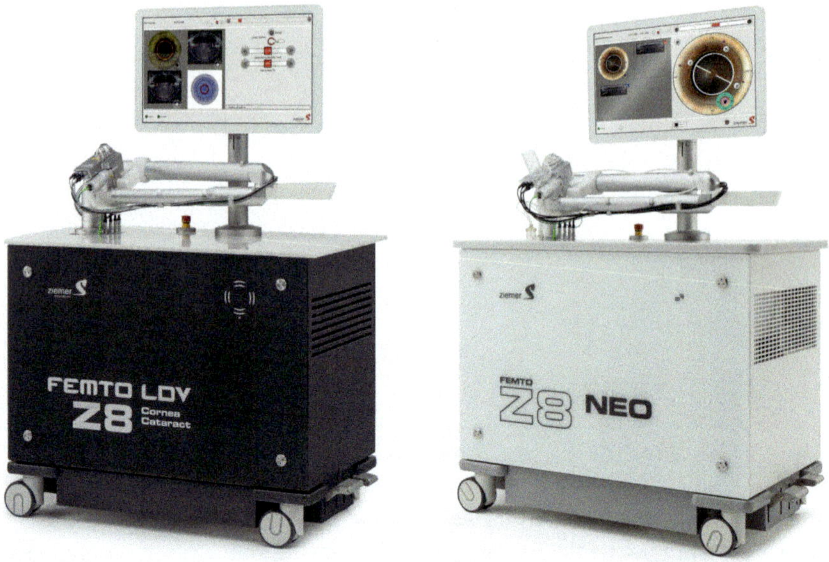

Fig. 26.1 Compact portable FEMTO LDV Z8 and FEMTO Z8 NEO laser systems

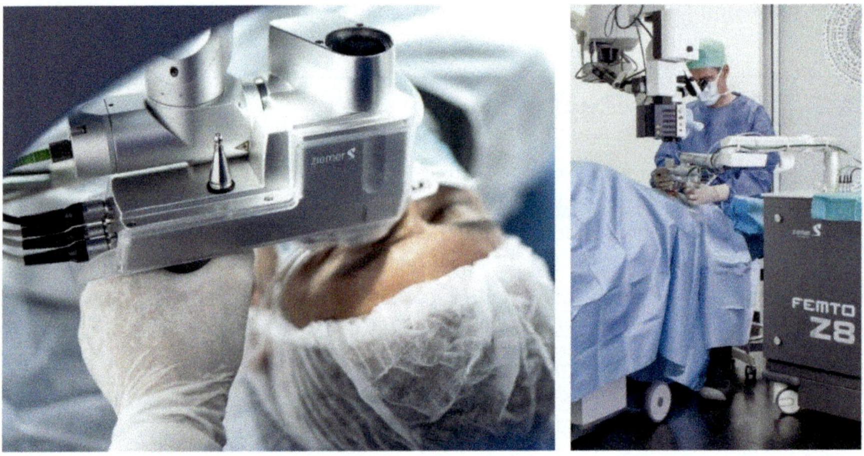

Fig. 26.2 Z8 laser applicator (left) and overall surgical setting (right)

In the same way that a surgeon moves a blade through tissue, a slow-scan system moves the fast-scan line through tissue (Fig. 26.3). With the Z8, the slow-scan system can freely orient and move the fast-scan line inside the eye tissue in three dimensions. This means that the Z8 has the capability of sculpting arbitrary

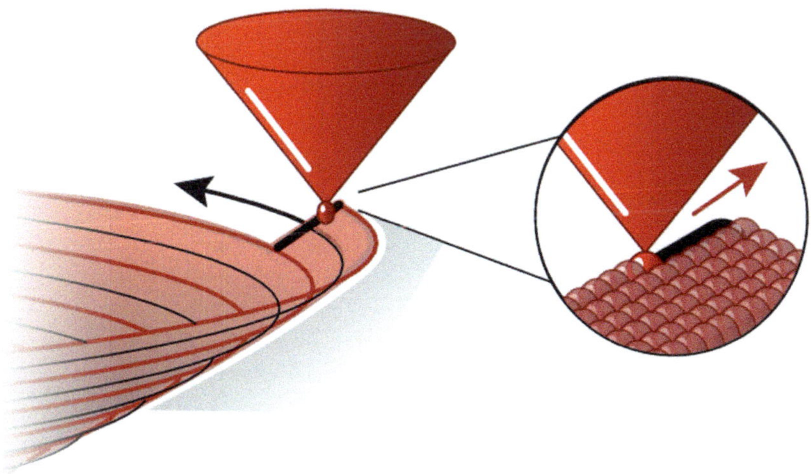

Fig. 26.3 Fast-scan line (bold black) moving along a trajectory to perform a curved cut, with the zoomed-in view showing the overlapping laser spots with an evenly spaced spot distance

shaped 3D surfaces similarly to a five-axis robotic manufacturing machine. In this analogy, the machining tool is a pattern of laser spots generated by a fast scanner.

The fast-scan-slow-scan scheme integral to the Ziemer femtosecond lasers was first presented at the AAO 2005 conference, where surgeons performed wetlabs with a pre-series device which received FDA clearance for the creation of flaps and lamellar corneal surgery in early 2006. The Ziemer femtosecond laser system was then continuously expanded to the full anterior eye segment in order to perform cataract surgeries. For lenticule resection, the pioneering work introduced by ZEISS with the VisuMax laser system could not be directly transferred to the Ziemer laser systems due to the fundamental differences between the scanning methods. Therefore, completely new scan patterns had to be developed from the ground up [2]. After two years of development, the first surgeries on humans [3] were performed and CE marking was obtained in 2020. The CLEAR lenticule extraction solution is the second on the market after SMILE from ZEISS.

26.3 Laser Process

Within the described fast-scan-slow-scan scheme, the Z8 applies laser pulses at high frequencies of up to 20 MHz in an overlapping manner. This allows a strong reduction of pulse energy depending on the temporal and spatial proximity of subsequent laser pulses (referred to as low energy-high frequency in [4]). In general, with an increasing repetition rate, the energy required for tissue separation is reduced (Fig. 26.4). In the same way, increasing the spot overlap also reduces the

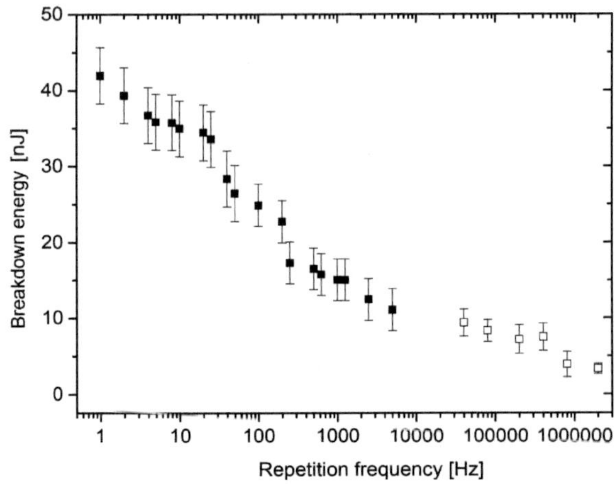

Fig. 26.4 Effect of repetition rate on the threshold energy of overlapping spots (adapted from [5])

required pulse energy. In the Z8 laser system, both effects are combined to enable low-energy laser eye surgery [5].

Tight spot spacing at high frequencies in combination with low pulse energy is beneficial for smooth cut surfaces and minimises the effects on the surrounding tissue. Additional factors on a microscopic level that influence clinical performance are summarised in Fig. 26.5 qualitatively. It is important to note that minimising or maximising a single parameter will not necessarily lead to improved clinical results. Inter-device comparison on isolated parameters is not conclusive. Similarly, it would be unscientific to compare, on a per-parameter basis, a *single-pulse process* with the fundamentally different *multi-pulse process with overlapping spots*, as used by the FEMTO LDV lasers. A comparison of macroscopic aspects of the entire laser process is more conclusive from a user perspective.

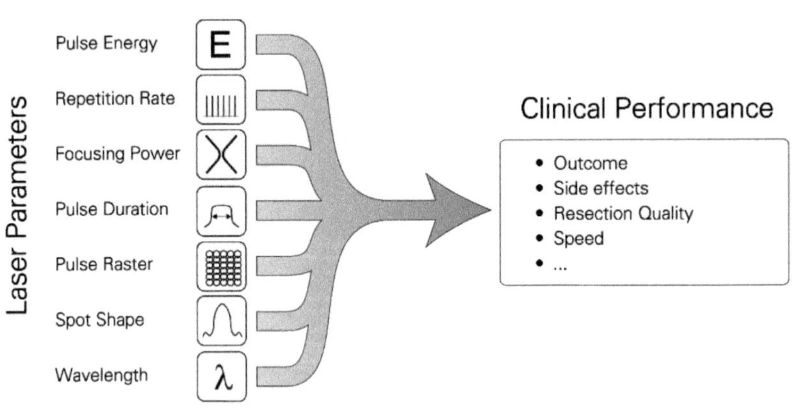

Fig. 26.5 Clinical performance of laser systems depends on a complex interrelation of laser parameters that cannot be compared on a simple per-parameter basis

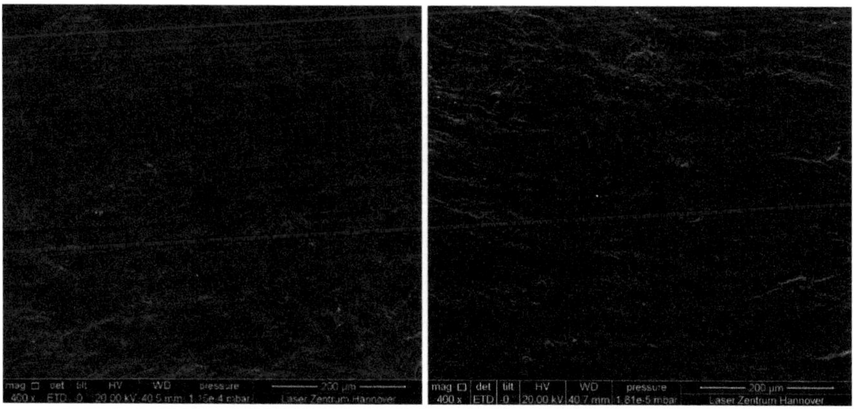

Fig. 26.6 Scanning electron microscope images of human lenticules from two sites

As it stands today, there are no quantitative relationships available that allow for a direct deduction of clinical performance from laser process parameters. Therefore, companies have to determine empirically, in collaboration with clinical experts, parameter sets for their laser systems and set their own optimisation objectives. For Ziemer, a key objective during the development of lenticular cuts was a similar surface quality to that of LASIK flaps. This could be achieved by a new spot pattern that has been optimised for lenticular contours and operates at about one-third of the pulse energy used for LASIK flap creation with the Z8.

Figure 26.6 shows two examples of scanning electron microscope images of human lenticules of 5 dpt correction after extraction from two different Z8 laser systems at two different sites. The surfaces appear homogenous with the absence of tags (indicators of tissue bridges). Undisturbed collagen lamellae are faintly visible in both samples. The difference in the overall appearance could be attributed to either different imaging angles or patient-dependent variability of the tissue. Differences in surgical techniques of lenticule separation could also be a contributing factor.

26.4 Patient Interface

Before the development of scan patterns, a decision needed to be made on the type of patient interface. Finite element analysis with various material models showed that the anterior part of the cornea intended for lenticular resection is under compression (right side in Fig. 26.7) and strains are homogenous (left in Fig. 26.7). While compression favourably stabilises the tissue during a cut, homogeneous strains result in a homogeneous state of the cornea when the cornea returns to its natural shape after undocking.

Theoretically, curved applanation results in less deformation, but the higher variability of the deformed state depends on how the curved patient interface

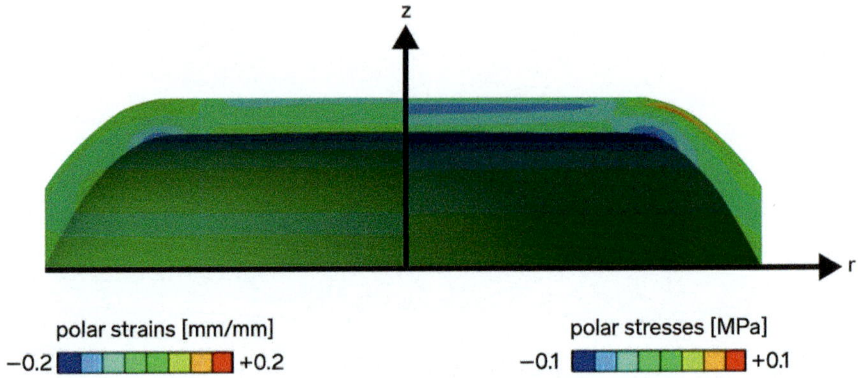

Fig. 26.7 Polar (radial) strains (left side) and stresses (right side) in the cornea during docking

matches the aspheric (and often asymmetric) shape of the individual eye. The practical importance of these two theoretical effects is not well understood. However, clinical experience of more than 15 years with lamellar resection, including more than 8 million flaps, supports the concept of flat applanation for refractive lenticule resection. In addition to LASIK flap creation, the Z8 is capable of resecting large homogenous grafts of less than 20 μm thickness [6] which strongly indicated its suitability for thin lenticule resection as well.

For lenticule extraction, the Z8 uses the standard applanating patient interface for corneal surgery. To attach the eye to the laser applicator, the patient interface applies suction to the sclera and the limbus using a design that was originally developed for the AMADEUS microkeratome, also designed and manufactured by Ziemer Ophthalmic Systems/Switzerland. The design was later used on predecessor models of the Z8, starting with the first LDV system (formerly named DaVinci) [4]. For the Z8, the design was adopted to enable two docking methods: a.) One-step docking: installation of the patient interface first on the laser applicator, followed by docking of the whole assembly to the eye or b.) Two-step docking: applying the patient interface first on the patient with suction and the subsequent docking of the laser applicator.

Favourably, the design leaves more space for the cornea to settle inside the suction ring and to conform with the applanation surface. This makes the patient interface compatible with eyes of different shapes and provides a larger tolerance for docking. Additionally, the cavity that is created between the peripheral cornea and the inner wall of the suction ring (Fig. 26.8, left) allows excess gas to be extracted if higher power settings are used.

Vacuum level and suction time are comparable to LASIK. Including the AMADEUS, in excess of 10 million cuts have been performed with this technology with a very low complication rate. The latest version of the software resects a lenticule in less than 18 s, which is about half of the mean flap cutting time of the technology at the time of its first clinical use in 2000. The suction is stable enough that the light handheld laser applicator can follow the movements made

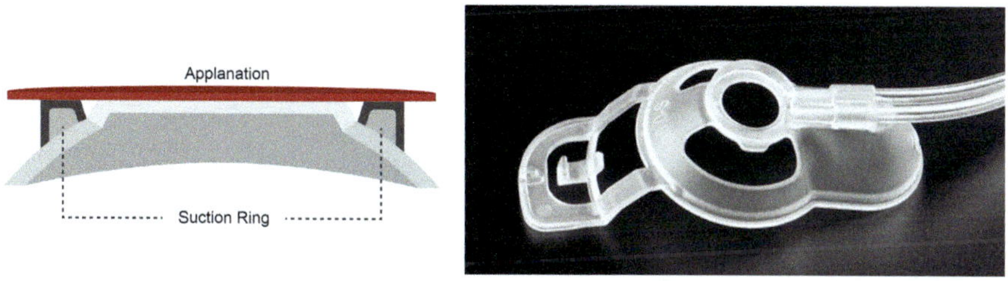

Fig. 26.8 Z8 applanating patient interface for corneal and refractive surgery

by the patient's head. Events of suction loss are rare, even when sudden movement occurs. A risk assessment in a regulatory context on 39,000 eyes undergoing CLEAR surgery could confirm that the patient interface-related complication rate is low: Suction loss was identified as the most frequent patient interface-related complication during CLEAR surgery, with a rate of 0.04% (data on file, Ziemer/Switzerland).

26.5 Scan Pattern

The main challenge in designing efficient scan patterns for a successful refractive procedure is enabling short cutting times while ensuring a high level of accuracy. The lenticule resection as performed by the Z8 laser has a circular shape when viewed from the top. The aim of this is to not introduce additional biomechanical asymmetries in the cornea, which an elliptic shape for astigmatic corrections would induce. A continuous spiral-shaped trajectory was chosen to cover this circular shape (see Fig. 26.9, bottom left) in a way that a tight spot spacing and a homogeneous distribution of laser spots are achieved.

The desired refractive correction results in a curved posterior cutting surface. To cut this curved surface, the focus position of the laser changes continuously during the spiral cut. The required depth change of the focus position is about 10–150 μm in total and therefore about two magnitudes smaller in scale than the lateral dimensions of the lenticule (5–9 mm in diameter). For pure myopic corrections, following this spiral leads to a smooth monotonic depth adjustment of the focus. For astigmatic lenticules, this is not the case anymore as an Archimedean spiral with evenly spaced lateral distances between spiral turns does not follow contour lines of equal cutting depth. To illustrate this, Fig. 26.9 compares a scan pattern following height contour lines and the spiral-shaped trajectory. The focusing system of the Z8 dynamically follows the undulated spiral in one continuous jerk-free movement [7]. This continuous spiral scan pattern preserves tight spot spacing and ensures homogeneous distribution of laser spots

The anterior surface of the lenticule is cut parallel to the applanation patient interface, resulting in a constant distance to the anterior cornea surface. We consider the parallel cut to the anterior surface to be crucial for the safety of lenticule

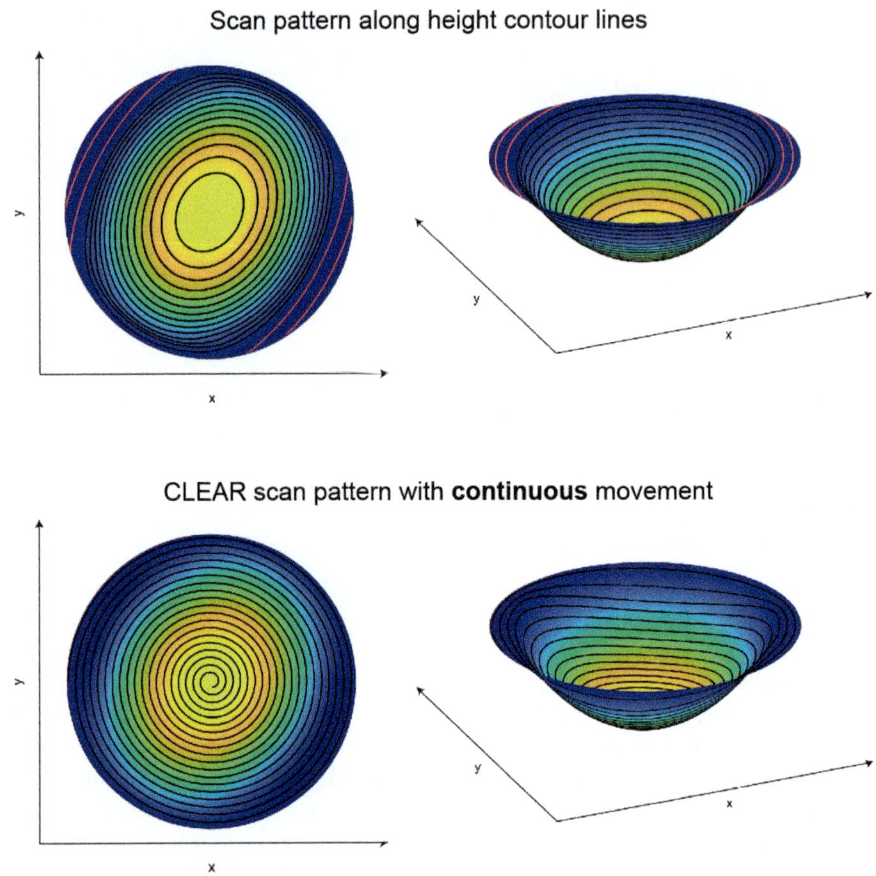

Fig. 26.9 Scan patterns for myopic astigmatic correction profiles. Profile depth is colour-coded. Left: Top view. Right: Side view of the same profile. **First row**: Illustration of a scan pattern following height contour lines of equal focus depth. A separate transition zone, shown in pink, is added to ensure a circular lenticule shape. **Second row**: Archimedean-spiral-shaped trajectory with integrated transition zones and the homogeneous distribution of laser spots

extraction in general, as it keeps the lenticule cap uniformly strong and enables straightforward re-treatments or rescue cuts, should these be required in rare circumstances.

To enable the extraction of the lenticule, up to two access tunnels can be freely positioned [8]. The use of two access tunnels helps surgeons without lenticule extraction experience to easily identify the anterior and posterior interfaces of the lenticule. In addition, it can help to separate the anterior cut in the event that the posterior cut has been accidently separated first.

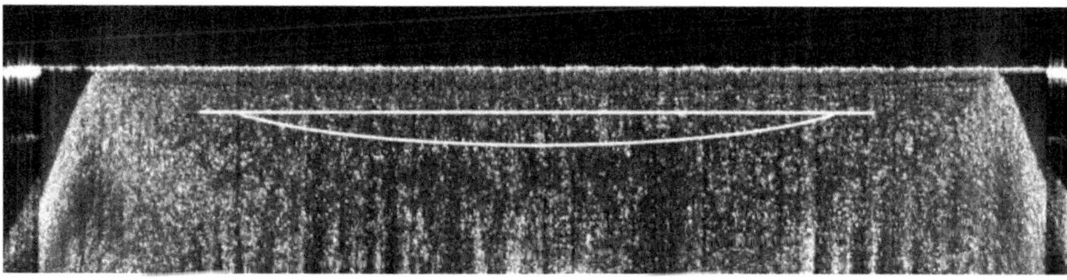

Fig. 26.10 Intraoperative Z8 OCT image of a human cornea with an overlaid lenticule shape to verify the positioning. Image with nonuniform scale in horizontal and vertical axis

26.6 Centration and Docking Control

The Z8 laser offers several centration methods to ensure precise alignment during the docking procedure.

In a first step, during docking, a fixation light in the laser applicator helps to align the handheld laser applicator with the visual axis of the patient eye.

In a second step, once suction has been applied, automatic image recognition methods detect eye features such as the pupil position or limbal/corneal markings that are applied by the surgeon pre-operatively. When used in combination with a compatible diagnostic device, notably the GALILEI (Ziemer Ophthalmic Systems/ Switzerland), centration can also be performed automatically using a diagnostic reference image. Cyclotorsion compensation is also performed in this step by automatic image processing on corneal markings or iris patterns.

It is important to note that the Z8's scanning technology with dynamic focus adjustment allows for the positioning and rotation of the treatment pattern even after suction has been applied. This includes manual corrections to the automatic positioning and rotation according to the surgeon's preferences.

Correct docking as well as the state of the cornea can also be verified using the integrated OCT to image the anterior segment (Fig. 26.10). This allows, for example, the adjustment of the distance from the anterior corneal surface to the lenticule according to the epithelium thickness or the detection of foreign bodies on the epithelium.

26.7 Conclusions

Overlapping low-energy pulses combined with a fast-scan-slow-scan scheme, originally conceived by Ziemer in 2003 for flap creation, have been successfully applied to refractive lenticule extraction on portable laser systems for anterior segment surgery.

References

1. Rathjen C. Ophthalmological apparatus for the breakdown of eye tissue. US8920408B2. (filed 2004)
2. Rathjen C. Apparatus for working on eye tissue by means of a pulsed laser beam. US10918523B2. (filed 2018)
3. Izquierdo L, Sossa D, Ben-Shaul O, Henriquez M. Corneal lenticule extraction assisted by a low-energy femtosecond laser. J Cataract Refract Surg. 2020;46(9):1217–1221
4. Lubatschowski H. Overview of commercially available femtosecond lasers in refractive surgery. J Cataract Refract Surg. 2008;24(1):102–7.
5. Lubatschowski H, Rathjen C. Apparatus for and method of refractive surgery with laser pulses. US8221400B2. (filed 2005)
6. Groeneveld-van. BE, van der Star. L, Ghaly. M, Laouani. A, Melles. G, Kocaba. V. Laser assisted Bowman layer graft preparation. EBAA (Eye Bank Association of America). 2022, Chicago
7. Rathjen. C, Steinlechner. M. Ophthalmological device for processing a curved treatment face. US2023201039. (filed 2022)
8. Steinlechner. M, Bernau. W. Ophthalmological device for surgical treatment of a cornea. EP3988063B1. (filed 2020)

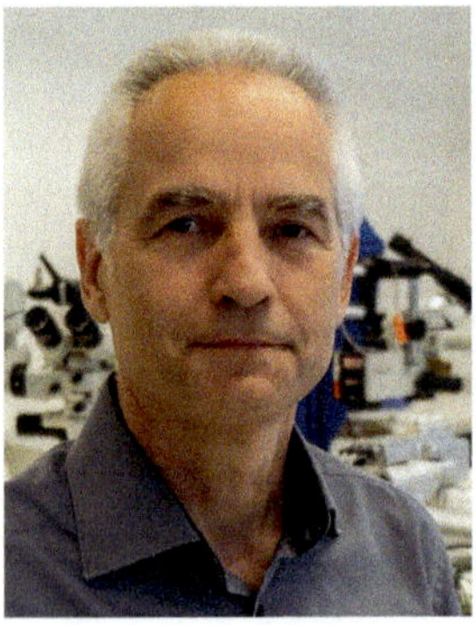

Christian Rathjen, PhD, is the Vice President for Technology and Strategy at Ziemer Ophthalmic System, Port Switzerland. He is a femtosecond lasers expert with more than 20 years of experience. Previously, he worked at CERN, Geneva Switzerland, developing equipment for superconducting magnets and ultra-high vacuum for the LHC accelerator. He studied engineering at the University of Hannover, Germany, where he also served as a research assistant. In parallel to his professional work, Dr. Rathjen earned a PhD in metrology, during which he invented and implemented a 3D scanning method for surface analysis. In addition to his academic role, he developed equipment to investigate the biomechanics of screw-bone connections, which led to the creation of automated surgical screwdrivers for the cervical spine. Dr. Rathjen's major contributions to ophthalmology include the invention of the Femto LDV Family of low energy femtosecond lasers and the Galilei Scheimpflug analyzer for anterior segment tomography and biometry. Recent contributions in which he plays a leading role include solid-state lasers for surface ablation and various femtosecond laser applications, such as lenticular extraction. His strong focus on innovation has resulted in over 350 granted patents.

Lenticule Extraction as Performed on the Ziemer FEMTO LDV Z8: CLEAR®

27

Shady T. Awwad, Yara Bteich, and Jad F. Assaf

Abstract

"This chapter provides an in-depth exploration of the CLEAR lenticule extraction procedure carried out on the Ziemer FEMTO LDV Z8 and its newer version FEMTO Z8 NEO, which are portable multipurpose surgical laser systems for the anterior chamber. The laser systems, their working principle, and laser process of overlapping low-energy laser spots create unique scan patterns. Descriptions of the patient interface, automatic image-based cut placement, and lenticule profiles are provided."

Keywords

Keratorefractive lenticule extraction (KLEX) • Ziemer FEMTO LDV Z8 • Corneal lenticule extraction for advanced refractive correction (CLEAR) • Small incision lenticule extraction (SMILE)

27.1 Keratorefractive Lenticule Extraction on the FEMTO LDV Z8

First introduced on the VisuMax femtosecond laser platform (Zeiss, Jena, Germany) in 2011 as small incision lenticule extraction (SMILE), keratorefractive lenticule extraction (KLEX) technology recently became available on several other platforms, including the Ziemer Z8 as corneal lenticule extraction for advanced refractive correction (CLEAR). We aim to familiarize the reader with lenticule extraction as performed on this platform, describing the technology and

S. T. Awwad (✉) · Y. Bteich · J. F. Assaf
Beirut, Lebanon
e-mail: sawwad@gmail.com

W. Sekundo and F. M. Wagner (eds.), *Femtosecond Laser Assisted Lenticule Extraction*,
https://doi.org/10.1007/978-3-031-60424-9_27

science behind it, highlighting its key features, describing the surgical steps, and summarizing our initial clinical outcomes while discussing the ones in the literature.

27.2 Surgical Procedure

The treatment plan is first entered into the CLEAR software (Fig. 27.1A). The latter allows adjustments for incision count and size, alongside programming options for target refraction, cap depth and width, optical zone (up to 8.0 mm), and energy settings, all necessary for tailoring treatment parameters to both surgeon preference and patient characteristics (Fig. 27.1B–D). Additionally, one incision can be programmed to lead to the anterior interface, while the second one can be designed to lead to the posterior interface (guiding tunnels), flattening the learning curve for the beginning surgeon. To be able to extract the lenticule easily, a minimum thickness called *handling offset* is automatically programmed into the treatment.

The procedure is performed under topical anesthesia following standard prepping and draping protocols, with the Z8 system positioned right next to the surgical or excimer laser microscope, depending on the available setting, and the Z8 handpiece extending right over the surgical field. Ziemer has implemented automatic centration and registration of the treatment plan based on imaging taken from the GALILEI ColorZ tomography device, obviating the need for manual marking. For people not using a GALILEI, we recommend limbal markings to be made using the slit-lamp (Fig. 27.2A). Subsequently, these markings are extended under the surgical or excimer laser microscope using a 3-prong instrument such as the Awwad 3-Blade Marker for CLEAR from Epsilon Ophthalmic Surgical Instruments, Irvine, USA (Fig. 27.2B). The 3-prong instrument extends the markings based on the fixation light reflex, which approximates the corneal vertex (Fig. 27.2C) Extending the preoperative markings onto the cornea facilitates their recognition by the surgeon and by the Z8's automatic centration and cyclotorsion system after initiating docking and suction. Once centered, the Z8 handpiece is docked and suction is applied, with full applanation of the cornea (Fig. 27.2D). Attention is directed to the LCD screen of the Z8 system. The automatic recognition system of the Z8 allows centration and rotation of the planned treatment based on the surgeon's centration marks. However, the surgeon has the freedom to manually re-adjust centration and rotation, if necessary *(described in a previous chapter)* (Fig. 27.2E). At any time, the built-in optical coherence tomography (OCT) system in the Z8 may be activated to ensure adequate applanation over the intended treatment zone.

The laser procedure is then initiated by creating the refractive interface posterior to the lenticule, which, at the time of writing, is performed in a concentric fashion followed by the larger cap interface anterior to it, in the same fashion, and subsequently, making one or two access incisions. Suction is then automatically discontinued and the surgeon resumes focusing through the eyepieces of the surgical or excimer laser microscope.

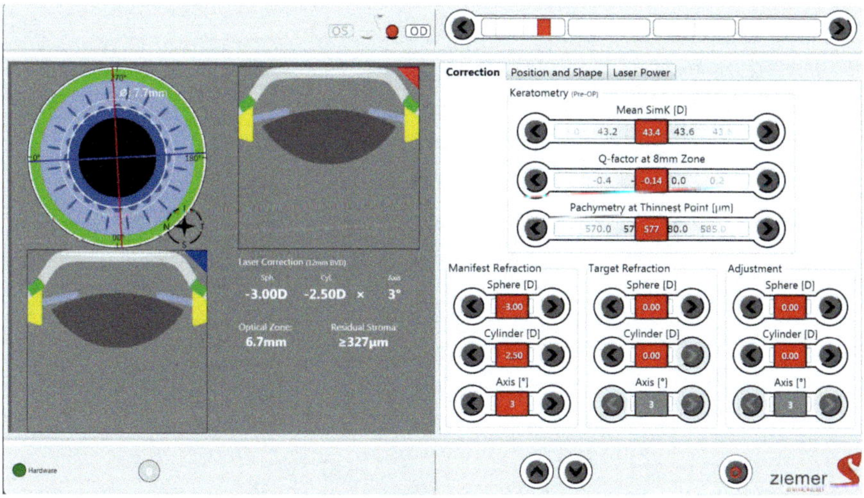

(A)

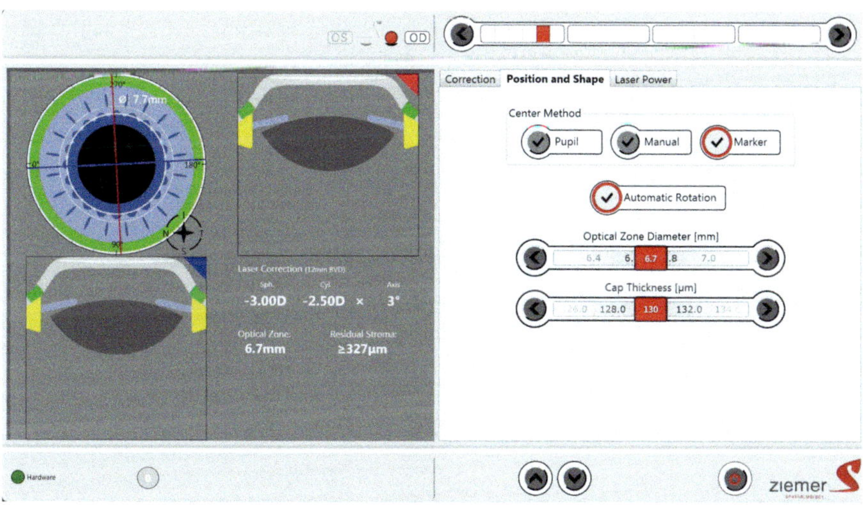

(B)

Fig. 27.1 (A–D) Snapshots from the software showing how refractive errors are entered into the system and how different settings can be adjusted

To isolate the lenticule for extraction, the surgeon utilizes a blunt-tipped lenticule separator. This involves opening one of the incisions to reach the cap interface first, followed by the lenticule interface by maneuvering the tip upward and downward, respectively. For the uninitiated surgeon, guiding tunnels can be helpful: one incision can be separated to access the anterior interface, while the second incision is used to access the posterior interface. Subsequently, the oval-tip end dissector is employed to separate the lenticule from the surrounding tissue. A microforceps

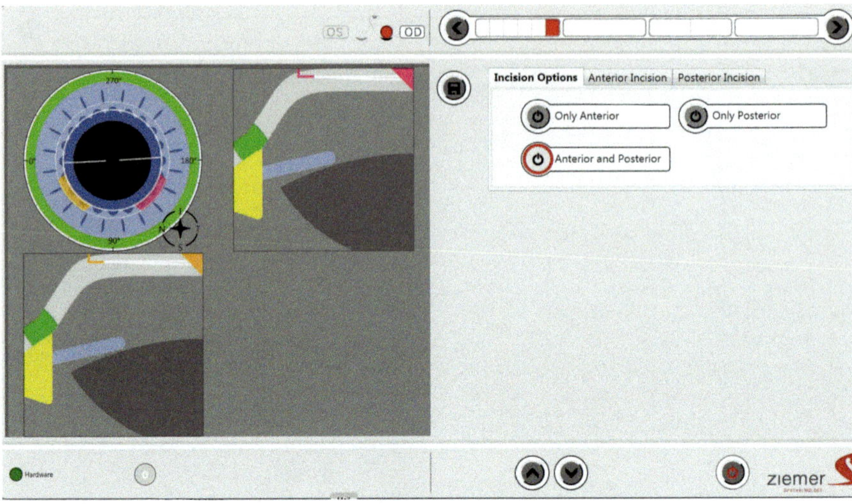

(C)

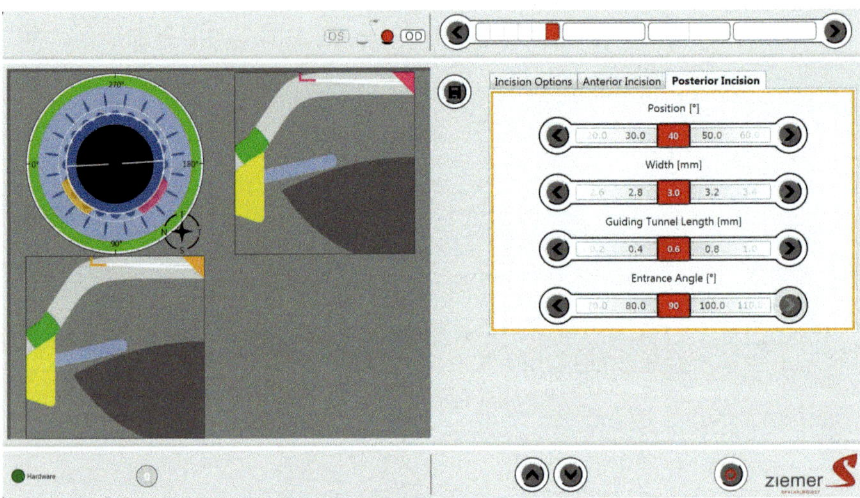

(D)

Fig. 27.1 (continued)

is employed to extract the lenticule, followed by a check of the lenticule integrity. Finally, the cap is smoothed gently using surgical micro-sponges to appose it to the stromal bed.

Postoperative medications include fourth-generation fluoroquinolones, administered four times daily for a week, prednisolone acetate four times daily for one week, then gradually tapered over three additional days, and preservative-free aqueous replacement eye drops as needed.

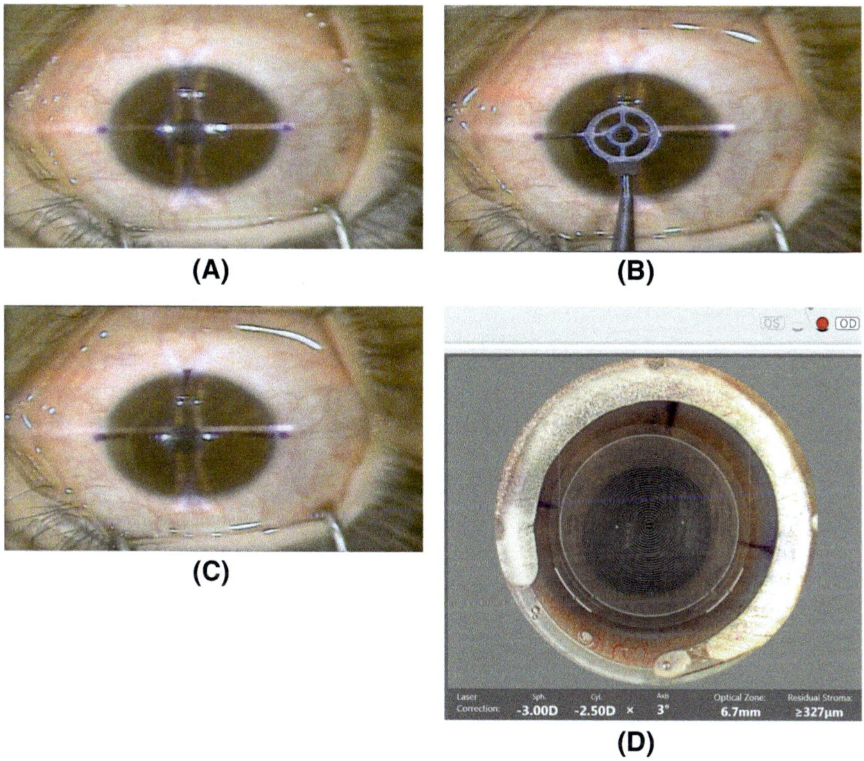

Fig. 27.2 (A) Limbal markings placed at the slit lamp, (B) Extension of the markings using the 3-prong marker, centered on the corneal vertex, (C) Extension of the preoperative markings into the cornea allows them to be recognized by the automatic centration and cyclotorsion system of the Z8, (D) Snapshot after suction has been applied, (E) Option of manual re-centration after suction. (F) Intraoperative OCT section

27.3 What This Platform Brings

The FEMTO LDV Z8 employs low-energy laser pulses, operating at a rapid repetition rate in the megahertz range, to achieve plasma-induced ablation. These precisely focused and overlapping pulses, each carrying energy levels typically below 50 nJ, effectively minimize stromal gas generation while ensuring precise laser focus. Due to the low energy per pulse, tissue is not disrupted and pulses must overlap to avoid tissue bridges. This technique minimizes mechanical stress on the tissue with subsequent inflammation and patient discomfort. Surgeons have the flexibility to adjust energy settings, optimizing the procedure for quicker visual recovery.

The full applanation induced by the docking interface allows the surgeon to make intraoperative adjustments for cyclotorsion and realign the treatment precisely on the visual axis, all without releasing suction. This accuracy is further

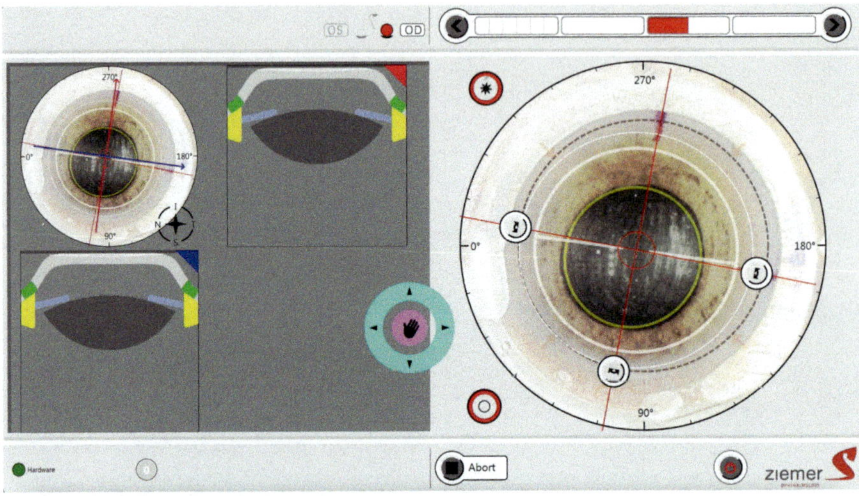

(E)

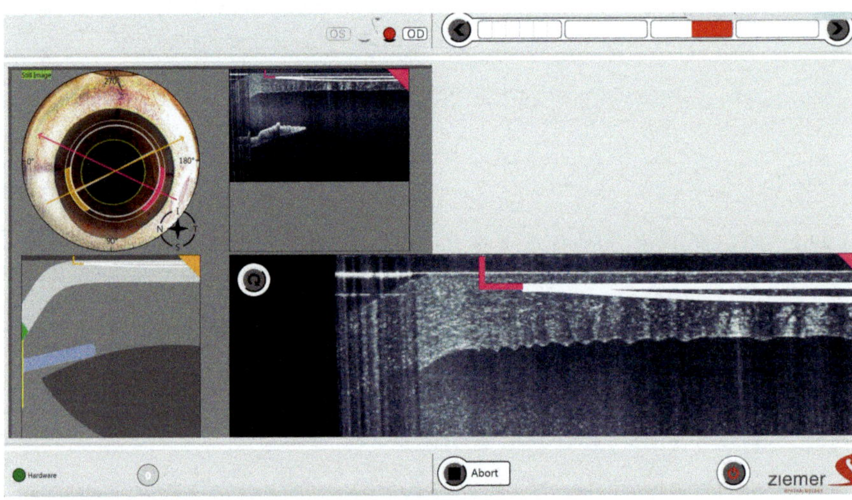

(F)

Fig. 27.2 (continued)

augmented by the automatic recognition and registration software. Additionally, the induced active suction is computerized, with an extremely low chance of suction loss, as evidenced by the Z8 long-track history of solid suction stability. Moreover, the use of intraoperative OCT allows the surgeon to observe the real-time corneal applanation generated by the system, ensuring that the planned lenticule remains within the applanation area and aligns precisely with the intended treatment zone (Fig. 27.2F).

The FEMTO LDV Z8 also has a lot of ergonomic advantages. Firstly, it allows the surgeon to operate under their microscope of choice, whether it is a standalone one or the one of an excimer laser. Secondly, its small size and mobility allow it to migrate from a laser room to an operating room in the same or different venue, where it fits in virtually any available space.

27.4 Clinical Results

In this chapter, we present the 6 months results from the first 117 consecutive eyes performed at the American University of Beirut Medical Center. The preoperative patient characteristics and lenticule and cap parameters are detailed in Table 27.1. Mean preoperative SEQ was −4.00 ± 1.73D ranging from −9.75D to −1.625D, and cap depth was 126.9 ± 5.67 μm [110, 140] with 6.59 ± 0.13 mm [6.3, 7.0] optical zone.

27.4.1 Visual and Refractive Outcomes

Postoperative UDVA was 20/20 in 97.4% of eyes at 6 months (Fig. 27.3A) with 47.3% of eyes gaining 1 or more CDVA lines (Fig. 27.3B). The average spherical equivalent (SEQ) decreased from −4.00 ± 1.73D preoperatively to −0.02 ± 0.22D 3 months postoperatively and was stable at 6 months (Fig. 27.3C). Additionally, there was no significant over- or under-correction of SEQ (Fig. 27.3D), with 98% of eyes being within ± 0.5D in SEQ and 97% within ± 0.5D of residual cylinder.

27.4.2 Corneal Higher-Order Aberrations

Figure 27.4 summarizes the corneal higher-order aberrations values at every post-operative visit. Spherical aberrations increased only mildly postoperatively, with a trend of increase in high myopia and an actual decrease in mild myopia. There was a slight increase in horizontal coma.

27.4.3 Safety

Loss of suction was not experienced in any case, and none of the lenticules were torn upon inspection postoperatively. Seven eyes (6.5%) lost 1 CDVA line 6 months postoperatively (Fig. 27.3B). One eye had an incision roof tear (eye #2 in the consecutive series), which healed by itself with a UDVA of 20/20 on day 1 postoperatively.

Table 27.1 Demographics and surgical parameters

Demographics	n	
No. of eyes	117	
No. of patients	60	
	Mean ± SD	Median [Range]
Age (y)	27 ± 6.10	27 [18, 43]
Gender (M:F)	29:31	
Visual parameters		
Sphere (D)	−3.61 ± 1.75	−3.25 [−9.75, −1.25]
Cylinder (D)	−0.77 ± 0.67	−0.5 [−3, 0]
MRSE (D)	−4.00 ± 1.73	−3.62 [−9.75, −1.625]
UDVA (logMAR)	0.93 ± 1.20	1.18 [−8, 1.6]
CDVA (logMAR)	−0.025 ± 0.04	0 [−0.12, 0.12]
Aberrometry (OZ at 6 mm)		
RMS total	1.23 ± 0.53	1.1 [0.45, 2.62]
Total HOA	0.40 ± 0.15	0.39 [−0.25, 1.18]
Vertical coma	−0.04 ± 0.15	−0.06 [−0.51, 0.39]
Horizontal coma	0.04 ± 0.15	0.03 [−0.3, 0.9]
Spherical aberration	0.21 ± 0.06	0.21 [0, 0.35]
Vertical trefoil	−0.02 ± 0.12	−0.02 [−0.39, 0.4]
Horizontal trefoil	−0.01 ± 0.13	0 [−0.51, 0.34]
Pachymetry		
Thinnest CCT (μm)	553.1 ± 32.9	553 [450, 659]
Surgical parameters		
Cap thickness (μm)	126.9 ± 5.67	130 [110, 140]
Optical zone (mm)	6.59 ± 0.13	6.6 [6.3, 7]
Suction ring (mm)	9.5 ± 0	

CCT: central corneal thickness
CDVA: corrected distance visual acuity
D: diopter
F: female
HOA: higher-order aberrations
logMAR: logarithm of the minimum angle of resolution
M: male
MRSE: manifest refraction spherical equivalent
OZ: optical zone
UDVA: uncorrected distance visual acuity

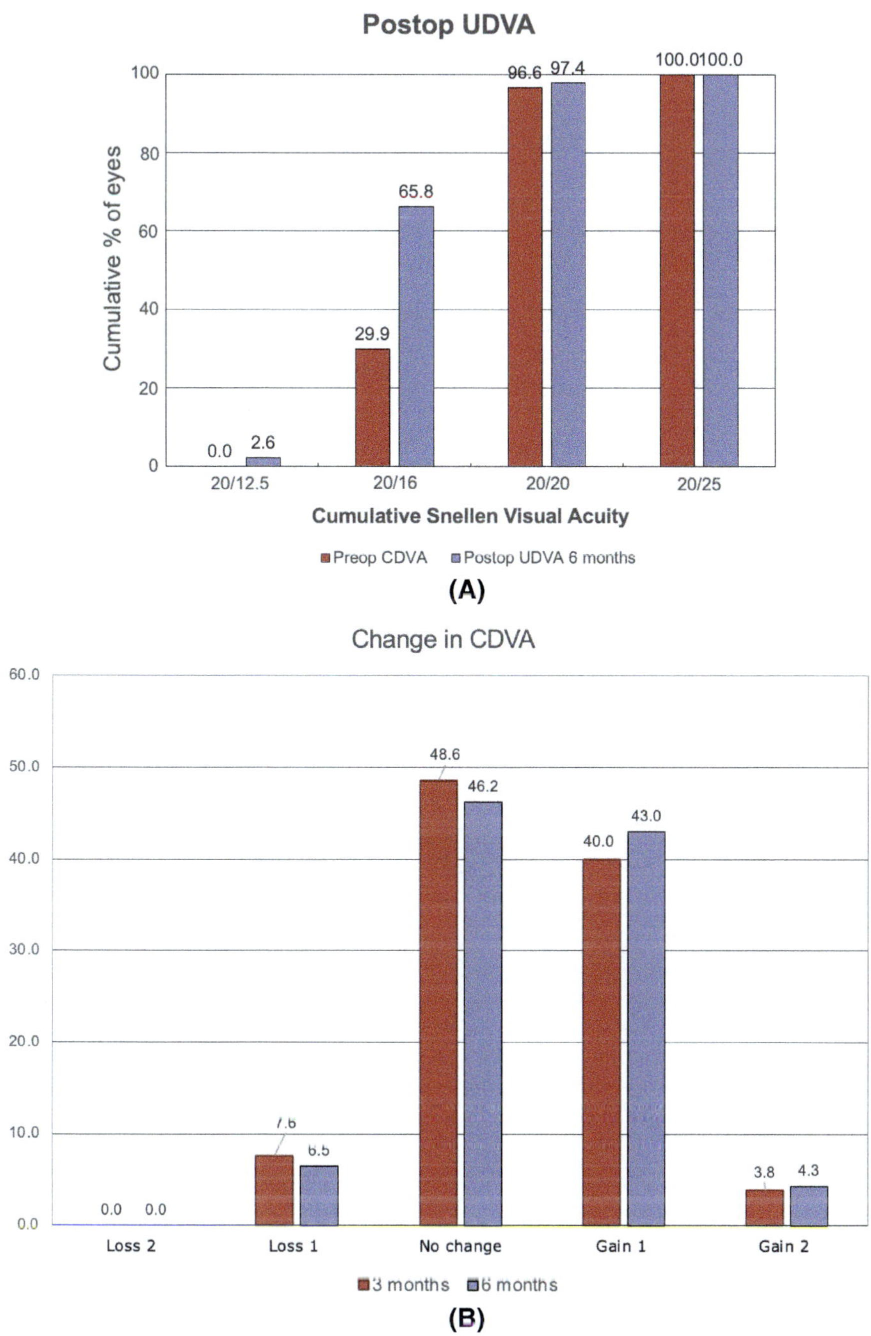

Fig. 27.3 (A) Postoperative uncorrected distance visual acuity (UDVA) versus preoperative corrected distance visual acuity (CDVA), (B) Gain or loss of CDVA lines, (C) Stability of spherical equivalent refraction over time, in months, (D) Attempted vs achieved spherical equivalent

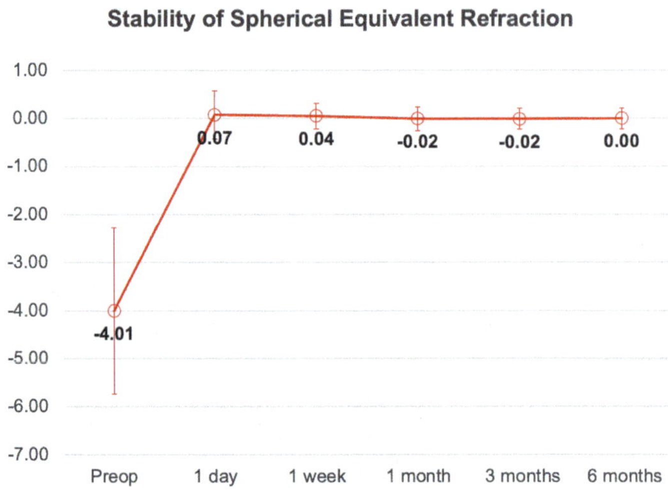

(C)

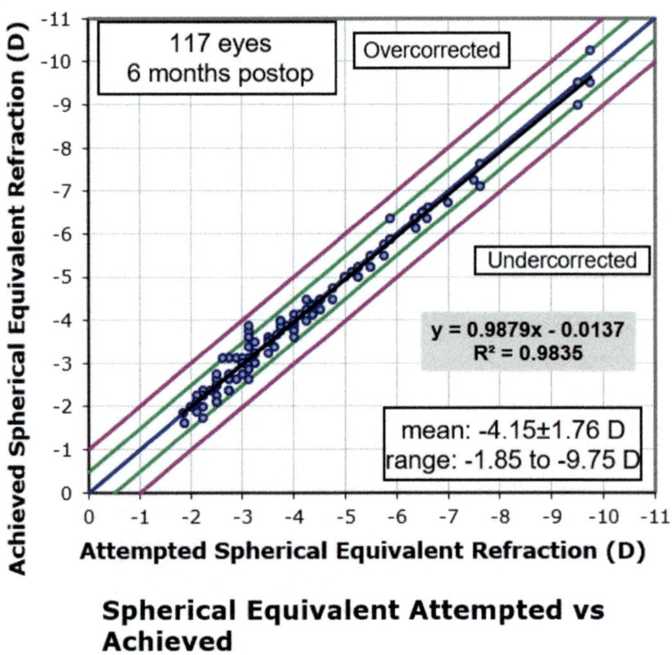

(D)

Fig. 27.3 (continued)

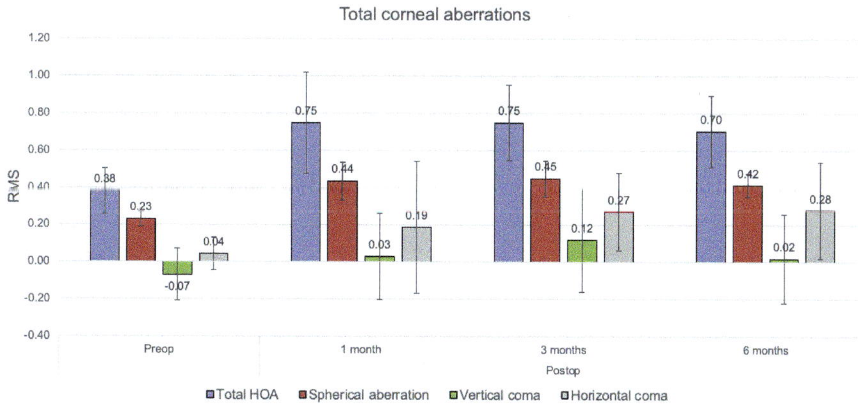

Fig. 27.4 Higher-order aberrations (HOA) over the different postoperative intervals: total HOA, spherical aberration, vertical and horizontal coma

27.4.4 Comparison

Izquierdo et al. demonstrated promising and comparable results but were limited to five eyes [1] and results by Leccisotti et al. showed good results. However, they were still inferior to our results. We believe our improved results stem from the new modifications implemented by Ziemer to the CLEAR procedure after Leccisotti's publication, including the endorsement of a larger suction ring and improvements to the posterior energy distribution [2]. We also believe that rigorous centration on the corneal vertex, and not the pupil center, especially in systems with full corneal applanation like the Z8, is key to minimize the induction of coma and maximize UDVA and CDVA.

Doga et al. demonstrated comparable results between the two different lenticule extraction platforms (VisuMax and FEMTO LDV Z8) in terms of efficiency, safety, and stability but with a limited follow-up of one month [3]. Other studies also show similar visual and refractive results to those reported following SMILE with 80–95% of eyes with postoperative UDVA of 20/20 or better [4–8].

27.5 Conclusion

Results from our first 117 eyes treated with corneal lenticule extraction using the FEMTO LDV Z8 femtosecond laser show great accuracy, effectiveness, stability, and safety. More data is sure to come from different centers across the globe evaluating the performance of CLEAR over a wider range of refractive errors and with longer follow-ups.

References

1. Izquierdo LJ, Sossa D, Ben-Shaul O, Henriquez MA. Corneal lenticule extraction assisted by a low-energy femtosecond laser. J Cataract Refract Surg. 2020;46(9):1217–21. https://doi.org/10.1097/j.jcrs.0000000000000236.
2. Leccisotti A, Fields SV, De Bartolo G. Refractive corneal lenticule extraction with the CLEAR femtosecond laser application. *Cornea.* Published online, 2022:https://doi.org/10.1097/ICO.0000000000003123
3. Дога АВ, Мушкова ИА, Майчук НВ, Образцова МР, Малышев ИС. Современные технологии рефракционной экстракции лентикулы: сравнительный анализ клинико-функциональных результатов. Офтальмология. 2022;19(2):291–8.
4. Lin F, Xu Y, Yang Y. Comparison of the visual results after SMILE and femtosecond laser-assisted LASIK for myopia. J Refract Surg. 2014;30(4):248–54. https://doi.org/10.3928/1081597X-20140320-03.
5. Sekundo W, Kunert KS, Blum M. Small incision corneal refractive surgery using the small incision lenticule extraction (SMILE) procedure for the correction of myopia and myopic astigmatism: results of a 6 month prospective study. Br J Ophthalmol. 2011;95(3):335–9. https://doi.org/10.1136/bjo.2009.174284.
6. Wang Y, Bao X liu, Tang X, Zuo T, Geng W li, Jin Y. [Clinical study of femtosecond laser corneal small incision lenticule extraction for correction of myopia and myopic astigmatism]. Zhonghua Yan Ke Za Zhi Chin J Ophthalmol. 2013;49(4):292–298.
7. Kamiya K, Shimizu K, Igarashi A, Kobashi H. Visual and refractive outcomes of femtosecond lenticule extraction and small-incision Lenticule extraction for myopia. Am J Ophthalmol. 2014;157(1):128-134.e2. https://doi.org/10.1016/j.ajo.2013.08.011.
8. Sekundo W, Gertnere J, Bertelmann T, Solomatin I. One-year refractive results, contrast sensitivity, high-order aberrations and complications after myopic small-incision lenticule extraction (ReLEx SMILE). Graefes Arch Clin Exp Ophthalmol. 2014;252(5):837–43. https://doi.org/10.1007/s00417-014-2608-4.

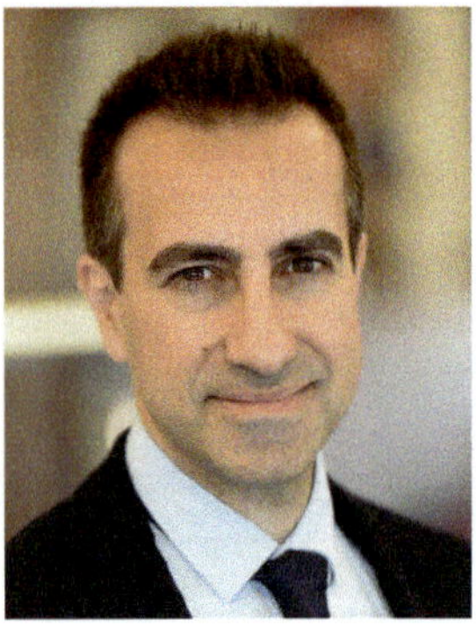

Shady Awwad is a professor of Ophthalmology and the head of the cornea & refractive surgery division at the American University of Beirut Medical Center. He received many international awards including the George Waring Medal for editorial excellence from the Journal of Refractive. He has founded many online analytical tools and software, and has several patents in computer vision machine learning. His clinical interests and research are focused on elective and therapeutic refractive surgery, analytical corneal imaging, machine learning and computer vision, and wavefront technology.

Part VII

Smooth Incision Lenticular Keratomileusis (SILK®)

Unique Features of the ELITA Laser for SILK®

28

Hong Fu and Tobin Island

Abstract

The chapter delves into the unique features of the ELITA femtosecond laser for smooth incision lenticular keratomileusis (SILK®), focusing on advancements in corneal lenticule procedures.

Keywords

ELITA femtosecond laser • Smooth Incision Lenticular Keratomileusis (SILK®) • Corneal refractive surgery • Femtosecond laser technology • Biconvex lenticule design • Lenticule extraction procedures

The ELITA femtosecond laser system is an innovative corneal refractive surgical system developed by Johnson & Johnson. Its **S**mooth **I**ncision **L**enticular **K**eratomileusis (**SILK**®) procedure is J&J's corneal lenticule removal procedure for refractive vision correction. In this chapter, we will describe the following unique ELITA features and design rationales that form the foundation for the SILK® technology and discuss future developments and concepts:

1. Ultra-thin tissue-bridge-free corneal incision technology
2. Femto-focus detection technology
3. Patient interface
4. Biconvex lenticule design
5. Future developments and concepts.

H. Fu (✉) · T. Island
Johnson-Johnson Surgical Vision Inc., Milpitas, USA
e-mail: hfu15@its.jnj.com

W. Sekundo and F. M. Wagner (eds.), *Femtosecond Laser Assisted Lenticule Extraction*,
https://doi.org/10.1007/978-3-031-60424-9_28

Background

The femtosecond laser has progressively become a major technology for ophthalmic surgery for over two decades. The AMO division of Johnson & Johnson Vision has been associated with the femtosecond laser technology since the acquisition of IntraLase, which first commercialized the femtosecond laser ophthalmic application with the IntraLase 600C Laser Keratome in 2001 [1, 2]. Today, among multiple femtosecond laser corneal surgeries, the two highest volume applications are the flap creation in the laser-assisted in situ keratomileusis (LASIK) procedure and the corneal lenticule removal procedure.

The LASIK procedure was first developed in early 1990 [3]. Modern LASIK procedures comprise two laser surgeries: First, a femtosecond laser is used to create a flap on the cornea, which is then mechanically folded back to expose the corneal stroma; second, the exposed stroma is ablated with an excimer laser, which reshapes the cornea and corrects the refractive error [4]. One well-known advantage of LASIK is that over 90% of patients gain 20/20 or better visual acuity on the day after the operation.

The concept for using a femtosecond laser to create a stromal lenticule for in situ keratomileusis was originally developed and demonstrated on ex vivo animal eyes by Kurtz et al. in 1998 [5]. It was first commercialized in 2009 when Zeiss launched the VisuMax 200 (shortly thereafter upgraded to VisuMax 500) and its small incision lenticule extraction (SMILE) procedure [6, 7], which uses the femtosecond laser to cut a lenticule in the cornea stroma with a 3 mm long entry cut for the lenticule extraction. Lenticular extraction is advantageous compared to LASIK in that it requires only one laser and is considered less invasive to the corneal biomechanics because the entry wound is much shorter than the arc length of the LASIK flap side cut which is about 24 mm. Today, the corneal lenticule extraction procedure has become a widely adopted corneal refractive surgery with millions of eyes having been treated. However, there remain important opportunities to improve the lenticule extraction procedure. For example, it is common that the lenticule surfaces, especially the posterior interface, adhere to the cornea due to uncut tissue bridges (incomplete dissection by the laser), so the surgeon must use a mechanical lenticule separation instrument to dissect and separate the interfaces. This manipulation can cause intraoperative challenges [8] and can compromise the tissue interface quality [9], which is one of the reasons that visual recovery for lenticule extraction is generally longer than for LASIK. For reference, the two published US FDA clinical studies for SMILE showed that 63% of eyes in pure myopia treatment [10] and 44% of eyes in myopia with astigmatism treatment [11] reached 20/20 or better at 1 week post-operation.

The ELITA next-generation femtosecond laser, as shown in Fig. 28.1 and Table 28.1, is designed with the aim to provide easier lenticule removal and superior visual outcome based on the femtosecond laser-tissue interaction physics.

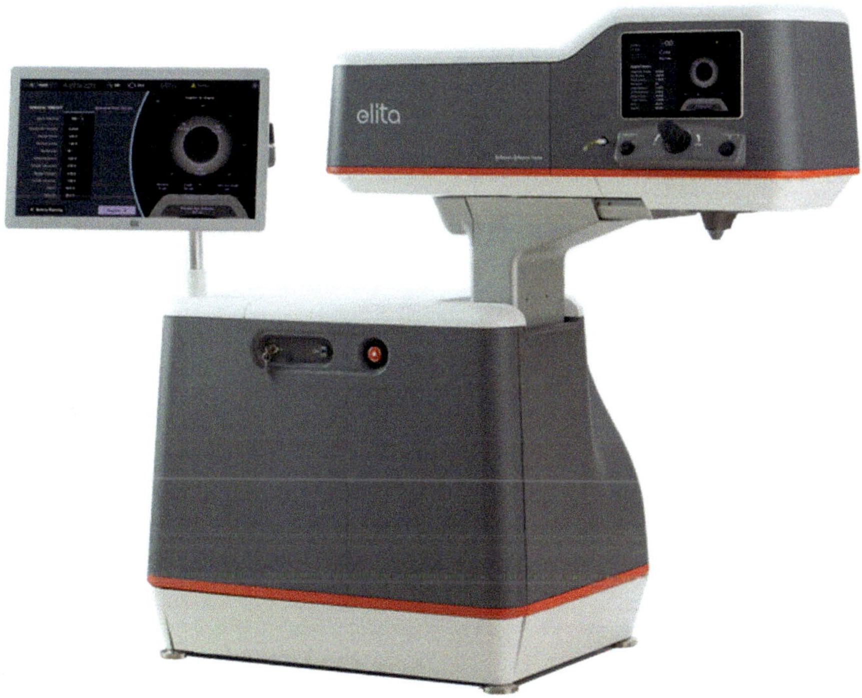

Fig. 28.1 ELITA femtosecond laser system for corneal refractive surgery

28.1 Ultra-Thin Tissue-Bridge-Free Lenticular Dissection Technology

The ELITA femtosecond laser is intended to provide a corneal lenticule procedure with easy lenticule removal and superior visual outcome. This requires ELITA to produce an ultra-thin tissue-bridge-free lenticular dissection. Based on the physics of photodisruption, the ultra-thin tissue dissection requires ultra-low pulse energy, and the tissue-bridge-free dissection requires contiguous laser spots.

An ophthalmic femtosecond laser generates ultra-short laser pulses with a pulse duration of several hundred femtoseconds (1 fs = 10^{-15} s). When the pulse is focused by the beam delivery optics to achieve a power density greater than the plasma threshold of cornea in the order of 10^{13} W/cm^2, the laser pulse induces a micron-scale incision in the tissue at the focus through a plasma-induced shock-wave and a cavitation bubble [12–14]. This laser-tissue interaction process is called photodisruption. The lower the pulse energy, the smaller the cavitation bubble and the thinner the interface of the tissue dissection [15, 16].

The power density of a laser pulse at the focus, $P(r, t)$, can be described by the product of a Gaussian function for its temporal profile and another Gaussian

Table 28.1 Key features of ELITA femtosecond laser system

Laser, optics, and scanning system nominal specifications	
Femtosecond laser type	Mode-locked, diode-pumped, ytterbium-doped fiber laser
Pulse duration	150 fs (in corneal tissue)
Pulse repetition rate	10 MHz
Center wavelength	1040 nm
Numerical aperture of optics	0.6
Focus spot diameter	1.0 μm (FWHM)
Pulse energy for lenticule incision	40–55 nJ
Contiguous spots pattern	1 μm mean center-to-center spot separation
Digital-encoder guided 3D scanning	Sub-μm trajectory control accuracy in depth direction
Fast blanking pulse control	30 μs switching transition time
Surgical volume	10 mm diameter, 750 μm depth
Visualization for dock/undock	13 mm field of view, real-time
Visualization during laser cutting	2 mm field of view, real-time
Patient interface nominal specifications	
Patient interface (PI) design	Flat PI lens
Automatic PI calibration	Each PI is calibrated with sub-μm accuracy
IOP increase under docking	52 mmHg
Real-time suction loss monitor	Yes. Cutting is paused in 0.1 s if suction loss is detected
Suction loss rate	<0.5%
System nominal specifications	
Ambient operating temperature	16–26 C
Ambient operating humidity	20–70%RH
System dimension	165 cm (W) × 70 cm (L) × 170 cm (H) 58″ (W) × 28″ (L) × 67″ (H)
System weight	265 kg
Preventive maintenance service	Annual
CDRH laser class (21 CFR 1040)	Class 4

function for its spatial cross-sectional distribution at the focus [17–20],

$$P(r,t) = P_0 \exp\left[-\left(\frac{2\sqrt{\ln 2}}{\tau}t\right)^2\right] \exp\left[-\left(\frac{2\sqrt{\ln 2}}{d}r\right)^2\right], \tag{28.1}$$

where t is time, τ is the laser pulse duration defined as full width at half maximum (FWHM), r is the distance to the center of the focus, and d is the FWHM focus spot diameter. The integration of the power density over the time and the focal plane gives the pulse energy, E:

$$E = 2\pi \int_{-\infty}^{\infty} \mathrm{d}t \int_{-\infty}^{\infty} P(r,t) r\mathrm{d}r = P_0 \left(\frac{\sqrt{\pi}}{2\sqrt{\ln 2}} \right)^3 \tau \cdot \mathrm{d}^2. \tag{28.2}$$

The peak power density is given by:

$$P_0 = \left(\frac{2\sqrt{\ln 2}}{\sqrt{\pi}} \right)^3 \frac{E}{\tau \cdot d^2} \approx 0.829 \frac{E}{\tau \cdot d^2}. \tag{28.3}$$

From Eq. (28.3), we see that using a shorter pulse duration τ and a smaller focus spot diameter d, one can achieve the same peak power density P_0 for photodisruption at a lower pulse energy E.

To achieve the shortest pulse duration, ELITA uses a custom-designed femtosecond fiber laser that has a spectral bandwidth-limited pulse duration of about 150 fs and has a pulse repetition rate of 10 MHz. Compared with all other ophthalmic femtosecond laser systems on the market, which have pulse durations ranging from 200 to 800 fs [21–24], ELITA uses the shortest pulse duration. Figure 28.2 shows a comparison between an ELITA laser pulse and an iFS laser pulse.

Since a shorter laser pulse consists of more laser cavity modes that are distributed over a wider wavelength spectrum than a longer pulse, a shorter pulse can be broadened significantly when it passes through the beam delivery optics. This is because the different wavelength modes travel at different velocities, thus stretching the pulse during propagation. This is called the pulse broadening effect due to

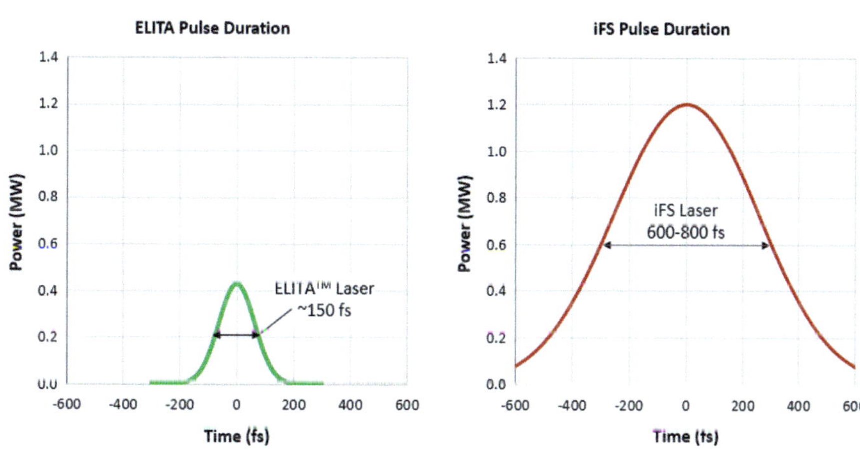

Fig. 28.2 Comparison of an ELITA laser pulse typically used for lenticular incision and an iFS laser pulse typically used for flap bed cut. The area under the pulse profile is the pulse energy, which is 50 nJ for the ELITA pulse and 700 nJ for the iFS pulse, respectively

group velocity dispersion (GVD). Let τ be the bandwidth-limited pulse duration at entrance of the beam delivery optics, $\Delta\tau$ be the amount of pulse duration increase at the exit, then we have the pulse duration $(\tau + \Delta\tau)$ at the exit [18]:

$$\tau + \Delta\tau = \sqrt{\tau^2 + 16(\ln 2)^2 \left(\frac{\text{GVD}}{\tau}\right)^2}. \tag{28.4}$$

One can prove from Eq. (28.4) that a bigger GVD and a smaller τ will lead to a greater $\Delta\tau$. To obtain the shortest pulse duration at the tissue, the ELITA laser source is built in with a negative GVD that exactly cancels out the positive GVD of the beam delivery optics, so the total GVD is zero. This technology is called "GVD precompensation". Figure 28.3 shows the pulse durations with and without GVD precompensation as a function of the bandwidth-limited pulse duration for the specific GVD of ELITA beam delivery optics. We see that without GVD precompensation, a pulse of 150 fs at the entrance of the beam delivery optics would have been broadened to about 350 fs at the exit. A pulse of 200 fs [24] at the entrance will become 300 fs at the exit, which is the minimum pulse duration that can be achieved without GVD precompensation. Figure 28.3 shows that the pulse broadening becomes less significant ($\Delta\tau/\tau \leq 10\%$) when the pulse duration is above 400 fs.

To obtain an extremely small focus spot size of 1.0 μm (FWHM), ELITA uses a beam delivery optics with high numerical aperture, NA = 0.6, which is defined by the formula:

$$\text{NA} = n \cdot \sin\theta, \tag{28.5}$$

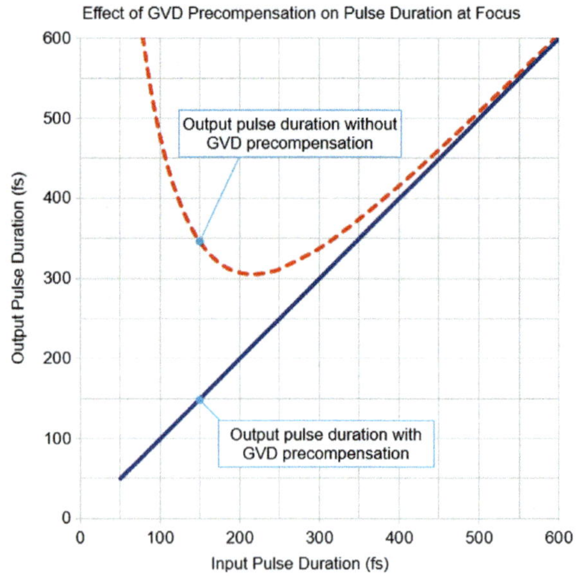

Fig. 28.3 Comparison of pulse durations at the focus (tissue) with (the straight blue line) and without (the red dashed curve) GVD precompensation as a function of the input bandwidth-limited pulse duration

where n is the refractive index of the medium, and θ is the half cone angle of the laser beam. Based on Snell's law, NA is a constant in any optical component throughout the beam path. For air, $n = 1$, $\theta = 36.9°$; for cornea, $n = 1.377$, $\theta = 25.8°$. In general, larger NA leads to tighter beam focus at the focal point and larger beam divergence elsewhere. The exact focus spot size depends on NA, the entrance beam size and shape, and the beam-lens filling factor [20].

From system design standpoint, it is impractical to achieve the desired sharp focus (NA = 0.6) with the conventional large field optics to cover the entire 10 mm diameter surgical field due to the bulkiness of the optics and the anatomic structure limit associated with human eye. Instead, ELITA uses a small moving focusing objective lens to cover the 10 mm surgical field. The optical field of view (FOV) of this moving objective lens is 2 mm. Because the moving objective lens blocks the visualization of the full field during laser treatment, ELITA uses a unique dual-channel video imaging system for procedure visualization. Before and after the laser treatment, the moving objective is parked outside the field and the imaging channel provides a 13 mm real-time FOV. During the laser treatment, the objective lens moves across the surgical field and the ELITA cutting imaging channel provides a 2 mm real-time FOV that moves together with the moving objective and shows the live photodisruption bubbles at the cutting location. During cutting, the suction pressure and the floating head movement are monitored, and the laser treatment will be paused if suction loss or significant head movement are detected.

Another key design choice for ensuring a 1.0 μm spot across the entire treatment field is to use a flat PI lens instead of a curved PI lens, because a curved PI will introduce significant wavefront aberrations to the laser focus at the peripheral areas of the surgical field (see the detailed discussion in Sect. 28.3).

With these three design options, i.e., high NA, moving objective lens and flat PI lens, ELITA achieves the design target to have a uniform low pulse energy plasma threshold across the entire 10 mm surgical field within measurement tolerance of sub-nJ.

The 1 μm spot diameter describes the tight confinement of the laser pulse energy in the focal plane (*XY* plane). Another critical parameter, which is related to the beam focus diameter but describes the confinement of the pulse energy in the beam propagation direction (Z-direction), is the depth of focus given by [19, 20]:

$$\Delta = \frac{n\pi w_0^2}{\lambda} = \frac{n\pi d^2}{(2\ln 2)\lambda}, \tag{28.6}$$

where n is the refractive index of medium ($n = 1.377$ for cornea), w_0 is the $1/e^2$ radius of Gaussian beam at the focus, $d = (2\ln2)^{1/2}\, w_0$ is the FWHM spot diameter, and λ is the laser wavelength in air. Let z be the beam propagation distance from the focus, the $1/e^2$ radius of the Gaussian beam, $w(z)$ is given by.

$$w(z) = w_0\sqrt{1 + \left(\frac{z}{\Delta}\right)^2}. \tag{28.7}$$

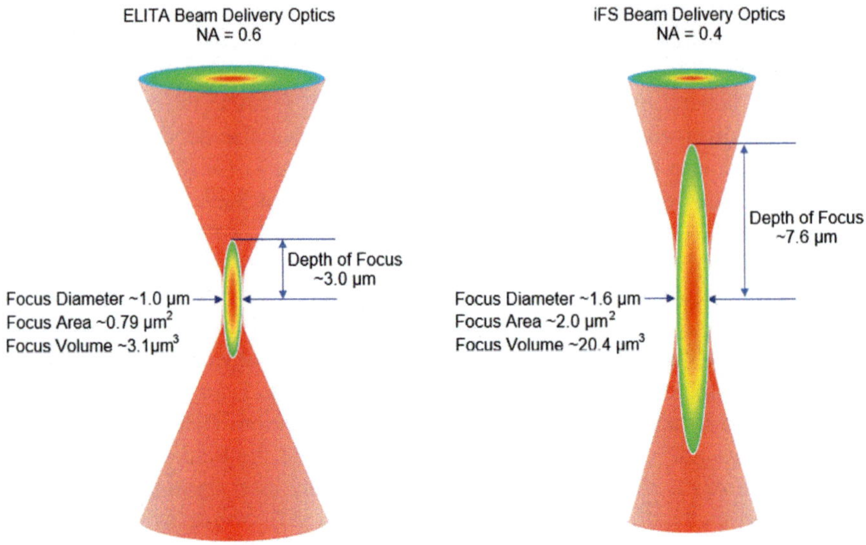

Fig. 28.4 Comparison of focus spot diameter, area, depth of focus, and focal volume in cornea for ELITA and iFS, where $n = 1.377$, $\lambda = 1.040\ \mu\text{m}$ for ELITA, and $1.053\ \mu\text{m}$ for iFS are used. Far from the focus, i.e., $|z| \gg \Delta$, the ELITA beam diverges faster (with a half cone angle of 25.8°) than the iFS beam does (16.9°) in the cornea

Since pulse energy density is inversely proportional to the cross-sectional area of the beam, at $z = \Delta$, the pulse energy intensity is half of that in the focal point. A comparison of the focus spot diameter, area, depth of focus, and focal volume for ELITA and iFS is shown in Fig. 28.4. It is seen that the region of high laser intensity at the focus is much more confined in ELITA than it is in iFS.

As a result of shortest pulse duration and small focus spot, ELITA reaches photodisruption threshold of about 30 nJ per pulse and achieves robust corneal dissection at 40–50 nJ per pulse without uncut dark spots. Of the 40–50 nJ energy per pulse, the portion that is converted to form plasma is estimated to be about 10–20 nJ, which contributes to the photodisruption. The rest of the pulse energy is either transmitted or scattered without interacting with the tissue. Based on Linz [16], an oscillating cavitation bubble is generated by the plasma and the volume of the cavitation bubble at the maximum radius, $R_{\text{Cavitation}}$, is universally proportional to the laser pulse energy when it is sufficiently above the plasma threshold. Because the radius is proportional to the cubit root of volume, we have:

$$R_{\text{Cavitation}} \propto (\text{Pulse Energy})^{\frac{1}{3}}. \tag{28.8}$$

Considering a cavitation bubble is centered at the tissue dissection plane, we can reasonably assume that the laser-affected zone thickness, LAZT, i.e., the laser-tissue interaction range perpendicular to the dissection interface, including both sides of the dissection plane, is proportional to the diameter of the cavitation bubble:

$$\text{LAZT} \propto 2R_{\text{Cavitation}}. \tag{28.9}$$

For a corneal lenticule procedure, after the lenticule removal, the total interface thickness, including the lower half from the posterior lenticular dissection and the upper half from the anterior dissection, is still equal to the full LAZT. In the case of LASIK, however, the lower half of the interface, i.e., the stromal bed surface, is smoothed out to a great extent by the excimer laser ablation [25], so the interface thickness becomes approximately half of the LAZT, which is primarily contributed by the upper half of the tissue interface on the flap. Therefore, for a lenticule procedure to produce an equal or thinner interface thickness than that of LASIK requires:

$$\text{LAZT}_{\text{Lenticule}} \leq \text{LAZT}_{\text{LASIK}} \approx \frac{\text{LAZT}_{\text{Flap}}}{2}. \tag{28.10}$$

Combining Eqs. (28.8–28.10), and using $E_{\text{Lenticule}}$ and E_{Flap} to represent the energy per pulse for lenticule dissection and flap bed creation, respectively, we find the necessary condition for a lenticular interface to be thinner than the LASIK interface:

$$E_{\text{Lenticule}} \leq \frac{E_{\text{Flap}}}{8}. \tag{28.11}$$

The ELITA lenticule procedure with $E_{\text{Lenticule}} \approx 50$ nJ meets this requirement when it is compared with iFS-LASIK procedure with $E_{\text{Flap}} \approx 700$ nJ. Equation (28.11) is a necessary but not a sufficient condition for a corneal lenticule procedure to produce an ultra-thin interface that is thinner than that of the LASIK. Another necessary condition is that the lenticule removal must be as easy as lifting a flap, so that the corneal interface is not compromised by the manually operated mechanic separation of the lenticular surfaces.

To produce a *tissue-bridge-free* lenticular dissection requires contiguous cutting spots, which in turn requires more laser pulses and faster scanning speed. ELITA uses a 10 MHz pulse repetition rate. To scan such high reprate pulses, ELITA uses a high frequency resonant scanner to produce a fast scanline, acting as the femto-cutting *blade*, then it uses a high-precision digital-encoder guided *XYZ-Φ* four-dimensional scanning system (where Φ is the azimuthal orientation of the fast scanline) to move the fast scanline to cut lenticule. This digital-encoder guided scanning system provides a sub-μm control accuracy between the target and the executed cutting trajectories in the depth direction. To achieve uniform photodisruption of the lenticular dissection, ELITA uses a proprietary fast *Laser Blanking* technology to control the photodisruption on and off quickly. It should be noted that the cavitation bubble formation takes less than 10 ns [12, 13], while the time interval between adjacent pulses for a 10 MHz pulse repetition rate is 100 ns, so a cavitation bubble can only be generated by a single pulse. A schematic

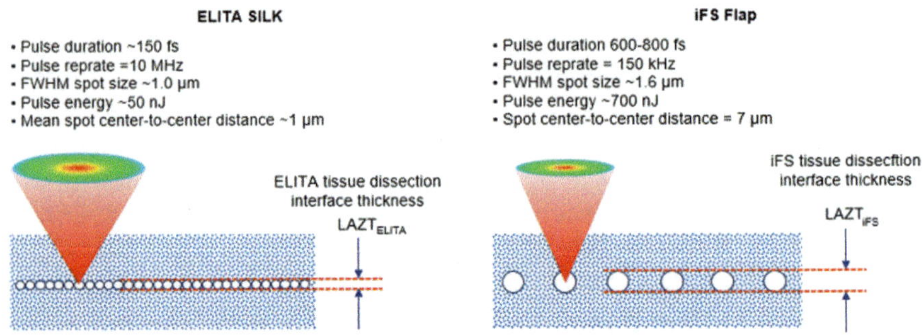

Fig. 28.5 Comparison of spot contiguity between ELITA and iFS lasers. In theory, because using ultra-low pulse energy, ELITA lenticular interface $LAZT_{ELITA}$ is smaller than half of the iFS flap interface thickness $LAZT_{iFS}$, i.e., less than the iFS-LASIK interface thickness

comparison of contiguous spot pattern for ELITA and the discrete spot pattern for iFS is shown in Fig. 28.5.

It is worth mentioning that the contiguity of the scanning spots is not as necessary for a flap creation as it is for a lenticular dissection, because the flap creation primarily *separates* the parallel lamellar fibrils, while the lenticule dissection *cuts* the lamellar layers of collagen fibrils. Therefore, a non-contiguous spot pattern for lenticular dissection is more prone to leave uncut tissue bridges and lead to difficult lenticule separation and removal.

Figures 28.4 and 28.5 show that, due to the smaller depth of focus and the smaller cavitation bubble, the laser-tissue interactions in an ELITA procedure, from both the laser intensity distribution standpoint and the range of mechanic disturbance standpoint, are more closely confined to the intended dissection location. Beyond this layer, the laser beam expands quickly as a function of z, and the energy intensity drops quickly to below the laser-tissue interaction threshold so that there is no laser-tissue interaction. For example, when cutting a lenticule at 110 μm depth for a typical cornea with an epithelium thickness of 50 μm, Bowman's layer thickness of 20 μm, the closest point at the Bowman's layer to the focus is $z = 110\ \mu\text{m} - 50\ \mu\text{m} - 20\ \mu\text{m} = 40\ \mu\text{m}$. Based on Eq. (28.7), the area of the beam cross section is $[w(z)/w_0]^2 = 1 + (40/3.0)^2 = 178$ times the area at focus. Assuming a typical pulse energy of 50 nJ is used for the lenticular incision, and the typical photodisruption threshold is 30 nJ, then the energy density at the Bowman's layer is $[50\ \text{nJ}/w^2(z)]/[30\ \text{nJ}/{w_0}^2] \approx 0.94\%$ of the photodisruption threshold: there is no laser-tissue interaction. In comparison, for a femtosecond laser system with NA = 0.4, $\Delta = 7.6\ \mu\text{m}$, pulse energy = 125 nJ, photodisruption threshold = 100 nJ, the beam area at the Bowman's layer will be 29 times that at focus, and the energy density at the Bowman's layer will be 4.3% of the photodisruption threshold, which is greater than the case of ELITA, but is also much below the laser-tissue interaction threshold. Therefore, even if the ELITA contiguous spot pattern may require higher total energy dosage, the energy is delivered to a more confined region at the intended tissue dissection plane; the undesired collateral impact beyond the intended dissection location is smaller. The understanding that higher energy dosage leads to higher collateral tissue damage is only correct when considering the same laser source, beam delivery optics, and the same spot scanning pattern.

In summary, with the shortest laser pulse duration, the extremely small focus spot size, the contiguous spot pattern, and the high-precision digital-encoder guided scanning system, ELITA is designed to create an ultra-thin tissue-bridge-free lenticular dissection with LASIK-like interface thickness based on the fundamental laser-tissue interaction physics.

28.2 Femto-Focus Detection Technology

By elegantly detecting, scanning, and analyzing the reflected light from the focus of the femtosecond laser beam, ELITA is designed with a high-precision, multi-purpose in situ femto-focus detection (FFD) system. The special design allows the FFD to be used in both confocal and non-confocal modes. The high-precision of the FFD comes from the high NA of the optics; the high-precision digital-encoder guided scanning system and the analysis algorithm. In the following, we describe three major applications.

Application 1: Submicron Patient Interface Calibration (Auto-Z Calibration)

The measurement principle is the confocal relation between the object distance of the focus and the image distance of the focus as illustrated on the left of Fig. 28.6. By scanning the laser focus in *Z*-direction, the depth of the contact surface of the PI lens can be measured with sub-μm accuracy. For each ELITA procedure, after the PI cone is mounted to the laser beam exit port, the depths at three *XY* locations are measured (see the highlighted green disks on the right of Fig. 28.6) from which the plane of PI lens, $Z_{PI}(x, y)$, is determined. The mean offset is measured with less than 1 μm precision, and the polar tilt angle is measured with less than 0.01° precision. The algorithm will adjust and place the cutting pattern at the intended target depth with respect to the PI surface at any *XY* location. Auto-Z corrects any depth error which may be contributed by the PI lens or by minute optical system drift to sub-μm accuracy. Auto-Z also detects misplacement of the PI.

Application 2: Sub-nanojoule Plasma Threshold Detection

Since the femtosecond laser-tissue interaction is initiated by plasma formation, the plasma threshold energy (the lowest pulse energy at which the plasma is initiated) is the single most relevant parameter that describes the combined performance of the femtosecond laser engine and the beam delivery optics. The lower the plasma threshold, the higher the photodisruption efficiency of the femtosecond laser system.

ELITA uses the FFD to measure the plasma threshold of the PI glass in a non-confocal mode. In this measurement, the laser focus is scanned from air to the glass surface. If the pulse energy is below the plasma threshold of the glass,

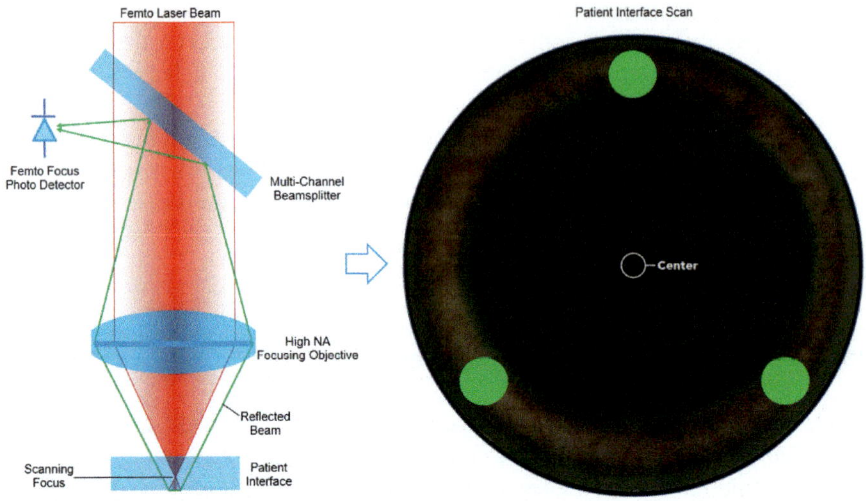

Fig. 28.6 ELITA PI calibration principle and implementation. The depths of the PI plane at three *XY* locations are measured with sub-μm accuracy. The PI offset and tilt are compensated for by adjusting the trajectory of the laser cutting pattern accordingly

the FFD signal is a continuous function when the focus passes through the glass surface. If the pulse energy is above the plasma threshold, the FFD signal will drop sharply when the focus passes through the glass surface, because part of the light energy is converted to plasma and part of the light is scattered by the plasma. By adjusting the pulse energy, the plasma threshold can be measured within 1 nJ. We call this energy the glass-burn threshold (GBT). Although the plasma threshold of cornea is different from GBT, the ratio of the two for a given system is a constant for different ELITA systems. The peak power density for a given system which has a fixed temporal pulse profile and a fixed spatial distribution at the focal plane is determined by the pulse energy. Based on the clinically optimized relations between the pulse energy settings for different corneal incisions and the GBT of the systems, we can determine the energy settings for a newly ELITA system within just a few percent of its final clinically optimized settings. A manufacturing or service engineer can measure the GBT within minutes to judge the performance of the system, which is more accurate, more relevant, and more practical than measuring the laser pulse duration at the focus and measuring the focus spot size (Fig. 28.7).

Application 3: Real-Time Photodisruption Monitor

There are undesired but potentially possible situations where the laser-tissue interaction behaves unexpectedly, such as dark spots, i.e., no photodisruption, or when the contact between the patient interface and the cornea becomes compromised, i.e., loss of meniscus. As of now, no femtosecond laser on the market provides real-time photodisruption monitoring. Since the cavitation bubble reflects the laser

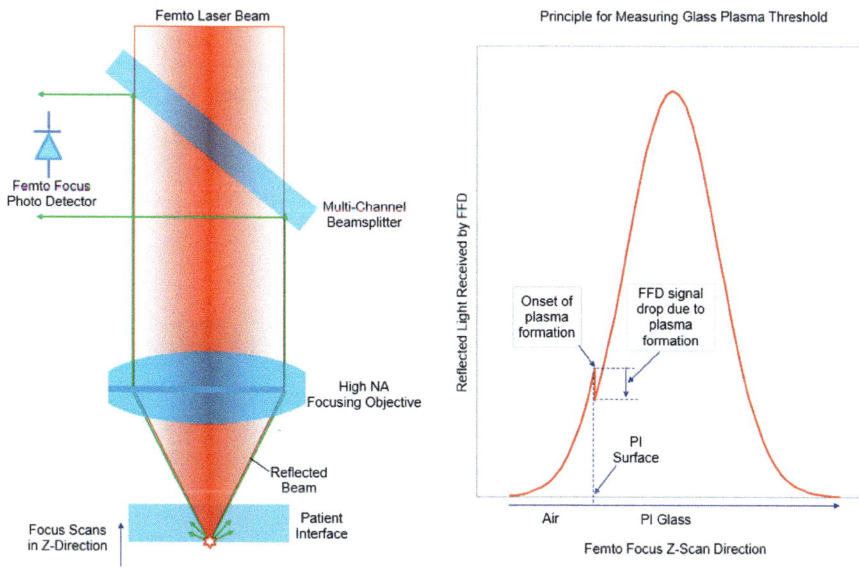

Fig. 28.7 Principle for measuring the GBT with the FFD in non-confocal mode. Based on the GBT, we can set the initial energy for surgery for a newly installed or a system after service based on clinically proven relations between GBT and energy settings

beam, the FFD signal can detect the strength of the photodisruption at the focus. Currently, ELITA records the FFD signal of every procedure for post-operative treatment analysis. It has been proven that the above-mentioned abnormal photodisruption situations can be detected. In principle, the FFD signal can be used to control the laser incision parameters to optimize the cutting, can be displayed on the GUI screen for surgeon to monitor, or can be used as an alarm to automatically pause the treatment. We will evaluate the needs (Fig. 28.8).

28.3 Patient Interface (PI)

A femtosecond laser for corneal refractive surgery always requires a PI to fix the cornea for precise laser pattern delivery. The PI also provides a sterile separation between the eye and the system. Figure 28.9 shows the ELITA PI kit. It consists of three components: the PI cone, the suction ring assembly, and the protective cap.

The *PI cone* consists of a plastic cone and a flat lens. For treatment of each eye, a new PI cone is attached and locked to the laser output port. The PI lens is measured and calibrated by the ELITA Auto-Z calibration system within sub-μm accuracy.

The *suction ring assembly* consists of a soft suction ring, a plastic gripper, and a vacuum tubing. During docking, the soft suction ring grabs an annulus area of the sclera by the vacuum pressure supplied by the vacuum pump system. The gripper

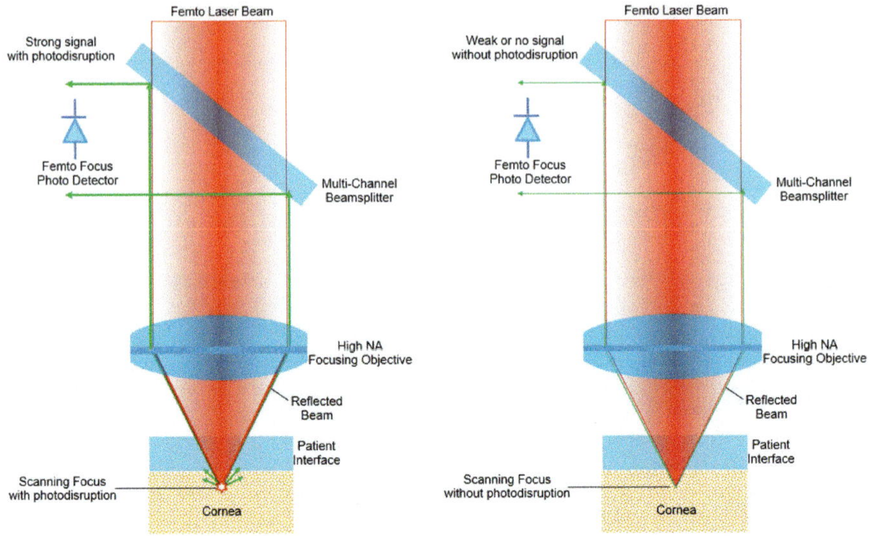

Fig. 28.8 Principle of real-time photodisruption monitoring with FFD in non-confocal mode. The FFD receives more reflected light when there is strong photodisruption (left), it receives little to no light when there is no photodisruption (right). Currently, ELITA records the FFD signal of each procedure for post-operative treatment analysis

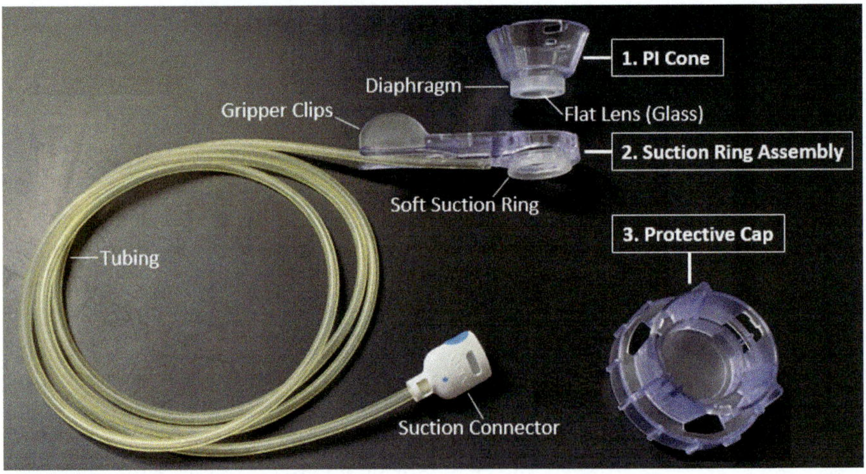

Fig. 28.9 ELITA patient interface kit. It consists of three components: the PI cone, the suction ring assembly, and the non-functional protective cap

is opened by squeezing the clips and the PI cone diaphragm shall be fully inserted into the gripper. When the PI lens applanates the cornea to reach a meniscus diameter of 10 mm, the clips are released so the gripper firmly holds the PI diaphragm. Now the eye is docked with the system. To undock, turn off the vacuum to disengage the suction ring from the eye, press the clips to disengage the PI cone from the gripper, and then use the protective cap to detach the PI cone from the system.

The *protective cap* is a cover to protect the PI lens from contamination during handling and an auxiliary tool for attaching the PI cone to or detaching the PI cone from the laser output port. After the PI cone is mounted firmly on the laser output port, the protective cap is removed prior to the laser treatment. The ELITA PI is referred to as a 2-piece design because the PI cone and the suction ring are two separate components.

Essentially, the ELITA PI adopted the proven iFS PI design with some modifications, see Table 28.1 for a comparison. Here we emphasize a few design choices. Like the iFS PI, the ELITA PI uses the soft suction ring on the sclera to provide sufficient lateral holding force ($\geq$ 2 N) to keep the eye stabilized against possible unintentional eye rolling movements driven by the extraocular eye muscles, which have a maximum force of 0.5–1 N [26]. The lateral eye holding force is proportional to the product of the suction pressure, the contact area between the suction ring and the sclera, and the coefficient of friction between the suction ring and the sclera. Since the coefficient of friction of human skin tissue is about 0.2 or greater [27], while that of cornea is in the range of 0.006–0.015 [28], the ELITA and IntraLase PI are designed to have sufficient contact area between the suction ring and the sclera. Any PI that only applies suction on the cornea will not provide sufficient force to overcome the extraocular muscle force of the eye if the muscle is unintentionally triggered during treatment (Table 28.2).

ELITA uses a vacuum pump as the source of suction. The vacuum pressure is 500 mmHg, which is basically the same pressure provided by the syringe as used in the IntraLase PI. The vacuum pressure is monitored by three vacuum meters at different locations in the vacuum supply. If there is a suction loss, the system will report an error and pause the treatment within 0.1 s.

Learning from the Catalys suction ring design [29], we introduced the sclera support structure inside the suction ring. This reduces eyeball deformation, and therefore reduces the intraocular pressure (IOP) increase. Under typical docking conditions with specified suction pressure, load force, and full applanation, the ELITA PI induces a ΔIOP $\approx$ 52 mmHg (ΔIOP = IOP under docking − IOP before docking), while the IntraLase PI, which does not have the sclera support structure, induces a ΔIOP $\approx$ 75 mmHg. Based on experiments with ex vivo porcine eyes, the maximum docking load for ELITA was ΔIOP $\approx$ 79 mmHg compared with ΔIOP $\approx$ 92 mmHg for the IntraLase PI.

Like the iFS PI, the ELITA PI uses a flat but bigger fused silica lens. For achieving a uniform focus quality in the entire 10 mm diameter surgical field, a high numerical aperture (NA = 0.6) for ELITA beam delivery optics is important. A curved PI will introduce optical aberration to the laser beam which increases radially from the center of the PI to the periphery. For NA = 0.6, a curved PI with

Table 28.2 Comparison between ELITA PI and iFS PI

Parameters	iFS PI	ELITA PI
PI design	2-piece, flat PI lens	2-piece, flat PI lens
Suction ring material	Soft	Soft
Eye holding force, lateral	≥ 2 N	≥ 2 N
Eye holding force, vertical	≥ 3 N	≥ 3 N
Suction ring ID	12.6 mm	12.6 mm
Suction ring OD	21.3 mm	21.3 mm
Gripper OD	20.6 mm	22.5 mm
Cone height	27.9 mm	21.0 mm
Half cone angle	30°	21°
PI lens diameter	11.0 mm	13.0 mm
Surgical field diameter	9.5 mm	10.0 mm
Suction pressure	475 mmHg	500 mmHg
Suction source	Syringe	Vacuum pump
Sclera support	No sclera support	With sclera support
IOP increase	$\approx$75 mmHg	$\approx$52 mmHg
PI calibration	No calibration (MFG spec = ± 10 μm)	Auto calibration with sub-μm accuracy
Auto suction loss detection	No	Yes
Floating head motion detection	No	Yes
Suction loss rate	<0.5%	Design Target < 0.5%

a radius of curvature of 20 mm, which is used by several commercial femtosecond laser systems, will deteriorate the Strehl ratio of the focus (i.e., the ratio of actual peak intensity at the focus to the maximum peak intensity in ideal situation) by 23% when the focus is moved from the center to the periphery of the 10 mm diameter surgical field. Accordingly, the photodisruption threshold energy at the periphery will increase by 29% (1/0.77 $\approx$ 1.29) relative to the value at the PI center, see Fig. 28.10.

A flat PI allows post-docking centration adjustment, which is a valuable feature for achieving the best lenticule centration and therefore the best visual outcome. In contrast, if the lenticule center is moved away from the apex of a curved PI, the depth profile of the lenticule surface relative to the curved PI surface becomes asymmetric. Consequently, the off-center cutting requires high frequency modulation in the *Z*-direction, leading to increased error in lenticule shape.

We point out that the curved PIs as used on the market also have significant applanation effects on the cornea, because the radii of curvature of these PIs are about 20 mm, while that of cornea is only 7–8 mm. For example, to achieve a 10 mm meniscus, a flat PI will down press the cornea vertex by about 1.8 mm, while the curved PI will down press the vertex by about 1.2 mm. Another effect is

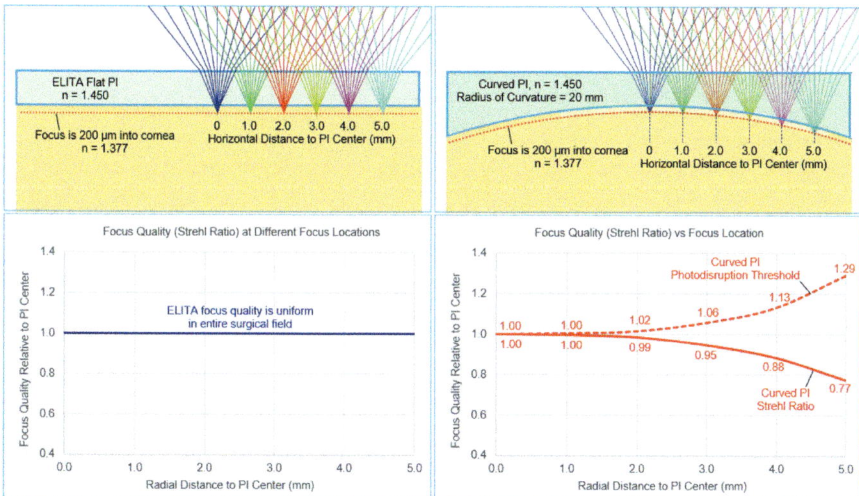

Fig. 28.10 Comparison of focus quality uniformity in surgical field between the ELITA flat PI design and a hypothetical curved PI design. The optical modeling is done for the focus at 200 μm depth in the cornea. The index of refraction for fused silica glass is $n = 1.450$ at wavelength 1040 nm. The index of refraction for the cornea is $n = 1.377$. The Strehl ratio is constant in the entire surgical field for the flat PI, but it drops significantly at the periphery with the curved PI

associated with the enlargement of the optical zone under applanation. This effect, if not compensated for, will cause 5.7% overcorrection for the flat PI and 5.0% overcorrection for the curved PI. This applanation effect has been compensated for in the ELITA lenticule shape design.

Both flat PI and curved PI are widely and successfully used in femtosecond laser refractive surgery. The curved PI design is biased toward more patient comfort during the surgery. The ELITA PI is designed to provide superior surgical performance, including extremely low rate of suction loss, ultra-low pulse energy photodisruption in the entire surgical field, post-docking centration adjustability, and sub-μm depth calibration. All these are important for ELITA SILK procedure to achieve easy lenticule removal and the best visual outcome.

28.4 Biconvex Lenticule Design

Unlike all other corneal lenticule procedures which use plano-convex lenticule incision shape in the same fashion as LASIK, ELITA uses a proprietary biconvex lenticule incision shape, see Fig. 28.11.

The basic principle for corneal refractive correction, including LASIK and corneal lenticule procedures, whether they use plano-convex or biconvex shape

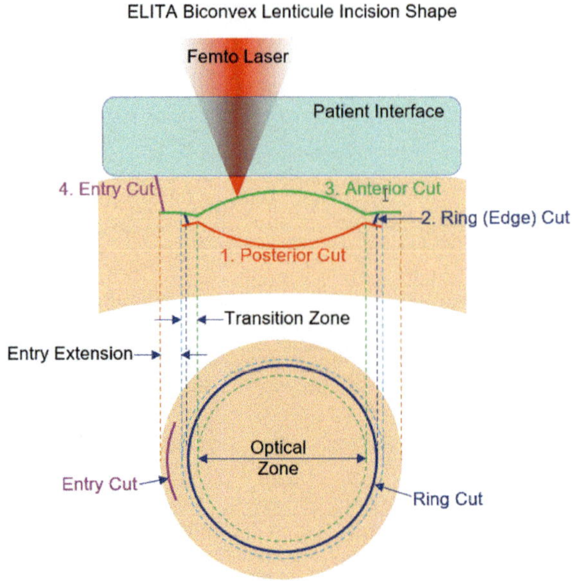

Fig. 28.11 ELITA uses a biconvex lenticular incision shape for cornea under applanation. The incision is performed in four steps: a) The posterior lenticular cut, b) the ring lenticular edge cut, c) the anterior lenticular cut, and d) the entry cut

of the removed tissue, is described by the Munnerlyn equation [4]:

$$\Delta D = (n - 1)\left(\frac{1}{R_2} - \frac{1}{R_1}\right), \tag{28.12}$$

where ΔD is the refractive error to be corrected, $n = 1.377$ is the refractive index of cornea, R_1 and R_2 are the radii of curvature of the anterior corneal surface before and after correction, respectively. The Munnerlyn equation is derived from the standard focal length formula $f = R/(n - 1)$ for a spherical surface with radius R. For pure myopia, R_1 is independent of the meridian angle and the anterior cornea is a spherical surface. For myopia with astigmatism, R_1 is a function of the meridian angle, ϕ, and the corneal shape is a toric surface. Mathematically, a toric surface can always be expressed as sum of a pure spherical surface plus a pure cylindrical surface. R_1 and R_2 can be calculated from the keratometry values K_1 and K_2 for the cornea, and from the intended correction usually expressed in the form of SPH/CYL × θ, where SPH, CYL, and θ are the sphere, cylinder, and cylinder axis orientation of the refractive error to be treated.

In essence, a refractive corneal surgery, including both LASIK and corneal lenticule procedures, is to vacate a space in cornea which has a specific *Z*-displacement profile, $\Delta Z(\rho, \phi)$, such that the original anterior corneal surface, $Z_1(\rho, \phi)$, will be displaced to the desired corneal surface, $Z_2(\rho, \phi)$, after the surgery, see Fig. 28.12.

It should be noted that the *Z*-displacement function is determined by the original and the desired anterior corneal surface functions,

$$\Delta Z(\rho, \varphi) = Z_1(\rho, \varphi) - Z_2(\rho, \varphi). \tag{28.13}$$

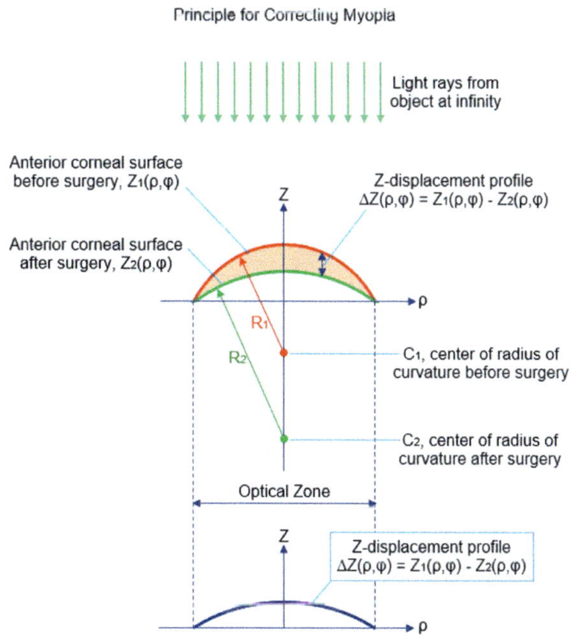

Fig. 28.12 Corneal refractive surgery is to vacate a tissue volume with the desired *Z*-displacement profile (blue) such that the original anterior corneal surface (red) will displace to the desired location (green) as described by the Munnerlyn formula

However, a given *Z*-displacement function does not uniquely determine the anterior lenticule shape, $Z_A(\rho, \phi)$, and the posterior lenticule shape, $Z_P(\rho, \phi)$, but only requires their difference to be equal to the desired *Z*-displacement function,

$$\Delta Z(\rho, \varphi) = Z_A(\rho, \varphi) - Z_P(\rho, \varphi). \tag{28.14}$$

This gives freedom to choose the individual anterior and posterior lenticular shapes. LASIK and most corneal lenticule procedures use the plano-convex shape for the removed tissue, which is inherited from the flap creation with a microkeratome or with a femtosecond laser. ELITA uses the biconvex lenticule incision shape under applanation. The shapes under various stages during the procedure are illustrated Fig. 28.13.

Both biconvex and plano-convex lenticule shapes are required to produce the same *Z*-displacement profile. The volumes of the two shapes are the same which is equal to the volume integration of the *Z*-displacement function $\Delta Z(\rho, \phi)$. The anterior interface depth for the plano-convex shape is a constant, which is the cap depth for lenticule procedures or the flap thickness for LASIK. The anterior interface depth for biconvex lenticule is not a constant: it is equal to anterior depth input parameter at the apex of the lenticule and becomes deeper when moving to the periphery. The depth of the lenticule periphery depends on the manifest correction and the optical zone diameter. For example, to correct a − 4.00 D sphere with anterior depth setting of 110 μm, the anterior depth at lenticule apex is 110 μm, and it becomes 133, 137, 143 μm at the periphery for optical zone

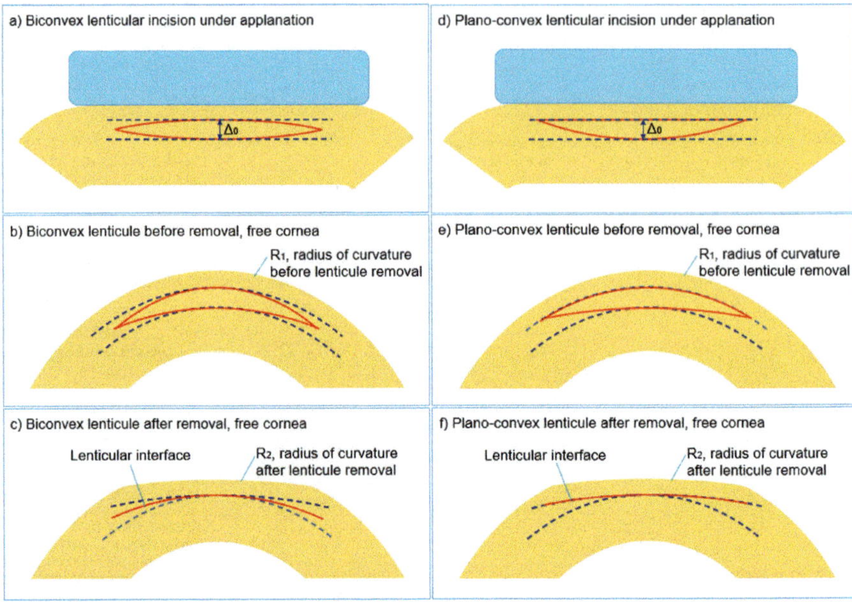

Fig. 28.13 Illustration of biconvex and plano-convex lenticule incision shapes. For clarity, transition zone, entry extension, and entry cut are not shown here. a) ELITA biconvex lenticule incision (red curves) under applanation, where the dashed blue lines indicate two lamellar layers that touch the apex of anterior and posterior lenticular incisions. b) The biconvex incision shape becomes convex concave in free cornea. c) After the lenticule is removed, the interface has a variable depth relative to anterior corneal surface. d) A plano-convex lenticule incision under applanation. e) The plano-convex incision also becomes convex concave in free cornea. f) After the lenticule is removed, the interface has equal depth relative to the anterior cornea

= 6.0, 6.5, and 7.0 mm, respectively. For treating myopia with astigmatism, the depth of the periphery varies as a function of the meridian angle.

ELITA chooses the biconvex lenticule incision shape with the purpose to cut less collagen fibrils and corneal nerves, because both are denser at the anterior stroma than they are at the posterior [6]. The first advantage is that the biconvex incision starts at a deeper depth in the cornea where there are less collagen fibrils and less opaque-bubble-layer (OBL) generated. Combining the advantages of the biconvex lenticule design, the low pulse energy, which produces smaller cavitation bubbles, and contiguous spots pattern, which provides better connectivity for the photodisruption-induced pressured gas to distribute in the intended dissection plane, ELITA SILK procedure produces almost none or very little OBL in both anterior and posterior lenticular incisions, which is important for achieving easier lenticule removal. In contrast, a study of OBL in SMILE showed that $11.70\% \pm 7.35\%$ area had OBL in the anterior lenticular surface for cap thickness = 110 μm, $6.6\% \pm 4.68\%$ for cap thickness = 140 μm [30]. Since OBL can distribute both below and above the intended dissection surface [31], the portion that is above the dissection surface can block the laser beam during cutting, causing adhesion. Theoretically, cutting less collagen fibrils implies that the biomechanics of the remaining cornea is stronger. The biconvex incision also theoretically cuts less corneal nerves, leading to better nerve preservation and faster nerve regeneration in comparison with a plano-convex incision shape. This will be shown in the following chapter in this book.

In addition to the biconvex shape design, ELITA SILK is designed with a 0.3 mm transition zone with a ramp up (for anterior) or ramp down (for posterior) angle of about 1°. The ring lenticule edge cut with a 60° side cut angle is placed in the transition zone, about 0.1 mm beyond the optical zone boundary, ensuring that the optical zone is not compromised by the edge cut. For pure myopia treatment, the lenticule edge thickness is equal to the flat-add thickness plus about 3 μm contributed by the ramp of the transition zone, allowing the use of thinner flat add to save the tissue while achieving sufficient edge strength for lenticule removal without tear. For myopia with astigmatism, the lenticule edge thickness varies around the circumference. It reaches minimum = Flat add + about 3 μm at the maximum refractive meridian of SPH + CYL, (the meridian of $\theta_{AXIS} + 90°$, when using the negative cylinder sign convention), and reaches maximum at the meridian of θ_{AXIS}, see Fig. 28.14.

To place the entry cut sufficiently far away from the visual field of the eye and to allow the lenticule separation tool to go over the lenticule edge for easier access and separate the edge, an anterior annulus outside the transition zone, called entry extension, is dissected. The width of the annulus is called entry-to-edge distance and can be selected within 0.2–1.0 mm, depending on the surgeon's preference and considerations of other lenticule parameters such as optical zone. From top view, the entry cut is located about 0.1 mm inside the periphery of the entry extension, see Fig. 28.11. From cross-sectional view, the entry cut is connected to the anterior lenticular surface, which should guide the lenticule separation instrument to first separate anterior lenticular surface with minimum ambiguity, see Fig. 28.14 a. To minimize the gas bubble blocking the laser beam, the cut is performed from bottom up in the following sequence: Posterior cut → Ring cut → Anterior cut → Entry cut. The 60° side cut angle is chosen to minimize the interference between the laser beam and the side cut gas bubble.

Unlike all other corneal lenticule procedures that use spiral scanning patterns to create lenticular dissections, ELITA uses a proprietary radial scanning approach. With the high-precision digital-encoder guided scanning system and fast blanking, ELITA radial scan pattern can achieve sub-μm cutting trajectory control and uniform photodisruption. The top view of the radial lenticular scan is schematically shown in Fig. 28.15.

ELITA supports post-docking, corneal-mark-based lenticule centration, and cyclotorsion axis adjustments, see Fig. 28.16.

Let's first review the basics of centration. Eye optics consists of the following refractive elements: the anterior and posterior corneal surfaces, the anterior and posterior crystalline lens surfaces, and the gradient refractive index of the crystalline lens. Each element has its own different optical axis [32]. The pupil

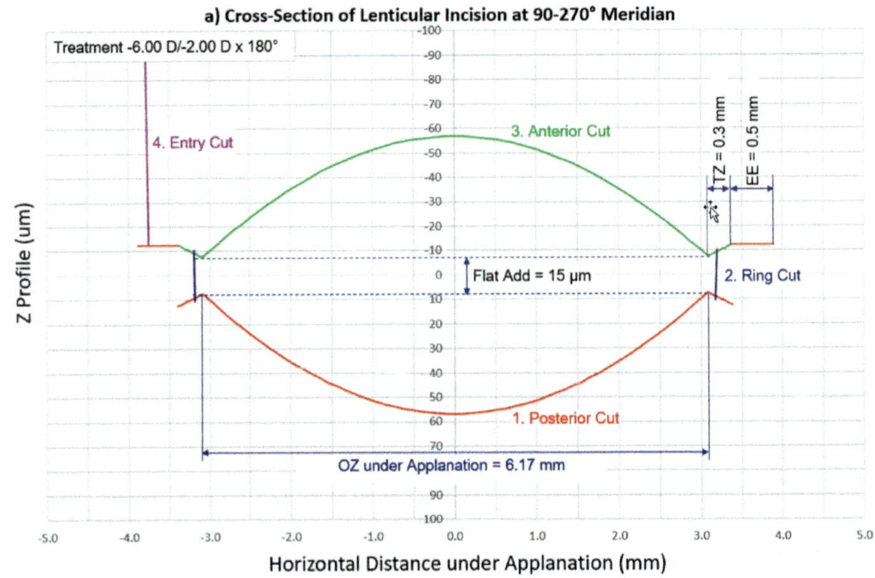

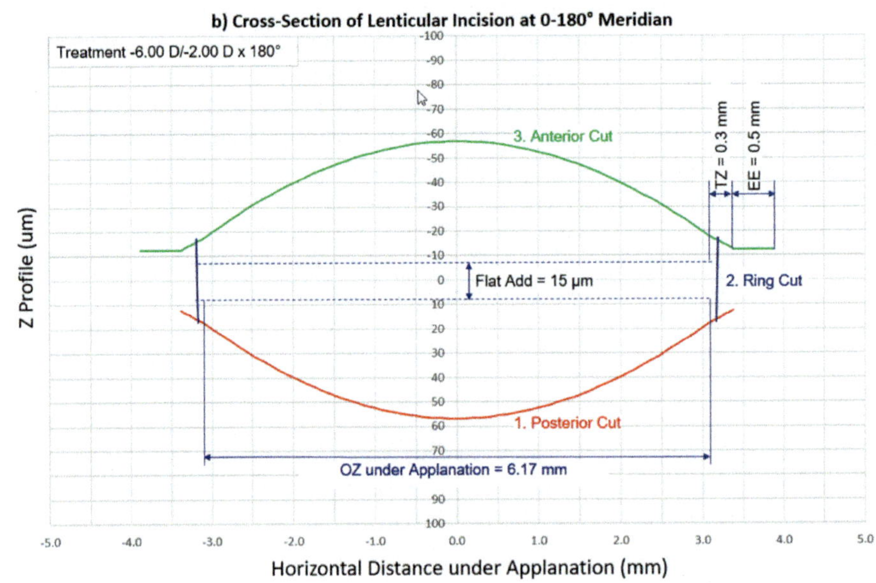

Fig. 28.14 Example of lenticule target treatment shape. a) Cross-sectional view of lenticular incisions at the meridian with the largest correction of SPH + CYL. At this meridian, the lenticule edge thickness is minimum and is equal to flat add + about 3 μm. The ramp up angle of the transition is only 0.96°; it looks bigger in the graph because the unit for *Z*-axis is μm and that for *XY* is mm. b) Cross section at the meridian with the least correction of SPH and thickest lenticule edge. The optical zone under applanation is slightly bigger than OZ = 6.0 mm for free cornea due to the applanation compensation

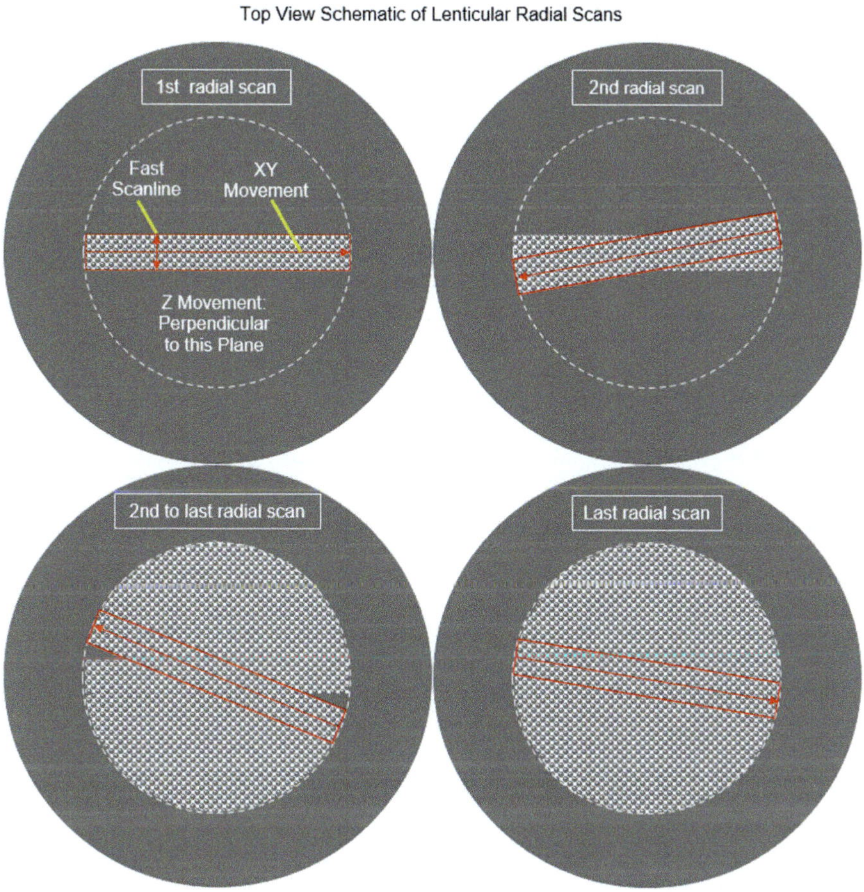

Fig. 28.15 Top view schematic of the radial scans for generating posterior and anterior lenticular dissections. The fast scanline is always oriented perpendicular to the *XY* movement as digitally controlled by the scanline rotator. The *Z* movement of the radial scan (not shown here) follows the posterior and anterior profiles, respectively, as shown in Fig. 28.14

controls the amount of light contributing to the retinal image, as well as influencing the image quality through its effects on diffraction, aberration, and depth of focus. The fact that the pupil center usually shifts when pupil dilates suggests that the pupil selects a certain part of the collective eye optics to achieve the optimal visual outcome [33]. The visual axis is the effective optical axis of this selected part of the collective eye optics.

The ideal centration for a refractive treatment is to correct the magnitude of refractive power but keep the visual axis unchanged, which is associated with the selected part of the collective eye optics by the pupil before treatment, so the best corrected retinal image quality is preserved and the image location at fovea remains the same. However, there are no physical landmarks for identifying

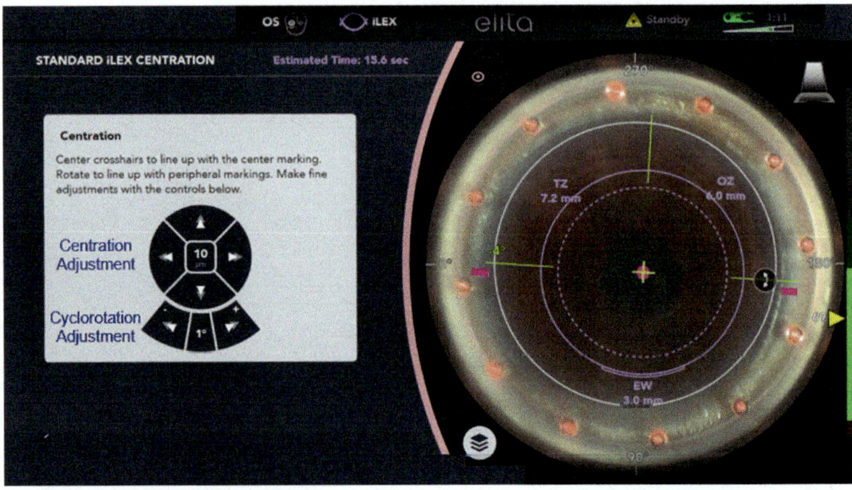
OS
iLEX
elita
Standby
STANDARD iLEX CENTRATION
Estimated Time: 13.6 sec
Centration
Center crosshairs to line up with the center marking. Rotate to line up with peripheral markings. Make fine adjustments with the controls below.
Centration Adjustment
10
Cyclorotation Adjustment
1°
TZ
7.2 mm
OZ
6.0 mm
EW
3.0 mm

Fig. 28.16 Post-docking lenticule centration adjustment and cyclorotation axis alignment based on the corneal marks

the visual axis. In addition, refractive surgery, while only reshaping the anterior corneal surface, will alter the collective optics and hence the visual axis. On the other hand, the anterior corneal surface has the largest refractive power of about 48 D (the refractive power of the entire eye is about 60 D), and the largest impact on the collective eye optics.

Two centration locations are widely used for corneal refractive surgeries. Both are determined when the eye is not under docking and is fixated to the fixation beam: (a) The corneal vertex—which is the location of the first Purkinje reflection [34]. At this location, the fixation beam is normally incident onto the cornea and does not change direction, which, by definition, is the optical axis of the anterior corneal surface. (b) The pupil center—which is the location on the cornea above the pupil center on the iris plane. In most cases, the distance between the two locations is small [35]. There is no statistically significant difference between the two centration methods [36]. In some cases, the two locations can be far apart ($\geq$ 0.6 mm), commonly referred to as large angle kappa. In such a case, the lenticule center should be placed between the two locations (corneal vertex and pupil center) to minimize the potential off-center side effects associated with each of the two centration methods. During lenticule centration, it is always important to ensure that any part of the lenticule edge is outside the pupil so the patient does not see the scattered light that may be produced by the tissue discontinuity at the lenticule edge.

With the current release of ELITA, we recommend surgeons to gently ink-mark their preferred centration location. We point out that the apparent pupil center under applanation is usually shifted from the pupil center mark in the free eye, as the eye may have rolled during docking and because of the optical parallax effect due to applanation. By using the pupil center marking method, ELITA demonstrated small centration error: 0.33 mm (mean) ± 0.16 mm (SD) (from min = 0.05 mm to max = 0.56 mm). In SMILE, the subjective fixation method yields 0.36 mm ± 0.19 mm (from 0.02 to 0.95 mm) [34].

For treating astigmatism, we recommend surgeons to ink-mark two peripheral locations horizontally: (1) when the patient is in sitting position to trace the 0–180° meridian as used in the manifest measurement for cylinder axis, and (2) when the patient is lying down for treatment, the eye usually has some cyclotorsion rotation. The 0–180° axis of the lenticule overlay on the GUI screen should be adjusted to be parallel to the hypothetical line connecting the two marks.

Based on the Zernike polynomials expansion for wavefront errors or the corresponding tissue shapes, the sum (or difference) of any two second-order terms is also a second-order term, and any second-order term is a sum of a spherical term and a cylindrical term. For a manifest refractive error expressed in the form of $\mathrm{SPH}_m/\mathrm{CYL}_m \times \theta_m$, the refractive power associated with the second-order shape is a function of the meridian angle θ,

$$P_m(\theta) = \mathrm{SPH}_m + \mathrm{CYL}_m \cdot \sin^2(\theta - \theta_m). \tag{28.15}$$

To correct the manifest refractive error, a refractive surgery must remove a second-order tissue shape, corresponding to a treatment refraction:

$$P_t(\theta) = \mathrm{SPH}_t + \mathrm{CYL}_t \cdot \sin^2(\theta - \theta_t). \tag{28.16}$$

In theory, the targeted postoperative refraction, $P_p(\theta)$, is given by:

$$P_p(\theta) = P_m(\theta) - P_t(\theta) = \mathrm{SPH}_p + \mathrm{CYL}_p \cdot \sin^2\left(\theta - \theta_p\right). \tag{28.17}$$

It is well known that, when the cylinder axes are different, the sphere and cylinder values cannot be subtracted directly. However, the functions as shown in Eqs. (28.15) and (28.16) can be subtracted directly, because the local thicknesses of the two shapes can be subtracted directly.

From Eq. (28.17), we can calculate $\mathrm{SPH}_p/\mathrm{CYL}_p \times \theta_p$ for any given $\mathrm{SPH}_m/\mathrm{CYL}_m \times \theta_m$ and $\mathrm{SPH}_t/\mathrm{CYL}_t \times \theta_t$. We point out that Eq. (28.17) does not include hidden variables that may contribute to the refractive outcome for each individual treatment. Such hidden variables can come from the manifest measurement errors, treatment cylinder axis alignment error, and error in lenticular scanning, which is extremely small for ELITA because of the high-precision digital-encoder guided scanning system, and postoperative tissue response. Some of the variables can be systematic and can be corrected through nomogram adjustments.

Using Eq. (28.17) with basic trigonometric calculations, we can show that, if the magnitudes of the treatment are correct, i.e., $\mathrm{SPH}_t = \mathrm{SPH}_m$, $\mathrm{CYL}_t = \mathrm{CYL}_m$, but the treatment axis is misaligned with the preop axis with an error $\Delta\theta = \theta_t - \theta_m$, then the treatment will induce an overcorrection for the sphere, ΔSPH, an undercorrection for the cylinder, ΔCYL, with an axis 45° away from the center line between the treatment axis and the manifest axis, closer to the manifest axis, and the spherical equivalent will not be affected:

$$\begin{aligned}\Delta\text{SPH} &= |\text{CYL}_m \cdot \sin(\Delta\theta)| \\ \Delta\text{CYL} &= -2|\text{CYL}_m \cdot \sin(\Delta\theta)| \\ \Delta\text{SE} &= \Delta\text{SPH} + \frac{\Delta\text{CYL}}{2} = 0 \\ \theta_P &= \frac{\theta_t + \theta_m}{2} - \text{sign}(\Delta\theta) \cdot 45^\circ (\text{in deg}). \end{aligned} \tag{28.18}$$

For example, to treat a refractive error of − 3.75 D/− 1.50 D × 26°, if the actual treatment has the correct magnitudes, but the treatment axis is placed at 33°, then, based on Eq. (28.18), this axis error will cause an overcorrection in sphere, ΔSPH = 1.50 D × sin(7°) ≈ + 0.18 D, an undercorrection in cylinder, ΔCYL = − 2 × 1.50 D × sin(7°) ≈ − 0.37 D, and the axis of the residual cylinder will be at θ_P = −15.5°, equivalent to 164.5° following the 1–180° convention for axis. There is no error induced to SE by the axis error.

From Eq. (28.18), we can calculate the refractive errors induced by the axis misalignment (see Fig. 28.17a) and calculate the tolerance for the misalignment corresponding to − 0.25 D undercorrection of the cylinder (see Fig. 28.17b). As expected, the tolerance depends on the magnitude of the cylinder to be treated. The peripheral marking and treatment axis alignment are always recommended for treating a cylinder of magnitude greater than 0.5 D. The manifest axis measurement, the peripheral marking, and the treatment axis alignment should be done as accurately as practical possible.

To summarize, we list the basic elements of the ELITA SILK algorithm in Table 28.3, and the treatment parameter ranges in Table 28.4. Compared with other corneal lenticule technologies, ELITA SILK technology features ultra-thin tissue-bridge-free dissection, the biconvex lenticular incision shape, and the high-precision digital-encoder guided radial scanning pattern.

28.5 Future Developments and Concepts

To address unmet needs and to benefit from technological advancements, ELITA technology is developed from the ground up. Here, we briefly introduce the following cadence projects which are at different development stages, including the 1-piece patient interface (clinical evaluation stage), automatic lenticule centration and cyclotorsion alignment (clinical evaluation stage), SILK for hyperopia and mixed astigmatism (preclinical ex vivo tissue evaluation), and wavefront guided SILK procedure (algorithm development stage).

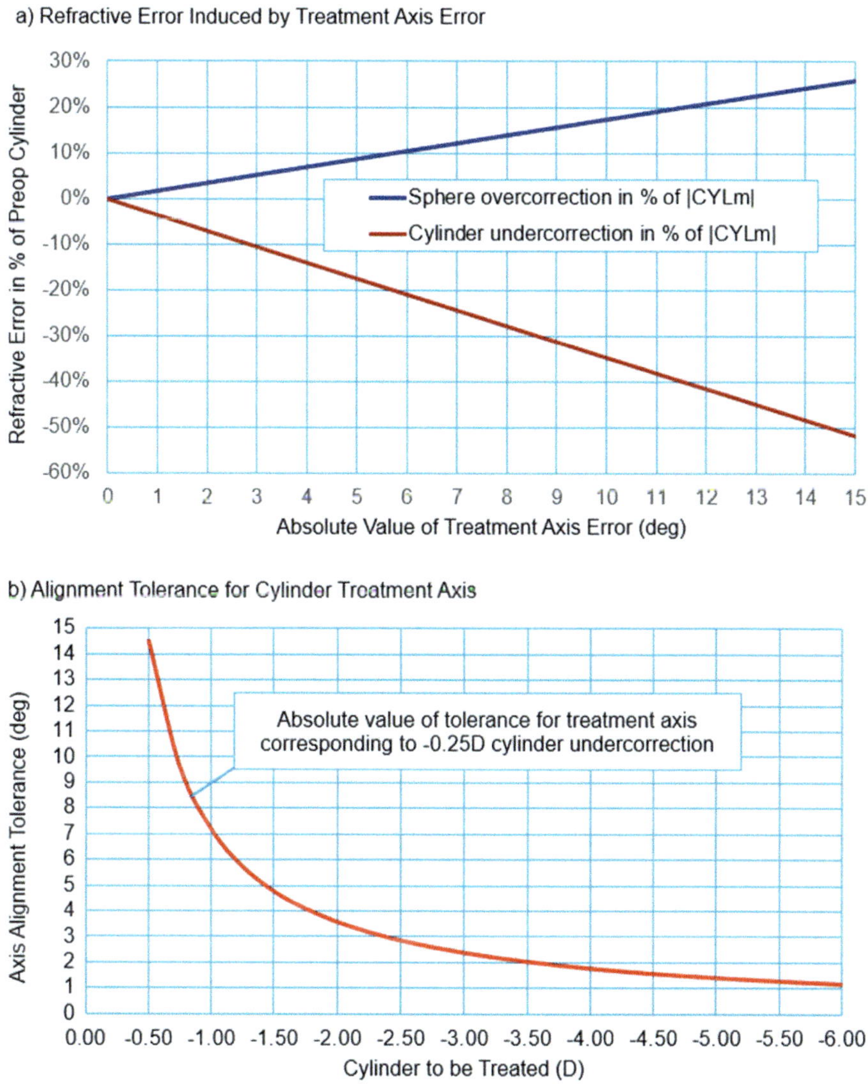

Fig. 28.17 a) Sphere overcorrection and cylinder undercorrection in percentage of the magnitude of the cylinder to be treated as a function of treatment axis error. b) Tolerance for the treatment axis misalignment as a function of the manifest cylinder to be treated

Single-Piece Patient Interface (1-piece PI)

Surgeons experienced with different femtosecond lasers usually have different preferences for the PI design, some prefer the 2-piece PI design as ELITA currently offers, others prefer a 1-piece PI. To meet this need and to better fit smaller eyes, we are developing the ELITA 1-piece PI (see Fig. 28.18). The similarities and the differences between the 2-piece PI and 1-piece PI are listed in Table 28.5.

Table 28.3 Summary of the basic elements of ELITA SILK algorithm

1	Input data: • The user inputs patient-related treatment parameters and nomogram • The user inputs pulse energies, lenticule parameters, and lane length (i.e., the optical path length between the eye chart and the eye) and vertex distance (i.e., the distance between the phoropter lens and the cornea) used in the manifest measurement • System inputs the Auto-Z PI calibration result, the post-docking adjustments for lenticule centration and cyclotorsion axis
2	Calculate the lenticule shape for cornea under applanation: • Apply lane length and vertex distance correction: The algorithm converts the nomogram-adjusted manifest refractive correction to the correction on cornea for optical infinity based on the lane length and vertex distance • Calculate Z-displacement function for free cornea based on the Munnerlyn equation and the keratometry values K_1 and K_2 • Apply applanation compensation: The algorithm performs a mathematical shape transfer to transfer the Z-displacement function from free cornea into the biconvex shape for cornea under applanation. This shape transfer ensures that, when the applanation is removed, the incision shape produces the Z-displacement function as intended for the free cornea • Apply flat-add compensation: The algorithm corrects the effect of the flat-add layer on refraction • Apply eyeball axial length correction: After the lenticule removal, the eyeball axial length becomes shorter. The algorithm corrects the Munnerlyn equation for this difference
3	Generate the lenticular scanning trajectory: • The algorithm incorporates all the geometric inputs to generate the target scanning trajectory including posterior, ring, anterior, and entry cuts • The algorithm generates a time series for the fast blanking to ensure uniform photodisruption • The digital-encoder guided scanning system will follow the target trajectory with closed-loop motion control • The real-time digital-encoder readings are recorded (Note: based on the intended target cutting trajectory and the executed cutting trajectory, we find that the error between the target lenticular Z-profile and the executed lenticule Z-profile is less than 1 μm)

Both PI designs are compatible with the ELITA system. Surgeons can choose one or use both interchangeably.

Automatic Centration and Cyclotorsion Alignment

We are testing a center-mark-free automatic lenticule centration and cyclotorsion adjustment software. This approach comprises three steps as shown in Fig. 28.19. Step-1: ink-mark three peripheral marks, M1, M2, and M3, on the cornea when the patient is in the sitting position. The M1 and M2 marks are aligned with the horizonal 0–180° axis, the M3 mark should be at about 270° location. There is no accuracy requirement for M3 location. The three marks form a triangle which is used as a coordinate system moving with the cornea. Step-2: ELITA takes a white light image of M1, M2, and M3 on cornea and then takes an IR light image of the pupil when the eye fixates at the fixation target before placing the suction ring on the eye. From the IR image, ELITA finds the pupil center and calculates

Table 28.4 ELITA SILK treatment parameter ranges

Treatment range	
Manifest sphere	0.00 D to – 12.00 D
Manifest cylinder	0.00 D to – 6.00 D
Manifest sphere + Manifest cylinder	– 1.00 D to – 12.00 D
Manifest axis	0–180°
Minimum residual bed thickness	250 μm
Lenticule parameters	
Optical zone diameter	5.5–7.0 mm
Anterior depth for lenticule apex	100–130 μm
Transition zone width	0.3 mm fixed
Ring cut (lenticule edge cut) location	0.2 mm inside the transition zone OD (fixed)
Actual diameter of removed lenticule	Optical zone + about 0.3 mm
Entry-to-edge distance	0.2–1.0 mm
Flat-add thickness	15–30 μm
Edge thickness parameter	10 μm (fixed)
Actual lenticule edge thickness	Minimum edge thickness ≈ flat add + about 3 μm; varies with meridian when cylinder ≠ 0
Entry position (top view)	0–180°
Entry width (arc length)	3–5 mm
Entry side cut angle	60° (fixed)
Entry cut ending position (cross section)	Top (the entry cut is channeled to the anterior lenticular surface)
Lang length	2–8 m
Vertex distance	0–16 mm
Posterior lenticule energy	40–90 nJ
Anterior lenticule energy	40–90 nJ
Ring energy	40–90 nJ
Entry energy	40–90 nJ

the coordinate of the pupil center in the coordinate system determined by M1, M2, and M3 locations. Step-3: ELITA takes the image of M1, M2, and M3 on the applanated cornea and determines the pupil center based on the coordinate in the coordinate system of the 3 marks. Docking usually changes the positional relation between cornea and iris, and the apparent pupil center of cornea under applanation is not an accurate target for lenticule centration. The cyclotorsion axis of the treatment is automatically placed in parallel to the line connecting M1 and M2 under applanation.

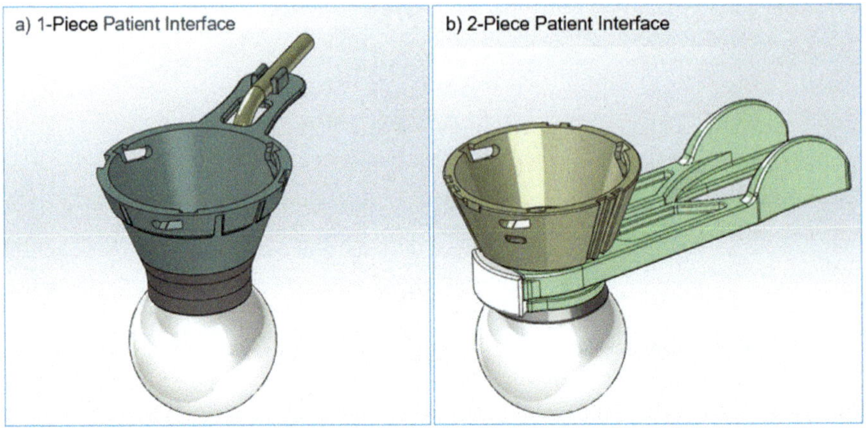

Fig. 28.18 Illustration of ELITA 1-piece PI design and the currently released 2-piece PI design. The 1-piece PI has a smaller suction ring and no gripper to fit better small or deep-set eyes as well as for normal and big eye anatomy conditions

SILK for Hyperopia and Mixed Astigmatism

ELITA with its large surgical field (10 mm diameter) and post-docking centration capability is particularly suitable for treating hyperopia and mixed astigmatism, because these treatments involve thick lenticule edges, large optical zones, and large transition zones [6]. A preliminary evaluation of SILK procedure for hyperopia and mixed astigmatism on ex vivo porcine eyes was done by an ophthalmologist. The treatment parameters used are listed in Table 28.6. Figures 28.20 and 28.21 show the screenshots of the cutting process and of the lenticule removal process, respectively, whereas Fig. 28.22 shows the recorded scanning trajectory for treating hyperopia with and without astigmatism.

Table 28.7 lists the treatment parameters used for treating mixed astigmatism. The cutting process and ease of lenticule removal are similar to that of hyperopia treatment. Figure 28.23 shows the recorded scanning trajectory for treating mixed astigmatism. In all cases, the thickness differences between the actual and the target scanning trajectories are within 0.3 μm. In comparison with the 16 μm tissue removal per diopter for a 7 mm optical zone, the accuracy of the scanning trajectory is excellent.

Wavefront Guided SILK

Wavefront guided visual correction provides the potential to achieve super vision, i.e., vision better than emmetropia, due to typical higher-order aberration (HOA) (RMS $\approx$ 0.3 μm) in emmetropic eyes [37, 38]. Although wavefront guided LASIK produces excellent visual outcomes, because of its interface quality and registration, in comparison with corneal lenticule procedures, it has not achieved super vision potential. We believe that the flap-induced corneal shape regression may be one of the fundamental variables that limits further improvement.

Table 28.5 Comparison of ELITA 1-piece PI design with the current 2-piece PI design

Parameters	2-piece PI (current)	1-piece PI (to be released)
Suction ring and cone optics	2 separate pieces	*1 molded piece*
PI lens	Flat PI lens	Flat PI lens
Suction ring material	Soft	Soft
Eye holding force, lateral	≥2 N	≥2 N
Eye holding force, vertical	≥3 N	≥3 N
Suction area	Sclera	*Sclera and cornea*
Suction ring OD	21.3 mm	*19.0 mm*
Gripper OD	22.5 mm	*No gripper*
Cone height	21.0 mm	21.0 mm
Half cone angle	21°	21°
PI lens diameter	13.0 mm	13.0 mm
Surgical field diameter	10.0 mm	10.0 mm
Suction pressure	500 mmHg	500 mmHg
Suction source	Vacuum pump	Vacuum pump
Sclera support	With sclera support	With sclera support
IOP increase	≈52 mmHg	≈38 mmHg
PI calibration	Auto calibration with sub-μm accuracy	Auto calibration with sub-μm accuracy
Auto suction loss detection	Yes	Yes
Floating head motion detection	Yes	Yes
Suction loss rate	Design target < 0.5%	Design target < 0.5%

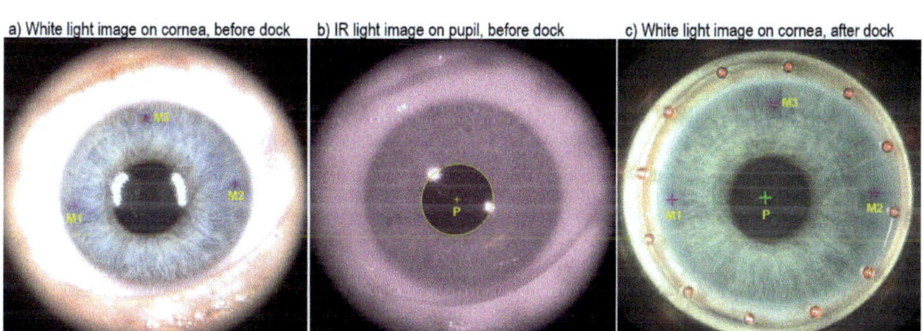

Fig. 28.19 Human docking study (without laser treatment) verified the feasibility of the center-mark-free auto-centration and cyclotorsion adjustment method. As can be seen on the right picture, the apparent pupil center under applanation is shifted from the pupil center of free cornea

Table 28.6 Parameters for treating hyperopia with astigmatism used in the preclinical evaluation

Manifest sphere	+4.00 D	Entry position	90°
Manifest cylinder	+1.00 D	Entry width	3.0 mm
Manifest axis	180°	Entry-to-edge distance	0.0 mm
Flat K1	43.50 D	Anterior depth	160 μm
Steep K2	43.50 D	Optical zone	7.0 mm
Posterior energy	55 nJ	Transition width	0.7 mm
Anterior energy	55 nJ	Flat add	30 μm
Ring energy	65 nJ	Additional edge thickness	0 μm
Entry energy	65 nJ	Laser treatment time	22.0 s

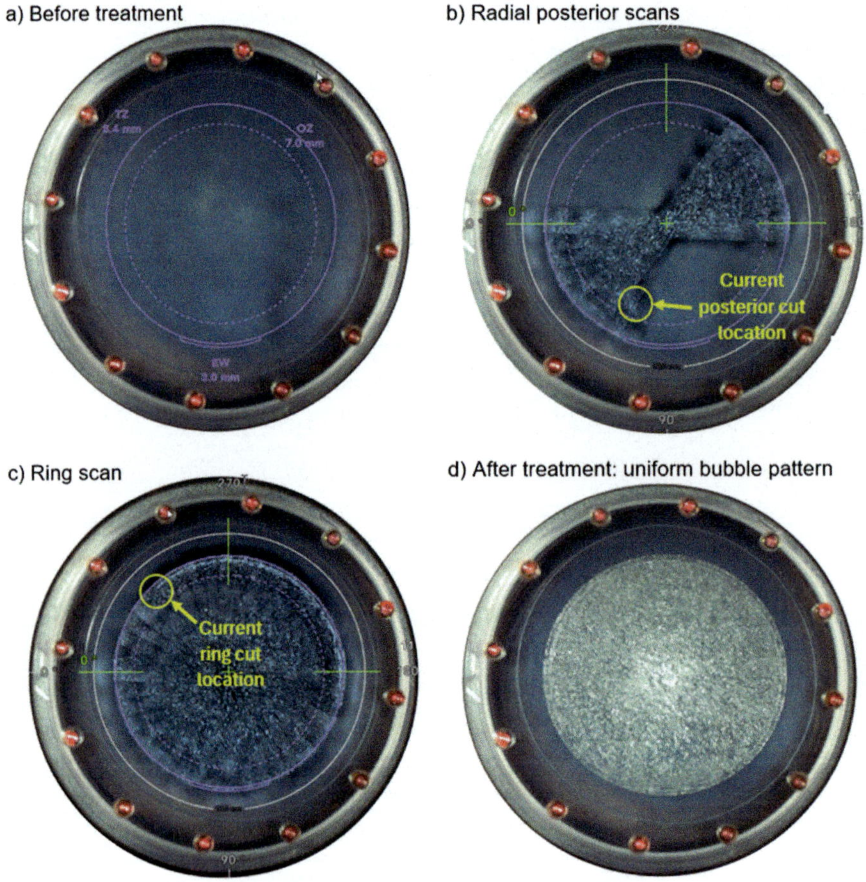

Fig. 28.20 Screenshots of SILK cutting process for treating hyperopia with astigmatism. The GUI screen displays a stitched image consisting of the stationary large FOV image taken before pressing the footpedal, the live concurrent 2mm moving FOV, and a series of small FOV images taken during the cut

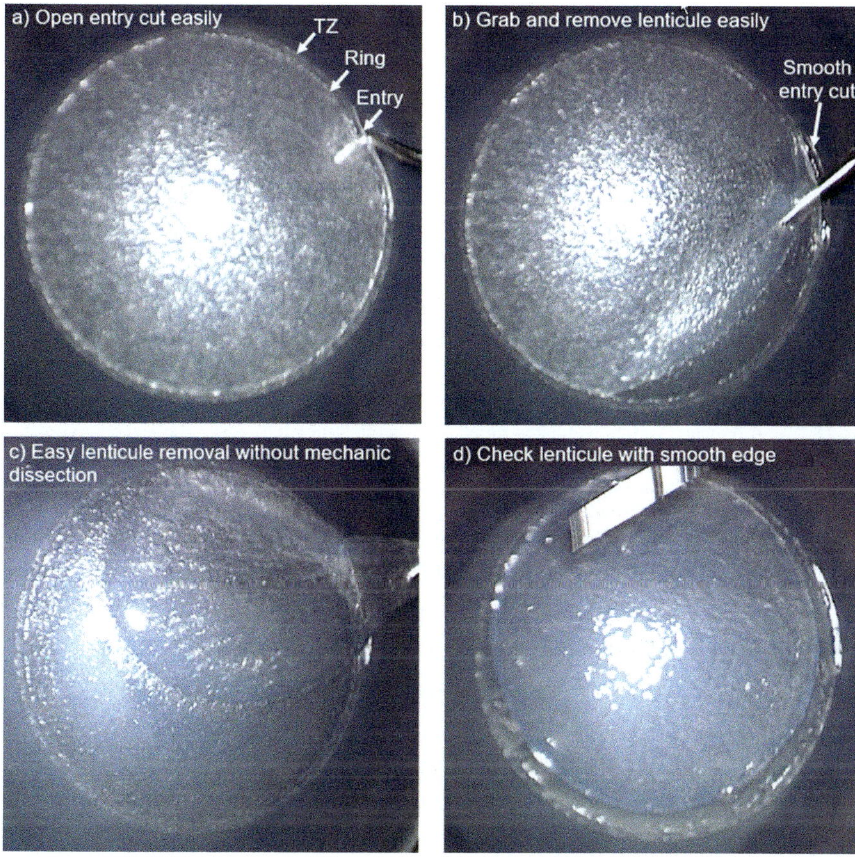

Fig. 28.21 Screenshots of lenticule removal process for treating hyperopia with astigmatism

The physics for wavefront guided refractive treatment is to reshape the cornea such that through eye wavefront (for light emitting from retina to exiting cornea) will become a plane wave. Let $W(x, y)$ be the wavefront error before treatment, $T(x, y)$ the thickness of the corneal tissue to be removed, and $n = 1.377$ the index of refraction of cornea, then [37, 38]:

$$T(x, y) = \frac{W(x, y)}{n - 1} \tag{28.19}$$

Equation (28.19) is called the thin phase plate model for treating the wavefront error. It states that, if a local wavefront is behind the leading wavefront, the amount of tissue at this location must be removed according to Eq. (28.19) for the local wavefront to catch the leading wavefront after surgery as light propagates at a slower speed in tissue than in air. Figure 28.24 illustrates the basic principle for wavefront guided treatment.

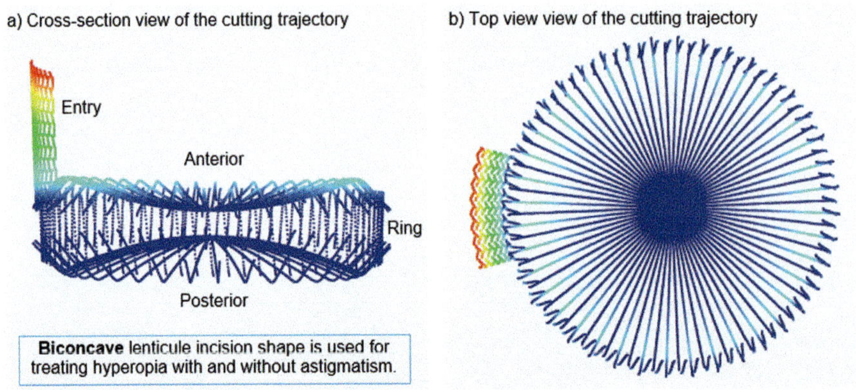

Fig. 28.22 Biconcave lenticule incision trajectory is reconstructed based on the real-time readings from the digital encoders of the scanning system. Within the optical zone, there are a total of 9480 points on the target trajectory, $\{Z_{t,n}\}$ ($n = 1, 2, \ldots, 9480$), and an equal number of actual recorded values, $\{Z_{r,n}\}$. Let $\{\varepsilon_n\}$ be the error between the achieved and target trajectories, $\{\varepsilon_n = Z_{r,n} - Z_{t,n}\}$, then the mean, standard deviation, minimum, and maximum of $\{\varepsilon_n\}$ are 0.001, 0.151, –0.287, and 0.277 μm, respectively. The digital-encoder guided scanning is extremely accurate

Table 28.7 Lenticule parameters for treating mixed astigmatism used in the preclinical evaluation

Manifest sphere	– 1.50 D	Entry position	90°
Manifest cylinder	+3.00 D	Entry width	3.0 mm
Manifest axis	180°	Entry-to-edge distance	0.0 mm
Flat K1	43.50 D	Anterior depth	160 μm
Steep K2	43.50 D	Optical zone	7.0 mm
Posterior energy	55 nJ	Transition width	0.7 mm
Anterior energy	55 nJ	Flat add	30 μm
Ring energy	65 nJ	Additional edge thickness	0 μm
Entry energy	65 nJ	Laser treatment time	22.0 s

The thin phase plate model is an approximation because the corneal surface is not flat but a curved phase plate. The ELITA wavefront guided lenticule treatment algorithm considers and corrects this difference. Therefore, when the wavefront is solely contributed by the lower-order refraction SPH/CYL $\times$ θ, the removed thickness profile will be the same as that derived from the Munnerlyn equation.

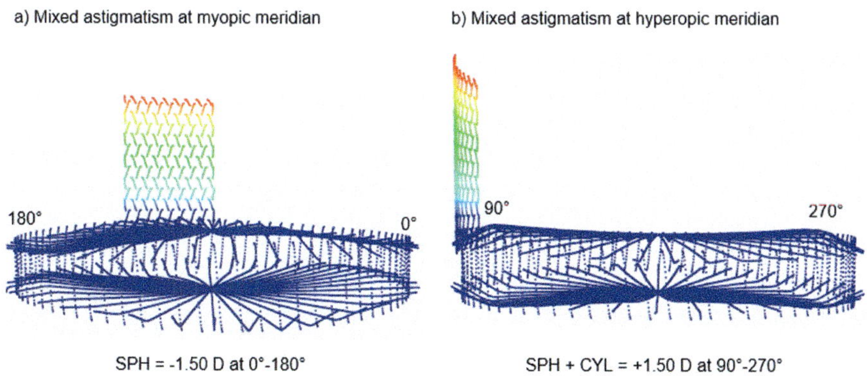

Fig. 28.23 Cross-sectional view of the lenticule incision trajectory for treating mixed astigmatism reconstructed from real-time recorded data of the digital encoders of the scanning system. The difference between the achieved thickness and the target thickness at lenticule center and at optical zone boundary at meridian angles 0°, 90°, 180°, and 270° are – 0.01, 0.01, 0.07, 0.01, – 0.03 μm, respectively. These are negligible in comparison with about 16 μm tissue removal per diopter for 7 mm optical zone

Fig. 28.24 Illustration of the relation between the wavefront error and the lenticule thickness based on the thin phase plate model

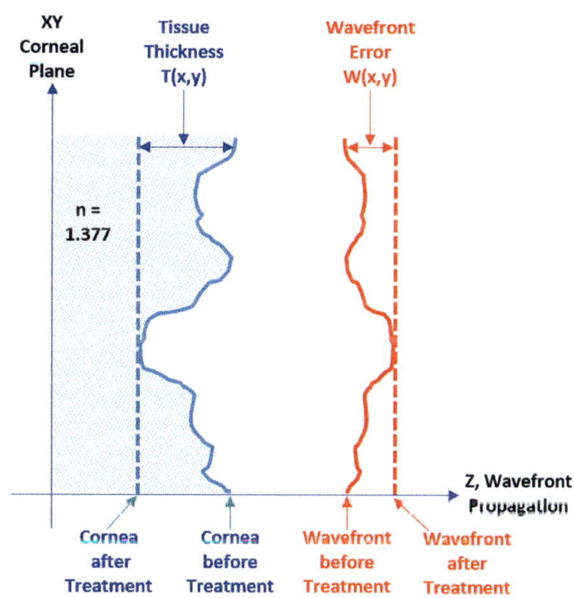

The reason that ELITA with sub-μm cutting precision can treat sub-μm HOA RMS is that the maximum thickness of the tissue shape $T(x, y)$ for treating any specific high-order Zernike term is much greater than the RMS value associated with this term. Let γ_{nm} be defined as the following ratio for treating a specific high-order Zernike term $Z_n{}^m$ (ρ, ϕ):

$$\gamma_{\mathrm{nm}} \equiv \frac{\max\{T_{\mathrm{nm}}(x, y)\} - \min\{T_{\mathrm{nm}}(x, y)\}}{\mathrm{RMS}_{\mathrm{nm}}}. \tag{28.20}$$

Based on Eq. (28.19), bearing in mind that $\mathrm{RMS}_{\mathrm{nm}}$ is equal to the coefficient of term $Z_n{}^m$ (ρ, ϕ) in the Zernike expansion series for the wavefront error $W(x, y)$, we have:

$$\gamma_{\mathrm{nm}} = \frac{\max\left\{Z_n^m(\rho, \varphi)\right\} - \min\left\{Z_n^m(\rho, \varphi)\right\}}{n - 1}. \tag{28.21}$$

The values of $\{\gamma_{\mathrm{nm}}\}$ for third-order and fourth-order Zernike terms are shown in Table 28.8. They range from 8.9 to 16.8. For example, to treat a spherical aberration of RMS $=$ 0.3 μm, the corresponding corneal incision has a peak-to-valley thickness of $0.3 \times 8.9 = 2.7$ μm; to treat a vertical coma of RMS $=$ 0.3 μm, the corresponding corneal incision peak-to-valley thickness is $0.3 \times 15 = 4.5$ μm. ELITA has sufficient precision to treat these terms. To achieve the best accuracy, ELITA will only use the posterior incision to correct the HOA terms. The fact that the SILK procedure induces very low total HOA RMS $\approx$ 0.13 μm (mean)$\pm$0.13 μm (SD) for 6 mm pupil (including all third-order to sixth-order terms) [39] is strong evidence that ELITA can treat HOA. In addition, the ELITA lenticule scanning technique, consisting of radial lenticular scans at different meridian angles, is particularly suited for correcting the HOA wavefront error because the Zernike polynomials are expressed as functions of the radius and the meridian angle.

Another key enabling factor is that ELITA is designed with IR illumination and autofocusing imaging optics for taking high-quality iris image for iris registration. A clinical study to verify iris registration (without laser treatment) has been conducted on 33 volunteers/eyes. All iris images taken with ELITA have been matched successfully with the respective iDesign iris images. Figure 28.25 shows one example.

In summary, with the sub-μm scanning trajectory precision, iris registration, and post-operative corneal biomechanical stability (e.g., no regression due to the long flap side cut as in a LASIK procedure), we expect that ELITA can perform wavefront guided lenticule procedure and deliver superior visual outcome.

Table 28.8 Ratio of the corneal incision thickness for treating an HOA RMS to the HOA RMS for third-order and fourth-order wavefront errors

j	n	m	$Z_j(\rho,\theta) = Z_n^m(\rho,\theta), j = [n(n+2)+m]/2$	Name of aberration	Wavefront error (um)				γ_{nm} = Ratio of Corneal Incision PV to HOA RMS
					RMS	Peak	Valley	PV	
6	3	−3	$Z_3^{-3}(\rho,\theta) = \sqrt{8}\cdot\rho^3\cdot\sin(3\theta)$	Vertical trefoil	1.0	2.8	− 2.8	5.7	15.0
7	3	−1	$Z_3^{-1}(\rho,\theta) = \sqrt{8}\cdot\left(3\rho^3-2\rho\right)\cdot\sin\theta$	Vertical coma	1.0	2.8	− 2.8	5.7	15.0
8	3	1	$Z_3^{1}(\rho,\theta) = \sqrt{8}\cdot\left(3\rho^3-2\rho\right)\cdot\cos\theta$	Horizontal coma	1.0	2.8	− 2.8	5.7	15.0
9	3	3	$Z_3^{3}(\rho,\theta) = \sqrt{8}\cdot\rho^3\cdot\cos(3\theta)$	Oblique trefoil	1.0	2.8	− 2.8	5.7	15.0
10	4	−4	$Z_4^{-4}(\rho,\theta) = \sqrt{10}\cdot\rho^4\cdot\sin(4\theta)$	Oblique quadrafoil	1.0	3.2	− 3.2	6.3	16.8
11	4	−2	$Z_4^{-2}(\rho,\theta) = \sqrt{10}\cdot\left(4\rho^4-3\rho^2\right)\cdot\sin(2\theta)$	Oblique secondary astigmatism	1.0	3.2	− 3.2	6.3	16.8
12	4	0	$Z_4^{0}(\rho,\theta) = \sqrt{5}\cdot\left(6\rho^4-6\rho^2+1\right)$	Spherical	1.0	2.2	− 1.1	3.4	8.9
13	4	2	$Z_4^{2}(\rho,\theta)\sqrt{10}\cdot\left(4\rho^4-3\rho^2\right)\cdot\cos(2\theta)$	Vertical secondary astigmatism	1.0	3.2	− 3.2	6.3	16.8
14	4	4	$Z_4^{4}(\rho,\theta) = \sqrt{10}\cdot\rho^4\cdot\cos(4\theta)$	Vertical quadrafoil	1.0	3.2	− 3.2	6.3	16.8

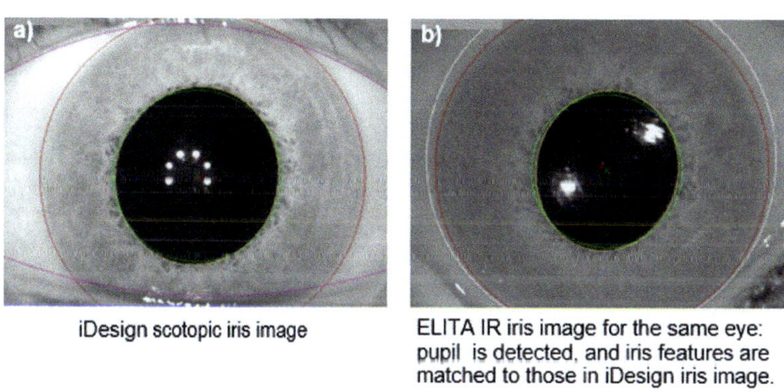

Fig. 28.25 a) iDesign iris image. b) ELITA iris image for the same eye. ELITA iris registration algorithm successfully found the features and matched them with the iDesign images for all the 33 patients/eyes in the study

Acknowledgements ELITA is the result of enduring teamwork among Johnson-Johnson Vision R&D, clinical, medical, marketing, manufacturing, service, and the management teams, the optics and laser suppliers, and many worldwide renowned refractive surgeons. The authors deeply appreciate the opportunity to represent them in writing this chapter.

References

1. US FDA Premarket Notification for IntraLase 600C Laser Keratome, Decision Date 12/17/1999. 510(k) Number K993153.
2. Kurtz R. The story of IntraLase—how developers of the femtosecond ophthalmic surgical lasers took a chance and built a company. Cataract & Refractive Surgery Today, Up Front; 2002.
3. Pallikaris IG, Papatzanaki ME, Stathi EZ, Frenschock O, Georgiadis A. Laser In Situ Keratomileusis. Lasers in Surg Med. 1990;10:463–8.
4. Munnerlyn CR, Koons SJ, Marshall J. Photorefractive keratectomy: a technique for laser refractive surgery. J Cataract Refract Surg. 1988;14:46–52.
5. Kurtz RM, Horvath C, Liu HH, Krueger RR, Juhasz T. Lamellar refractive surgery with scanned intrastromal picosecond and femtosecond laser pulses in animal eyes. J Refract Surg. 1998;14:541–8.
6. Editor SW. Small Incision Lenticule Extraction (SMILE). Springer International Publishing Switzerland; 2015.
7. Reinstein D, Archer TJ, Carp GI. The surgeon's guide to SMILE. SLACK Incorporated; 2018.
8. Ivarsen A, Asp S, Hjortdal J. Safety and complications of more than 1500 small-incision lenticule extraction procedures. Ophthalmology. 2014;121:822–8.
9. Agca A, Ozgurhan EB, Yildirim Y, et al. Corneal backscatter analysis by in vivo confocal microscopy: fellow eye comparison of small incision lenticule extraction and femtosecond laser-assisted LASIK. J Ophthalmol. 2014; Article ID 265012.
10. US FDA. Summary of Safety and Effectiveness Data (SSED), for VisuMax Femtosecond Laser for refractive correction for pure myopia, PMA Number: P150040; 2016.
11. US FDA; Summary of Safety and Effectiveness Data (SSED), for VisuMax Femtosecond Laser for refractive correction for myopia with astigmatism, PMA Number: P150040/S003; 2018.
12. Juhasz T, Kastis G, Suarez C, Bor Z, Bron WE. Time-resolved observations of shock waves and cavitation bubbles generated by femtosecond laser pulses in corneal tissue and water. Lasers Surg Med. 1996;19:23–31.
13. Vogel A, Busch S, Parilitz U. Shock wave emission and cavitation bubble generation by picosecond and nanosecond optical breakdown in water. J Acoust Soc Am. 1996;100(1):148–65.
14. Vogel A, Venugopalan V. Mechanisms of pulsed laser ablation of biological tissues. Chem Rev. 2003;103:577–644.
15. Vogel A, Linz N, Freidank S, Paltauf G. Femtosecond-laser-induced nanocavitation in water: implications for optical breakdown threshold and cell surgery. Phys Rev Lett. 2008;100. Article 038102.
16. Linz N. Controlled nonlinear energy deposition in transparent dielectrics by femtosecond and nanosecond optical breakdown. Toenning, Luebeck, and Marburg: Der Andere Verlag. ISBN: 978-3-86247-076-1.
17. Linz N, Freidank S, Liang XX, Vogel A. Wavelength dependence of femtosecond laser-induced breakdown in water and implication for laser surgery. Phys Rev B. 2016;B94. Article 024113.
18. Fundamental Optics. CVI Melles Griot 2009 Technical Guide, vol 2, issue 1.

19. Mansuripur M. The physical principles for magneto-optical recording. Cambridge : Cambridge University Press; 1998.
20. Gaussian Beam Optics. CVI Melles Griot 2009 Technical Guide, vol 2, issue 1.
21. Technical Specification. Zeiss Brochure for VisuMax 500.
22. Technical Specification. Zeiss Brochure for VisuMax 800.
23. Technical Specification. Schwind Brochure for OTAS.
24. Technical Specification. Ziemer Brochure for LDV Z Models.
25. Canones-Zafra R, Gros-Otero J, Garcia-Gonzales M, et al. Atomic force microscopy for the evaluation of corneal surface roughness after femtosecond laser flap creation and excimer ablation. Int Ophthalmol. 2023; Article s10792-023-02821-z.
26. Collins CC, Carlson MR, Scott AB, Jampolsky A. Extraocular muscle forces in normal human subjects. Invest Ophthalmol Vis Sci. 1981;20(5):654–64.
27. Vilhena L, Ramalho A. Friction of human skin against different fabrics for medical use. Lubricants. 2016;4(1):6.
28. Wilson T, Aeschlimann R, Tosatti S, et al. Coefficient of friction of human corneal tissue. Cornea. 2015;34(9):1179–85.
29. Talamo JH, Gooding P, Angeley D, et al. Optical patient interface in femtosecond laser-assisted cataract surgery: contact corneal applanation versus liquid immersion. J Cataract Refract Surg. 2013;39(4):501–10.
30. Wu D, Li B, Huang M, Fang XJ. Influence of cap thickness on opaque bubble layer formation in SMILE: 100 versus 140 μm. J Refract Surg. 2020;36(9):592–6.
31. Marino GK, Santhiago MR, Wilson SE. OCT study of the femtosecond laser opaque bubble layer. J Refract Surg. 2017;33(1):18–22.
32. Atchison D, Smith G. Optics of the human eye. Butterworth-Heinemann, Elservier Science Limited; 2002.
33. Charman WN. Optics of the eye. In: Handbook of optics. Editor in Chief Bass M. McGRAW-HILL Inc.; 1995, vol I.
34. Kang SY, Lee H, Reinstein DZ, et al. Comparison of the distribution of lenticule decentration following SMILE by subjective patient fixation or triple marking centration. J Refract Surg. 2018;34(7):446–52.
35. Reinstein DZ, Archer T, Rowe EL, Gobbe M. Distribution of pupil offset and angle kappa in a refractive surgery preoperative population of 750 myopic, emmetropic, and hyperopic eyes. J Refract Surg. 2021;37(1):49–58.
36. Neal D, Raymond TD, Copland RJ, Xiong W. Laser refractive surgery centration: visual axis or line-of-sight? ARVO 2015; Poster 3939.
37. Krueger RR, Applegate RA, MacRae SM. Editors for wavefront customized visual correction—the quest for super vision II. SLACK Inc.; 2004.
38. Dai GM. Wavefront optics for vision correction. Bellingham: SPIE Press; 2008. ISBN: 9780819469663.
39. Chen L, Fu H. Evaluation of high-order aberrations after corneal lenticule removal with a new femtosecond laser system. ARVO 2023; Poster 4814.

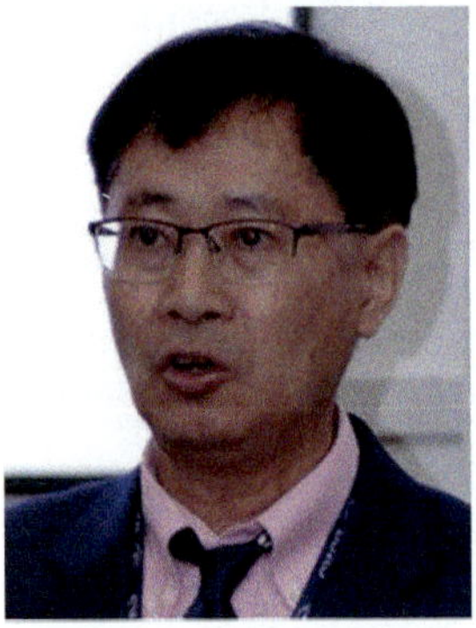

Hong Fu has been the principal inventor for ELITA Femtosecond Laser System and the industry first biconvex lenticule algorithm for corneal refractive surgery. He holds 40 patents or patent applications in laser related fields. He has been a primary contributing author on 25 peer-reviewed papers on laser, optics, and physics before joining industry. He has deep passion to apply mathematics and physics to improve the clinical outcome. Hong Fu is a Research Fellow and Senior R&D Manager at Johnson-Johnson Vision in Silicon Valley, California, USA. Prior to Johnson-Johnson, he worked at various positions, including engineer, manager, director, VP for R&D and Engineering, and VP for manufacturing. Hong Fu earned Ph.D. in laser physics at University of Stuttgart, Germany; did graduate study at the Institute of Theoretical Physics of Chinese Academy of Sciences, Beijing; and earned BS degree in nuclear physics at Sichuan University, Chengdu, China. He pursued postdoctoral research at the Optical Sciences Center, University of Arizona, Tucson, USA.

Lenticule and Interface Properties in SILK® 29

Rohit Shetty, Pooja Khamar, Ritica Mukherji, and Anushree Bhatkal

Abstract

This chapter delves into keratorefractive lenticule extraction (KLEx) procedures, focusing on the novel smooth incision lenticule keratomileusis (SILK®) technique designed for the ELITA™ femtosecond laser platform by Johnson & Johnson. Against the backdrop of the global myopia surge and the growing demand for refractive surgery, the chapter explores the unique features of SILK®, comparing it to established procedures like laser-assisted in situ keratomileusis (LASIK) and photorefractive keratectomy (PRK).

Keywords

Keratorefractive Lenticule extraction (KLEx) • Smooth incision lenticule keratomileusis (SILK®) • ELITA™ femtosecond laser platform • Refractive surgery • Laser-assisted in situ keratomileusis (LASIK)

29.1 Introduction

The recent boom in the prevalence of global myopia can only mean a greater demand for refractive surgery. The demand for refractive procedures is expected to grow at a compound annual rate of 4% from 2019 to 2024 [1].

Keratorefractive **L**enticule **Ex**traction (KLEx) procedures are emerging as the current game changers in the world of refractive surgery. With a wide array of new lenticular-based refractive procedures coming into the industry, it becomes imperative to understand how these newer techniques are unique and how they compare to the tried and tested procedures like LASIK and PRK.

R. Shetty · P. Khamar (✉) · R. Mukherji · A. Bhatkal
Narayana Nethralaya Eye Institute, Bangaluru, India
e-mail: dr.poojakhamar@gmail.com

W. Sekundo and F. M. Wagner (eds.), *Femtosecond Laser Assisted Lenticule Extraction*,
https://doi.org/10.1007/978-3-031-60424-9_29

We must also consider the advancement in ophthalmological innovation which has been used to overcome the shortcomings of current laser-based refractive procedures. The modifications in laser energy settings and the lenticule shape of the KLEx procedures have an impact on post-operative healing and visual recovery. In addition, features like automated centration, static cyclotorsion compensation (SCC) and variation in laser cut patterns can influence the surgeon's experience as well.

Low-energy femtosecond lasers have wavelengths in the range of 1015–1065 nm, which is hardly absorbed by transparent corneal tissue, so it can be focused to produce incisions on any layer in the cornea. Additionally, they have the following physical properties:

- High pulse repetition rates (MHz) and low-energy pulses (nJ)
- Accurate laser focus
- Decreased stromal gas generation
- More precise tissue cuts.

ELITA™ SILK® platform utilizes a low-energy femtosecond laser for lenticule creation. Interestingly, there is minimal spot-to-spot separation (mean spot separation is < 1 μm), which is achieved through a combination of shorter pulse duration, smaller spot size, high pulse repetition rate, and fast scanning.

In this chapter, we will discuss the origin and advantages of KLEx as well as elucidate the features of Smooth Incision Lenticule Keratomileusis (SILK®), a new KLEx procedure designed for the ELITA™ femtosecond laser platform by Johnson & Johnson (Irvine, CA, USA). We will highlight the laser settings and lenticule shape of SILK® to try to understand how the former can impact early post-operative wound healing in terms of epithelial remodeling and keratocyte changes. We will also look at the visual recovery and effect of the novel lenticular shape on aberrations and visual quality parameters such as depth of focus.

29.2 Past, Present and Future

In the year 1999, the precursor to modern refractive lenticular extraction (ReLEx) was first described, which used a picosecond laser to construct a lenticule which would be manually removed after lifting a flap. In 2007, following the introduction of the VisuMax femtosecond laser (Carl Zeiss Meditec, Jena, Germany), the femtosecond lenticule extraction (FLEx) procedure was reintroduced. The next stage following FLEx was a new procedure called small incision lenticule extraction (SMILE) which included removal of the refractive lenticule from a small incision of about 2–3 mm [2].

SMILE gained popularity as it was a flapless and minimally invasive form of laser vision correction for the treatment of myopia and myopic astigmatism [2]. In various studies, SMILE fared better than laser in situ keratomileusis (LASIK) as lesser nerves are severed in SMILE resulting in lesser incidence of post-operative dry eye. It also has no flap-related complications [3].

SMILE also results in a biomechanically stronger cornea as compared to LASIK because the stronger anterior and peripheral collagen fibers are left relatively intact. Additionally, vertical cuts in SMILE have a greater biomechanical effect in comparison to horizontal cuts, with greater weakening for deeper incisions [4].

Due to the mentioned advantages and an acceptable visual recovery as compared to LASIK, lenticular extraction procedures are largely being preferred globally.

Refractive surgery procedures are continuously evolving with time and technology, to provide better and more precise patient outcomes. SMILE was FDA-approved in 2016, and since then, there has been an enormous development in the KLEx procedures to improve on the approach. Various companies are coming up with different platforms to carry out KLEx procedures. Apart from SMILE by Carl Zeiss, there is the SmartSight by SCHWIND ATOS, CLEAR by Ziemer and the ELITA SILK by Johnson & Johnson.

With so many newer options in the market available, it is difficult to decide which machine or method is the best for our patients. To decide the success of a surgery, apart from the visual recovery, wound healing also plays an important role in long-term outcomes. In this chapter, we attempt to discuss SILK in detail, starting from the difference in the machine parameters, the lenticule shape and its impact on visual recovery and wound healing, and also how each has an impact on the long-term outcome.

29.3 Biconvex Lenticule Shape Before and After Lenticule Removal

Photoablation on a prolate myopic cornea results in loss of negative asphericity as the cornea becomes more oblate (periphery is steeper). Greater depths of tissue must be ablated in order to preserve the corneal asphericity with conventional laser ablation procedures [5, 6].

Reduced antero-posterior diameter of a biconvex lenticule could help preserve the corneal asphericity without additional tissue ablation. Preservation of corneal asphericity could lead to superior visual outcomes.

The thickness and shape of the lenticule primarily depend upon the degree of refractive error and the cutting capability of the laser employed in the machine. The myopic lenticule created by the VisuMax® femtosecond system for SMILE has a *"plano-convex"* shape. In contrast, the myopic lenticule created by the ELITA™ femtosecond laser has a *"biconvex"* shape, (Fig. 29.1) which is cut with ELITA's tissue bridge-free incision.

To prove this, we performed the initial steps of the SILK® procedure for one eye each of a patient, i.e., the laser was fired and lenticule was created. Thereafter, the eye was imaged on ASOCT (after resolution of the opaque bubble layer) to determine shape of the lenticule. (Fig. *29.2*) Dissection and lenticule extraction was done four hours later.

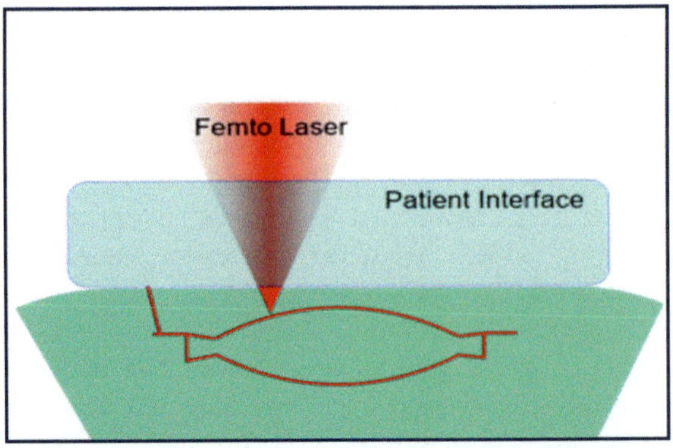

Fig. 29.1 Illustration of biconvex SILK lenticule

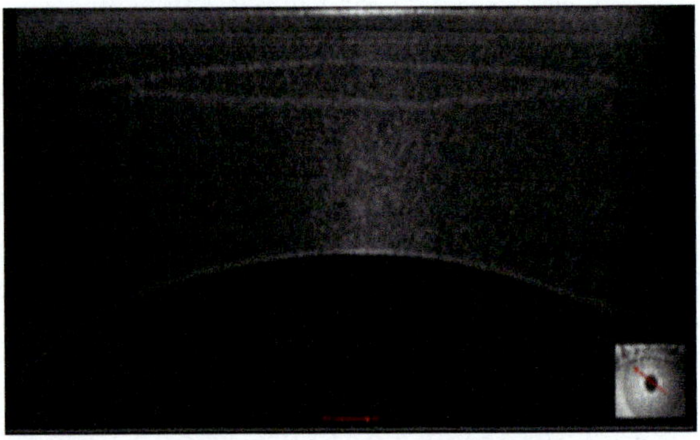

Fig. 29.2 Anterior segment OCT cross-sectional images depicting biconvex SILK lenticule

Using the “applanation-like cornea” ASOCT images from MS-39 (Costruzione Strumenti Oftalmici (CSO), Firenze, Italy), image processing was done to enhance the lenticular edges followed by edge tracking. This gave us the 3D rendering of the lenticules further confirming the biconvex shape. (Figs. 29.2 and 29.3).

The three-dimensional (3D) lenticule profile was developed using 10 mm radial optical coherence tomography (OCT) images from MS-39. The images were captured intra-operatively just after the cap cut and before lenticule extraction. The captured OCT image of the cornea (Fig. 29.4a) was flattened at the air-epithelium interface using “applanation-like cornea” mode (Fig. 29.4b) in the Phoenix software (v4.0.0.36, CSO, Firenze, Italy). The flattened image was then exported into custom-built software (built using Python 3.7.9, Python Software Foundation, USA). The software starts by enhancing the edges in the image (Fig. 29.4c).

The software then detects the relevant edges from the image such as the air-epithelium interface (yellow line, Fig. 29.4d), anterior cap cut (red dash line, Fig. 29.4d) and posterior cap cut (blue dash line, Fig. 29.4d). These steps were repeated for all the 12 captured radial frames which were 15 degrees apart in eyes undergoing SILK. All 12 anterior and posterior edges were fitted with respective smooth surfaces to get the 3D structures. The final 3D structure view for SILK is shown in Fig. 29.4e.

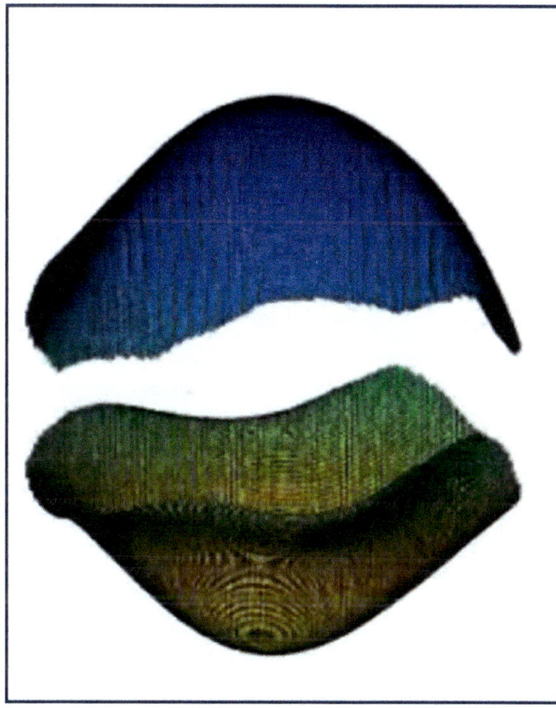

Fig. 29.3 3D reconstruction of lenticule profile: Biconvex configuration of SILK lenticule

The tissue bridge-free incision of the biconvex SILK® lenticule allows easy separation and extraction of lenticule. Furthermore, the biconvex shape lenticule protects a majority of the corneal nerve trunks from getting cut during lenticule formation. (Fig. 29.6).

29.4 Bowman's Layer Changes in SILK®

At times, microdistortions can be observed in the Bowman's layer after SMILE, especially for high myopia owing to the longer arc length of the cap than the stromal bed after removing the lenticule. Quantitative evaluation of the microdistortions on optical coherence tomography (OCT) has found that there is a positive correlation between the magnitude of the refractive error corrected and the Bowman Roughness Index (BRI). The BRI is defined as the enclosed area between the actual and ideal smooth layer to quantify microdistortions. The microdistortions, however, are reported to remain stable after a week, with no impact on long-term visual performance. The post-operative BRI in SMILE eyes is also reported to be similar to the pre-operative BRI in comparison to LASIK eyes, indicating earlier wound healing after SMILE.

An irregular Bowman's layer after refractive lenticule extraction can result in irregular optics and subsequent poor quality of vision. SILK appears to create

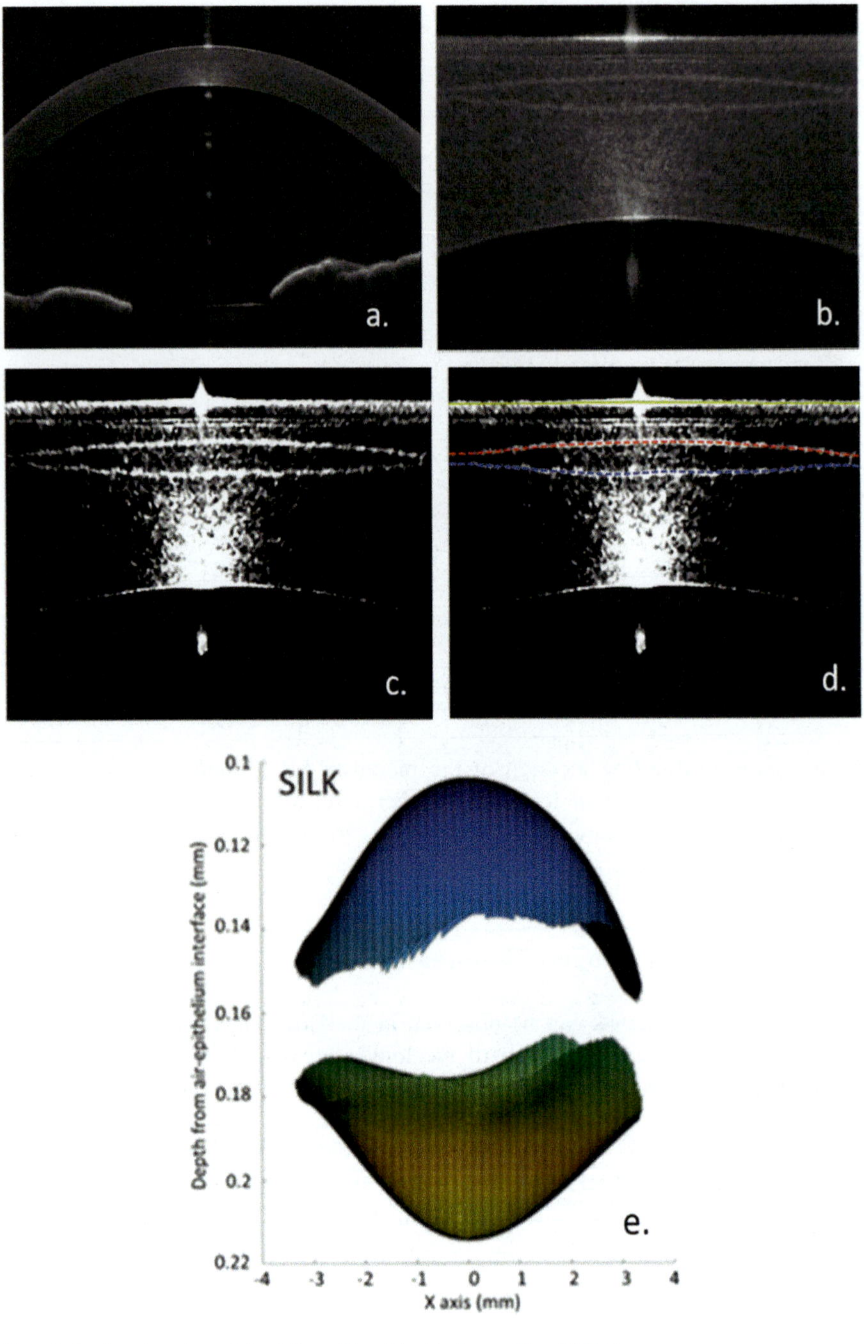

Fig. 29.4 Construction of the 3D profile of lenticule profile of SILK

only a few or no microdistortions at all. However, this needs to be elucidated in a comparative study. (Fig. 29.5) This could be due to greater approximation of identical interface surfaces by virtue of its novel shape.

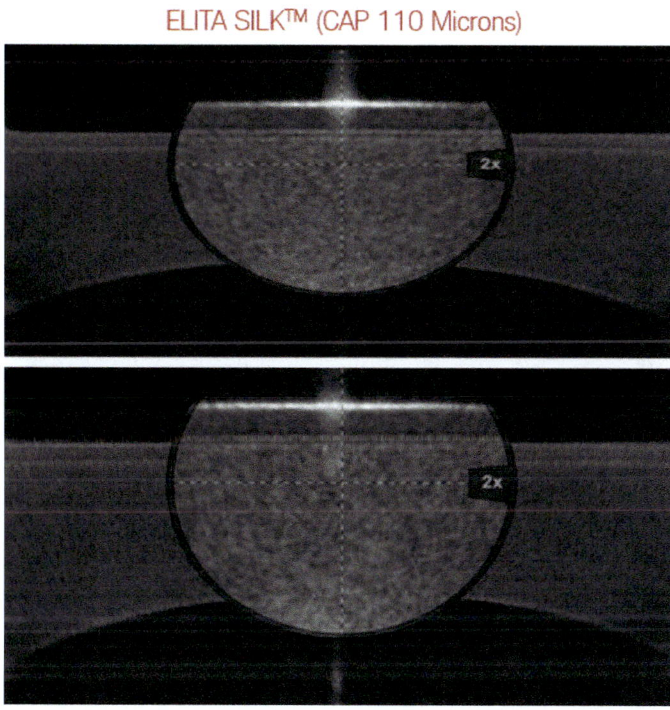

Fig. 29.5 Depiction of Bowman's layer status post-SILK: Regular and straight

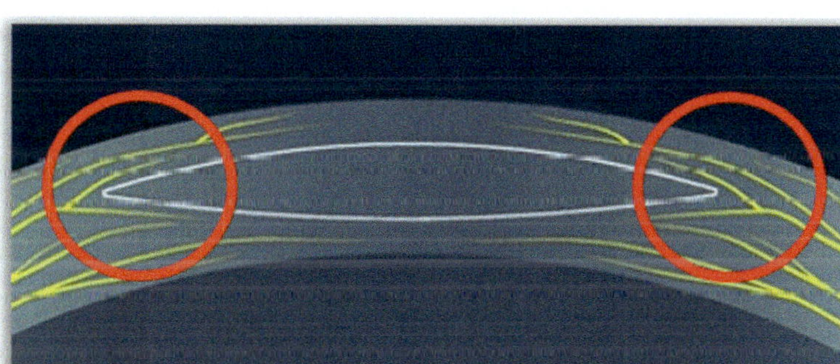

Fig. 29.6 Depiction of the pattern of nerves severing in SILK: Presumed preservation of nerve trunks due to the biconvex shape of SILK lenticule

29.5 Comparing Corneal Nerve Regenerations and Changes Between SILK® and LASIK®

Corneal nerve regeneration after a refractive surgery is an essential healing process. The number of nerve trunks cut during flap creation for LASIK is higher in the immediate post-operative period [7]. SMILE procedure is known to sever lesser number of corneal nerves as compared to LASIK owing to its small incision site. However, the shape of the lenticule may also play a role in nerve damage. Since the biconvex SILK lenticule leaves more residual cap at the periphery of the lenticule, the number of nerves cut may be lesser than in LASIK (Fig. 29.6) which could be responsible for faster nerve regeneration post-surgery. However, further studies concentrating on the comparison of wound healing and nerve regeneration after SILK and other KLEx procedures at similar cap depths are needed to confirm this.

The nerve regeneration post-LASIK and SILK were studied using confocal microscopy on the HRTIII RCM Confocal Microscopy at one-month, three-month, six-month post-operative follow-ups. (Fig. 29.7). In the confocal images in Fig. 29.7, we can see that the nerves started regenerating at post-operative one month and were nearly completely regenerated by six months for SILK. The regeneration of nerves was faster and superior for SILK as compared to LASIK at all-time points.

Earlier and faster nerve regeneration is stressed upon as the nerve growth factors are responsible for a healthy ocular surface milieu. The most common cause of dryness and ocular discomfort post-operatively is the destruction of nerves. There is always a crosstalk between the nerves and the ocular surface (particularly the epithelium). Poor nerve regeneration results in an unhealthy/inflamed ocular surface and patient is uncomfortable for longer period of time post-surgery.

29.6 Epithelial Remodeling in SILK®

Healthy nerve regeneration translates to healthy ocular surface. The nerve growth factors are crucial for ocular surface healing and reducing the ocular surface inflammation [8]. MMP-9 (Matrix Metallo Proteinase-9) is an inflammatory marker which is a marker for epithelial disease, and thus, ocular surface inflammation will have an effect on epithelial remodeling post-refractive surgery.

In turn, epithelial remodeling has an impact on visual clarity. A healthy, regular epithelium makes a smooth refracting surface which is responsible for a clear vision as opposed to an irregular, unhealthy surface which results in an unclear vision.

We evaluated the epithelial healing in SILK by imaging the epithelium on the Optovue (Visionix, France). It was observed that the epithelial remodeling after SILK was regular, i.e., the difference between peripheral and central epithelial thickness was less than 5μ. (Fig. 29.8) which could be the result of healthier nerve regeneration after the surgery.

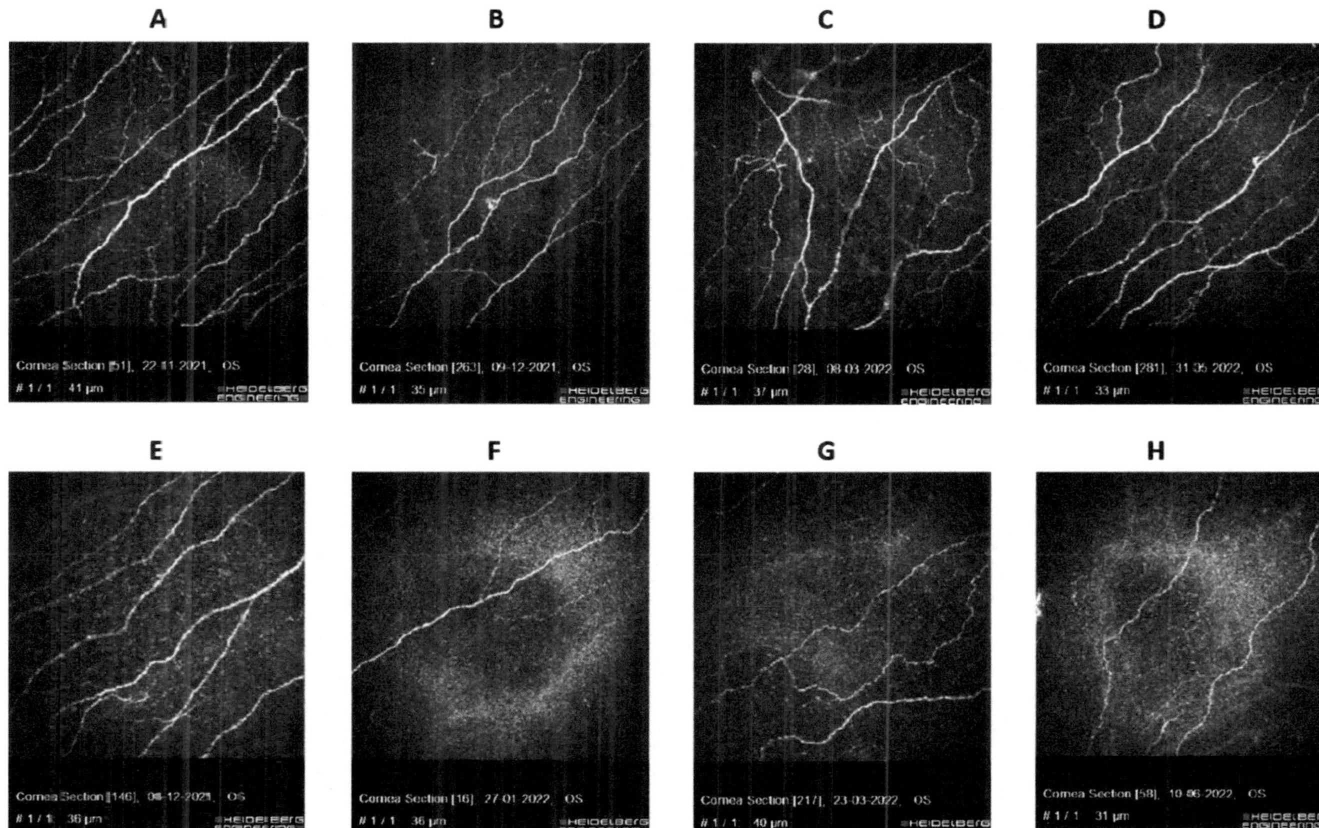

Fig. 29.7 IVCM images depicting post-operative nerve regeneration after (TOP ROW) SILK and (BOTTOM ROW) LASIK procedure. Figure 29.7A and E depicts pre-operative sub-basal nerves before SILK and LASIK, respectively. Figure 29.7B and F shows sub-basal nerve plexus 1-month post-surgery. Figure 29.7C and G shows faster regeneration of sub-basal nerves three-month post-SILK as compared to LASIK. Figure 29.7D and H shows nerve regeneration at six-month post-SILK and post-LASIK, respectively

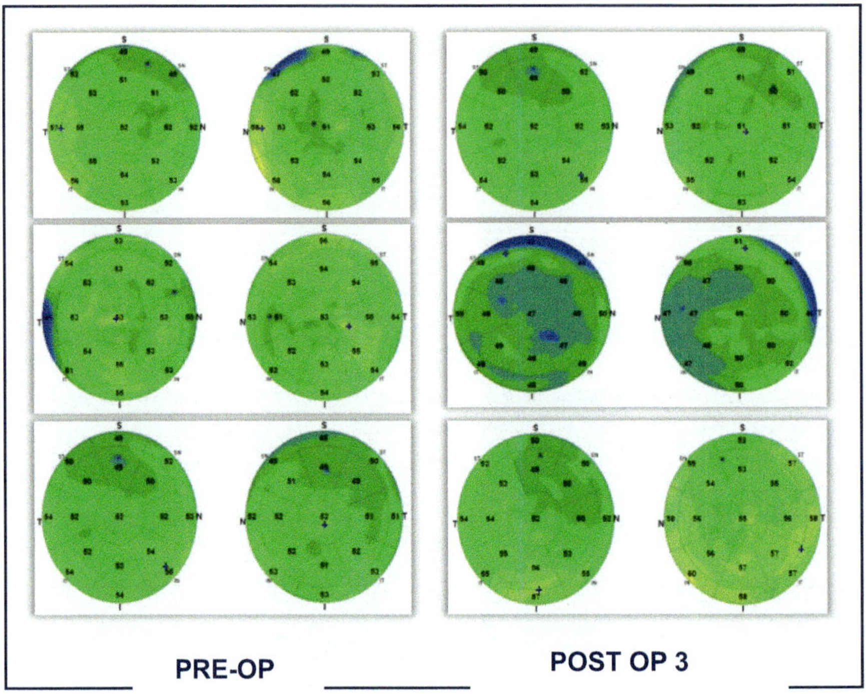

Fig. 29.8 Regular epithelial healing (at three-month post-surgery) after SILK surgery of MRSE of −6.75 D

The visual quality was assessed in patients undergoing SILK by looking at the Ocular Scatter Index. There was significantly lesser scatter observed in patients who underwent SILK procedure post-operatively as compared to pre-operative OSI, reinforcing the fact the epithelium was healthier after a nerve sparing refractive surgery. (Fig. 29.9).

29.7 Stromal Wound Healing and Structural Changes at the Level of Collagen in SILK®

Corneal wound healing after a refractive surgery has an important impact on the safety, efficacy, predictability and stability of laser vision correction; hence, it affects the clinical outcomes. [9] With the introduction of variable energy delivery across different KLEx platforms, it becomes important to understand how this variation in energy affects the keratocyte changes and stromal wound healing that occur after refractive surgery at an ultrastructural level.

Keratocytes play a crucial role in carrying out the wound healing after any refractive surgery. Corneal wound healing after refractive surgery mainly comprises of keratocyte apoptosis immediately after surgery, followed by the

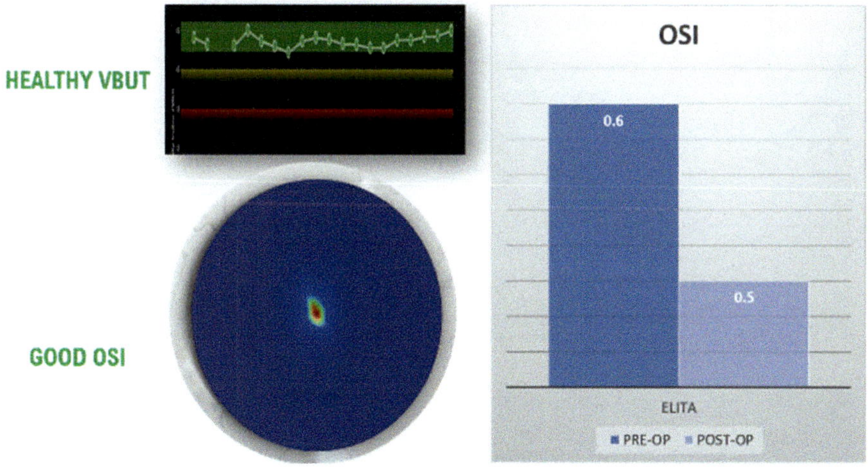

Fig. 29.9 Lesser incidence of post-operative ocular surface scatter with SILK translating to better visual quality

appearance of activated myofibroblastic cells which lay down healthy collagen and other substances for wound healing response [10]. Ultimately, there is repopulation of normal (quiescent) keratocytes usually by 4 weeks after surgery [11].

Aberrant corneal wound healing is associated with aberrant collagen being laid down which will lead to poor visual outcomes and also post-surgery regression.

Keeping the above things in mind, we looked at the keratocytes using the IVCM (HRTIII RCM) at one-month, three-month and six-month post-operatively to study the wound healing response. We observed that the activated keratocytes persist longer, as late as till six months in LASIK as compared to SILK. These patients had a repopulation of healthy keratocytes by six months. (Fig. 29.10). This might have visual implications in visual recovery after these new KLEx procedures.

29.8 Impact of Aberration Profile on Depth of Focus in SILK®

SMILE has previously been shown to induce lesser change in Q value on the anterior corneal surface as compared to LASIK. Furthermore, changes in corneal Q value have been demonstrated to significantly impact corneal higher-order aberrations after refractive surgery such as LASIK and SMILE [12].

An oblate cornea refracts peripheral rays more anteriorly as compared to the central rays, passing through a flattened corneal surface thereby diminishing the contrast of the retinal image. This becomes more apparent with increasing pupil size. Therefore, a greater change in anterior corneal asphericity could impact functional vision of the patient resulting in suboptimal outcomes after refractive surgery [5].

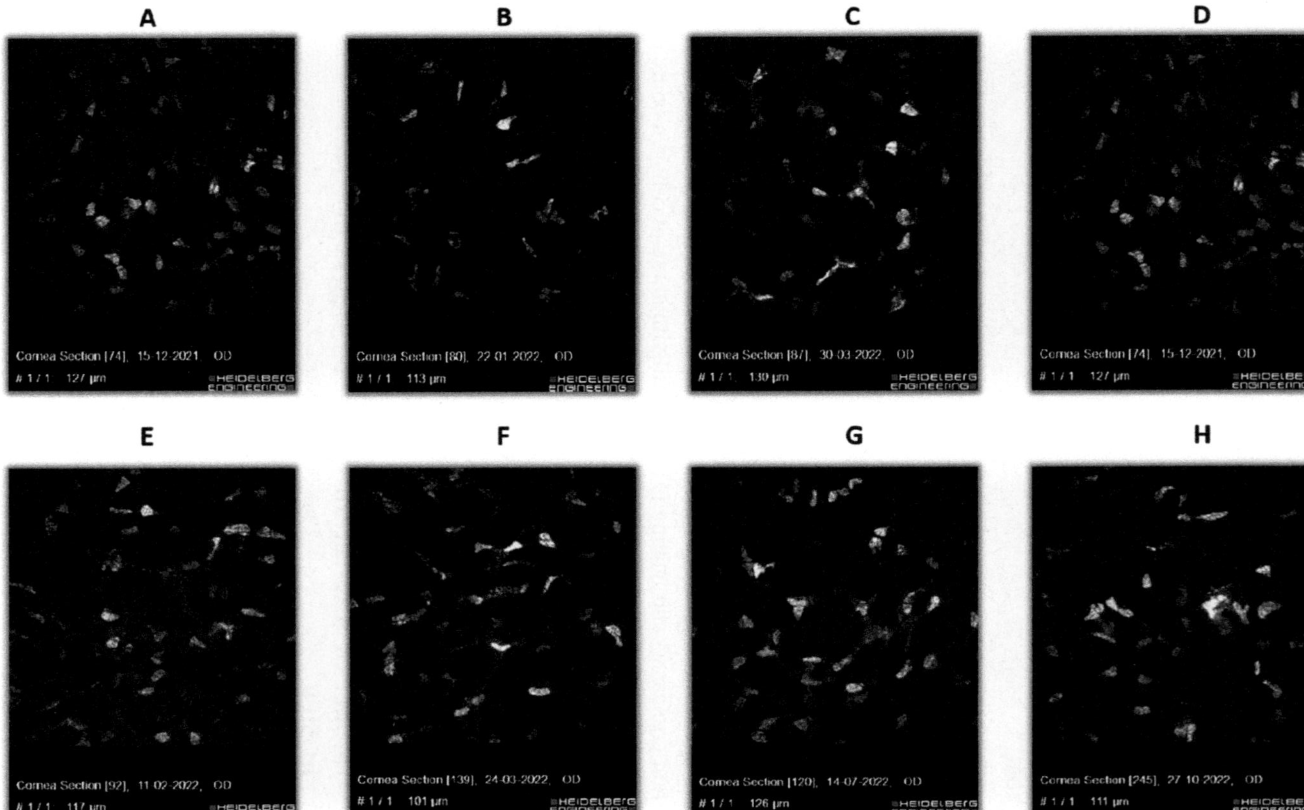

Fig. 29.10 Wound healing keratocyte response as seen on IVCM in (TOP ROW) SILK and (BOTTOM ROW) LASIK procedures. Figure 29.10A and E shows pre-operative keratocytes at the level of interface in SILK and LASIK, respectively. Figure 29.10B and F shows post-operative activated keratocytes at the level of interface in SILK and LASIK, respectively, at one month. Figure 29.10C and G shows faster recovery of keratocytes at three-month post-SILK as compared to LASIK. Figure 29.10D and H shows return of a higher number of normal keratocytes in SILK eye at six months as compared to LASIK

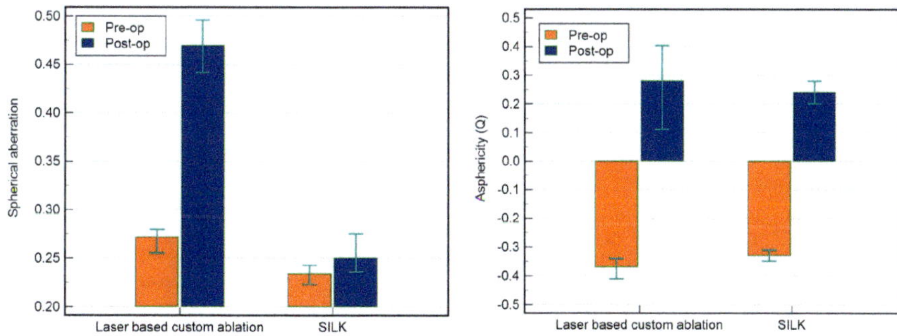

Fig. 29.11 Comparison of change in SA and asphericity between SILK and other laser-based custom ablation (pre-op to post-op three months). SILK shows a minimal change in SA values as compared to pre-operative values

As discussed in the previous section, the novel biconvex lenticular shape of the SILK® could allow the maintenance of corneal asphericity (Q value) after myopic laser ablation. In a study comparing asphericity and consequently, the spherical aberration (SA) between SILK® and other excimer laser-based custom ablation treatment in 125 eyes *[extrapolatable to a larger population]*, we found a minimal change in SA at three months from pre-op value, in the eyes undergoing SILK®. (Fig. 29.11) This could be responsible for good depth perception and subsequently help give the patient a "*perfect*" night vision.

Preservation of spherical aberration of either sign can help in attaining depth of focus [13, 14]. Myopic/hyperopic ablation-induced change in SA can alter depth of focus. In a study conducted by Shetty et al., it was established that aberrometric and refractive status of eyes that underwent LASIK was closest to emmetropic eyes [15].

In addition to depth of focus, we also compared the ocular aberrations as measured on Tracey iTrace® Wavefront Aberrometer. The spherical aberration for distant, intermediate and near targets in SILK was similar to emmetropes. (Fig. 29.12 (A). At distance (Fig. 29.12 (B), the SILK eyes showed slightly higher defocus as compared to emmetropes ($p > 0.05$) whereas it was comparable for near and intermediate targets. However, LORMS was comparable between the groups ($P > 0.05$). (Fig. 29.12D).

RMS higher-order aberrations and Coma RMS were also similar between the groups ($P > 0.05$). (Fig. 29.12 (C)

This proved that depth of focus post-Elita SILK is similar to depth of focus in an emmetropic eye and there was better preservation of DOF with Elita SILK.

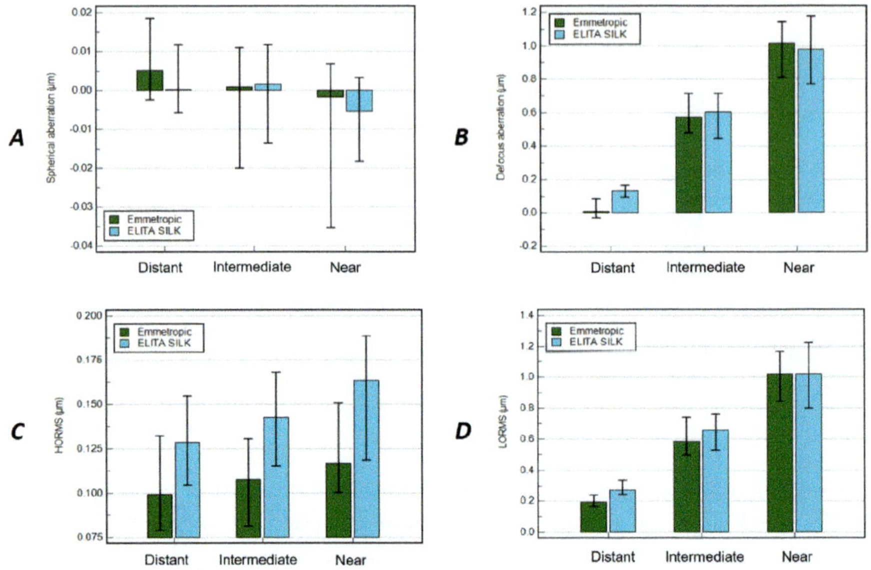

Fig. 29.12 Assessment of SA, defocus, HORMS and LORMS in emmetropic [50 eyes] and post-SILK [70 eyes]

29.9 Conclusion

The unique laser settings and lenticule shape of SILK® allow better preservation of corneal nerves post-refractive surgery and thereby promoting healthy ocular surface healing and faster stromal healing compared to flap-based procedures. Future studies will also show, if the unique lenticule shape has advantages over other KLEx procedures. Healthy ocular surface in turn could impact visual clarity post-surgery. In addition, we found good preserved depth of focus in patients undergoing SILK®. We believe that this could be attributed to the minimal change in SA as a result of the biconvex lenticular shape.

References

1. Honavar SG. Refractive surgery—the 20/happy game changer. Indian J Ophthalmol. 2020;68(12):2639–2640. https://doi.org/10.4103/ijo.IJO_3503_20. PMID: 33229630; PMCID: PMC7857008.
2. Ganesh S, Brar S, Arra RR. Refractive lenticule extraction small incision lenticule extraction: A new refractive surgery paradigm. Indian J Ophthalmology. 2018;66(1):10–19, https://doi.org/10.4103/ijo.IJO_761_17
3. Michelle Stephenson PUBLISHED 15 APRIL 2021 The Current State of SMILE versus LASIK.

4. Sachdev GS, Ramamurthy S. Decade—long journey with small incision lenticule extraction: The learnings. Indian J Ophthalmology.2020;68(12):2705–2710, https://doi.org/10.4103/ijo.IJO_2622_20
5. Holladay JT, Dudeja DR, Chang J. Functional vision and corneal changes after laser in situ keratomileusis determined by contrast sensitivity, glare testing, and corneal topography. J Cataract Refract Surg. 1999;25(5):663–9. https://doi.org/10.1016/s0886-3350(99)00011-5.
6. Gatinel D, Malet J, Hoang-Xuan T, Azar DT. Analysis of customized corneal ablations: theoretical limitations of increasing negative asphericity. Invest Ophthalmol Vis Sci. 2002;43(4):941–8.
7. Lee BH, McLaren JW, Erie JC, Hodge DO, Bourne WM. Reinnervation in the Cornea after LASIK. Invest Ophthalmol Vis Sci. 2002;43(12):3660–4.
8. Lambiase A, Micera A, Pellegrini G, Merlo D, Rama P, De Luca M, Bonini S. Stefano Bonini; In Vitro Evidence of Nerve Growth Factor Effects on Human Conjunctival Epithelial Cell Differentiation and Mucin Gene Expression. Invest Ophthalmol Vis Sci. 2009;50(10):4622–30. https://doi.org/10.1167/iovs.08-2716.
9. Azar DT, Chang JH, Han KY. Wound healing after keratorefractive surgery: Review of biological and optical considerations. Cornea. 2012;31:S9-19.
10. Wilson SE. Everett Kinsey Lecture. Keratocyte apoptosis in refractive surgery. CLAO J. 1998;24(3):181–5. PMID: 9684078.
11. Liu YC, Ang H, Teo E, et al. Wound healing profiles of hyperopic-small incision lenticule extraction (SMILE). Sci Rep. 2016;6:29802. https://doi.org/10.1038/srep29802.
12. Zhang H, Wang Y, Li H. Corneal Spherical Aberration and Corneal Asphericity after Small Incision Lenticule Extraction and Femtosecond Laser-Assisted LASIK. J Ophthalmol. 2017;2017:4921090. https://doi.org/10.1155/2017/4921090.
13. Yi F, Robert Iskander D, Collins M. Depth of focus and visual acuity with primary and secondary spherical aberration. Vision Res. 2011;51(14):1648–58.
14. Rocha KM, Vabre L, Chateau N, Krueger RR. Expanding depth of focus by modifying higher-order aberrations induced by an adaptive optics visual simulator. J Cataract Refract Surg. 2009;35(11):1885–92. https://doi.org/10.1016/j.jcrs.2009.05.059.
15. Shetty N, Dadachanji Z, Narasimhan R, et al. Status of Residual Refractive Error, Ocular Aberrations, and Accommodation After Myopic LASIK, SMILE, and TransPRK. J Refract Surg. 2019;35(10):624–31. https://doi.org/10.3928/1081597X-20190916-02.

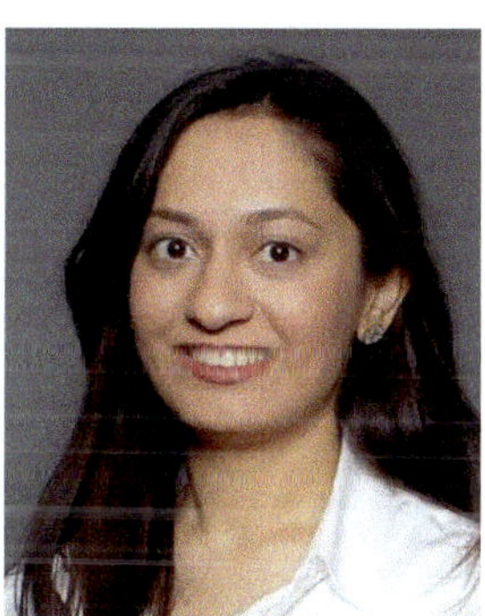

Pooja Khamar is a distinguished consultant in cataract and refractive services at Narayana Nethralaya Eye Institute. With extensive clinical and research experience, she has significantly advanced ophthalmology, particularly through her Ph.D. research on wound healing in refractive surgery at Maastricht University. Her specialized training includes a CORE fellowship at Narayana Nethralaya, Bangalore, focusing on cataract and refractive surgery, dry eye, and keratoconus. Dr. Khamar is actively involved in translational research at the GROW and IBMS Lab, working on projects that benefit patients and the medical community. Recognized through numerous publications and as a faculty member at prestigious conferences, Dr. Khamar has been named one of the Top 10 Rising Stars of Ophthalmology and awarded the Troutman Award for her exceptional contributions to refractive surgery. Her work has been honored on both national and international platforms. With her extensive knowledge, clinical expertise, and research contributions, Dr. Khamar is a trusted authority in ophthalmology, dedicated to improving patient care and advancing scientific understanding.

Clinical Results in Myopia/Myopia with Astigmatism Correction Using SILK®

30

Mahipal S. Sachdev, Raghav Malik, Rohit Shetty, Pooja Khamar, Jodhbir S. Mehta, Ivan Gabric, Brian L. Schwam, Ying Wang, and Michal Laron

Abstract

"This chapter presents the initial clinical results of myopia and myopia with astigmatism correction using the ELITA™ smooth incision lenticular keratomileusis (SILK) procedure, a novel keratorefractive lenticule extraction (KLEx) technology. Conducted in two Indian centers, the prospective study involved 170 eyes of 85 subjects. The procedure showcased an easy lenticule removal, with 85.3% of cases graded as "no dissection needed" or "mild dissection needed." At six-month post-operative, 63% of eyes achieved uncorrected visual acuity (UCVA) of 20/16 or better, and 92% had residual astigmatism of 0.50 D or less. The ELITA™ SILK procedure, blending laser-assisted in situ keratomileusis (LASIK) advantages with KLEx features, proves to be

M. S. Sachdev · R. Malik
Centre for Sight, New Delhi, India

R. Shetty · P. Khamar
Narayana Nethralaya Eye Institute, Bengaluru, India

J. S. Mehta
Department of Cornea and External Eye Diseases, Singapore National Eye Centre, Singapore, Singapore

Cornea and Refractive Surgery Group, Singapore Eye Research Institute, Singapore, Singapore

Duke-NUS Graduate Medical School, Ophthalmology Academic Clinical Program, Singapore, Singapore

I. Gabric
Specialty Eye Hospital Svjetlost, School of Medicine University of Rijeka, Zagreb, Croatia

B. L. Schwam · Y. Wang · M. Laron (✉)
Johnson-Johnson Surgical Vision Inc., Milpitas, USA
e-mail: mlaron@its.jnj.com

W. Sekundo and F. M. Wagner (eds.), *Femtosecond Laser Assisted Lenticule Extraction*,
https://doi.org/10.1007/978-3-031-60424-9_30

a promising approach for laser refractive correction, offering high precision and rapid visual recovery. Further refinement of the nomogram could enhance post-operative outcomes, solidifying the potential of ELITA™ SILK in myopia correction."

Keywords

ELITA SILK • Keratorefractive lenticule extraction (KLEx) • Myopia correction • Astigmatism correction • Clinical outcomes • Refractive surgery • Laser-assisted in situ keratomileusis (LASIK)

30.1 Introduction

The principles and the properties of the newest KLEX procedure SILK have been explained in detail in previous chapters. This chapter reports on the first clinical outcomes obtained from a prospective, multicenter, single-arm, open-label clinical study conducted at two sites in India (Centre for Sight in New Delhi and Narayana Nethralaya Eye Hospital in Bangalore). The study has an Ethics Committee approval and the usual inclusion and exclusion criteria as described in the original publication [1]

Data from 170 eyes of 85 subjects is presented. Preoperative mean MRSE was −4.14 D ± 1.32 D (range, −1.38 D to −8.88 D); preoperative mean MRS was −3.75 D ± 1.27 D (range −1.25 D to −8.00 D) and mean MRC was −0.77 D ± 0.62 D (range 0.00 D to −3.00 D). The lenticule optical zone was set in all cases to 6.0 mm. Data from 158, 130, 138 and 124 eyes were available from the one-week, one-, three- and six-month visits, respectively.

30.2 Ease of Lenticule Removal

The ease of lenticule removal was graded by surgeons based on the scale described in Table 30.1. In 85.3% of cases, surgeons graded the ease of lenticule removal as "no dissection needed" or "mild dissection needed." No cases were graded as "unable to dissect" (Fig. 30.1).

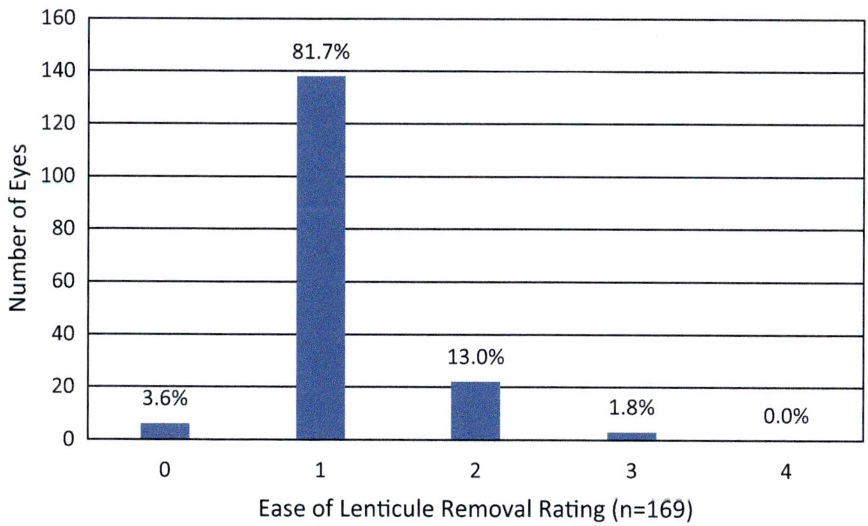

Fig. 30.1 Ease of lenticule removal surgeon ratings ($n = 169$), where 0 = no dissection needed and 4 = unable to dissect

Table 30.1 Ease of lenticule removal rating scale

Grade	Description
0	No dissection needed
1	Mild dissection required (< 50% of lenticule)
2	Moderate dissection needed (50–75% of lenticule)
3	Significant dissection needed (76–100% of lenticule)
4	Unable to dissect

30.3 Effectiveness

At three- and six-month post-operatively, 54% and 63% of eyes had uncorrected visual acuity (UCVA) of 20/16 or better, respectively (Figs. 30.2A and B). UCVA of 20/20 or better was achieved by 96% of eyes at both three- and six-month post-operatively (Figs. 30.2A and B).

30.4 Safety

In terms of safety, at six months, there was no loss of lines of corrected distance visual acuity (CDVA) for any eye. Further, in 59% of cases, there was an improvement of 1 or 2 lines of CDVA (Fig. 30.3).

All eyes showed high levels of refractive stability from one month through six-month post-operatively (Fig. 30.4). Both Figs. 30.4 and 30.5 A and B demonstrate a mild systematic under-correction of refractive error of approximately −0.33 D with a trend of larger under-correction for higher myopic refractive errors. The mild under-correction can be reduced in the future with a nomogram refinement. As shown in the figures, stability was generally achieved within one-month post-operatively.

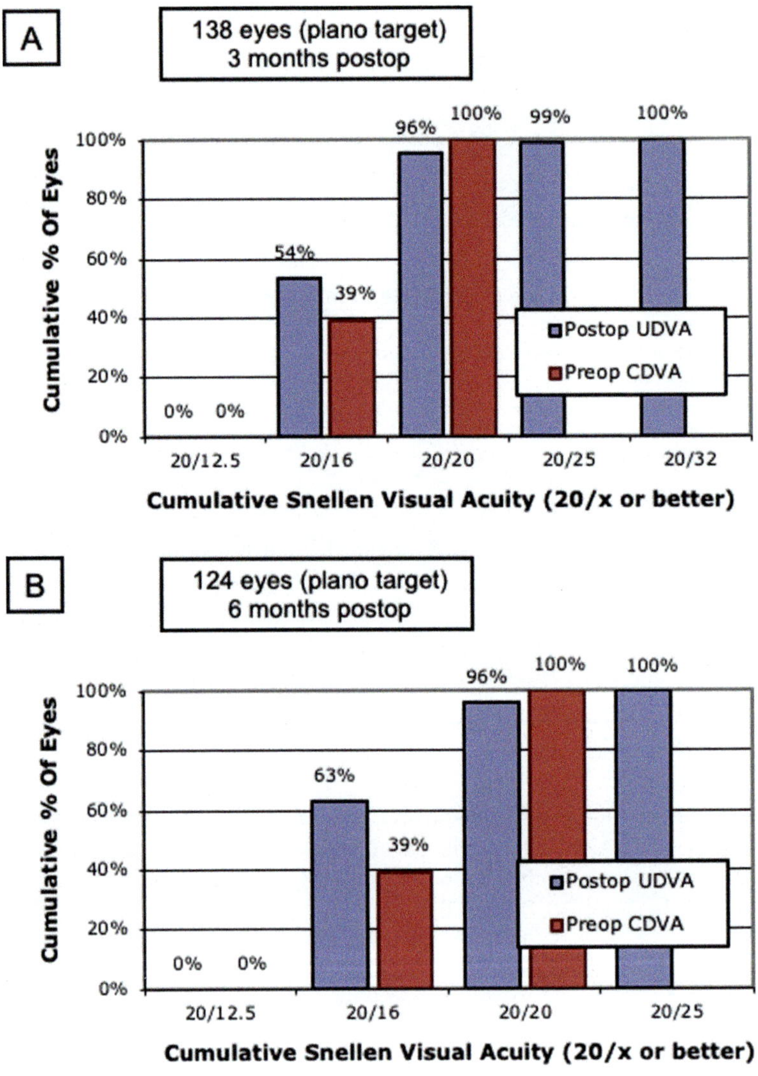

Fig. 30.2 Cumulative Snellen visual acuity (20/x or better) comparing post-operative (post-op) uncorrected distance visual acuity (UDVA) with preoperative (preop) corrected distance visual acuity (CDVA) at A three months and B six months

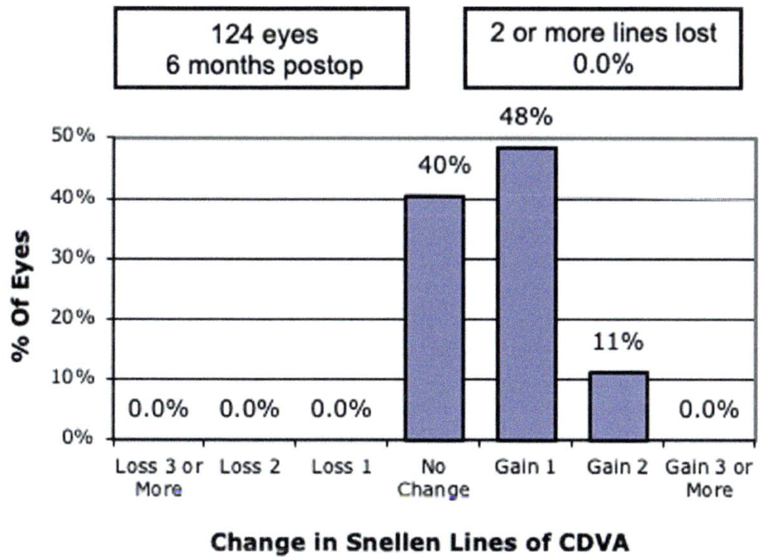

Fig. 30.3 Change in corrected distance visual acuity (CDVA) at six months compared to preoperative

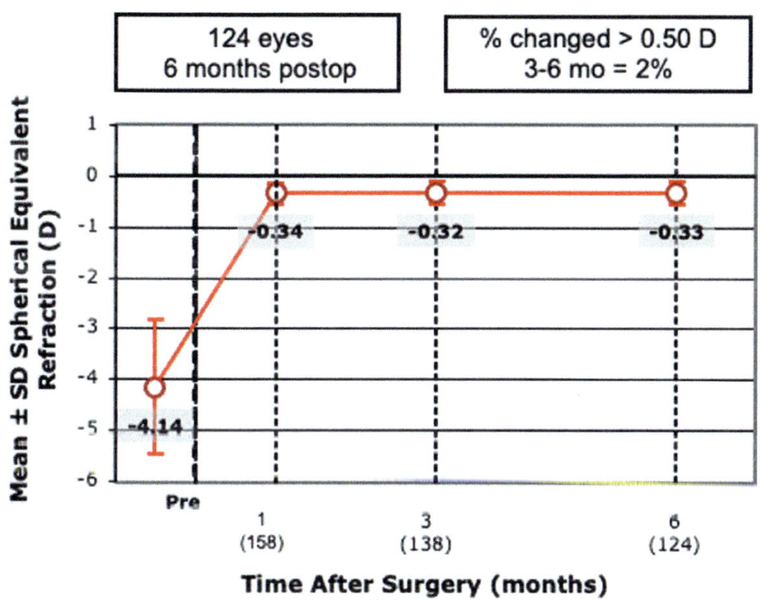

Fig. 30.4 Stability of spherical equivalent refraction over six months

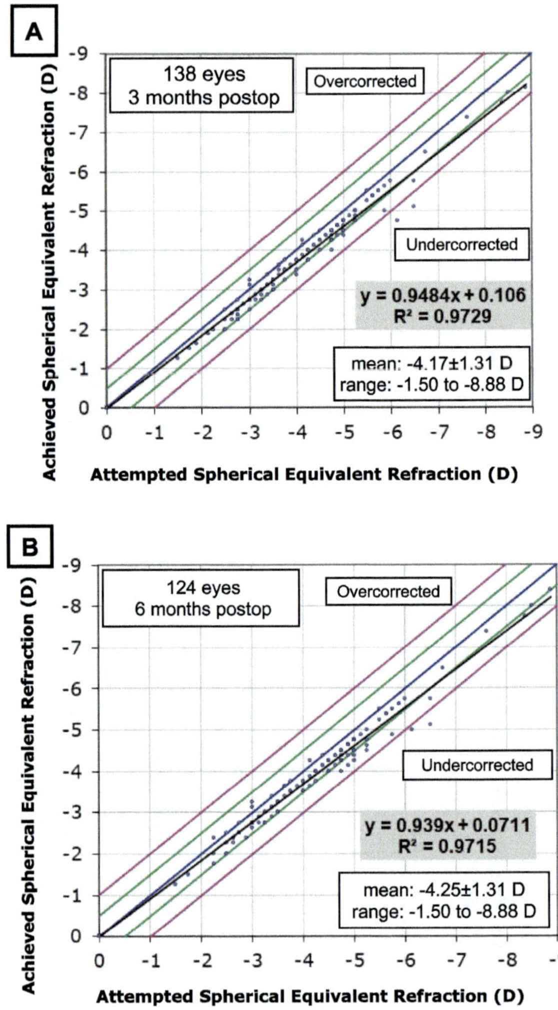

Fig. 30.5 Attempted versus achieved spherical equivalent refraction at A three and B six months. The blue line indicates a perfect result, and the green and pink lines depict over- and under-correction of 0.50 D and 1.00 D, respectively

30.5 Astigmatism Correction

The distribution of astigmatism preoperatively and post-operatively is presented in Fig. 30.6. At six-month post-operatively, 92% of eyes had residual astigmatism of 0.50 D or less. Of those, 69% had residual astigmatism of 0.25 D or less.

The highest astigmatism included in this cohort was -3.00 D. The details below present this subject's astigmatism correction by ELITA™ SILK procedure:

The preoperative manifest refraction and keratometry readings were:

OD: −6.75/−1.75 × 10 Keratometry: 40.2/42.1 × 96
OS: −5.25/−3.00 × 170 Keratometry: 40.0/42.6 × 79

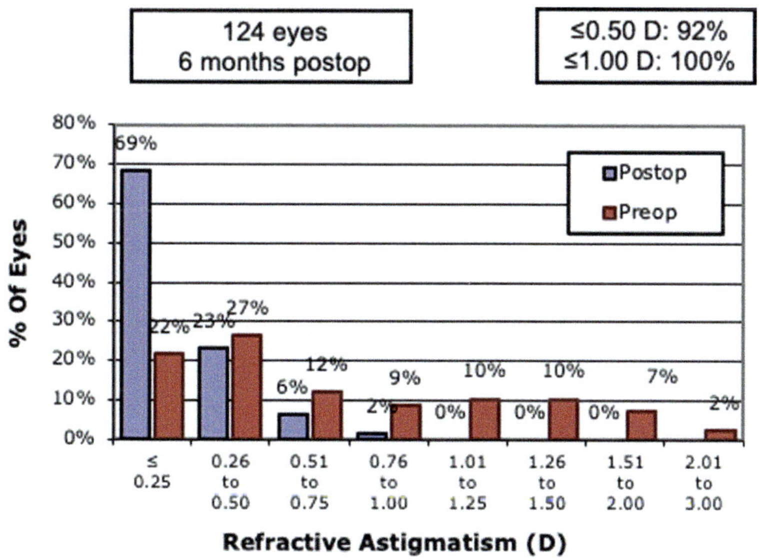

Fig. 30.6 Distribution of refractive astigmatism at six months (post-op) compared to preoperative (preop)

At three-month post-operatively, the residual manifest refraction for this subject was:

OD: −0.25 D sph Keratometry: 35.3/35.3 × 58
OS: −0.25 D sph Keratometry: 36.0/36.0 × 35

The uncorrected visual acuity for this subject at three-month post-operatively was 20/20 + 1 and 20/20 for OD and OS, respectively.

30.6 High Astigmatism Correction Example

The study cohort did not include eyes with astigmatism greater than 3.00 D. The following is one case not included in this cohort as an example of the ability of the ELITA™ system to correct for higher levels of cylinder. Of note, the ELITA™ system allows for cyclotorsion correction during centration and after docking is completed. This case had preoperative manifest refraction of:

OD: −1.50/−4.00 × 010 Keratometry: 41.4/44.5 × 97
OS: −2.25/−3.50 × 160 Keratometry: 41.5/44.2 × 73

At three-month post-operatively (last available visit at the time of writing this chapter), the residual manifest refraction for this subject was:

OD: −0.50/−0.25 × 170 Keratometry: 39.5/40.6 × 83
OS: −0.50/−0.25 × 180 Keratometry: 38.8/39.4 × 116

The uncorrected visual acuity for this subject at three-month post-operatively was 20/20 -1 and 20/20 -2 for OD and OS, respectively.

30.7 Conclusion

The ELITA™ SILK procedure is a new KLEX technology and procedure designed to provide a tissue bridge-free lenticule removal procedure that combines the advantages of LASIK (fast visual acuity recovery) and KLEX (single laser, minimally invasive) procedures.

Early clinical outcomes demonstrate ease of lenticule removal and high levels of safety, efficacy and stability for the ELITA™ SILK laser refractive correction procedure. Fine tuning the accuracy of refractive correction with a refined nomogram will provide even higher levels of post-operative UCVAs.

Reference

1. Sachdev MS, Shetty R, Khamar P, Malik R, Schwam BL, Fu H, Voorhees AP, Laron M. Safety and effectiveness of smooth incision lenticular keratomileusis (SILK™) Using the ELITA™ femtosecond laser system for correction of myopic and astigmatic refractive errors. Clin Ophthalmol. 2023;17:3761–73.

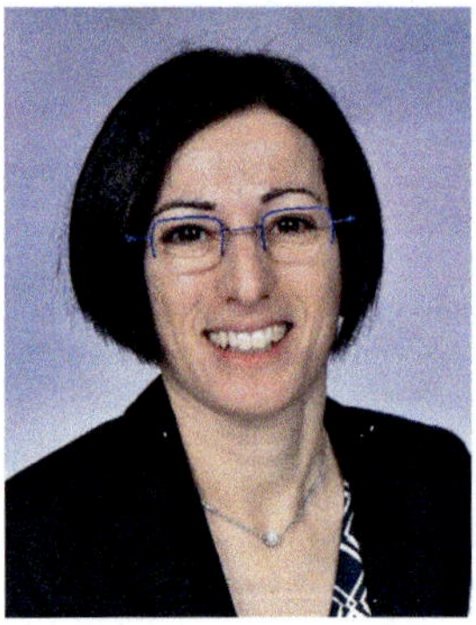

Michal Laron, PhD is Senior Principal Clinical Research Scientist at Johnson & Johnson Vision, Milpitas, California, USA. Dr. Laron has over 20 years of clinical studies experience in both academia and industry involving cutting edge ophthalmic devices, imaging, and electro-diagnostic techniques. She studied Optometry at the Hadassah College in Jerusalem, Israel, and practiced for several years. She received her PhD in Physiological Optics and Vision Science from the University of Houston, Texas, USA, with a dissertation titled: "The multifocal Visual Evoked Potential (mfVEP) as a Clinical Tool in Detecting Visual Pathway Abnormalities in Multiple Sclerosis." Later she served as Post-Doctoral Scholar at the University of California, Berkeley, School of Optometry, where she investigated functional and structural changes of the retina in adolescents with Type I diabetes using electrophysiology and other imaging techniques. After publishing three papers as a first author during her PhD, and two additional papers during her postdoctoral scholarship with podium presentations and invited talks, she turned to industry and continues to collaborate on numerous abstracts and manuscripts.

Part VIII

Marketing and Patient Communication

How to Promote SMILE Procedures

31

Bertram Meyer and Jean-Francois Faure

Abstract

This chapter guides refractive surgeons in promoting small incision lenticule extraction (SMILE) amidst increased competition in the refractive surgery market. It emphasizes SMILE's unique features—flapless, bladeless, and all-femtosecond laser procedure—and introduces key marketing focal points.

Keywords

Small incision lenticule extraction procedure (SMILE) • Refractive surgery market • All-femtosecond laser procedure

31.1 Introduction

In the current landscape of increased competition within the refractive surgery market, surgeons undertaking SMILE procedures must be well-prepared, particularly in addressing the needs of increasingly informed patients. At the beginning of SMILE era, the claims were restricted to the comparison with excimer laser-based procedures, mainly Lasik. Over a decade later, SMILE established itself as an excellent refractive procedure throughout the entire world. The best proof is the introduction of other KLEx procedures also represented in this book. This will inevitably lead to commercial claims in which KLEx procedure is superior, but

B. Meyer (✉)
Eye Center Cologne, Cologne, Germany
e-mail: Meyer@augencentrumkoeln.de

J.-F. Faure
Paris, France

W. Sekundo and F. M. Wagner (eds.), *Femtosecond Laser Assisted Lenticule Extraction*,
https://doi.org/10.1007/978-3-031-60424-9_31

this will take time as newer procedures still have to find their place in the market. Since the authors of this chapters have no personal experience with any other KLEx procedures but SMILE, this chapter is crafted to assist surgeons in their daily practice of SMILE surgery. It offers insights to empower them in devising effective marketing strategies for all-femtosecond refractive surgery.

SMILE stands out as a 100% femtosecond refractive treatment, distinguished by its flapless nature and a single-step procedure. The femtosecond laser is instrumental in reshaping the cornea, making the surgery bladeless, flapless, and an all-femtosecond laser procedure.

When promoting this cutting-edge laser technology, three keywords serve as key focal points for an impactful marketing strategy:

1. **Bladeless**: Emphasize the absence of traditional surgical blades in the SMILE procedure. Highlight the precision and safety offered by the femtosecond laser, providing patients with the reassurance of a minimally invasive approach.
2. **Flapless**: Communicate the advantage of SMILE being a flapless procedure, eliminating concerns associated with flap complications. Position this feature as a distinct benefit, offering reduced risk and a smoother recovery experience for patients.
3. **All-femtosecond laser procedure**: Accentuate the comprehensive use of femtosecond laser technology throughout the entire SMILE procedure. Illustrate how this advanced technology contributes to increased accuracy, enhanced predictability, and an overall superior surgical experience.

By using these keywords into the marketing strategy, surgeons can effectively communicate the unique and compelling aspects of SMILE, fostering patient trust and differentiation in the competitive refractive surgery market.

31.2 Tools for Patient Recruitment

Medical advertising varies significantly among countries, necessitating careful consideration of legal obligations before initiating clinic communications. Ensuring compliance with local regulations and liaising with relevant public authorities is crucial when crafting promotional strategies for SMILE. It is imperative to align the dissemination of information about SMILE with the legal framework in the respective country of practice.

Refractive surgeons bear an ethical responsibility to furnish accurate and truthful information in their promotional efforts. In instances where direct advertising may pose legal challenges, alternative materials and methods can be employed. Several tools have been identified to assist refractive surgery centers in generating interest in SMILE among potential patients.

Legal Compliance Check:

- Carry out a thorough review of legal frameworks governing medical advertising in the specific country.
- Ensure that all promotional activities adhere to established regulations and guidelines.
- Seek legal counsel to navigate complexities and mitigate risks associated with advertising compliance.

Educational Seminars and Workshops:

- Host informative sessions to educate the public about SMILE, its benefits, and the procedure itself.
- Collaborate with reputable speakers, including surgeons and industry experts, to enhance credibility.
- Use multimedia presentations, case studies, and interactive Q&A sessions to engage the audience.

Online Presence:

- Develop a professional and user-friendly website that provides comprehensive information about SMILE.
- Leverage social media platforms to share success stories, patient testimonials, and educational content.
- Utilize search engine optimization (SEO) strategies to enhance online visibility and reach a broader audience.

Printed Materials:

- Produce brochures, pamphlets, and informational materials that can be distributed at the clinic or relevant community events.
- Ensure that printed materials comply with regulatory requirements and are designed to captivate the reader's interest.

Collaboration with Optometrists and Ophthalmologists.

- Forge partnerships with local optometrists and ophthalmologists to promote SMILE within the professional network.
- Provide educational materials and conduct joint seminars to enhance awareness and referrals.

Patient Testimonials and Success Stories:

- Showcase real patient experiences and success stories through various channels.
- Obtain consent and adhere to privacy regulations when featuring patient testimonials.

Community Engagement:

- Participate in community events, health fairs, or local sponsorships to increase visibility.
- Offer free informational sessions or consultations to address questions and concerns.

These tools, when deployed thoughtfully and ethically, can significantly contribute to patient recruitment and foster positive perceptions of SMILE within the target demographic.

31.2.1 In Your Center: Building Brand Awareness

To establish brand awareness about the superior technology available in your premium center, consider the following strategies:

1. **Leaflet:**
   - Design informative brochures accessible to patients in the refractive surgery center or distributed during seminars.
   - Include subtopics such as details and advantages of the SMILE technique, qualifications of surgeons and staff, and information about femtosecond laser technology and other surgical equipment.
   - Emphasize the advanced equipment and the high qualifications of the staff.
2. **Video Support:**
   - Create short video clips explaining the surgery technique and its benefits, featuring patient testimonies who have chosen the SMILE technique.
   - Display these informative videos on screens in the waiting room and consider sharing them on prominent public platforms like YouTube.
   - Leverage the versatility of video clips for seamless integration with online information dissemination.
3. **The Waiting Room:**
   - Transform the waiting room into a reflection of the "New Technology" spirit, ensuring a modern design and furnishings.
   - Use videos and brochures to engage and inform patients, reducing perceived waiting time and generating interest in SMILE surgery.
   - Make the waiting room a showcase for the refractive center, creating an environment that sparks curiosity and desire to learn more about SMILE.
4. **Qualified Staff:**
   - Recognize that surgeons and staff serve as the most influential advertising for the center.
   - Emphasize the importance of a positive image reflected by the surgeon's personality and the professionalism of the staff.
   - Ensure staff members are highly qualified and well-versed in various refractive surgery methods, including SMILE.

- Staff behavior, expertise, and awareness of the latest technologies contribute to the overall positive perception of the clinic and the quality of patient care

These key points underscore the importance of various tools in reinforcing brand awareness about the superior technology offered in your premium center. By use of a combination of informative materials, visual content, an inviting waiting room environment, and a highly qualified staff, your center can effectively communicate the advantages of the SMILE technique and position itself as a leader in refractive surgery.

31.2.2 Outside of Your Center: Campaigns and Incentives

To extend your reach and increase patient numbers, engage in comprehensive campaigns and offer incentives across various channels, with a special focus on targeting the youth:

1. **Website:**
   - Invest in a website that effectively communicates your clinic's offerings, including details on SMILE surgery, surgeon profiles, and pricing information.
   - Use animations and figures to illustrate the SMILE technique, and include a section for frequently asked questions.
   - Allow for user interaction, such as submitting questions via email or scheduling a first check.
   - Maintain an updated section with scientific papers about SMILE for credibility.
   - Consider adding a forum for patient experiences, moderated by qualified administrators.
   - Invest in advertising campaigns for improved search engine results (SEO) and consider delegating web management to specialized companies.
2. **Social Networks:**
   - Leverage platforms like Facebook, Xing, Google + , Instagram, TikTok, etc., to encourage patient interactivity and positive comments.
   - Encourage patients to share positive experiences and recommend your clinic on these platforms.
   - Leverage the power of social networks in targeting the younger generation.
3. **Traditional Media:**
   - Consider traditional print media, radio, and TV for editorials or advertorials.
   - Develop smart and appealing TV and radio spots, keeping in mind the younger, Internet-focused generation.
   - Acknowledge the expense and potential dead loss associated with traditional media, focusing on their effectiveness for specific demographics.
   - Recognize that the younger generation, the primary target, is more Internet-focused than traditional media-oriented

4. **Network of SMILE Experts:**
   - Create, manage, and develop a network of health professionals likely to refer patients for refractive surgery.
   - Include ophthalmologists, opticians, optometrists, and general practitioners in this network.
   - Implement visits to introduce SMILE surgery to these professionals, emphasizing technical details and postoperative results.
   - Integrate referrals into the refractive care pathway and maintain relationships through newsletters and occasional meetings.
5. **Phone Calls:**
   - Use phone calls as an additional support to other communication channels.
   - Ensure staff answering calls are well-informed about the SMILE technique to address potential patients' questions.
6. **Price Policy:**
   - Position the price of SMILE surgery at the top of the pyramid, reflecting its status as the most sophisticated refractive surgery technique.
   - Emphasize the state-of-the-art concept and avoid positioning it as a low-cost option.
7. **Vouchers and Incentives**:
   - Introduce a referral system where recommending patients receive financial vouchers or discounts for successful referrals leading to refractive procedures.
   - Exercise sensitivity and tact in managing such marketing strategies
8. **Word of Mouth**:
   - Encourage satisfied patients to share their experiences with their social environment.
   - Consider engaging well-known individuals or influencers for postoperative testimonials and video clips, enhancing the credibility of SMILE.
   - Request testimonials or short video clips from well-known individuals who have undergone SMILE.

By deploying a combination of online and offline tools, you can effectively extend your campaigns and incentives beyond the walls of your center, reaching a wider audience and establishing SMILE as a leading refractive surgery option.

31.3 Tools to Convince Patients

31.3.1 Tools to Convert Refractive Candidates into SMILE Refractive Patients

Converting LASIK patients to SMILE is a strategic move, particularly as up-to-date patients prefer premium services and more advanced surgical techniques. To achieve this conversion, it is essential to believe in the technology and effectively communicate the benefits to potential patients. Here are strategies for different scenarios:

1. **First Sample: Patient Unaware of Refractive Surgery**:
   - Directly introduce SMILE without discussing other procedures like LASIK or PRK.
   - Educate the patient on the benefits and advantages of SMILE, emphasizing its uniqueness and effectiveness.
2. **Second Sample: Patient Aware of LASIK or PRK but Not SMILE**:
   - Provide evidence and detailed information about the SMILE procedure to convert patients.
   - Highlight the superior outcomes, safety, and unique advantages of SMILE compared to LASIK or PRK.
   - Emphasize technological advancements and the precision of the femtosecond laser used in SMILE.
3. **Third Sample: Patient Interested in SMILE**:
   - Explore how the patient discovered SMILE and use this information to tailor your communication.
   - Reinforce the patient's interest by elaborating on the specific benefits of SMILE.
   - Address any questions or concerns the patient may have and provide additional information to solidify their decision.

Several tools can help surgeons in converting SMILE interest into actual procedures among potential refractive patients:

- **Educational Materials**:
  - Design informative brochures, leaflets, and videos specifically focused on SMILE.
  - Highlight the advanced technology, safety, and benefits of the SMILE procedure.
  - Use visual aids, illustrations, and animations to simplify complex concepts for better understanding.
- **Scientific Research and Evidence**:
  - Reference and discuss relevant scientific papers and studies supporting the efficacy and safety of SMILE.
  - Provide data on postoperative results, patient satisfaction, and long-term outcomes.
- **Patient Testimonials**:
  - Showcase testimonials and success stories from previous SMILE patients.
  - Feature before-and-after photos to visually demonstrate the positive impact of SMILE on patients' lives.
- **Interactive Consultations**:
  - Utilize interactive consultations to address individual patient concerns and preferences.
  - Customize the discussion based on the patient's unique situation, providing personalized information about SMILE.

- **Comparative Analysis**:
  - Communicate a comparative analysis between SMILE, LASIK, and PRK, emphasizing the distinct advantages of SMILE.
  - Clearly outline the reasons why SMILE may be a superior choice for certain patients.
- **Digital Presence**:
  - Optimize your clinic's website to include detailed information about SMILE, its benefits, and the expertise of your surgical team.
  - Leverage social media platforms to share educational content, patient stories, and updates about SMILE.
- **Patient Education Events**:
  - Host educational events or webinars specifically focused on SMILE.
  - Encourage potential patients to attend these events to learn more about the procedure and address any questions.

By utilizing these tools and strategies, surgeons can effectively convert refractive candidates into SMILE refractive patients, ensuring that patients are well-informed and confident in their choice of this advanced surgical technique.

31.3.2 Discussion with Future Patients: Key Points for SMILE Surgery

Convincing patients of the benefits of SMILE surgery requires thorough and patient-oriented explanations. The surgeon should communicate in simple terms, utilizing explicative supports such as brochures. Here is a mixed bag of key points to discuss with future patients:

1. **The Future of Laser Vision Correction**:
   - Emphasize that SMILE represents the future of laser vision correction with its 100% bladeless, 100% flapless, and 100% all-femtosecond laser procedure.
2. **Equipment Qualities**:
   - Highlight the importance of trusting both the surgeon and the surgical facilities.
   - Create a confidential climate and underscore the advantages of using advanced technical devices for SMILE surgery.
3. **Femtosecond Laser (VisuMax®)**:
   - Discuss the unique benefits of the VisuMax® femtosecond laser, including predictability, efficacy, stability, and precision.
   - Position the laser as the third generation in laser refractive surgery, contributing to the success of SMILE surgery.
4. **Minimal Incision Size**:
   - Emphasize the minimally invasive nature of SMILE with a less than 2.5 mm incision.
   - Highlight how this preserves corneal biomechanical stability and offers maximum protection.

5. **Less Ocular Dryness**:
    - Address postoperative comfort by explaining that minimal reaction in the cornea leads to less severe dry eye syndrome.
    - Preserve corneal nerves, reducing disturbances in lacrimal secretion and postoperative dryness.
6. **Single-Step Procedure**:
    - Emphasize that SMILE is a single-step procedure, reducing stress for the patient by eliminating the need to move to another bed.
7. **Flapless**:
    - Highlight the flapless nature of SMILE, reducing the risk of vision quality loss due to flap accidents.
    - Discuss how this minimizes complications associated with lifting and re-putting human tissue.
8. **Ultra-fast Laser Action**:
    - Reassure patients about the quick procedure, with the creation of the lenticule taking only 8–10 s (for VisuMax 800).
9. **Natural Design of Contact Glass**:
    - Explain how the curved design of the contact glass fits the ocular surface's anatomy, avoiding complications during lenticule creation.
10. **Soft Corneal Suction**:
    - Contrast SMILE with other lasers, highlighting the short and discomfort-free corneal suction time.
    - Emphasize the reduced risk of intraocular pressure complications.
11. **Safety Assets and Permanent Surgeon Control**:
    - Stress the safety provided by the surgical microscope equipped with a digital video camera, ensuring visual control throughout the procedure.
    - Discuss the femtosecond precision and high-precision optics contributing to accuracy and predictability.
12. **Noiseless and Odorless**:
    - Position the VisuMax® as allowing noiseless and odorless surgery, enhancing patient comfort.
13. **Peri-operative Technical Devices**:
    - Discuss the quality of the topographer and wavefront analyzer, ensuring precision in measurements before surgery.
14. **Quick Vision Recovery**:
    - Highlight the fast vision recovery after SMILE, comparable to LASIK and faster than PRK.
15. **Quick Return to Sports**:
    - Stress that the flapless and less invasive nature of SMILE allows patients to return to sports almost immediately after surgery.
16. **Real Alternative to PRK**:
    - Position SMILE as a real alternative to PRK, especially for individuals whose professions or lifestyles prohibit LASIK surgery.
17. **Immediate Resumption of Daily Activities**:
    - Emphasize that patients can resume daily activities almost immediately after SMILE with minimal risk of complications.

SMILE not only revolutionizes the technological aspect of refractive surgery but also enhances patients' postoperative quality of life, allowing them to return to their daily activities with minimal constraints and maximum comfort.

31.4 Eventual Adverse Events: Communicating Risks and Avoiding Marketing Mistakes

In refractive surgery marketing, it is crucial to not only highlight the advantages but also discuss potential adverse events. This transparency makes patients feel safer, knowing their surgeon is prepared to manage difficulties. While SMILE is a sophisticated technique, it is important to communicate that no surgical procedure is entirely risk-free.

31.4.1 Peri-Operative Adverse Events

31.4.1.1 Suction Loss

- This occurs in around 0.5% of cases (with VisuMax 800 almost impossible)
- Suction loss can lead to restarting the SMILE procedure in most cases.
- In very few cases where completion is not possible, rescheduling for PRK or LASIK is a safer alternative.

31.4.1.2 Dissection in the Wrong Layer

- Affects around 0.6% of lenticule preparations.
- May increase surgery time but does not cause long-term vision loss.

31.4.1.3 Secondary Fracture Line Close to the Incision

- Happens in less than 0.3% of all preparations.
- Requires standard follow-up to ensure complete healing.

31.4.1.4 Epithelial Cells Remaining in the Interface

- Occurs in around 0.3% of lenticule extractions.
- If vision is disturbed, removal can be done through Nd:YAG or simple irrigation of the interface.

31.4.2 Common Postoperative Adverse Events

- Recovery period lasts 5–6 h.
- Some patients may experience blurred vision, dry eyes, or increased light sensitivity, common to both LASIK and SMILE surgery.

- These events are temporary and do not result in long-term visual loss or corneal damage.

31.4.3 Classical Mistakes in the SMILE Marketing

1. **Confusing Surgeon's View with that of a Patient:**
   - Emphasize excellent visual outcomes and safety, focusing on the overall future experience for the patient rather than just technological proofs.
2. **Clinical Trial Image:**
   - Present SMILE as a refined way to perform surgery with a newer, but proven refractive tool, not as a new concept. Highlight over 30 years of experience in refractive laser surgery.
3. **Introducing SMILE as a Niche Market:**
   - Clarify that SMILE is the reference treatment for myopia from −1.00 to −10.00 diopters and astigmatism up to −5 diopters, with hyperopia and presbyopia to be introduced in near future (as of the time of writing)
4. **Bashing LASIK or PRK Procedure:**
   - Acknowledgements LASIK and PRK as good refractive techniques with over 30 years of clinical results.
   - Assure patients that SMILE is state-of-the-art but not a replacement; all myopia patients can benefit from SMILE.

Key Point: Do not alarm patients with the "new" SMILE procedure; communicate it as a more accurate, predictable, and safer laser use, emphasizing that all myopia patients treated benefit from SMILE now.

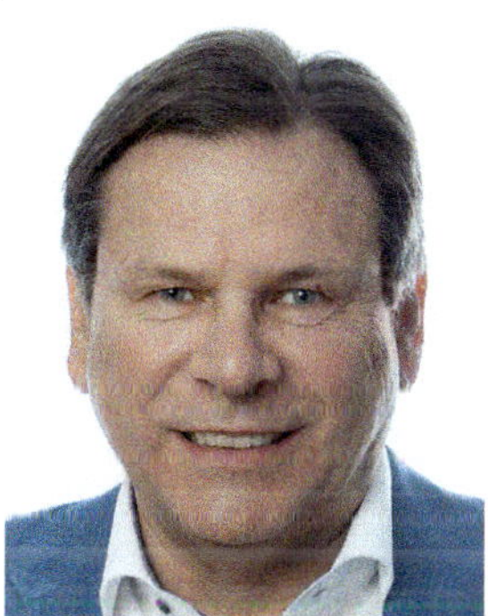

Bertram Meyer is a specialist in laser refractive surgery, with a career spanning over three decades since he began his practice in 1992. Notably, he has been performing SMILE (Small Incision Lenticule Extraction) procedures since 2010. Bertram Meyer offers his expertise in private clinics located in Cologne, Germany, and Dubai, UAE.

His professional contributions extend beyond clinical practice. Bertram Meyer regularly shares his knowledge and advancements in the field through lectures and updates at prominent annual meetings, including those organized by the German Ophthalmological Society (DOG), the German Society of Cataract and Refractive Surgery (DOC), the German-speaking Society of Intraocular Lens Implantation (DGII), and the European Society of Cataract and Refractive Surgeons (ESCRS). These presentations primarily focus on Femto-Lasik and Laser-Assisted-Lenticule-Extraction e.g. ReLEx®SMILE, reflecting his deep expertise and commitment to advancing laser refractive surgery.

Index

W. Sekundo and F. M. Wagner (eds.), *Femtosecond Laser Assisted Lenticule Extraction*, https://doi.org/10.1007/978-3-031-60424-9